Ultrasound THE REQUISITES

SERIES EDITOR   **James H. Thrall,** M.D.
Radiologist-in-Chief
Department of Radiology
Massachusetts General Hospital
Boston, Massachusetts

Ultrasound

THE REQUISITES

ALFRED B. KURTZ, M.D.
Professor of Radiology
Vice Chairman of the Department of Radiology
Jefferson Medical College
Thomas Jefferson University
Philadelphia, Pennsylvania

WILLIAM D. MIDDLETON, M.D.
Associate Professor of Radiology
Chief of Ultrasound
Mallinckrodt Institute of Radiology
Washington University School of Medicine
St. Louis, Missouri

with **1000** illustrations
with **56** color plates

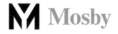

St. Louis Baltimore Boston
Carlsbad Chicago Naples New York Philadelphia Portland
London Madrid Mexico City Singapore Sydney Tokyo Toronto Wiesbaden

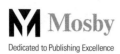
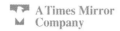

Mosby

Dedicated to Publishing Excellence

A Times Mirror
Company

Editor-in-Chief: Susan Gay
Managing Editor: Elizabeth Corra
Project Manager: Linda McKinley
Production Editor: Catherine Bricker
Manufacturing Manager: Linda Ierardi

Printed in the United States of America
Composition by Top Graphics
Printing/binding by Maple-Vail Book Manufacturing Group

Mosby–Year Book, Inc.
11830 Westline Industrial Drive
St. Louis, Missouri 63146

Library of Congress Cataloging in Publication Data

Kurtz, Alfred B.
   Ultrasound: the requisites/Alfred B. Kurtz, William D. Middleton
      p. cm.—(The requisites)
   Includes bibliographical references and index.
   ISBN 0-8016-8096-4
    1. Diagnosis, Ultrasonic. 2. Ultrasonics in obstetrics.
3. Generative organs, Female—Ultrasonic imaging. I. Middleton,
William D. II. Title. III. Series. IV. Series: Requisites series.
   [DNLM: 1. Ultrasonography. WN 208 K96u 1995]
RC78.7.U4K87   1995
616.07′543—dc20
DNLM/DLC
for Library of Congress   95-11324
                                        CIP

96 97 98 99 00 / 9 8 7 6 5 4 3 2 1

To my parents,
whose support and love of learning were the unspoken
forces that led me into medicine and then into academics.
They took pleasure in my successes, which they were in
large part responsible for, and they lived long enough to see me
achieve many of my goals.

*To **Dr. Harold Jacobson** and the late **Dr. Tom Beneventano***
of Montefiore Medical Center of Albert Einstein College of Medicine,
from whom I learned the art of radiology.
They taught me to push my diagnostic capabilities to their limits.

*To **Dr. Barry Goldberg***
of Jefferson Medical College of Thomas Jefferson University,
who encouraged me to do research and helped me discover the
almost limitless uses of ultrasound.
His friendship and support opened doors in radiology
which permitted my rapid advancement in this field.

*To **Dr. David Levin***
of Jefferson Medical College of Thomas Jefferson University,
who I thank for creating an atmosphere in which research
and writing flourish.

*To my wife **Barbara** and my three daughters, **Dana, Liza,** and **Amy,***
who are the lights of my life.
Without their unflagging support and love,
I would never have had the time or peace of mind to have even
considered this project.

A.B.K.

*To the late **Dr. Lee Melson,***
my mentor, colleague, and friend, who taught me most of what I
know about ultrasound, but most importantly taught me and others
of compassion, the love of family, and the joy of life.

*To my wife, **Mary,***
a devoted, loving spouse and an excellent radiologist.
She fine-tuned much of my writing and offered unique insights such as,
"You weren't very alert when you wrote this chapter, were you?"

*To my children, **B.I.** and **Dana,***
my current works in progress and the two biggest joys in my life.

*To my parents, **Bill** and **Joyce,***
whose support, guidance, and unconditional love have made me all
that I am.

To all the radiology residents I have been privileged to work with at
the Mallinckrodt Institute of Radiology,
whose interest in learning ultrasound was the primary incentive for
me to co-author this book.

W.D.M.

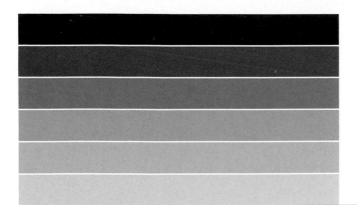

Foreword

Ultrasound: The Requisites is the fifth book in an ongoing series designed to provide core material in major subspecialty areas of radiology for residents during their training and for the practicing radiologist seeking a concise review.

The diversity between departments of radiology in how diagnostic ultrasound is both practiced and taught makes developing a concise text especially challenging. In some institutions, diagnostic ultrasound is practiced as a modality embracing all applications. In other departments, ultrasound is incorporated into an organ system approach to specialization. Drs. Kurtz and Middleton have done a wonderful job in producing a text that will serve the radiology resident and practicing radiologist equally well in both circumstances by designing each chapter as a self-contained unit that covers both relevant technical material and clinical applications.

The Requisites series has emphasized the use of tables and boxes to highlight and emphasize important material including differential diagnoses. Drs. Kurtz and Middleton have used this approach well in *Ultrasound: The Requisites,* and they have also added another innovative approach which highlights important material for the reader. Basic material in every chapter is highlighted in a *Key Features* box that gives the essence of what should be known and understood about each topic. The *Key Features* can be read alone as a first introduction for each chapter or read as a rapid review.

High-quality illustrations are a sine qua non of effective textbooks in radiology. Drs. Kurtz and Middleton have done an outstanding job in selecting a substantial number and wide breadth of images that illustrate all major normal structures and important pathological findings. A special feature of *Ultrasound: The Requisites* is the large number of color illustrations including, most importantly, color-Doppler images.

I believe residents in radiology will find *Ultrasound: The Requisites* to be an excellent vehicle for introducing themselves to the subject. The text provides both basic and state-of-the-art information in all chapters. In keeping with the philosophy of The Requisites series, the book can be easily read and reread during successive ultrasound rotations during a residency program. Physicians in practice and in fellowship programs should find *Ultrasound: The Requisites* attractive for the same reason—it is a concise way to expand or refresh their knowledge in the area.

In some sense, people entering training in radiology are forced to "start over" in terms of their medical knowledge base. The fundamental principles of basic science and clinical medicine learned in medical school provide the necessary background for training in radiology. However, the task of obtaining the specific knowledge and skills required to correctly interpret radiologic images is left almost entirely to residency training. Thus a resident entering a subspecialty rotation in a radiology training program has the formidable task of going from a minimal knowledge base of subspecialty specifics to a working knowledge of radiology in a very short period of time.

This observation was the basis for creating the Requisites in Radiology series. One book will be written to specifically cover each of the major subspecialty areas. The length of each particular book will be dictated by the material requiring coverage, but the goal is to provide the resident with a text that may be reasonably read within several days at the beginning of each subspecialty rotation.

The books are not intended to be exhaustive but instead should still provide the basic conceptual, factual, and interpretive material required for clinical practice. The reader should also note that, to provide a concise overall presentation of material, breast ultrasound and evaluation of the neonatal brain are covered in other books of the Requisites series.

Each book is written by internationally recognized authorities in their respective subspecialty areas. Since this is a completely new series, each author presents material within the context of today's contemporary radiology practice, as opposed to grafting new information onto old text material.

I congratulate Drs. Kurtz and Middleton for their outstanding contribution to the Requisites in Radiology series.

James H. Thrall, M.D.
Radiologist-in-Chief
Massachusetts General Hospital
Professor of Radiology
Harvard Medical School
Boston, Massachusetts

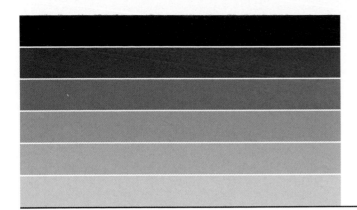

Preface

The technology of using sound to locate underwater objects was developed by the British in World War I. Called *sonar*, as an acronym for *so*und *na*vigation *r*anging, it was first used at sea in 1921. Its potential was so great that it was kept a secret and used effectively in World War II.

Attempts to use sonar in diagnostic medicine began in the late 1940s and became an accepted medical tool by the 1950s. Because it was used at high frequencies in the megahertz range, it was renamed *ultrasound*. Its power could be lowered, so it was even safe for pregnant women.

However, ultrasound's beginnings were modest, and only the largest and most obvious structures could initially be detected. Since that time, a series of technological breakthroughs have created a rapid and almost uninterrupted period of growth. These innovations took ultrasound from A Mode to bistable B Mode and then to gray scale. Scanning changed from single pictures to multiple real-time images. Doppler technology (to study particle movement) developed—first continuous wave and then pulsed and color Doppler. Transducer technology modified the size and types of transducers, making them small enough to be used at ends of intracavitary probes and at the tips of catheters.

Most of these advances have taken place since the 1970s. In the less than three decades since then, ultrasound has evolved from a fledgling modality to an integral part of many diagnostic and treatment plans. Diagnostic ultrasound is unique in its portability, relative ease of application, and ability to evaluate any soft-tissue area, both close to or far away from the transducer. It can be used from the skin surface, in an intracavitary position, and can now even be used intraoperatively. This explosion in technology has come with a proliferation of writing, resulting in hundreds of articles and textbooks on the subject. The standard textbooks in the field of diagnostic ultrasound are now multiple volumes in size.

The goal of this Requisites series book, as with the previous volumes in the series, is two-fold. First, it is intended to serve as introductory material that can be read in three to four weeks by a radiology resident or practitioner while they are first being exposed to diagnostic ultrasound. Therefore we have tried to emphasize the basic information and fundamental principles of ultrasound. In addition, the book is intended to serve as a review for senior residents studying for boards and for experienced practitioners who encounter specific diagnostic problems. For this reason, we have incorporated more advanced information and more sophisticated techniques, such as color Doppler.

The book has been organized to make it as easy to read and to learn from as possible. It has been divided by organ system into sections covering the abdomen, obstetrics, gynecology, and superficial parts and the vascular system. Individual chapters are broken down into subsections that are listed on the first page of each chapter. Information is then presented in the text, tables, and figures. In addition, a *Key Features* summary is listed at the ends of chapters.

We have put a great deal of ourselves into writing this book. We hope that it will impart both the basic and advanced aspects of all areas of diagnostic ultrasound. We also hope that our enthusiasm for ultrasound is apparent and that this book will pique your interest for and understanding of this remarkable diagnostic modality. The versatility of ultrasound, with its ease and accuracy of diagnosis, will hopefully become an integral part of your diagnostic armamentarium.

Alfred B. Kurtz, M.D.
William D. Middleton, M.D.

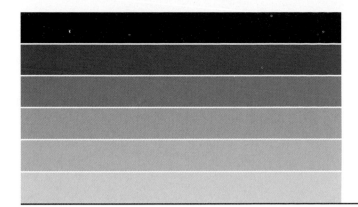

Acknowledgments

Writing a book is an undertaking that requires both time and dedication. It is impossible to do this task alone, and although it is not possible to acknowledge everyone who contributed their time, we would like to thank select individuals for making this project possible and seeing it to its completion. First and foremost, we would like to thank our secretaries, Emily Pompetti and Lynn Losse, for their tireless help in typing, organizing, proofreading, and editing. Without their constant dedication to this task, their continued support, and their sense of humor, we could not have finished this book in a timely manner.

We would also like to thank the photographers in our departments: Ken Goodman, Fred Ross, Michelle Wynn, and Tom Murry. They were always available to make prints, to redo incorrect prints, and to make illustrations. Their devotion to detail is one of the primary reasons that the final figures are of such a high quality.

Finally, we asked for and received help from many of our radiology colleagues in clarifying select points of information and in providing images. We want to thank them all, and they are appropriately recognized throughout the book. We particularly want to thank Dr. Larry Needleman of Jefferson Medical College of Thomas Jefferson University, Dr. Harris Finberg of Phoenix Perinatal Associates, and Dr. Sherry Teefey of the Mallinckrodt Institute of Radiology. Their invaluable contributions and appropriate critiques strengthened important chapters.

CONTENTS

ABDOMEN

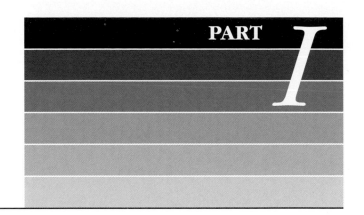

PART *I*

CHAPTER 1

Liver

For a Key Features summary see p. 33.

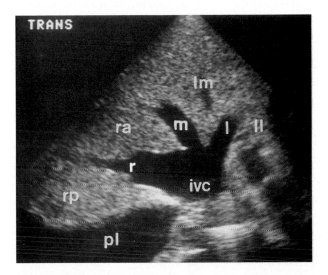

Fig. 1-1   Normal hepatic venous anatomy. Transverse view of the hepatic vein confluence shows the right hepatic vein *(r)*, middle hepatic vein *(m)*, and left hepatic vein *(l)* draining into the inferior vena cava *(ivc)*. These veins separate the right posterior *(rp)*, right anterior *(ra)*, left medial *(lm)*, and left lateral *(ll)* hepatic segments. The veins and IVC are enlarged in this patient due to heart failure. A right pleural effusion *(pl)* is also present.

ANATOMY

The liver is the largest organ in the normal abdomen, occupying most of the right upper quadrant. It is divided into a right lobe that contains an anterior and posterior segment and a left lobe that contains a medial and lateral segment. The right hepatic vein runs between the anterior and posterior right lobe segments, the left hepatic vein runs between the medial and lateral left lobe segments, and the middle hepatic vein runs between the medial left lobe segment and the anterior right lobe segment (Fig. 1-1). Whereas the hepatic veins separate the hepatic segments, the portal veins run through the middle of the segments, and each branch is named according to the seg-

ment it supplies. The exception is the umbilical segment of the left portal vein, which runs between the left medial and lateral segments. The portal veins can be distinguished from the hepatic veins by the periportal fibrofatty tissue, which produces brighter echoes around the portal veins (Fig. 1-2).

The ligamentum teres travels between the medial and lateral segments of the left lobe and is a useful landmark for separating them. The interlobar fissure is an indentation on the posterior aspect of the liver that separates the right and left lobes (Fig. 1-3) and identifies the location of the gallbladder fossa. The caudate lobe is a small segment of the liver located immediately anterior to the inferior vena cava (IVC). It is contiguous with the right lobe and

3

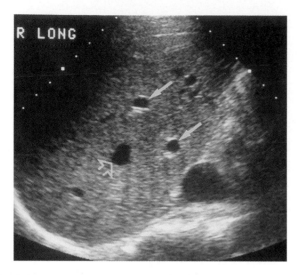

Fig. 1-2   Normal intrahepatic portal veins and hepatic vein. Longitudinal view of the liver demonstrates the increased periportal echogenicity associated with intrahepatic portal veins *(arrows)* contrasted to the lack of perivascular echogenicity associated with hepatic veins *(open arrow)*.

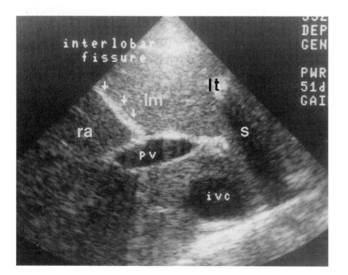

Fig. 1-3   Normal interlobar fissure. Transverse view of the liver near the region of the portal venous bifurcation *(pv)* demonstrates the interlobar fissure *(arrows)* separating the left medial *(lm)* from the right anterior *(ra)* hepatic segments. The interlobar fissure is unusually prominent in this case. The ligamentum teres *(lt)* separates the medial and lateral left lobe segments. Shadowing *(s)* is behind the ligamentum teres because of the prominent fatty components. The inferior vena cava *(ivc)* is also shown.

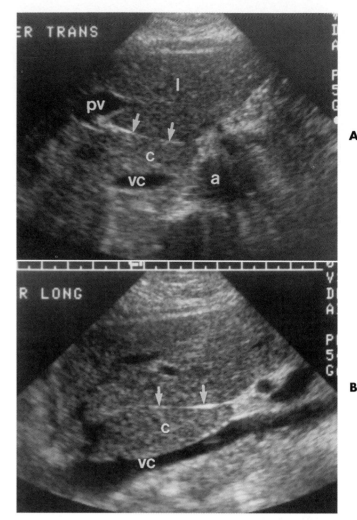

Fig. 1-4   Normal caudate lobe. **A,** Transverse view of the liver shows the caudate lobe *(c)* anterior to the inferior vena cava *(vc)*. It is separated from the left lobe *(l)* by the fissure for the ligamentum venosum *(arrows)*. The left portal vein *(pv)* and the aorta *(a)* are also visualized. **B,** Longitudinal view of the liver demonstrating similar structures in the sagittal plane.

Table 1-1 Hepatic segmental landmarks	
Segments	**Separating landmarks**
Left lateral/left medial	Ligamentum teres
	Umbilical segment of left portal vein
	Left hepatic vein
Left medial/right anterior	Interlobar fissure
	Gallbladder
	Middle hepatic vein
Right anterior/right posterior	Right hepatic vein
Caudate lobe/left lobe	Fissure for ligamentum venosum

Table 1-2 Characteristics of normal liver	
Characteristic	**Appearance**
Size	<15 cm
Echogenicity	≥ Right kidney
	< Pancreas
	< Spleen
Parenchyma	Homogeneous
Surface	Smooth

separated from the left lobe by the fissure for the ligamentum venosum (Fig. 1-4; Table 1-1).

The size of the liver can be difficult to gauge on sonography because it is often too large to be seen on a single real time image. Normal upper limits of liver length measured in the midclavicular line range from 13 to 17 cm (15 cm is used most frequently). Indirect signs of hepatomegaly include extension of the right lobe below the lower pole of the kidney (in the absence of a Riedels lobe), rounding of the inferior tip of the liver, and extension of the left lobe into the left upper quadrant above the spleen.

The liver parenchyma is normally homogeneous and is only interrupted by the portal triads and the hepatic veins. Echogenicity of the liver should be slightly greater than or equal to that of the right kidney but less than that of the pancreas. Previously, the liver was considered iso-echoic or hyperechoic in comparison to the spleen, but now it is clear that the liver is actually less echogenic than the spleen (Table 1-2).

TECHNIQUE

The liver is usually best scanned with a sector or a curved array transducer with center frequency ranging from 2 to 5 MHz. Linear array transducers are useful for imaging superficial abnormalities and the surface of the liver. The left lobe can be imaged effectively in most patients from an anterior subxyphoid approach, whereas the right lobe should be scanned from both a subcostal and intercostal approach to optimize detection and characterization of focal lesions. Intercostal scans are most effective with the patient supine during normal respiration so that the right lung base and its associated shadowing are not obscuring the superior aspects of the liver. Rib shadowing can be minimized by imaging in an oblique plane that is parallel to the long axis of the intercostal spaces. Once this orientation is achieved, the transducer should be angled anteriorly and posteriorly to visualize as much liver parenchyma as possible from that particular intercostal space. Subcostal scanning should be per-

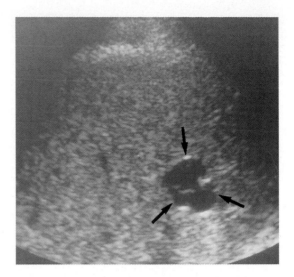

Fig. 1-5   Hepatic cyst. Transverse view of the liver demonstrates an anechoic lesion *(arrows)* with increased through transmission and well-defined back wall. The wall of the cyst is "puckered" and a thin septation is visualized. These findings are not unusual in cysts of the liver.

formed with the patient in a left lateral decubitus or left posterior oblique position so that the liver rotates inferiorly. More inferior displacement of the liver and further enhancement of subcostal scanning can be achieved by imaging during deep patient inspiration. It is important to angle the transducer superiorly while scanning from a subcostal approach, so that the dome of the liver can be visualized.

FOCAL LESIONS

Cysts

Hepatic cysts are the most common focal liver lesions. Because the liver is such a homogeneous organ, cysts are easy to detect and generally display the three classic sonographic criteria of an anechoic lumen, increased through transmission and a clear back wall. However, most hepatic cysts have at least a partial septation that disturbs the normally smooth contour of uncomplicated cysts (Fig. 1-5). Vascular lesions such as aneurysms, arterioportal fistulas, and portal-hepatic vein fistulas can simulate cysts on gray-scale sonography but are easily distinguished with Doppler analysis. Complex cystic lesions include hematomas, abscesses, and cystic metastases. Biliary cystadenomas and cystadenocarcinomas are rare neoplasms that appear as multiseptated cystic masses (Box 1-1).

The liver is involved in up to 50% of the cases of autosomal dominant polycystic disease. Despite extensive involvement, liver function remains normal in the vast major-

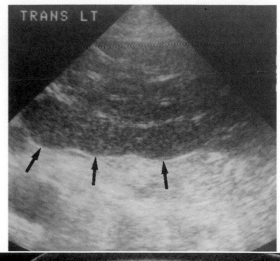

A

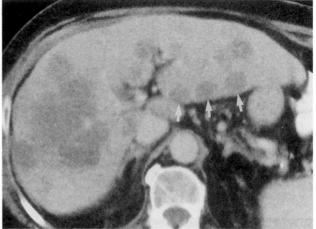

B

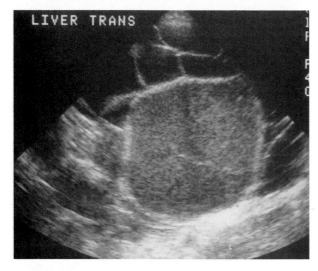

Fig. 1-6   Polycystic disease. Transverse view of the liver shows complete replacement with multiple cysts. One central cyst has internal echogenicity due to hemorrhage.

Fig. 1-8   Isoechoic metastases. **A,** Transverse view of the left hepatic lobe demonstrates three adjacent areas of nodularity along the posterior surface *(arrows)* but no definable focal lesions. **B,** CT scan of this area confirms three low attenuation hepatic metastases *(arrows)* along the posterior surface of the left lobe as well as multiple other metastatic lesions throughout the liver. None of these abnormalities were defined as focal lesions on sonography.

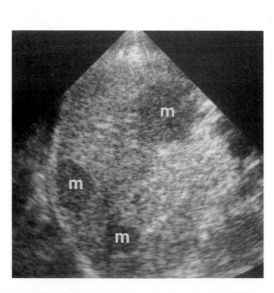

Fig. 1-7   Hypoechoic hepatic metastases. Longitudinal view of the liver demonstrates multiple hypoechoic masses *(m)*. Percutaneous biopsy revealed metastatic adenocarcinoma. A primary site was never identified in this patient.

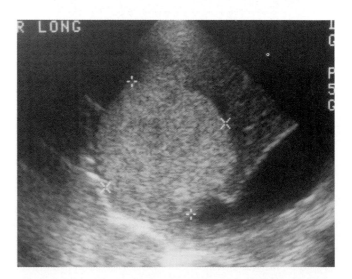

Fig. 1-9   Hyperechoic metastasis. Longitudinal view of the liver demonstrates a large homogeneous hyperechoic mass *(cursors)*. Other similar hyperechoic masses were seen elsewhere in the liver. Percutaneous biopsy revealed metastatic neuroendocrine tumor.

ity of patients. Symptoms arise from the mass effect of the numerous cysts or result from cyst hemorrhage (Fig. 1-6).

Metastases

Metastases are the most common cause of focal or multifocal solid liver lesions in North America. Their sono-

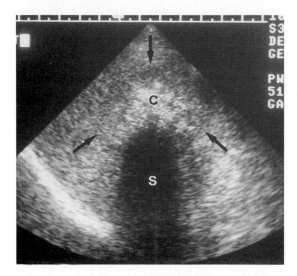

Fig. 1-10   Calcified hepatic metastasis. Transverse view of the liver demonstrates a poorly-defined hypoechoic lesion *(arrows)* with central calcification *(c)* producing a prominent posterior acoustic shadow *(s)*. Percutaneous biopsy revealed metastatic adenocarcinoma identical in histology to this patient's primary colon carcinoma.

graphic appearance varies from hypoechoic (Fig. 1-7), to isoechoic (Fig. 1-8), to hyperechoic (Fig. 1-9) and from homogeneous to heterogeneous. All primary malignancies can produce a wide spectrum of abnormalities in the liver, and although it is not possible to predict the primary based on the sonographic appearance of the liver metastases, the following trends are useful. Hyperechoic metastases tend to arise from the GI tract, most commonly from the colon. The colon is also the most common source for calcified metastases (Fig. 1-10), although mucinous primaries of the ovary (Fig. 1-11), breast, and stomach can also calcify (Box 1-2).

Many metastatic lesions have a target appearance with an echogenic center and a hypoechoic halo (Fig. 1-12). Although the halo was initially reported to represent compressed liver parenchyma, a recent study has shown that it usually represents proliferating tumor. Secondary to metastases, the most common cause of target lesions is hepatocellular carcinoma; hemangiomas only rarely have a target appearance. Adenomas and focal

Box 1-2   Calcified Hepatic Masses

LARGE, WITH OR WITHOUT MASS	SMALL, WITHOUT MASS
Metastases	Granulomas
Fibrolamellar hepatocellular cancer	Pneumocystis
Old hematoma	Biliary stones
Old abscess	

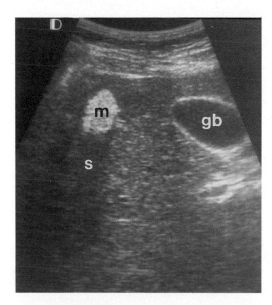

Fig. 1-11   Calcified hepatic metastasis. Transverse view of the liver demonstrates a uniformly hyperechoic mass *(m)* in the periphery of the liver. There is a faint posterior acoustic shadow *(s)*. This lesion corresponded to a hyperdense mass on CT and percutaneous biopsy confirmed that this represented metastatic ovarian cancer. The gallbladder *(gb)* is also seen on this view.

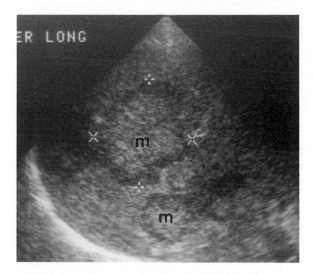

Fig. 1-12   Hepatic metastases with a target appearance. Longitudinal view of the liver in a patient with breast carcinoma reveals two metastatic lesions *(m)*. They both have a typical target appearance with a slightly hyperechoic central region and a hypoechoic rim.

Box 1-3 Hepatic Target Lesions

COMMON	UNCOMMON
Metastases	Lymphoma
Hepatocellular cancer	Adenoma
	Focal nodular hyperplasia
	Fungal microabscesses

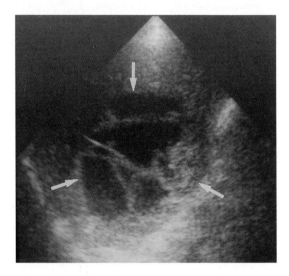

Fig. 1-13   Cystic hepatic metastasis. Longitudinal view of the liver demonstrates a large complex cystic mass *(arrows)* with multiple thick septations and solid components arising from the wall. This patient had a history of ovarian carcinoma and this is a typical sonographic appearance of metastatic ovarian cancer.

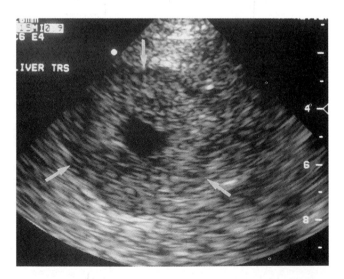

Fig. 1-14   Cystic hepatic metastasis. Transverse view of the liver demonstrates a large hypoechoic mass *(arrows)* with a central cystic component. This patient had a primary carcinoma in the parotid gland and histology of the liver lesion obtained from percutaneous biopsy was consistent with metastatic disease from the parotid. The central cystic region likely reflects tumor necrosis.

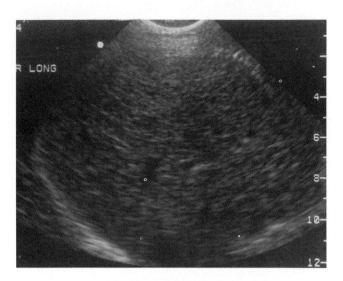

Fig. 1-15   Diffuse hepatic metastases. Longitudinal view of the liver demonstrates a diffuse inhomogeneity and coarsening of the hepatic echotexture. This patient had a history of breast carcinoma and multiple random liver biopsies were all positive for metastatic disease consistent with a breast primary.

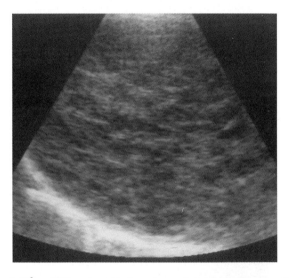

Fig. 1-16   Diffuse hepatic lymphoma. Longitudinal view of the liver demonstrates diffuse inhomogeneity and nodularity to the hepatic parenchyma. This was an immunocompromised renal transplant patient, and percutaneous biopsy revealed hepatic lymphoma.

Box 1-4 Diffuse Hepatic Inhomogeneity

COMMON	UNCOMMON
Cirrhosis	Hepatocellular cancer
Metastases	Hepatic fibrosis
Fatty infiltration	Lymphoma

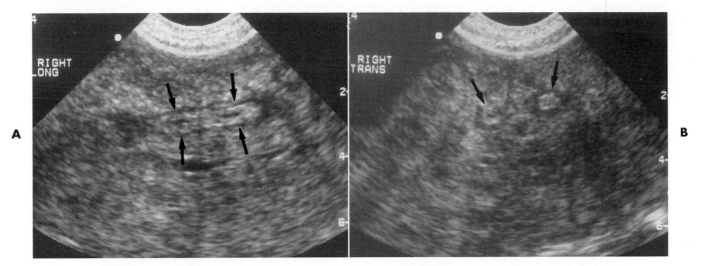

Fig. 1-17   Metastatic Kaposi's sarcoma. **A,** Longitudinal view of the right lobe of the liver in this patient with Acquired Immune Deficiency Syndrome demonstrates a markedly thickened portal triad *(arrows)*. **B,** Transverse view of the liver demonstrates two thickened portal triads seen in cross-section *(arrows)*. This patient had cutaneous Kaposi's sarcoma and the sonographic findings in the liver are typical of metastatic Kaposi's sarcoma.

nodular hyperplasia frequently appear as target lesions but both are very unusual lesions. Therefore target lesions are most often caused by either a primary or secondary hepatic malignancy (Box 1-3).

Cystic hepatic metastases are unusual but do occur. They generally have either thick walls, thick septations, or obvious solid components and therefore do not mimic simple hepatic cysts (Fig. 1-13). Cystic spaces in metastases may result from a cystic primary tumor (ovary) or from necrosis, such as squamous cell carcinomas, sarcomas, and large lesions from any primary (Fig. 1-14).

In addition to focal lesions, hepatic metastases may also cause a diffuse inhomogeneity in the liver, which is particularly typical for breast cancer (Fig. 1-15). The differential diagnosis for this appearance includes cirrhosis, hepatic fibrosis, hepatic lymphoma (Fig. 1-16), fatty infiltration, and diffuse hepatocellular carcinoma (Box 1-4).

A number of tumors can produce unusual appearances when they spread to the liver. Because of its tendency to infiltrate along the portal triads, Kaposi sarcoma can produce periportal thickening and increased periportal echogenicity (Fig. 1-17). Although it is solid, hepatic lymphoma can produce lesions that are anechoic because of tumor homogeneity and lack of internal acoustic interfaces. Generally, lymphomatous lesions can be differentiated from true cysts by lack of appropriate through transmission. In addition, hepatic lymphoma may also have a target appearance or produce diffuse inhomogeneity. Finally, peritoneal based metastases frequently localize to the right upper quadrant adjacent to the liver. When ascites is present, it is usually possible to distinguish peritoneal lesions from true intrahepatic lesions. In the absence of as-

cites, peritoneal lesions can look surprisingly intrahepatic. Therefore peripherally based lesions that appear intrahepatic are more likely to be peritoneal if the primary has a greater chance of going to the peritoneum than the liver, which is especially true in ovarian cancer (Fig. 1-18).

Hemangiomas

Hemangiomas are the most common benign liver lesion, occurring in approximately 7% of adults. They are composed of multiple, small, blood-filled spaces that are separated by fibrous septations and lined by endothelial cells. They are most common in women and frequently occur near the periphery of the liver; approximately 10% are multiple. With the exception of cysts, they are the most common incidental lesion detected on hepatic sonography.

Although it is unusual for hemangiomas to cause symptoms, giant hemangiomas (defined as greater than 4 cm) may have enough of a mass effect to be symptomatic. Hemangiomas rarely bleed enough to cause symptoms. Platelet sequestration and destruction by hemangiomas has been reported as a rare cause of thrombocytopenia (Kasabach-Merritt syndrome).

The classic sonographic appearance, seen in approximately 60% to 70% of hemangiomas, is homogeneous and hyperechoic (Fig. 1-19), and the majority are less than 3 cm in size. Atypical appearances tend to occur in larger lesions as a result of fibrosis, thrombosis, and necrosis. A significant percentage of the atypical hemangiomas have a hyperechoic periphery and a hypoechoic center (Fig. 1-20). A recent study indicates that this "atypical" appearance is fairly characteristic of hemangiomas and is rarely seen in metastatic disease. An additional finding occasionally seen in hemangiomas is increased through transmission. Despite the vascular nature of hemangiomas, blood flow is generally too slow to be detected with Doppler techniques. Therefore detection of arterial flow within a hepatic mass makes metastatic disease and he-

patocellular carcinoma more likely than hemangioma (Box 1-5).

The majority of hemangiomas are stable in both size and sonographic appearance. However, approximately 10% will undergo a decrease in echogenicity (Fig. 1-21), and 5% will regress partially or completely. Only 2% of hemangiomas enlarge on follow-up scans. Occasionally a he-

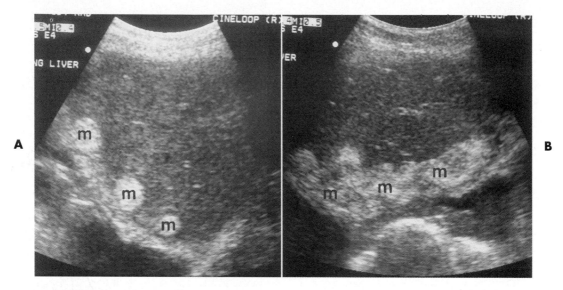

Fig. 1-18   Peritoneal-based perihepatic metastases from ovarian cancer. **A,** Longitudinal view of the liver shows three apparently intrahepatic hyperechoic peripheral masses *(m)*. **B,** Transverse view shows more extensive and confluent hyperechoic masses distorting the surface of the liver. The extrinsic nature of the masses is easier to appreciate on this view.

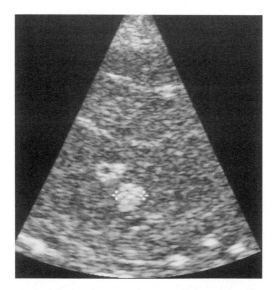

Fig. 1-19   Typical hemangioma. Magnified view of the liver shows a small homogeneous hyperechoic mass *(cursors)* consistent with a hemangioma.

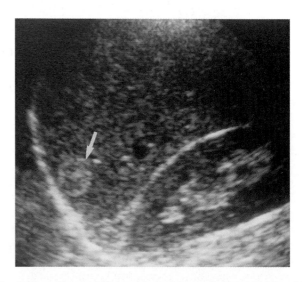

Fig. 1-20   "Atypical" hemangioma. Longitudinal view of the right lobe of the liver demonstrates a small lesion that has an isoechoic central component and a hyperechoic rim *(arrow)*. Although considered atypical for a cavernous hemangioma, the appearance is very suggestive of the diagnosis.

mangioma will change its sonographic appearance during the course of a single examination (Fig. 1-22); no other hepatic lesion is known to do this.

Since the sonographic appearance of most hemangiomas is characteristic but not pathognomonic, it is generally recommended that a patient at low risk for malignancy have a 6 month follow-up ultrasound to ensure stability of any homogeneous hyperechoic hepatic mass. However, some authorities would argue that this is not necessary, and others would recommend that the diagnosis of hemangioma be confirmed with magnetic resonance imaging (MRI) or Tc-99m tagged red blood cell

Box 1-5	Homogeneous Hyperechoic Lesions	
COMMON		**RARE**
Hemangioma		Adenoma
		Focal nodular hyperplasia
UNCOMMON		
Metastases		
Fatty infiltration		
Hepatocellular cancer		

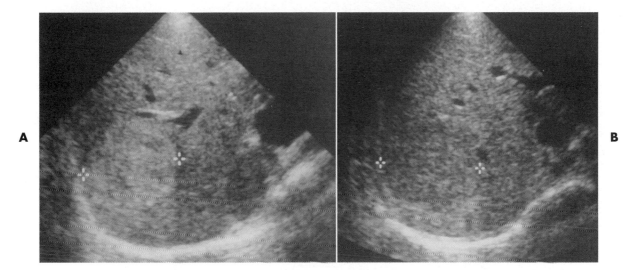

Fig. 1-21   Hemangioma changing appearance on follow-up scans. **A,** Transverse view of the liver demonstrates a homogeneously hyperechoic mass *(cursors)* in the right lobe. There is minimal increased through-transmission. **B,** Similar view taken 5 months later shows that the lesion has changed from a hyperechoic appearance to a slightly hypoechoic appearance. This occurs in approximately 10% of hemangiomas. (Courtesy Holly Burge MD, Raleigh, N.C.)

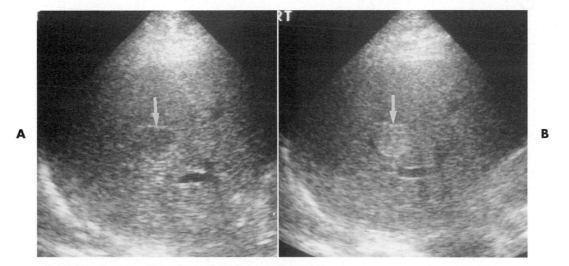

Fig. 1-22   Hepatic hemangioma changing rapidly over time. **A,** Longitudinal view of the right lobe of the liver demonstrates a slightly hypoechoic lesion *(arrow).* **B,** Similar image obtained approximately 90 seconds later demonstrates rapid change to a hyperechoic appearance.

(RBC) scintigraphy. Certainly, in a patient at risk for hepatic malignancy (one who has a known primary tumor elsewhere or a predisposition to forming hepatocellular carcinomas), a correlative study should be performed. Because scintigraphy is so specific for the diagnosis of hemangioma, it should be the preferred method in most patients, whereas MRI should be reserved for small lesions (less than 1 to 2 cm) and larger lesions adjacent to the heart or major hepatic vascular structures.

Occasionally, noninvasive tests will not establish the diagnosis of hemangioma and a biopsy is needed. This can be performed safely; however, the needle should pass through normal parenchyma before entering the hemangioma to achieve some tamponade effect. Fine needle aspirations generally obtain only blood and are not sufficient to make the diagnosis. Twenty-gauge core biopsy needles can obtain sufficient tissue for diagnosis in the majority of cases.

Hepatocellular Carcinoma

Primary cancer of the liver is sometimes referred to as "hepatoma" but the preferred terminology is *hepatocellular carcinoma (HCC)*. Although HCC can occur in nor-

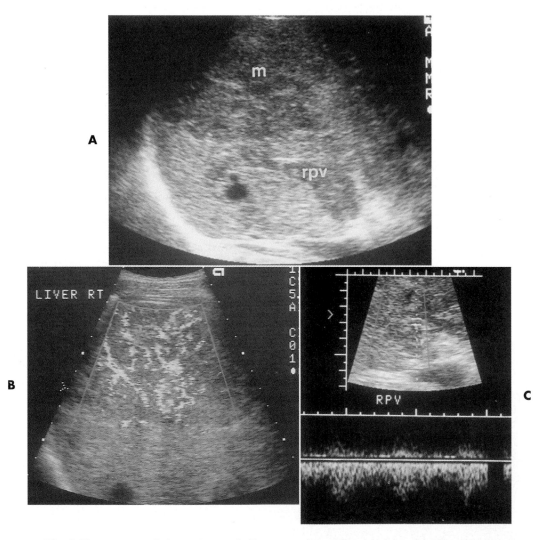

Fig. 1-23   Hepatocellular carcinoma. **A,** Transverse view of the right lobe of the liver demonstrates a large hypoechoic mass *(m)* replacing most of the anterior segment. The posterior branch of the right portal view *(rpv)* is filled with hypoechoic solid tissue similar in echogenicity to the hepatic tumor. **B,** Transverse color Doppler scan of the mass in the right lobe of the liver demonstrates marked hypervascularity of this lesion. Hypervascularity is characteristic of hepatocellular carcinoma, although this degree of detectable increased flow is unusual on color Doppler (see color insert, Plate 1). **C,** Pulsed Doppler waveform from the right portal vein demonstrates hepatofugal arterial signal arising from the thrombosed vein. This is highly suggestive of hepatocellular cancer that has invaded the portal vein.

mal livers, it is strongly associated with chronic liver disease, especially hepatitis B infection and cirrhosis. In fact, HCC is a major health problem in Asia due to the high prevalence of hepatitis B. In non–Asian populations, alcoholic cirrhosis is the most important condition predisposing to HCC. Other predisposing factors include hemochromatosis, Wilson's disease, and type I glycogen storage disease.

Cirrhotic livers pathologically display a spectrum of nodular lesions. Regenerating nodules form because of replication of hepatocytes and resulting compression and distortion of adjacent stroma and fibrous tissue. Adeno-

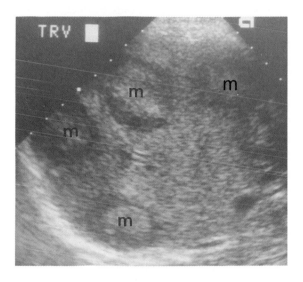

Fig. 1-24 Multifocal hepatocellular carcinoma. Transverse view of the liver demonstrates multiple masses *(m)* that have a target appearance.

matous hyperplasia (also known as *nodular hyperplasia, adenomatous hyperplastic nodules,* and *macroregenerative nodules*) is defined as a nodule that is significantly larger than the other regenerative nodules in a cirrhotic liver. They are usually larger than 1 cm and may contain atypical cells or actual malignant foci. In the latter case they are considered early HCC. It is believed that many HCCs develop from the following sequence: regenerative nodule, adenomatous hyperplasia, atypical adenomatous hyperplasia, to HCC.

The growth pattern of HCC is quite variable—it may be solitary (Fig. 1-23) [for Fig. 1-23, *B*, see also color insert, Plate 1]), multifocal (Fig. 1-24), or diffuse and infiltrating (Fig. 1-25). Echogenicity is also variable, and the general sonographic appearance is nonspecific. Most HCCs are hypervascular (Fig. 1-23), and arterial-portal shunts are characteristic. HCC has a strong tendency to invade hepatic vasculature, including both the portal veins (30% to 60%) and hepatic veins (15%). Therefore detection of intravenous soft tissue in a patient with hepatic mass(es) should raise suspicion for HCC (Fig. 1-23). Because bland portal vein thrombus can occur in cases of metastatic disease to the liver, hepatic vein thrombosis is more specific for HCC. Regardless of the thrombus location, if arterial flow is detected within the thrombus, then a reliable diagnosis of tumor invasion can be made (Fig. 1-23).

Fibrolamellar HCC is an unusual variant that occurs in younger patients without coexistent liver disease and has a much better prognosis than typical HCC. It is usually solitary and is more likely to contain calcification than typical HCC (Fig. 1-26). The central scar that is often present histologically is only occasionally seen sonographically.

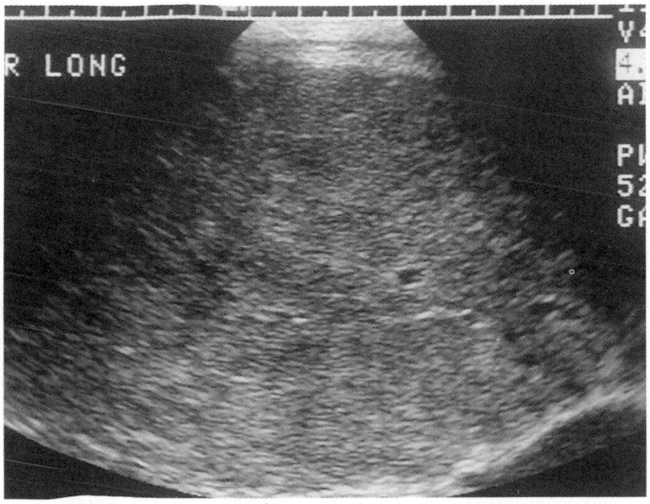

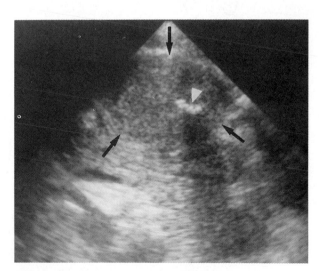

Fig. 1-25 Diffuse infiltrating hepatocellular carcinoma. Longitudinal view of the liver demonstrates diffuse inhomogeneity of the liver. Discrete focal lesions are difficult to identify.

Fig. 1-26 Fibrolamellar hepatocellular carcinoma. Transverse view of the left lobe of the liver demonstrates a solid mass *(arrows)* with a focal region of calcification *(arrowhead)*. This was a 23-year-old man with no history of previous liver disease.

Sonography is widely used in Asia to screen patients at risk for HCC, with a reported sensitivity of 80% to 90%. In North America, sensitivity is lower due to the larger body habitus of the patient population. In addition, sensitivity is lowered to approximately 50% in the setting of advanced cirrhosis with diffuse hepatic inhomogeneity. Despite the low sensitivity in advanced cirrhosis, sonography is still useful because it is highly specific. Therefore any focal mass detected sonographically in a patient with advanced cirrhosis should be considered malignant until proved otherwise.

Hepatic Adenoma

Adenomas are focal lesions that contain normal (or occasionally slightly abnormal) hepatocytes but that are largely devoid of Kupffer cells and bile ducts. They are frequently encapsulated and occur most commonly in women on birth control pills, although they also occur in men taking anabolic steroids and in patients with type I glycogen storage disease. Although their histology is benign, hepatic adenomas are considered surgical lesions because of their propensity to bleed. As with other solid focal lesions, their sonographic appearance is varied and nonspecific (Fig. 1-27). Internal hemorrhage may appear as a complex cystic component, and free intraperitoneal fluid may be seen in cases of intraperitoneal rupture. Adenomas are rare lesions, so they are usually not suspected in a patient unless the clinical history includes known use of oral contraceptives or previous bleeding episodes.

Focal Nodular Hyperplasia

Like adenomas, focal nodular hyperplasia (FNH) is a rare, focal, benign liver lesion. It is composed of hepatocytes, Kupffer cells, and bile ducts, and although it is usually well defined, it is not encapsulated. A central stellate scar is a characteristic gross finding. Unlike adenomas, there is minimal if any association between FNH and oral contraceptives, and bleeding complications are rare. However, studies show that oral contraceptives increase the risk of bleeding for both adenomas and FNH. The sonographic appearance of FNH ranges from hypoechoic to hyperechoic to mixed. The central scar seen pathologically is only occasionally seen sonographically (Fig. 1-28).

Because of the presence of Kupffer cells, approximately half of FNH lesions will show uptake of sulfur colloid that is equal to normal adjacent liver. Approximately 10% will appear hot on sulfur colloid scans due to increased accumulation of radionuclide compared with normal liver. Therefore sulfur colloid scans can be useful in distinguishing FNH from other focal liver lesions, since other lesions are almost always cold.

Focal Hepatic Infections

Pyogenic liver abscesses are most often a secondary development of seeding from intestinal sources, such as appendicitis or diverticulitis; as a direct extension from cholecystitis or cholangitis; or from endocarditis. Like abscesses elsewhere in the body, hepatic abscesses appear as complex fluid collections. Their echogenicity is usu-

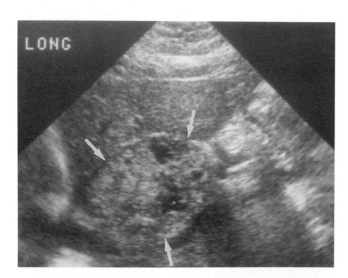

Fig. 1-27 Hepatic adenoma. Longitudinal view of the liver demonstrates an inhomogeneous but predominantly hyperechoic mass *(arrows)* that is replacing most of the caudate lobe of the liver. The cystic internal regions likely represent focal internal hemorrhage.

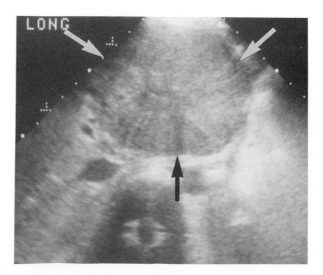

Fig. 1-28 Focal nodular hyperplasia. Transverse view of the liver demonstrates a large solid lesion *(arrows)* replacing much of the left lobe. The stellate configuration to the central aspect of this lesion suggests the diagnosis. Although this configuration is present in this lesion, it is not detected sonographically in most cases of focal nodular hyperplasia.

ally mixed, and although they may mimic solid hepatic masses, the presence of through transmission will often provide a clue to the cystic nature of the mass (Fig. 1-29). Abscesses may also appear as thick-walled cystic lesions or as cysts with fluid-fluid levels. Gas may also result in highly reflective regions with shadowing or ring down artifacts. Abscesses may calcify with healing. The differential for these various appearances primarily includes hematoma, hemorrhagic cyst, and necrotic or hemorrhagic tumor.

Fungal infections of the liver usually occur in immunocompromised patients; the most common organism is *Candida*. Although it usually causes very small lesions (referred to as *microabscesses*), larger lesions occasionally occur. The typical sonographic appearance is a target lesion with a central echogenic region and a peripheral hypoechoic halo. Early lesions may have a hypoechoic focus in the central hyperechoic region caused by necrosis and fungal elements; this appearance has been termed "wheel within a wheel." With healing, candidal abscesses become uniformly hyperechoic and ultimately may calcify.

Pneumocystis carinii infection of the liver is becoming increasingly common in patients with acquired immunodeficiency syndrome. Aerosolized pentamidine controls the infection in the lungs but does not achieve the sufficient systemic concentration necessary to prevent dissemination to other organs, including the liver, spleen, pancreas, and kidneys. Pathologically the lesions in these various organs are granulomas that may or may not show calcification. Sonographically the appearance is very characteristic and consists of multiple echogenic foci scattered throughout the liver (Fig. 1-30). The same appearance has been reported in a very limited number of cases of mycobacterium avium intracellulare and cytomegalovirus infection of the liver.

Parasitic infections of the liver include amebic abscesses, echinococcal disease, and schistosomiasis. Amebic abscesses result from primary colonic involvement with hepatic seeding through the portal vein and are indistinguishable from pyogenic abscesses. *Echinococcus granulosus* causes hydatid disease in the liver. The disease appears as cystic lesions that contain low level internal debris, internal daughter cysts, or a detached internal endocystic membrane. Schistosomiasis is rare in the United States but quite common worldwide. Ova reach the peripheral portal triads and cause a granulomatous reaction. The resulting periportal fibrosis appears as thickened echogenic portal triads.

Hepatic Infarcts

Liver infarcts are uncommon because of the dual arterial and portal blood supply. They usually occur in the setting of underlying vascular disease of the liver. The sonographic appearance of liver infarcts depends on their age; acute infarcts are hypoechoic and chronic infarcts are hyperechoic. Although a wedge shape is characteristic, it is not always seen sonographically (Fig. 1-31).

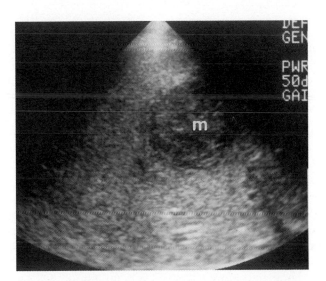

Fig. 1-29   Hepatic abscess. Transverse view of the liver demonstrates an inhomogeneous hypoechoic mass *(m)*. The appearance of the mass itself is nonspecific but the presence of increased through-transmission posterior to the mass suggests that this represents a complex fluid collection which was subsequently proven to be an abscess with percutaneous drainage.

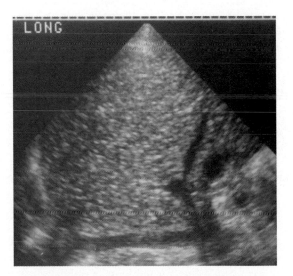

Fig. 1-30   Pneumocystis carinii infection of the liver. Longitudinal view of the liver demonstrates multiple diffuse nonshadowing small hyperechoic foci throughout the liver. Similar foci were seen in the kidneys bilaterally. Patient had Acquired Immune Deficiency Syndrome and pneumocystis carinii pneumonia. These hepatic findings are almost pathognomonic for this condition.

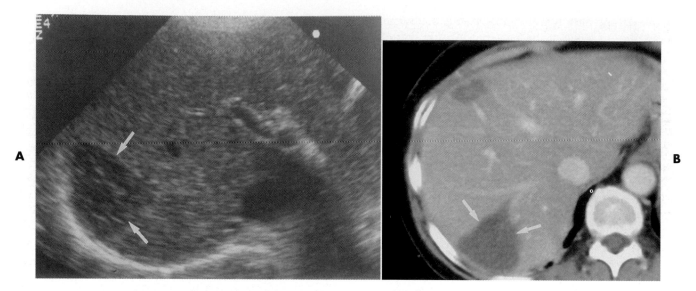

Fig. 1-31   Hepatic infarct. **A,** Transverse view of the liver shows a peripherally-based hypoechoic lesion *(arrows)* that has a wedge shape. **B,** CT scan at a similar level confirms a wedge-shaped region of nonenhancement *(arrows).* Another small infarct is seen anteriorly.

DIFFUSE PARENCHYMAL DISEASE

Hepatitis

Hepatitis usually results in no detectable sonographic abnormality. In a limited number of patients it can cause increased echogenicity of the portal triads (Fig. 1-32), but this is often a subtle finding. Hepatitis can also produce marked thickening of the gallbladder wall, contraction of the gallbladder lumen, and periportal lymphadenopathy.

Fatty Infiltration

Fatty infiltration of the liver is characterized pathologically by intracellular deposition of triglycerides within hepatocytes. It is extremely common in North America and is usually due to obesity. Other common causes include alcohol abuse and certain chemotherapy drugs. In addition, steroids, diabetes, malnutrition, total parenteral nutrition, and toxins, such as carbon tetrachloride, are potential causes.

Fatty infiltration most often manifests in a diffuse distribution and results in uniform increased echogenicity of the liver. Since the normal liver is only slightly more echogenic than the kidney, the diagnosis of fatty infiltration is best made by noting a marked discrepancy between the hyperechoic liver and the less echogenic kidney (Fig. 1-33). In addition, since the normal pancreas is more echogenic than the liver, fatty infiltration should be

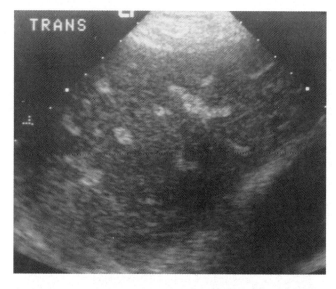

Fig. 1-32   Hepatitis. Transverse view of the liver demonstrates multiple unusually echogenic portal triads. This is a dramatic finding in this patient—the finding is usually more subtle.

considered whenever the liver appears hyperechoic compared to the pancreas (Fig. 1-34). Pancreatitis can cause decreased pancreatic echogenicity that may be mistaken for increased hepatic echogenicity when the two organs are compared. More advanced fatty infiltration will cause significant sound beam attenuation and will make the hepatic vessels, and in some cases the diaphragm, hard to visualize (Fig. 1-35).

In many cases of otherwise diffuse fatty infiltration, there will be focal areas of normal spared liver paren-

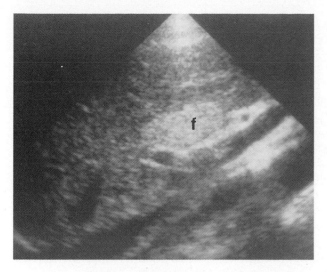

Fig. 1-40   Focal fatty infiltration of the liver. Longitudinal view through the region of the porta hepatis demonstrates an ovoid-shaped hyperechoic region of fatty infiltration *(f)* anterior to the porta hepatis. As in the previous figure, this is a typical site for focal fatty infiltration.

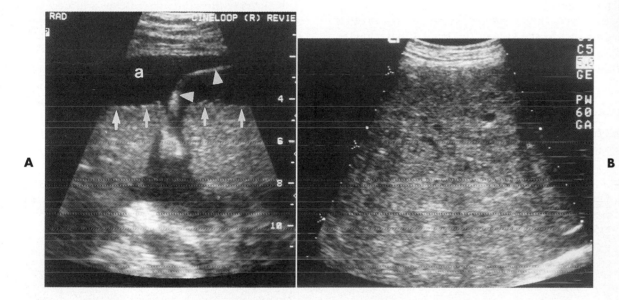

Fig. 1-41   Cirrhosis. **A,** Transverse view of the left lobe of the liver in a patient with alcoholic cirrhosis demonstrates perihepatic ascites *(a).* Nodularity to the anterior surface of the liver *(arrows)* is readily apparent. The ligamentum teres and falciform ligament *(arrowheads)* are outlined by the perihepatic ascites. **B,** Longitudinal view of the right lobe of the liver in another patient with primary biliary cirrhosis demonstrates coarsening and inhomogeneity of the hepatic echotexture.

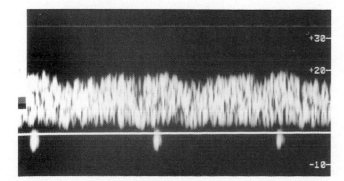

Fig. 1-42   Normal portal venous flow. Pulsed Doppler waveform of the portal vein demonstrates continuous antegrade flow into the liver with essentially no pulsations. This is typical of portal venous flow.

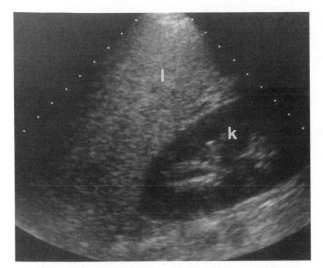

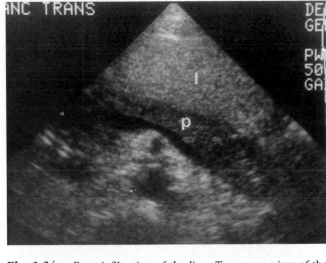

Fig. 1-33   Diffuse fatty infiltration of the liver. Longitudinal view of the right lobe of the liver *(l)* and right kidney *(k)* demonstrates marked discrepancy in echogenicity between the hepatic and renal parenchyma. The gain settings have been adjusted so that the hepatic parenchyma will appear normal, and by doing so the renal parenchyma is almost anechoic. This is a characteristic finding in diffuse fatty infiltration.

Fig. 1-34   Fatty infiltration of the liver. Transverse view of the epigastric region demonstrates pancreatic parenchyma *(p)* that is less echogenic than the hepatic parenchyma in the left lobe of the liver *(l).* This indicates either increased hepatic echogenicity or decreased pancreatic echogenicity. In the absence of a history suggestive of pancreatitis, fatty infiltration of the liver should be suspected in such cases.

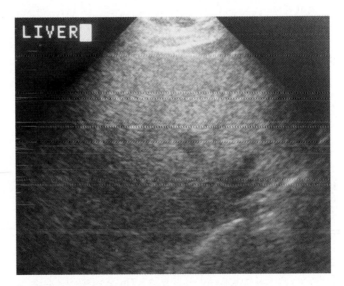

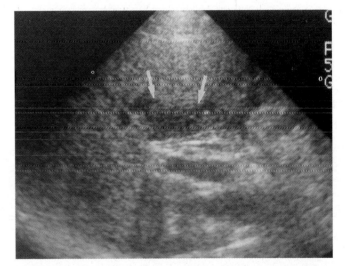

Fig. 1-35   Marked fatty infiltration of the liver. Transverse view of the liver demonstrates markedly increased echogenicity in the anterior aspect of the liver with progressively decreased echogenicity in the deeper portions of the liver due to sound beam attenuation. There is also loss of detectability of the diaphragm and of the intrahepatic vascular structures.

Fig. 1-36   Diffuse fatty infiltration with focal sparing. Longitudinal view through the porta hepatis demonstrates a focal hypoechoic region of hepatic parenchyma *(arrows)* located anterior to the porta hepatis. This represents normal hepatic parenchyma in a liver that is otherwise diffusely hyperechoic secondary to diffuse fatty infiltration.

chyma that appear hypoechoic with respect to the fatty infiltrated parenchyma. If the fatty infiltration is not recognized, the spared areas of normal parenchyma may be mistaken as focal hypoechoic lesions. Fortunately, the spared parenchyma is usually located in front of the right portal vein or portal bifurcation (Fig. 1-36) or around the

gallbladder (Fig. 1-37). Recognition of the typical locations and the fact that focal sparing is usually not spherically shaped generally leads to a confident diagnosis. In fact, when the presence or absence of fatty infiltration in the liver is uncertain, it is often possible to detect the characteristic areas of focal sparing, which allows for a more confident diagnosis of fatty infiltration in the remainder of the liver.

In cases where fatty infiltration of the liver is quite patchy, the geographic margins of the abnormally echogenic fatty infiltrated liver and the lack of mass effect on hepatic vessels serve as clues to the diagnosis (Fig. 1-38). Occasionally, fatty infiltration will be focal and nodular in appearance, which frequently occurs in the an-

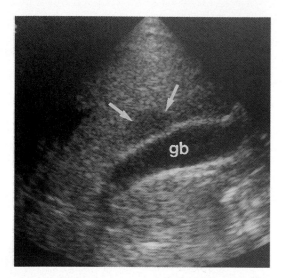

Fig. 1-37 Fatty infiltration with focal sparing. Longitudinal view of the gallbladder *(gb)* demonstrates a focal hypoechoic region of hepatic parenchyma *(arrows)* adjacent to the gallbladder. As in the previous figure, this is a typical site for focal hepatic sparing in a liver that is otherwise diffusely fatty infiltrated.

terior aspect of the medial segment of the left lobe immediately adjacent to the falciform ligament (Fig. 1-39). Another typical location for focal fatty infiltration is anterior to the portal vein bifurcation (Fig. 1-40), which is exactly where focal fatty sparing also typically occurs. The paradoxical deposition and lack of deposition of fat in this location is not well understood but may be related to relative differences in perfusion to this area. Regardless of the etiology, if an elongated hyperechoic lesion is seen in these typical locations in patients with no known primary malignancy, the diagnosis of focal fatty infiltration is almost certain; no further evaluation is necessary.

Cirrhosis

Cirrhosis is caused by hepatocellular death and resulting fibrosis and regeneration. It occurs most commonly due to alcohol abuse, which causes micronodular changes (less than 1 cm in size). Hepatitis is the next most common cause and it results in macronodular cirrhosis (nodules between 1 and 5 cm). Surface nodularity can easily be detected sonographically in the presence of ascites and is a fairly reliable sign of cirrhosis (Fig. 1-41, *A*). In the absence of ascites, surface nodularity is best detected using a high resolution linear or curved array transducer focused on the liver surface. Coarsening of the liver echotexture and inhomogeneity of the liver parenchyma are less specific abnormalities seen with cirrhosis (Fig. 1-41, *B*). Although in advanced disease the liver shrinks, prior to this there is frequently a redistribution of liver volume toward the caudate lobe and the lateral segment of the left lobe.

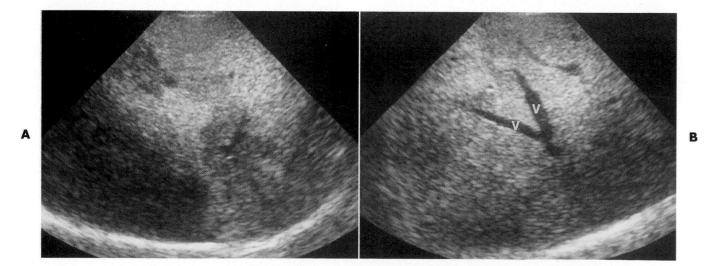

Fig. 1-38 Patchy fatty infiltration of the liver. **A,** Transverse view of the liver demonstrates patchy areas of increased echogenicity in the liver which are poorly marginated in areas and have geographic margins in other areas. **B,** Transverse view of the liver demonstrates a branching hepatic vein *(v)* that passes through a hyperechoic region of the liver without any displacement or distortion.

VASCULAR DISEASE

Normal Hemodynamics

The portal vein normally supplies 75% of the blood flow to the liver. Because it is isolated from the systemic veins and the right atrium, it is relatively unaffected by the pressure changes that occur during cardiac contraction and relaxation. Therefore portal flow is usually characterized by little if any pulsatility (Fig. 1-42). Normal flow velocities average about 20 to 30 cm/sec. Antegrade portal flow into the liver is referred to as hepatopetal.

The hepatic veins drain directly into the inferior vena cava near the right atrium, and the flow is very dependent on right atrial activity. Figure 1-43 illustrates the normal hepatic venous waveform and describes its relationship to atrial contraction and relaxation. Antegrade hepatic venous flow is away from the liver and is referred to as hepatofugal.

Hepatic arterial flow is similar to arterial flow to other solid organs such as the kidney and brain. It has a low resistance arterial waveform with well maintained antegrade flow throughout diastole (Fig. 1-44).

Portal Hypertension

Portal hypertension can be divided into intrahepatic, extrahepatic, and hyperdynamic categories (Box 1-6).

Intrahepatic portal hypertension is the most common type in North America due to the prevalence of alcoholic cirrhosis. In this disease, hepatocellular death results in scarring, which causes increased resistance to flow in the hepatic sinusoids and the small centrilobular veins that drain the sinusoids. Initially, the portal venous pressure increases so that total portal flow to the liver is maintained. However, the resistance to flow into the liver eventually becomes equal to resistance in potential portosystemic collaterals and some of the portal flow becomes diverted into those collaterals. As portal flow decreases, hepatic arterial flow increases to partially compensate for the diminished portal inflow. Eventually, resistance to flow in the sinusoids and central veins becomes so great that even the high pressure hepatic arterial flow has difficulty getting through the normal channels into the hepatic veins. At this point, some of the hepatic artery flow gets diverted into the portal system via microscopic collaterals at the level of the peribiliary plexus and vasa vasorum of the portal vein. When this occurs, flow in the portal vein reverses. This is called *hepatofugal flow* and it indicates advanced portal hypertension.

There are a number of sonographic findings that are seen with portal hypertension. On gray-scale, they include enlargement of the portal vein, splenomegaly, and ascites. Unfortunately, none of these is sufficiently sensitive or specific to be of much diagnostic value. Detection of portosystemic collaterals is the most specific sign of por-

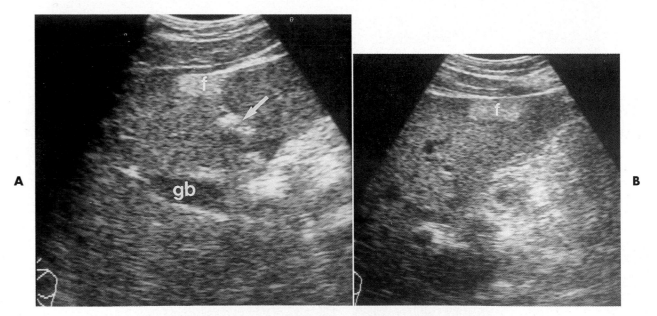

Fig. 1-39 Focal nodular fatty infiltration of the liver. **A,** Transverse view of the liver demonstrates a focal hyperechoic lesion due to fatty infiltration *(f)* in the most anterior aspect of the medial segment of the left lobe. It is positioned immediately adjacent to the lateral segment of the left lobe. The ligamentum teres *(arrow)*, which separates these two segments, is visualized posterior to the lesion. The gallbladder *(gb)* is also seen on this view. **B,** Longitudinal view of the medial segment of the left lobe again demonstrates the hyperechoic lesion *(f)* and displays the typical ovoid shape of focal fatty infiltration in this region.

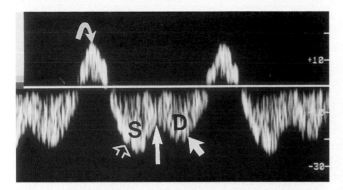

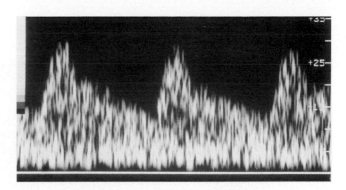

Fig. 1-43   Normal hepatic venous flow. Pulsed Doppler waveform of a normal hepatic vein demonstrates marked variation in the direction and velocity of hepatic venous flow. During right atrial contraction *(curved arrow),* flow is in a retrograde direction back into the liver, which is displayed above the Doppler baseline. After right atrial contraction, there is a phase of rapid right atrial filling and rapid outflow of blood from the hepatic veins into the right atrium, which is visualized as a large pulse below the baseline *(open arrow).* As the right atrium gets progressively fuller, flow out of the hepatic veins starts to slow and the Doppler waveform starts to return toward the baseline. At this point, the tricuspid valve opens up *(long arrow)* and blood from the right atrium starts to flow into the right ventricle. This promotes a second pulse of flow out of the hepatic veins and into the right atrium *(short arrow).* This second pulse of antegrade hepatic venous flow out of the liver is smaller in magnitude than the first pulse. Following this second antegrade pulse, the right atrium contracts again and the cycle repeats itself. The first antegrade pulse corresponds to ventricular systole *(S)* and the second smaller pulse corresponds to ventricular diastole *(D).*

Fig. 1-44   Normal hepatic arterial flow. Pulsed Doppler waveform from an intrahepatic artery demonstrates an arterial signal with a broad systolic peak and well-maintained diastolic flow throughout the cardiac cycle. This is characteristic of a low resistance type arterial bed such as the one that supplies the liver or other types of solid parenchymal organs.

Box 1-6 Classification of Portal Hypertension		
INTRAHEPATIC **Postsinusoidal**	**EXTRAHEPATIC** **Prehepatic**	**HYPERDYNAMIC** **Arterio-portal Fistula**
Cirrhosis	Portal vein thrombosis	Posttraumatic
Veno-occlusive disease	Portal vein compression	Congenital
		Atherosclerotic
Presinusoidal	**Posthepatic**	
Hepatic fibrosis	Hepatic vein thrombosis	
Schistosomiasis	IVC obstruction	
Lymphoma	Constrictive pericarditis	
Sarcoidosis		

hypertension. The easiest collateral to detect sonographically is the recanalized paraumbilical vein. This communicates with the umbilical segment of the left portal vein located between the medial and lateral segment of the left lobe of the liver. It travels in the ligamentum teres and communicates with abdominal wall collaterals (Fig. 1-45 [see also color insert, Plate 2]). It can range in size from 2 mm to greater than 1 cm. In some patients, the fibrous band of the obliterated umbilical vein is seen as a hypoechoic tubular structure in the ligamentum teres and is confused with a collateral on gray-scale. Therefore, detection of hepatofugal venous flow on Doppler is required to establish patency of this potential collateral. The next most easily detected collateral on sonography is the coronary vein. It can be seen behind the left lobe of the liver extending superiorly from the splenic vein (near the portosplenic confluence). It normally has blood flow directed into the splenic vein but may have flow directed away from the splenic vein in patients with portal hypertension (Fig. 1-46 [see also color insert, Plate 3]). Many other potential portosystemic collaterals exist but are more difficult to detect sonographically. These include

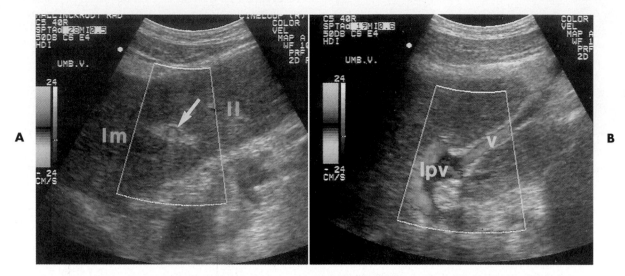

Fig. 1-45   Recanalized paraumbilical vein (see color insert, Plate 2). **A,** Transverse Doppler image of the left lobe of the liver shows a round vessel *(arrow)* in the region of the ligamentum teres between the left medial *(lm)* and left lateral *(ll)* segment. **B,** Longitudinal Doppler image through the ligamentum teres shows a 6 mm vessel *(v)* arising from the left portal vein *(lpv)* and extending out of the liver towards the anterior abdominal wall. Flow towards the transducer indicates hepatofugal flow away from the liver and is consistent with a recanalized paraumbilical vein (see color insert, Plate 2).

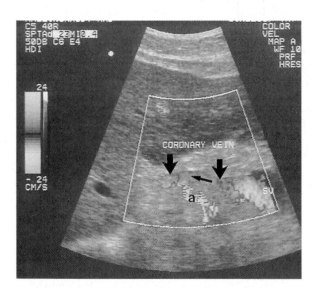

Fig. 1-46   Coronary vein collateral. Longitudinal view of the epigastric region using the left lobe of the liver as an acoustic window shows the splenic vein *(SV)* in cross-section. The coronary vein *(large arrows)* is seen arising from the splenic vein and coursing superiorly in front of an arterial branch of the celiac axis *(a)*. Flow direction in the coronary vein is away from the splenic vein *(small arrow)*, which is strong evidence of portal hypertension (see color insert, Plate 3).

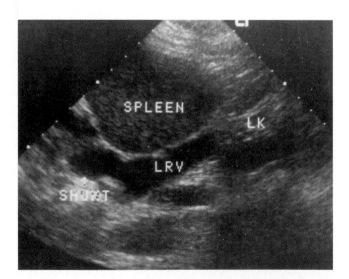

Fig. 1-47   Spontaneous spleno-renal shunt. Transverse view of the left upper quadrant demonstrates the spleen and the mid pole of the left kidney *(LK)*. An enlarged left renal vein *(LRV)* is seen exiting the left kidney and communicating with a vascular structure *(SHUNT)* that could be traced back to the splenic hilum. This is consistent with a spontaneous spleno-renal shunt.

splenorenal (Fig. 1-47), splenoretroperitoneal, superior mesenteric, and inferior mesenteric venous collaterals.

Detection of hepatofugal (retrograde) flow in the portal vein is another relatively specific sign of portal hypertension that occurs in advanced cases. Initially, it occurs in the peripheral branches of the portal vein (Fig. 1-48 [see also color insert, Plate 4]) but it eventually involves the central right and left portal branches and the main portal vein itself (Fig. 1-49 [see also color insert, Plate 5]). It can be recognized when portal flow is going in the opposite direction of the hepatic arteries (Fig. 1-48; Box 1-7).

Extrahepatic causes of portal hypertension are divided into prehepatic and posthepatic. Prehepatic causes include portal vein thrombosis and portal vein compression. Portal vein thrombosis frequently occurs in patients with preexisting portal hypertension resulting from flow

stasis. It also occurs in patients with hypercoaguable states and intestinal infection or inflammation (i.e., appendicitis, diverticulitis, inflammatory bowel disease). On gray-scale, detection of thrombosis depends on identification of an intraluminal filling defect (Fig. 1-50) or abnormal intraluminal echoes (Fig. 1-51). The latter finding

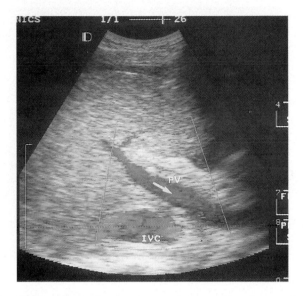

Fig. 1-49   Hepatofugal main portal venous flow. Longitudinal view of the main portal vein *(PV)* demonstrates flow away from the transducer *(arrow)* and therefore away from the liver. This indicates advanced portal hypertension. The inferior vena cava *(IVC)* is seen posterior to the portal vein (see color insert, Plate 5).

Box 1-7	Sonographic Signs of Portal Hypertension

Ascites	Portosystemic collaterals
Splenomegaly	Enlarged hepatic arteries
Portal vein enlargement	Hepatofugal (reversed) portal flow

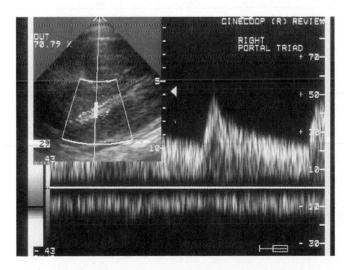

Fig. 1-48   Intrahepatic hepatofugal portal venous flow in a peripheral right portal triad. Longitudinal view of the right lobe of the liver demonstrates a portal triad that has two parallel vessels. One has flow towards the transducer, representing hepatopetal flow, and the other has flow away from the transducer, representing hepatofugal flow. The corresponding pulsed Doppler waveform from this portal triad indicates that the hepatopetal flow (above the baseline) is arising from the hepatic artery and that the hepatofugal flow (below the baseline) is arising from the portal vein (see color insert, Plate 4).

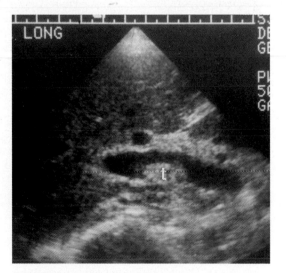

Fig. 1-50   Echogenic portal vein thrombosis. Longitudinal gray scale image of the portal vein demonstrates an echogenic intraluminal thrombus *(t)* that is only partially occluding the lumen.

may be difficult to distinguish from the artifactual low level echoes that often appear in the portal vein. Thrombus can appear hypoechoic (Fig. 1-52) or completely anechoic (Fig. 1-53). In the latter case it will be undetectable with gray-scale sonography, therefore color and duplex Doppler are important adjunctive tools. On color Doppler, portal vein thrombosis appears as a localized flow void or as complete lack of detectable intraluminal flow. When no flow is detected but no thrombus is seen on gray-scale, then the possibility of a patent vein with very slow flow should be considered. In such cases another imaging study, such as contrast enhanced CT or MRI, should be performed to document thrombosis or establish portal vein patency. The overall accuracy of color Doppler in diagnosing portal vein thrombosis is high, with a sensitivity and specificity of approximately 90%. False negatives are very uncommon and the negative predictive value is 98%. One potential cause of a false negative exam is when a large periportal collateral is confused with a patent portal vein (Fig. 1-54 [see also color insert, Plate 6]). On the other hand, the positive predictive value is only 60%, primarily because of false positives due to slow flow.

In addition to bland thrombus, tumors can invade the portal vein and produce intraluminal tumor thrombus. In general, tumor thrombus tends to expand the lumen of the vein more than bland thrombus. Tumor thrombus can confidently be diagnosed if blood flow is seen within the thrombus on color Doppler (Fig. 1-55 [for Fig. 1-55, *B*, see also color insert, Plate 7]). As mentioned earlier, hepatocellular carcinoma is the tumor most likely to invade the portal vein.

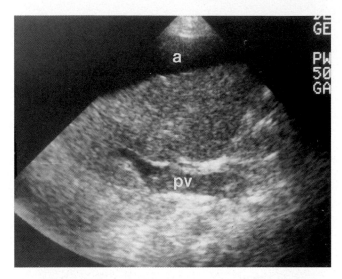

Fig. 1-51   Isoechoic portal vein thrombosis. Longitudinal view of the liver and porta hepatis demonstrates a small cirrhotic liver with perihepatic ascites *(a)*. The portal vein *(pv)* is filled with intraluminal echoes and is isoechoic to the liver, which is consistent with portal vein thrombosis.

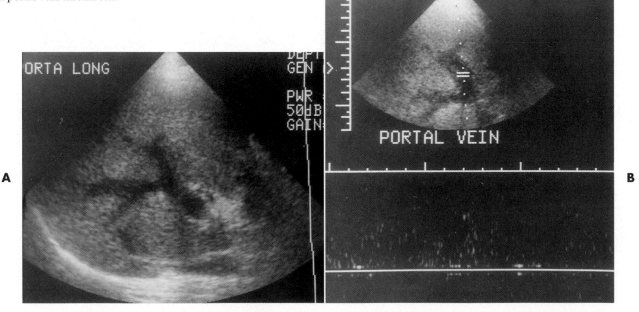

Fig. 1-52   Hypoechoic portal vein thrombosis. **A,** Longitudinal view of the porta hepatis and the right portal vein demonstrates low level internal echoes in the right portal venous system. **B,** Pulsed Doppler waveform from the anterior branch of the right portal vein demonstrates no detectable Doppler signal. A Doppler signal was readily detectable from the adjacent hepatic artery indicating that the lack of detectable flow in the portal vein was not likely a result of improper adjustment of Doppler technical parameters.

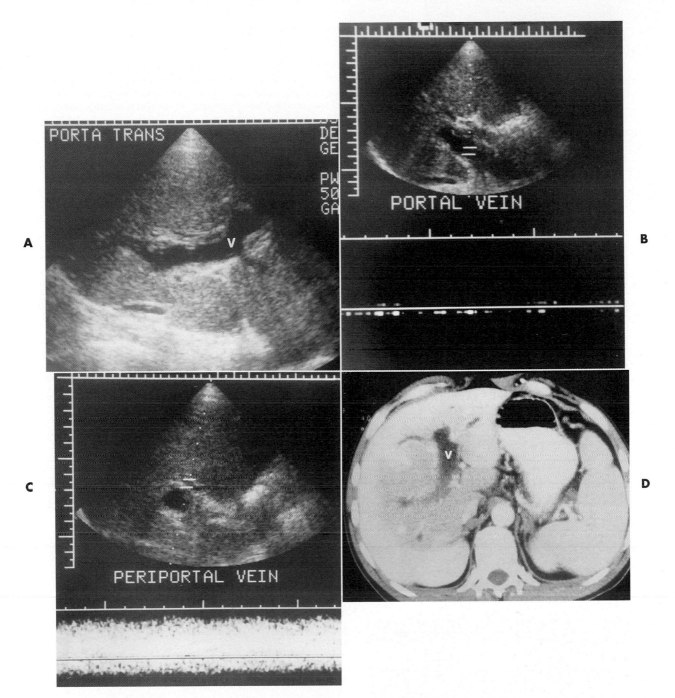

Fig. 1-53   Anechoic portal vein thrombosis with small periportal collaterals. **A,** Transverse ultrasound of the left portal vein *(v)* demonstrates no internal echoes. However, no flow was detected in this portal vein on pulsed Doppler waveform analysis. **B,** Gray scale image and pulsed Doppler waveform from the main portal vein demonstrates no detectable venous flow from the portal vein lumen. **C,** Gray scale image of the porta hepatis with pulsed Doppler sample volume placed adjacent to the portal vein demonstrates venous flow within a small periportal venous collateral. **D,** Contrast-enhanced CT scan shows lack of enhancement of the thrombosed left portal vein *(v)*. Multiple enhancing periportal collaterals are seen.

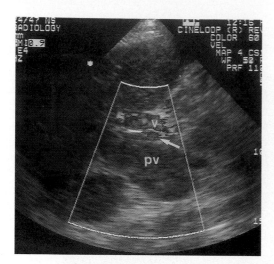

Fig. 1-54   Periportal collateral simulating a patent portal vein. Longitudinal view of the porta hepatis demonstrates a large vein *(v)* in the porta hepatis that looks like the portal vein. However, it is located in front of the hepatic artery *(arrow)*. The actual portal vein *(pv)* is located behind the hepatic artery and is thrombosed (see color insert, Plate 6).

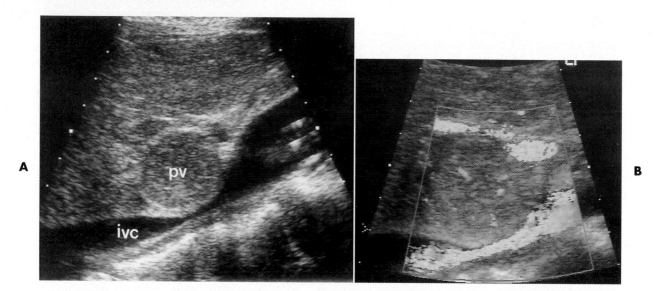

Fig. 1-55   Portal vein tumor thrombus. **A,** Sagittal gray scale image shows a dilated portal vein *(pv)* in cross-section. There is complete filling of the portal vein with intraluminal echoes isoechoic to the adjacent liver. The inferior vena cava *(ivc)* is seen posterior to the portal vein. **B,** Doppler image of the portal vein thrombus demonstrates multiple internal vessels consistent with a vascularized tumor, which was due to hepatocellular cancer (see color insert, Plate 7).

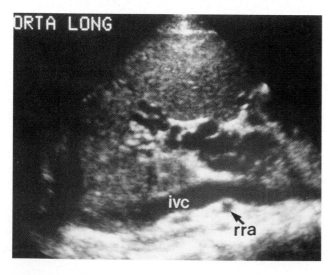

Fig. 1-56   Cavernous transformation of the portal vein. Longitudinal view of the porta hepatis demonstrates multiple tortuous vascular channels in the expected location of the portal vein. No normal portal vein is identified. Doppler analysis of these vessels demonstrated hepatopetal venous flow, consistent with periportal venous collaterals. Also seen is the inferior vena cava *(ivc)* and the right renal artery *(rra)*.

In some cases of portal vein thrombosis, prominent periportal collaterals with hepatopetal flow will form around the portal vein, which is referred to as cavernous transformation of the portal vein (Fig. 1-56). Cavernous transformation of the portal vein is actually a misnomer and should not be confused with recanalized portal vein thrombosis.

Posthepatic causes of portal hypertension include hepatic vein thrombosis, IVC thrombosis, IVC membranes, and constrictive pericarditis. Hepatic vein thrombosis, or the Budd-Chiari syndrome, can potentially produce all the signs of portal hypertension described earlier. In addition it can cause several characteristic changes in the hepatic vein flow. The most obvious is lack of flow in the hepatic veins despite clear identification of the veins on gray-scale (Fig. 1-57 [see also color insert, Plate 8]). In some cases the hepatic veins cannot be identified on gray-scale and no flow is detected on color Doppler. In many cases collateral drainage will develop to compensate for the occluded hepatic veins. This drainage may flow into a main hepatic vein or accessory hepatic vein that has been spared, or into subcapsular veins. When collaterals develop, the hepatic vein that supplies the collateral will have reversed flow (Fig. 1-58 [see also color insert, Plate 9]). In addition, since the hepatic veins are isolated from the right atrium, pulsatility will be blunted, and in most cases the waveform will be monophasic and flat. In the past a flat monophasic hepatic vein waveform was considered highly suggestive of Budd-Chiari syndrome, but it

is now clear that many other causes exist including cirrhosis, diffuse metastatic disease, extrinsic compression of the vein, liver transplant rejection, and other diffuse parenchymal diseases. In fact, a deep inspiration can also cause blunting and occasionally complete loss of hepatic vein pulsatility (Fig. 1-59). For this reason, hepatic vein waveforms should be obtained at normal end expiration.

The sensitivity of Doppler ultrasound in making the diagnosis of Budd-Chiari is quite high when relying on two criteria: (1) Hepatic vein(s) seen on gray-scale with no detectable flow or reversed flow on color Doppler; (2) hepatic vein(s) not seen on either gray-scale or color

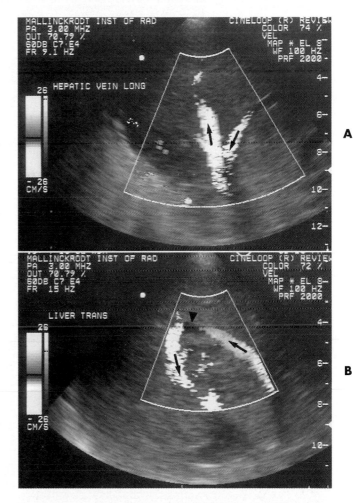

Fig. 1-58 Partial Budd-Chiari syndrome (see color insert, Plate 9). **A,** Longitudinal view of a hepatic venous confluence demonstrates normal direction of flow in one hepatic vein but reversed flow in an adjacent hepatic vein. Flow direction is indicated by the arrows. **B,** More peripheral view of the abnormal hepatic vein seen in **A** shows that this vein communicates with an intrahepatic collateral *(arrowhead),* which then communicates with a hepatic vein that has flow directed normally toward the inferior vena cava. Flow direction is indicated by the arrows. This patient had partial hepatic vein occlusion by a tumor thrombus in the inferior vena cava arising from a renal cell carcinoma.

Fig. 1-57 Budd-Chiari syndrome. Magnified longitudinal view of the liver demonstrates a hepatic vein *(HV, arrows)* and the inferior vena cava *(IVC).* No flow is detected within the hepatic vein despite ready detection of flow in the inferior vena cava. This patient went on to hepatic transplantation and Budd-Chiari syndrome was confirmed surgically (see color insert, Plate 8).

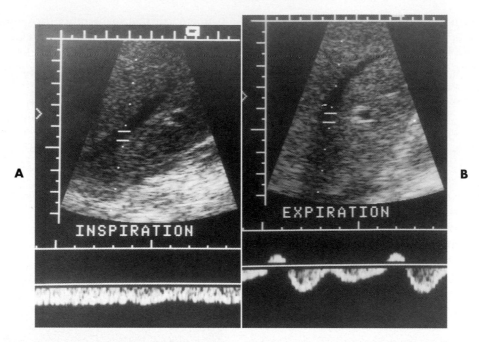

Fig. 1-59   Abnormal hepatic venous waveform due to deep inspiration. **A,** Gray scale image and pulsed Doppler waveform from a hepatic vein obtained during deep inspiration demonstrates flat monophasic flow with no pulsatility. **B,** Similar image obtained during normal end-expiration demonstrates normal triphasic hepatic venous pulsatility. This case illustrates the importance of obtaining hepatic venous waveforms during a normal end-expiration.

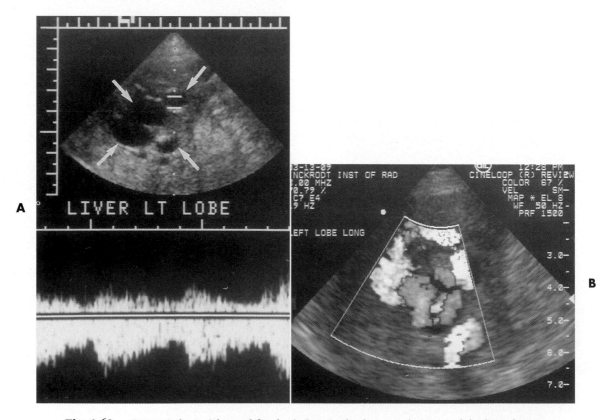

Fig. 1-60   Congenital arterial portal fistula. **A,** Longitudinal gray scale image of the liver demonstrates a multicystic appearing mass in the left lobe *(arrows)*. Doppler waveform analysis from one aspect of this mass demonstrates hepatofugal arterial flow. **B,** Longitudinal color Doppler image of the left lobe of the liver demonstrates color opacification throughout the cystic-appearing lesion, confirming its vascular nature (see color insert, Plate 10).

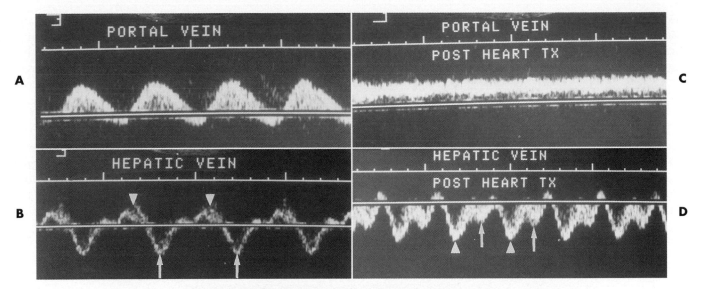

Fig. 1-61   Passive hepatic congestion due to cardiomyopathy. **A,** Pulsed Doppler waveform from the main portal vein demonstrates marked pulsatility with short periods of reversed flow below the baseline. **B,** Pulsed Doppler waveform from a hepatic vein demonstrates conversion of the systolic peak to a reversed direction *(arrowheads)* displayed above the baseline. The normal antegrade diastolic peak *(arrows)* continues to be preserved and displayed below the baseline. This inversion of the systolic peak indicates tricuspid regurgitation. **C,** Pulsed Doppler waveform from the portal vein following cardiac transplantation demonstrates conversion of flow to a normal nonpulsatile monophasic pattern. **D,** Pulsed Doppler waveform of the hepatic vein following heart transplant demonstrates return of normal antegrade systolic flow *(arrowheads)*. Antegrade diastolic flow *(arrows)* remains normal and displayed below the baseline.

Doppler ultrasound. Unfortunately, approximately 15% of patients with cirrhosis but no hepatic vein thrombosis will have one or more hepatic veins that cannot be identified on either gray-scale or color Doppler. Therefore the specificity of ultrasound is relatively poor.

The last category of portal hypertension is called hyperdynamic and it refers to arterio-portal fistulas. These fistulas may be congenital or posttraumatic (such as liver biopsy) and can also result from a hepatic artery aneurysm that erodes into the adjacent portal vein. They generally appear as a multilobulated, multicystic mass in the liver. Doppler analysis will reveal arterial flow within the lesion and reversal of flow in the draining portal vein (Fig. 1-60 [for Fig. 1-60, *B,* see also color insert, Plate 10]).

Passive Hepatic Congestion

Heart failure can result in passive congestion of the liver and resulting right upper quadrant pain and liver function abnormalities. It can be suggested by noting enlarged hepatic veins and inferior vena cava on gray scale. Pulsed Doppler waveforms from the portal vein will show prominent pulsatility related to the cardiac cycle. The minimum degree of portal vein pulsatility required to diagnose right heart dysfunction is not uniformly agreed upon. However, most would agree that when pulsatile portal flow reaches or goes below the Doppler

baseline, right heart dysfunction is almost certainly present (Fig. 1-61, *A*).

Right-sided heart failure will also produce increased pulsatility in the hepatic veins so that the antegrade and retrograde components are more equalized (Fig. 1-62).

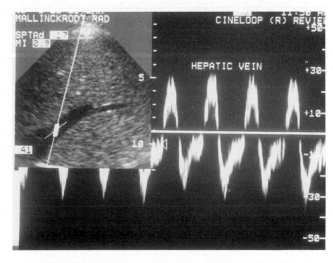

Fig. 1-62   Hepatic venous flow in a patient with right-sided heart failure. Gray scale image and pulsed Doppler waveform of the middle hepatic vein demonstrates increased pulsatility with large components of retrograde flow during right atrial contraction. This is referred to as the *W* pattern.

Tricuspid regurgitation causes the normally antegrade systolic hepatic vein flow to reverse and produces a waveform where there is only one antegrade pulse that occurs during diastole (Fig. 1-61, *B*).

Hepatic Transplant Complications

Improvements in surgical techniques have decreased, but not eliminated, the incidence of complications following liver transplantation. The major complications that sonography is capable of detecting are vascular and biliary. Identification of biliary obstruction and bile leaks depends on the same principles that apply to the native liver (see Chapter 3).

Vascular thrombosis and stenosis can affect the hepatic artery, portal vein, hepatic veins, and the IVC following transplantation. Arterial lesions are especially critical because the bile ducts are supplied exclusively by the hepatic arteries, and significant interruption of arterial flow results in biliary necrosis. Hepatic artery thrombosis is suspected when no arterial signal is detected on either duplex or color Doppler. Since thrombosis can affect the main hepatic artery or the right or left branch, all three vessels should be studied. In most cases an arterial signal excludes thrombosis. However, collateral arterial flow can develop in pediatric patients and result in a weak signal despite complete thrombosis of the main hepatic artery. Arterial stenosis is more difficult to detect. Peak

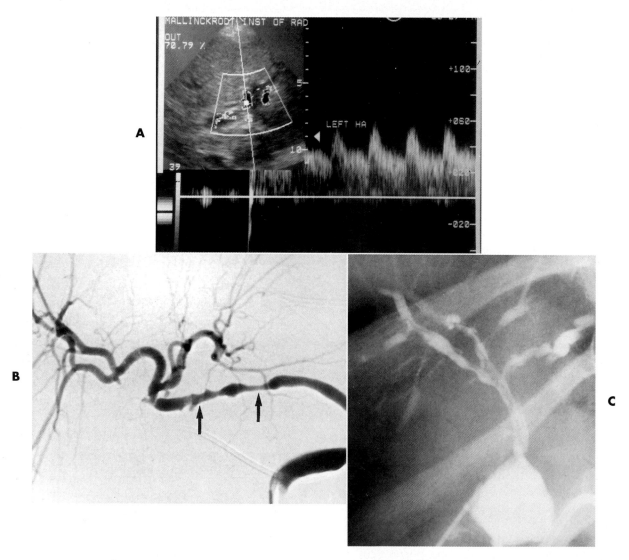

Fig. 1-63   Hepatic transplant artery stenosis. **A,** Pulsed Doppler waveform from the left hepatic artery demonstrates prominent diastolic flow. The resistive index measured 0.4, which is a finding consistent with more proximal hepatic artery stenosis. **B,** Hepatic arteriogram demonstrating a long irregular stricture of the main donor hepatic artery *(arrows)*. **C,** Cholangiogram demonstrating multiple strictures and irregularity of the intrahepatic bile ducts consistent with biliary ischemia.

systolic velocities greater than 200 cm/sec or focal increases in velocity of greater than threefold suggests a stenosis of greater than 50%. A more easily obtained and perhaps more accurate sign of proximal stenosis is a resistive index of less than 0.5 from an intrahepatic artery (Fig. 1-63):

$$\text{Resistive index} = \frac{(\text{systole} - \text{diastole})}{\text{diastole}}$$

As with other stenotic arteries, turbulent flow can cause perivascular soft tissue vibration that may be visible both on color Doppler and on pulsed Doppler.

Portal vein, hepatic vein, and IVC thrombosis appear as they would in native livers. Portal vein stenosis can occur at the anastomosis and should be suspected when there is a threefold to fourfold focal increase in the flow velocity in the portal vein. Stenosis of the IVC at the superior anastomosis causes focal velocity elevation, loss of pulsations in the hepatic veins and in the proximal IVC, and hepatic vein flow reversal. Loss of hepatic vein pulsatility has also been reported in rejection.

Portosystemic Shunts

A variety of portosystemic shunts can be created surgically to decompress the portal system in patients with portal hypertension. These generally involve a shunt between the portal vein or superior mesenteric vein and the inferior vena cava or between the splenic vein and the left renal vein. Of the surgical shunts, the portocaval shunts are in general the easiest to evaluate sonographically for shunt patency (Fig. 1-64 [see also color insert, Plate 11]). Splenorenal shunts are more difficult due to left upper quadrant bowel gas.

Intrahepatic shunts can be created percutaneously using expandable metallic stents. These are referred to as transjugular intrahepatic portosystemic shunts (TIPS). TIPS are very easy to evaluate for patency because the liver provides an acoustic window and overlying bowel gas is not a problem as it often is with surgical shunts. In fact, it is possible in most cases to detect shunt malfunction before the patients become symptomatic by performing regular Doppler evaluations of the shunt and the portal veins. In most normal cases there will be reversal of portal flow above where the stent enters the portal vein (Fig. 1-65 [see also color insert, Plate 12]). If this normal reversal converts to antegrade flow on follow-up scans, then there is probably decreased flow going through the shunt. This may be due to either a stenosis at the hepatic vein level or neointimal hyperplasia in the stent itself. Other signs of stent malfunction are a focal increase in velocities across the narrowed segment on a given examination (Fig. 1-66) or a temporal decrease in velocities proximal to the narrowing on sequential exams. In some patients neointimal hyperplasia and hepatic vein stenosis can also be imaged directly. It is seen as a narrowing in the flow lumen (Box 1-8; Fig. 1-67 [see also color insert, Plate 13]).

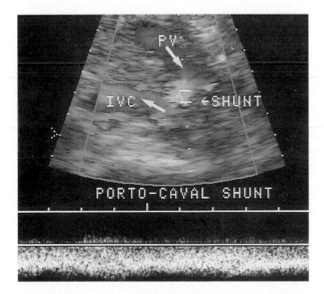

Fig. 1-64   Portocaval shunt. Longitudinal view of the porta hepatis demonstrates communication between the portal vein *(PV)* and inferior vena cava *(IVC)* via a surgically created shunt. The shunt is widely patent on the color Doppler image and monophasic flow is seen on the pulsed Doppler waveform. Flow direction in the portal vein and vena cava is indicated by the arrows. As expected, portal venous flow is reversed (see color insert, Plate 11).

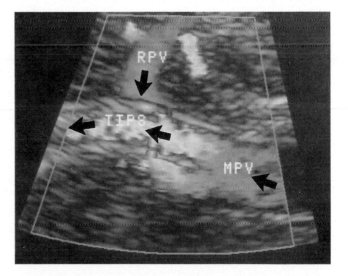

Fig. 1-65   Normal transjugular intrahepatic portosystemic shunt. Longitudinal view of the intrahepatic stent demonstrates intraluminal flow in the stent *(TIPS)* and main portal vein *(MPV)* away from the portal vein and towards the inferior vena cava. Flow in the right portal vein *(RPV)* above the entrance site of the shunt is reversed (i.e., directed towards the shunt). Flow direction is indicated by the arrows (see color insert, Plate 12).

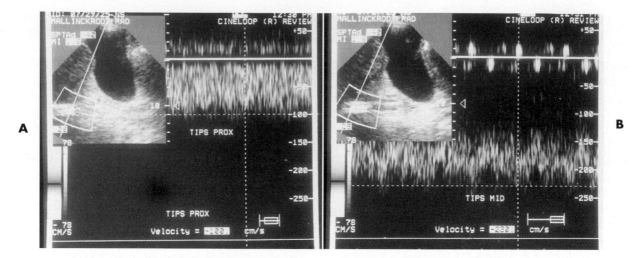

Fig. 1-66   Transjugular intrahepatic portosystemic shunt stenosis. **A,** Pulsed Doppler waveform from the proximal stent demonstrates a flow velocity of 100 cm/sec. **B,** Pulsed Doppler waveform from the midportion of the stent demonstrates a velocity of 230 cm/sec. This increase in velocity reflects faster flow across a narrowed segment of the stent. Neointimal hyperplasia was confirmed on a subsequent venogram.

Box 1-8   Signs of TIPS Malfunction

Change in intrahepatic portal flow from hepatofugal to hepatopetal

Flow void next to stent wall on color Doppler

Reversal of hepatic venous flow

Drop in stent velocity from one exam to the next

Focal increase in stent velocity on a single exam

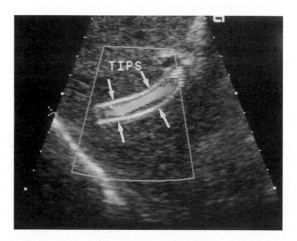

Fig. 1-67   Neointimal hyperplasia. Longitudinal color Doppler view of a TIPS stent shows a patent lumen but incomplete color opacification from wall-to-wall because of excessive neointimal hyperplasia along the posterior surface of the stent. The corrugated, echogenic walls of the stent *(arrows)* are well shown on this image (see color insert, Plate 13).

Key Features

Echogenicity of the liver should be equal or slightly greater than that of the right kidney, equal or less than that of the pancreas, and less than that of the spleen.

The segments of the liver are divided by the hepatic veins, the gallbladder, the interlobar fissure, and the ligamentum teres.

Focal liver lesions can exhibit a variety of appearances, none of which is absolutely specific for a particular etiology. Lesions with hypoechoic rims are usually malignant. Homogeneous hyperechoic lesions and lesions with hyperechoic rims are usually hemangiomas.

Fatty infiltration is usually diffuse and causes increased hepatic echogenicity. Fatty infiltration often localizes adjacent to the ligamentum teres or portal bifurcation. Focal sparing frequently localizes around the gallbladder and portal bifurcation.

Cirrhosis causes the hepatic parenchyma to be coarsened and inhomogeneous and the liver surface to be nodular.

The sonographic signs of portal hypertension are splenomegaly, ascites, portal systemic collaterals, and reversal of portal venous flow.

The diagnosis of portal vein thrombosis requires the combined use of gray-scale analysis and color-Doppler imaging and relies on the absence of detectable blood flow or the visualization of intraluminal filling defects.

Budd-Chiari syndrome may appear as an intraluminal hepatic vein thrombus, reversal of hepatic vein flow, no detectable hepatic vein flow, and hepatic vein collaterals.

SUGGESTED READINGS

Abu-Yousef MM: Duplex Doppler sonography of the hepatic vein in tricuspid regurgitation, *AJR* 156:79-83, 1991.

Abu-Yousef MM: Normal and respiratory variations of the hepatic and portal venous duplex Doppler waveforms with simultaneous electrocardiographic correlation, *J Ultrasound Med* 11:263-268, 1992.

Abu-Yousef MM, Milam SG, Farner RM: Pulsatile portal vein flow: a sign of tricuspid regurgitation on duplex Doppler sonography, *AJR* 155:785-788, 1990.

Atri M et al: Incidence of portal vein thrombosis complicating liver metastasis as detected by duplex ultrasound, *J Ultrasound Med* 9:285-289, 1990.

Birnbaum BA et al: Definitive diagnosis of hepatic hemangiomas: MR imaging versus Tc-99m-labeled red blood cell SPECT, *Radiology* 176:95-101, 1990.

Bolondi L et al: Liver cirrhosis: changes of Doppler waveform of hepatic veins, *Radiology* 178:513-516, 1991.

Bree RL et al: The varied appearances of hepatic cavernous hemangiomas with sonography, computed tomography, magnetic resonance imaging, and scintigraphy, *Radiographics* 7:1153-1175, 1987.

Cho KJ, Lunderquist A: The peribiliary vascular plexus: the microvascular architecture of the bile duct in the rabbit and in clinical cases, *Radiology* 147:357-364, 1983.

Cronan JJ et al: Cavernous hemangioma of the liver: role of percutaneous biopsy, *Radiology* 166:135-138, 1988.

Dodd GD et al: Detection of malignant tumors in end-stage cirrhotic livers: efficacy of sonography as a screening technique, *AJR* 159:727-733, 1992.

Duerinckx AJ et al: The pulsatile portal vein in cases of congestive heart failure: correlation of duplex Doppler findings with right atrial pressures, *Radiology* 176:655-658, 1990.

Gibney RG, Hendin AP, Cooperberg PL: Sonographically detected hepatic hemangiomas: absence of change over time, *AJR* 149:953-957, 1987.

Gibson PR et al: A comparison of duplex Doppler sonography of the ligamentum teres and portal vein with endoscopic demonstration of gastroesophageal varices in patients with chronic liver disease or portal hypertension, or both. *J Ultrasound Med* 11:327-331, 1992.

Gibson RN et al: Identification of a patent paraumbilical vein by using Doppler sonography: importance in the diagnosis of portal hypertension. *AJR* 153:513-516, 1989.

Goyal AK, Pokharna DS, Sharma SK: Ultrasonic measurements of portal vasculature in diagnosis of portal hypertension. A controversial subject reviewed, *J Ultrasound Med* 9:45-48, 1990.

Marn CS, Bree RL, Silver TM: Ultrasonography of the liver. Technique and focal and diffuse disease, *Radiologic Clin North Am* 29:1151-1170, 1991.

Millener P et al: Color Doppler imaging findings in patients with Budd-Chiari syndromes: correlation with venographic findings, *AJR* 161:307-312, 1993.

Mostbeck GH et al: Hemodynamic significance of the paraumbilical vein in portal hypertension: assessment with duplex US, *Radiology* 170:339-342, 1989.

Nelson RC, Chezmar JL: Diagnostic approach to hepatic hemangiomas, *Radiology* 176:11-13, 1990.

Quinn SF, Gosink BB: Characteristic sonographic signs of hepatic fatty infiltration, *AJR* 145:753-755, 1985.

Ralls PW: Color Doppler sonography of the hepatic artery and portal venous system, *AJR* 155:517-525, 1990.

Tessler FN et al: Diagnosis of portal vein thrombosis: value of color Doppler imaging, *AJR* 157:293-296, 1991.

Want SS et al: Focal hepatic fatty infiltration as a cause of pseudotumors: ultrasonographic patterns and clinical differentiation, *J Clin Ultrasound* 18:401-409, 1990.

Weltin G et al: Duplex Doppler: identification of cavernous transformation of the portal vein, *AJR* 144:999-1001, 1985.

Wernecke K et al: Pathologic explanation for hypoechoic halo seen on sonograms of malignant liver tumors: an in vitro correlative study, *AJR* 159:1011-1016, 1992.

Wernecke K et al: The distinction between benign and malignant liver tumors on sonography: value of a hypoechoic halo, *AJR* 159:1005-1009, 1992.

White EM et al: Focal periportal sparing in hepatic fatty infiltration: a cause of hepatic pseudomass on US, *Radiology* 162:57-59, 1987.

Yates CK, Streight RA: Focal fatty infiltration of the liver simulating metastatic disease, *Radiology* 159:83-84, 1986.

Yoshikawa J et al: Focal fatty change of the liver adjacent to the falciform ligament: CT and sonographic findings in five surgically confirmed cases, *AJR* 149:491-494, 1987.

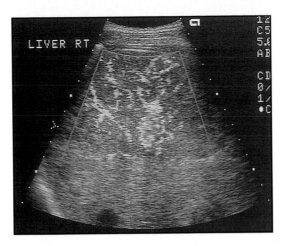

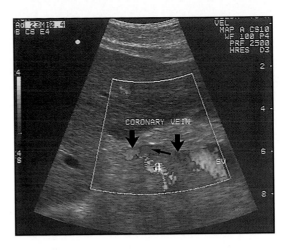

Plate 1 Hepatocellular carcinoma. Transverse color-Doppler scan of the mass in the right lobe of the liver demonstrates marked hypervascularity of this lesion. Hypervascularity is characteristic of hepatocellular carcinoma, but this degree of detectable increased flow is unusual on color Doppler (see also Fig. 1-23, *B*).

Plate 3 Coronary vein collateral. Longitudinal view of the epigastric region using the left lobe of the liver as an acoustic window shows the splenic vein *(SV)* in cross-section. The coronary vein *(large arrows)* is seen arising from the splenic vein and coursing superiorly in front of an arterial branch of the celiac axis *(a)*. Flow direction in the coronary vein is away from the splenic vein *(small arrow)*, which is strong evidence of portal hypertension (see also Fig. 1-46).

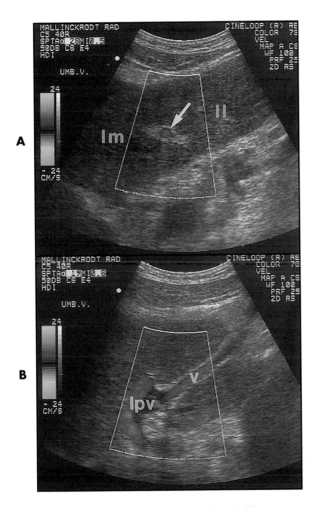

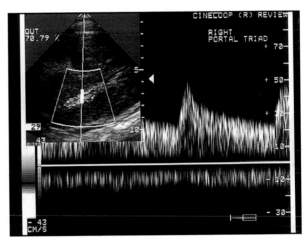

Plate 4 Intrahepatic hepatofugal portal venous flow in a peripheral right portal triad. Longitudinal view of the right lobe of the liver demonstrates a portal triad that has two parallel vessels. One has flow toward the transducer *(red)*, representing hepatopetal flow, and the other has flow away from the transducer *(blue)*, representing hepatofugal flow. The corresponding pulsed-Doppler waveform from this portal triad indicates that the hepatopetal flow (above the baseline) is arising from the hepatic artery and that the hepatofugal flow (below the baseline) is arising from the portal vein (see also Fig. 1-48).

Plate 2 Recanalized paraumbilical vein. **A**, Transverse color-Doppler image of the left lobe of the liver shows a round vessel *(arrow)* in the region of the ligamentum teres between the left medial *(lm)* and left lateral *(ll)* segment. **B**, Longitudinal color-Doppler image through the ligamentum teres shows a 6 mm vessel *(v)* arising from the left portal vein *(lpv)* and extending out of the liver toward the anterior abdominal wall. Flow toward the transducer indicates hepatofugal flow away from the liver and is consistent with a recanalized paraumbilical vein (see also Fig. 1-45).

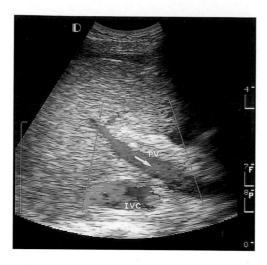

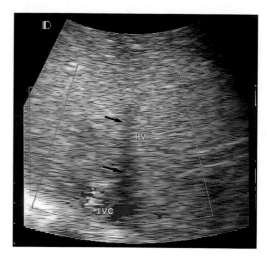

Plate 5 Hepatofugal main portal venous flow. Longitudinal view of the main portal vein *(PV)* demonstrates flow away from the transducer *(arrow)* and therefore away from the liver. This indicates advanced portal hypertension. The inferior vena cava *(IVC)* is seen posterior to the portal vein (see also Fig. 1-49).

Plate 8 Budd-Chiari syndrome. Magnified longitudinal view of the liver demonstrates a hepatic vein *(HV, arrows)* and the inferior vena cava *(IVC)*. No flow is detected within the hepatic vein despite ready detection of flow in the inferior vena cava. This patient went on to hepatic transplantation and Budd-Chiari syndrome was confirmed surgically (see also Fig. 1-57).

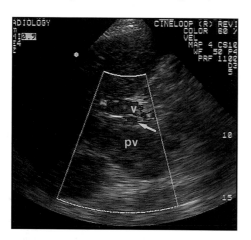

Plate 6 Periportal collateral simulating a patent portal vein. Longitudinal view of the porta hepatis demonstrates a large vein *(v)* in the porta hepatis that looks like the portal vein. However, it is located in front of the hepatic artery *(arrow)*. The actual portal vein *(pv)* is located behind the hepatic artery and is thrombosed (see also Fig. 1-54).

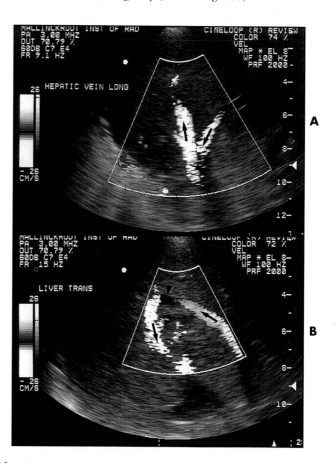

Plate 9 Partial Budd-Chiari syndrome. **A,** Longitudinal view of a hepatic venous confluence demonstrates normal direction of flow in one hepatic vein *(blue)* but reversed flow in an adjacent hepatic vein *(red)*. Flow direction is indicated by the arrows. **B,** More peripheral view of the abnormal hepatic vein seen in **A** shows that this vein communicates with an intrahepatic collateral *(arrowhead)*, which then communicates with a hepatic vein that has flow directed normally toward the inferior vena cava. Flow direction is indicated by the arrows. This patient had partial hepatic vein occlusion by a tumor thrombus in the inferior vena cava arising from a renal cell carcinoma (see also Fig. 1-58).

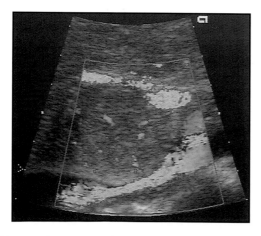

Plate 7 Portal vein tumor thrombus. Color-Doppler image of the portal vein thrombus demonstrates multiple internal vessels consistent with a vascularized tumor, which was due to hepatocellular cancer (see also Fig. 1-55, B).

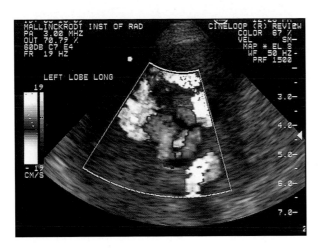

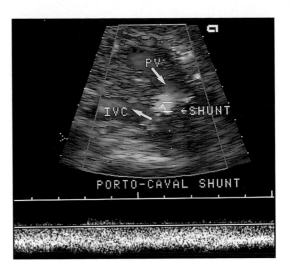

Plate 10 Congenital arterial portal fistula. Longitudinal color-Doppler image of the left lobe of the liver demonstrates color opacification throughout the cystic-appearing lesion, confirming its vascular nature (see also Fig. 1-60, *B*).

Plate 11 Portocaval shunt. Longitudinal view of the porta hepatis demonstrates communication between the portal vein *(PV)* and inferior vena cava *(IVC)* via a surgically created shunt. The shunt is widely patent on the color-Doppler image and monophasic flow is seen on the pulsed-Doppler waveform. Flow direction in the portal vein and vena cava is indicated by the arrows. As expected, portal venous flow is reversed (see also Fig. 1-64).

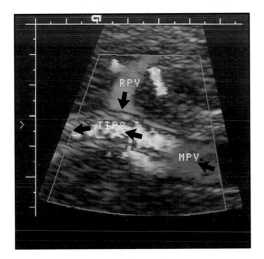

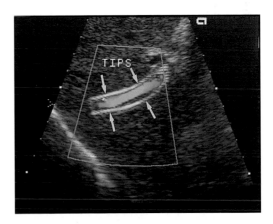

Plate 12 Normal transjugular intrahepatic portosystemic shunt. Longitudinal view of the intrahepatic stent demonstrates intraluminal flow in the stent *(TIPS)* and main portal vein *(MPV)* away from the portal vein and towards the inferior vena cava. Flow in the right portal vein *(RPV)* above the entrance site of the shunt is reversed (i.e., directed towards the shunt). Flow direction is indicated by the arrows (see also Fig. 1-65).

Plate 13 Neointimal hyperplasia. Longitudinal color-Doppler view of a TIPS stent shows a patent lumen but incomplete color opacification from wall-to-wall because of excessive neointimal hyperplasia along the posterior surface of the stent. The corrugated, echogenic walls of the stent *(arrows)* are well shown on this image (see also Fig. 1-67).

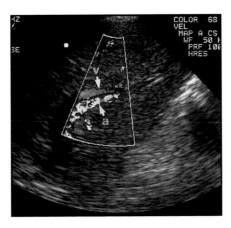

Plate 14 Enlarged hepatic artery simulating a dilated bile duct. Color-Doppler view shows that both of the parallel tubular structures are vascular. The enlarged hepatic artery *(a)* is seen posterior to the portal vein *(v)*. Flow is reversed in the portal vein secondary to severe portal hypertension (see also Fig. 3-12, *B*).

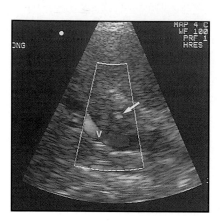

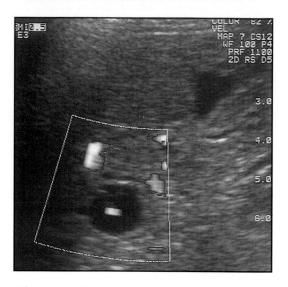

Plate 15 Cholangiocarcinoma. Color-Doppler view at the level of the mass demonstrates the hepatic artery *(arrow)* completely encased by this mass. This is generally regarded as a sign of non-resectability. The portal vein *(v)* is compressed by the mass (see also Fig. 3-20, *B*).

Plate 16 Caroli's disease with associated hepatic fibrosis. Color-Doppler view shows flow within the central echogenic focus ("central dot"), confirming its vascular nature (see also Fig. 3-31, *C*).

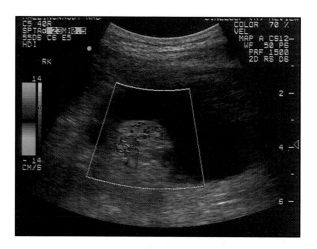

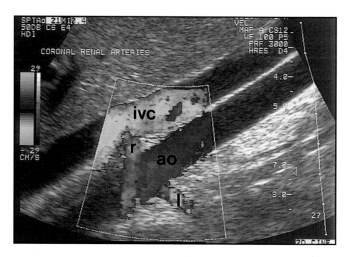

Plate 17 Cystic renal cell carcinoma. Longitudinal color-Doppler view of a cyst demonstrates vascularity within the mural nodule. This rules out the possibility of an adherent blood clot. Renal cell carcinoma arising from the wall of the cyst was confirmed surgically in this patient (see also Fig. 4-32, *B*).

Plate 18 Coronal view of the main renal arteries. Color-Doppler image obtained from the right lateral aspect of the abdomen demonstrates the inferior vena cava *(ivc)* and the aorta *(ao)* traveling side-by-side. The origins of the right *(r)* and left *(l)* renal arteries are well demonstrated. Views of this clarity are difficult to obtain in most patients (see also Fig. 4-71).

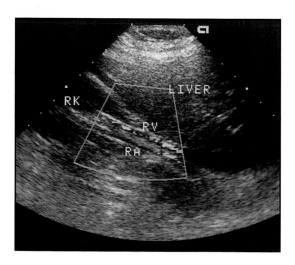

Plate 19 Normal relationship of the renal vein and renal artery. Transverse color-Doppler view of the right upper quadrant shows the liver and right kidney *(RK)* as well as the main renal artery *(RA)* and renal vein *(RV)*. The renal artery travels posterior to the renal vein (see also Fig. 4-72).

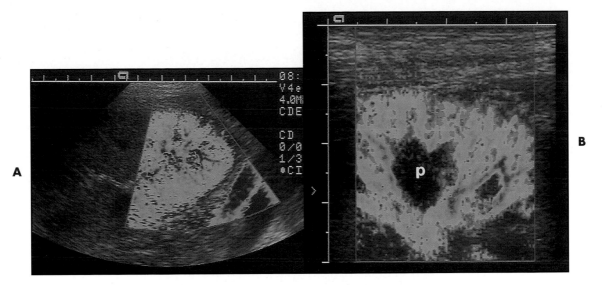

Plate 20 Normal renal parenchymal blood flow. **A,** Longitudinal power-Doppler view of a renal transplant demonstrates normal perfusion throughout the renal parenchyma with vessels extending from the renal sinus to the capsular surface. The iliac vessels are seen on the inferior aspect of the transplant. **B,** Transverse view of the superficial aspect of a renal transplant obtained with a 7.0-MHz linear array using power-Doppler imaging demonstrates a hypoechoic renal pyramid *(p)* exhibiting little detectable flow. There is readily detectable flow and multiple discrete identifiable vessels throughout the remainder of the cortex extending to the capsular surface of the transplant. This image graphically displays the difference in perfusion between the cortical tissue and the renal pyramids (see also Fig. 4-73).

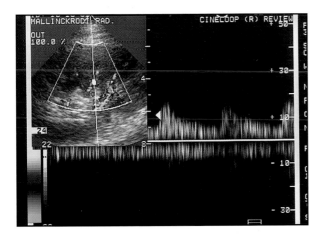

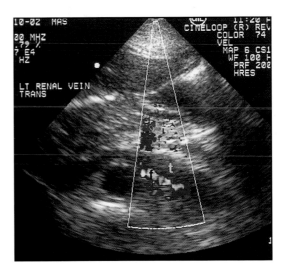

Plate 21 Right renal vein thrombosis. Longitudinal color-Doppler image and pulsed-Doppler waveform analysis of the right kidney demonstrates normal-appearing intrarenal blood flow on the color-Doppler study and normal arterial and venous waveforms on pulsed-Doppler analysis (see also Fig. 4-80, *A*).

Plate 22 Left renal vein thrombosis. Transverse color-Doppler image confirms that there is some residual flow *(f)* within the posterior aspect of the left renal vein, but that there is nonocclusive thrombus *(t)* in the anterior aspect of the renal vein. This indicates the difficulty in relying just on gray-scale imaging and pulsed-Doppler waveform analysis for the diagnosis of renal vein thrombosis (see also Fig. 4-81, *C*).

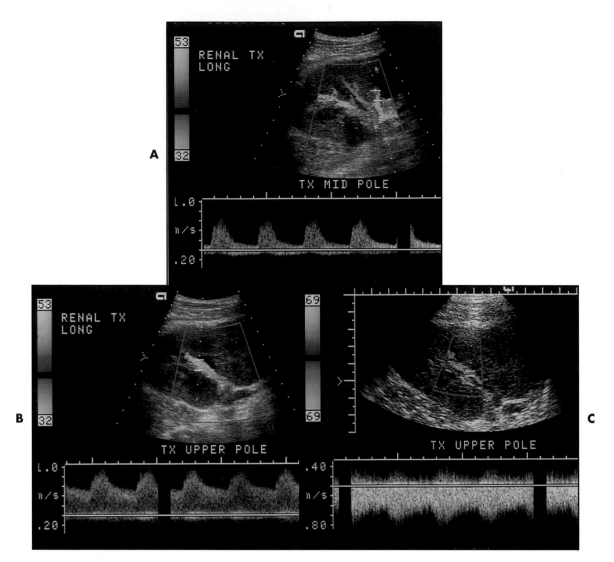

Plate 23   Renal arteriovenous fistula. **A,** Longitudinal color-Doppler image from the midpole of a renal transplant demonstrates several segmental vessels extending from the renal sinus into the renal parenchyma. The pulsed-Doppler sample volume is placed on a vessel in the midpole and the corresponding Doppler waveform shows slightly diminished diastolic flow but an otherwise normal appearance. **B,** Similar color-Doppler view, but in this case the pulsed-Doppler sample volume is placed on an artery leading to the upper pole. The corresponding waveform demonstrates increased flow velocities versus those in the vessel sampled in **A.** In addition, the diastolic flow is increased dramatically. These findings indicate a decreased resistance to flow in this vessel and are very suggestive of an arteriovenous fistula. **C,** Color-Doppler view of the upper pole of the transplant demonstrates the pulsed-Doppler sample volume positioned over an upper pole draining vein. The waveform from this vein is arterialized. This provides conclusive evidence of an arteriovenous communication in the upper pole (see also Fig. 4-82).

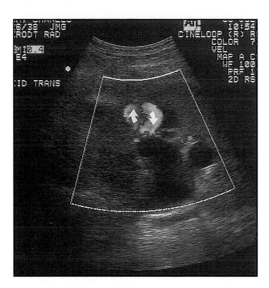

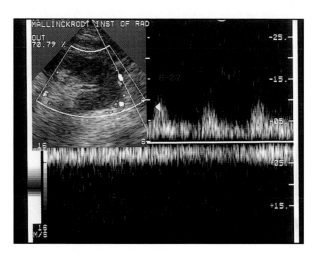

Plate 24 Pseudoaneurysm. Transverse view of the upper pole of a renal transplant shows blood flow in the lumen of a rounded structure. The swirling pattern of flow, with half of the lumen exhibiting flow traveling toward the transducer and the other half showing flow away from the transducer *(curved arrows)*, is characteristic of a pseudoaneurysm. Fig. 4-20 was also obtained from this patient (see also Fig. 4-83).

Plate 25 Renal transplant lower pole infarction. Color-Doppler image from the lower pole confirms the absence of parenchymal flow but the presence of collateral flow around the renal capsule. Both arterial and venous capsular flow is identified on pulsed-Doppler waveform analysis (see also Fig. 4-86, *C*).

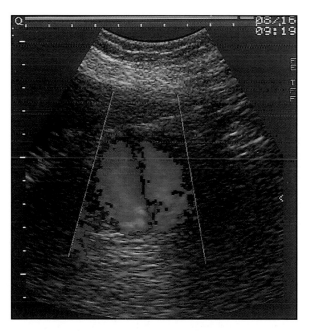

Plate 26 Splenic artery aneurysm simulating a pancreatic cyst. Longitudinal color-Doppler view of the left upper quadrant demonstrates flow within the lumen of this cystic structure. The swirling pattern with flow both toward and away from the transducer is typical of flow within an aneurysm. Arteriography subsequently proved this was a large splenic artery aneurysm (see also Fig. 5-15, *B*).

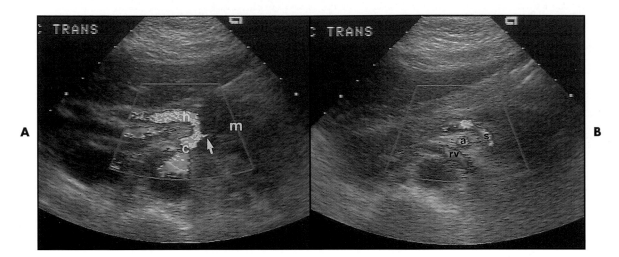

Plate 27 Pancreatic carcinoma that involves the celiac axis but spares the superior mesenteric artery. **A,** Transverse color-Doppler view of the upper abdomen demonstrates the celiac axis *(c)* and hepatic artery *(h).* A hypoechoic soft tissue mass *(m)* is seen obliterating the normal fat plane around these arteries. The soft tissue mass is also encasing and narrowing the origin of the splenic artery *(arrow).* In this patient the primary mass arose at the junction of the body and tail of the pancreas and extended posteriorly to involve these vessels. **B,** Transverse color-Doppler view slightly inferior to A shows the superior mesenteric artery *(a)* completely surrounded by echogenic fibrofatty tissue. At this level there is no evidence of arterial involvement. The splenic vein *(s)* and the left renal vein *(rv)* are also seen (see also Fig. 5-27).

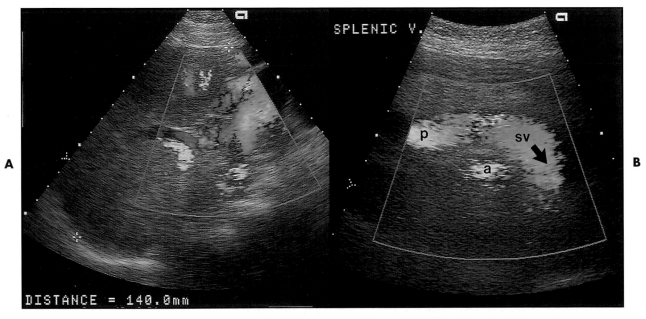

Plate 28 Splenomegaly. **A,** Longitudinal view of the left upper quadrant demonstrates mild splenomegaly with a splenic length of 14 cm. There are also prominent vessels in the splenic hilum displayed on a color-Doppler study. Based on the findings in this image, the splenomegaly could be due to a number of factors. The prominent hilar vascularity suggests portal hypertension, but splenomegaly stemming from other causes can also result in increased splenic blood flow and enlargement of the splenic hilar vessels. **B,** Transverse view of the epigastrium demonstrates the splenic vein *(sv)* and portosplenic confluence *(p).* Blood flow in the splenic vein is reversed *(arrow)* and traveling away from the portosplenic confluence. This is convincing evidence of portal hypertension with the development of splenic vein-to-systemic vein collaterals. A splenorenal shunt was subsequently identified in this patient. Also seen is the superior mesenteric artery *(a)* (see also Fig. 6-11).

CHAPTER 2

Gallbladder

For a Key Features summary see p. 53.

ANATOMY

The gallbladder is a pear-shaped organ that is positioned beneath the liver immediately adjacent to the interlobar fissure (Fig. 2-1). The fissure can be a useful landmark for locating small contracted gallbladders or gallbladders that are completely filled with stones (Fig. 2-2). Likewise, the gallbladder can be used as a landmark for identifying the junction between the left and right lobes of the liver. The upper limits of normal for the transverse dimension of the gallbladder is 4 cm. The length of the gallbladder is more variable but generally does not exceed 10 cm. The normal upper limit for the gallbladder wall thickness is 3 mm. When the gallbladder contracts, the echogenic mucosa and the hypoechoic muscularis become apparent and the wall may appear thickened (Fig. 2-3). However, even with gallbladder contraction, the wall usually remains less than 3 mm thick. See Table 2-1 for the characteristics of a normal gallbladder.

Variations in shape of the gallbladder are common. When the gallbladder fundus folds on itself it is referred to as a *phrygian cap*. There is frequently a junctional fold in the gallbladder neck and occasionally multiple folds. Gallbladder folds may mimic septations, but true septations are extremely rare, and in most cases it is possible to demonstrate communications between the folded segments of the gallbladder (Fig. 2-4). Variations in the location of the gallbladder are rare; intrahepatic gallbladders are probably the most frequently recognized. Most intrahepatic gallbladders are located immediately above the interlobar fissure (Fig. 2-5).

TECHNIQUE

Ideally, patients should fast after midnight before a gallbladder sonogram to ensure adequate gallbladder distention and to reduce upper abdominal bowel gas. A recent meal makes the examination harder to perform and interpret and decreases diagnostic sensitivity. However, in most cases diagnostic information can be obtained even in nonfasting patients, so a recent meal is not an absolute contraindication to performing a gallbladder sonogram.

Most gallbladder exams start with the patient in the supine position using a 3 or 5 MHz sector transducer. The gallbladder should be scanned from both a subcostal and intercostal approach whenever possible, since one of the approaches will usually display pathology and diminish artifacts more optimally. In most cases a deep inspiration allows better visualization of the gallbladder. Frequently there are low-level artifactual echoes in the gallbladder lumen resulting from reverberations, which can often be eliminated by scanning from a more lateral and superior approach and using more of the liver as a window. Scans should routinely be obtained with the patient in a variety of positions (left posterior oblique [LPO], left lateral decubitus [LLD], prone, upright) to document mobility of intraluminal structures, such as stones and sludge, and nonmobility of polyps and tumors. Although it is important to visualize the entire gallbladder, concentrate on the gallbladder neck, since stones can be missed if the entire neck is not visualized (Fig. 2-6) or if the stone is wedged in the neck (Fig. 2-7).

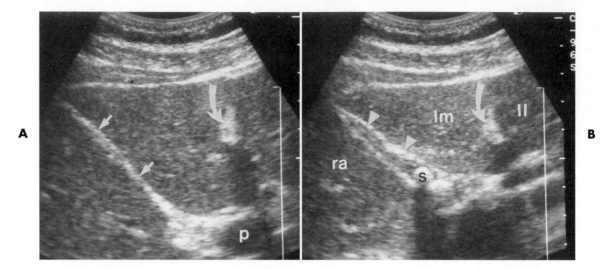

Fig. 2-1   Relationship of interlobar fissure to the gallbladder. **A,** Transverse view of the anterior aspect of the liver demonstrates the interlobar fissure *(arrows)* extending from the porta hepatis *(p).* The ligamentum teres *(curved arrow)* is also identified. **B,** Transverse view slightly inferior to **A** shows a contracted gallbladder *(arrowheads)* located immediately inferior to the interlobar fissure. A single gallstone *(s)* is seen in the gallbladder neck. The right anterior hepatic segment *(ra),* left medial segment *(lm),* and left lateral segment *(ll)* of the liver are separated by the ligamentum teres *(curved arrow),* interlobar fissure, and gallbladder fossa as indicated in these figures.

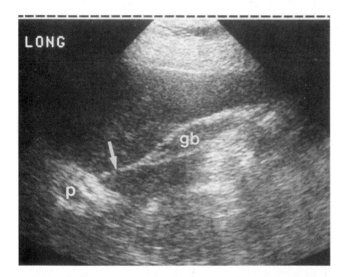

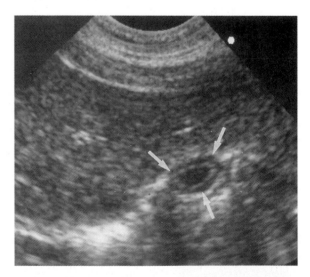

Fig. 2-2   Interlobar fissure localizing a contracted gallbladder. Longitudinal view of the right upper quadrant shows the interlobar fissure *(arrow)* extending from the portal vein *(p)* to an ovoid soft tissue structure *(gb).* Although this soft tissue structure has no lumen, its relationship to the interlobar fissure is strong evidence that it is a completely contracted gallbladder.

Fig. 2-3   Contracted gallbladder. Transverse view of the right upper quadrant demonstrates a contracted gallbladder *(arrows)* with good demarcation of the inner echogenic mucosal layer and the outer hypoechoic muscular layer of the gallbladder. Although the wall appears thickened in this image, it actually measured only 2.3 mm in thickness.

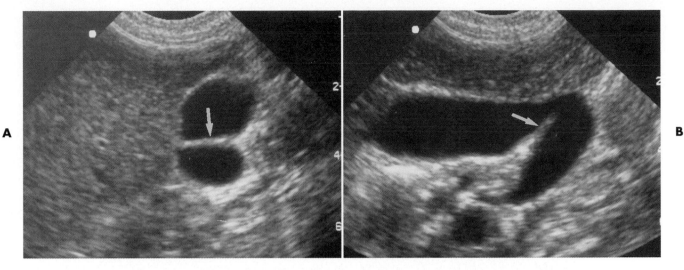

Fig. 2-4   Prominent gallbladder fold simulating a septation. **A,** Transverse view of the gallbladder demonstrates an apparent complete septation *(arrow)* separating the gallbladder into two compartments. **B,** Longitudinal view of the gallbladder shows that this actually represents a prominent gallbladder fold *(arrow)* and that the two apparently separate components actually communicate with each other.

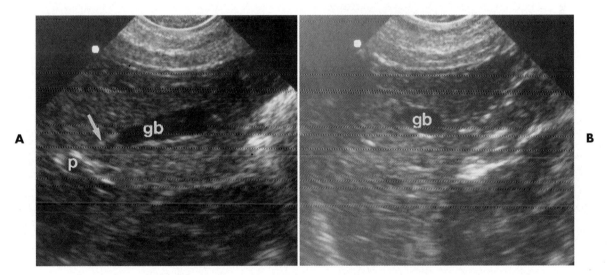

Fig. 2-5   Intrahepatic gallbladder. **A,** Longitudinal view of the gallbladder *(gb)* demonstrates the hepatic parenchyma completely surrounding the gallbladder lumen. The interlobar fissure *(arrow)* is seen running between the gallbladder and the portal vein *(p)*. **B,** Transverse view of the gallbladder *(gb)* demonstrates hepatic parenchyma completely surrounding the gallbladder lumen.

Table 2-1 Characteristics of the normal gallbladder	
Characteristic	**Appearance**
Location	Inferior to interlobar fissure
	Between left and right lobe
Size	<4 cm transverse
	<10 cm longitudinal
Wall thickness	<3 mm
Lumen	Anechoic

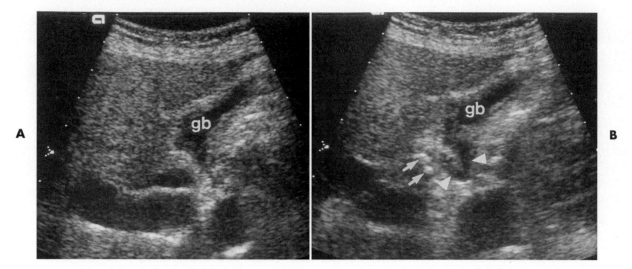

Fig. 2-6   Stones in the gallbladder neck that are difficult to visualize. **A,** Initial longitudinal view of the gallbladder *(gb)* shows that it is contracted but demonstrates no evidence of stones. **B,** Subsequent view better demonstrates a tortuous gallbladder neck *(arrowheads)* and two stones positioned in the neck *(arrows)*.

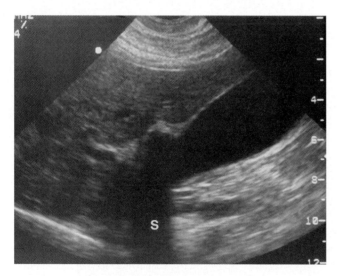

Fig. 2-7   Poorly visualized stone in the gallbladder neck. Longitudinal view of the gallbladder demonstrates an acoustic shadow *(s)* arising from the region of the gallbladder neck. This is because of a stone that is impacted in the gallbladder neck with no bile separating it from the gallbladder wall. Because of this, the anterior surface of the stone blends in with the anterior gallbladder wall and makes it difficult to perceive.

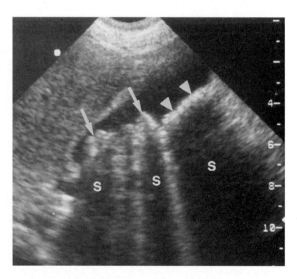

Fig. 2-8   Typical gallstones. Longitudinal view of the gallbladder demonstrates faceted stones *(arrows)* in the superior aspect of the gallbladder and multiple smaller stones *(arrowheads)* in the inferior aspect of the gallbladder. All of these stones cast acoustic shadows *(s)*.

GALLSTONES

Sonography has assumed an important role in evaluating the gallbladder because it is the most sensitive means of detecting gallstones. Multiple studies have documented sensitivities of greater than 90%. Even in obese patients sonography is better than oral cholecystography in detecting stones.

Gallstones appear as mobile, echogenic, intraluminal structures that cast acoustic shadows (Fig. 2-8). Shadowing occurs because of sound beam absorption by the stone. It is important to demonstrate shadowing because it distinguishes stones from other intraluminal abnormalities. Shadowing primarily depends on the size of the stone. Stones smaller than 3 mm may not cast a detectable shadow. In contrast, shadowing is largely independent of

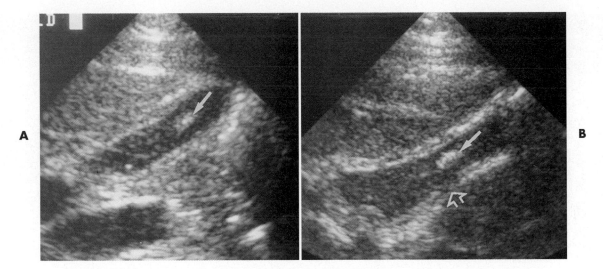

Fig. 2-9   Dependence of gallstone shadowing on transducer frequency. **A,** Longitudinal view of the gallbladder obtained with a 3 MHz transducer shows an echogenic focus *(arrow)* in the gallbladder lumen but no apparent shadow. Based on this image, the differential diagnosis would include a polyp or a sludge ball. **B,** Similar view obtained with a 5 MHz transducer shows the same echogenic focus *(arrow).* However, with this higher frequency transducer, the back wall of the gallbladder is clearly being obscured behind the echogenic focus *(open arrow)* because of acoustic shadowing. Detection of this shadowing allows for a confident diagnosis of cholelithiasis.

Table 2-2   Intraluminal abnormalities in the gallbladder

Ultrasound characteristics	Common	Uncommon
Shadowing and mobile	Stones	Nothing else
Nonshadowing and mobile	Sludge	Stones (<3 mm)
Nonshadowing and nonmobile	Polyps	Sludge

stone composition, and in particular, calcification is not necessary for shadow production.

Technical factors need to be optimized in order to demonstrate shadowing from small stones. Because sound absorption increases at higher frequencies, nonshadowing stones may be converted into shadowing stones by switching to a higher frequency transducer (Fig. 2-9). Another important factor is the focal zone. Since the beam profile is narrowest at the focal zone, it should be set at the depth of the stone so that the stone will absorb a greater percentage of the sound beam. If there are multiple small stones, shadowing may be best demonstrated by positioning the patient so that the stones are clumped together.

The major differential considerations are gallbladder polyps and sludge balls (Table 2-2). Polyps are small soft tissue structures that are adherent to the gallbladder wall. They do not move and do not shadow. Sludge balls (tumefactive sludge) are almost always mobile but do not produce a shadow.

When the gallbladder is completely filled with stones, all that is apparent is an echogenic shadowing structure in the right upper quadrant that could potentially be confused with a gas-filled loop of bowel. If an identifiable gallbladder is seen elsewhere, then the problem is solved. If not, then the character of the shadow is important, since in most cases stones produce a clean shadow and gas produces a dirty shadow (Fig. 2-10). Exceptions to this rule occasionally occur (Fig. 2-11) and are probably a result of differences in the surface characteristics of gallstones.

A stone-filled gallbladder will also frequently produce a *wall-echo-shadow (WES)* complex that consists of three, arc-shaped lines followed by a shadow (Fig. 2-12). The first line is echogenic and represents the interface between the gallbladder wall and the liver. The second is hypoechoic and represents the gallbladder wall itself. The third is echogenic and arises from the stones. Although a WES complex is a very reliable sign of a gallbladder filled with stones, it is not possible to demonstrate it in every case. Therefore it is a useful finding when seen but it is not useful when absent.

As mentioned earlier, the vast majority of gallstones fall to the dependent aspect of the gallbladder. When there are multiple small stones arranged in a layer along the dependent gallbladder wall, they may be confused with a thickened wall itself (Fig. 2-13). In such cases identification of the stones and detection of an acoustic shadow are easier on transverse views.

When the density of bile is increased by administration of oral cholecystographic agents, stones may float in a nondependent location. Rarely, a stone will float in the

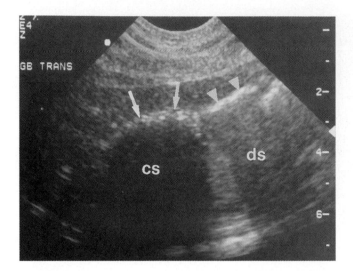

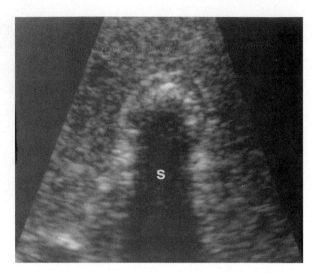

Fig. 2-10   Gallstones producing clean shadowing. Transverse view of the right upper quadrant demonstrates a clean shadow *(cs)* arising from the anterior surface of a gallbladder completely filled with stones *(arrows)*. A dirty shadow *(ds)* is seen arising from a gas-filled loop of bowel *(arrowheads)* adjacent to the gallbladder.

Fig. 2-12   Wall-echo-shadow complex. Magnified transverse view of the gallbladder demonstrates a series of curved lines with a clean posterior acoustic shadow *(s)*. The deep echogenic line represents the anterior surface of multiple gallstones in the gallbladder lumen. The adjacent hypoechoic line represents the gallbladder wall. The most superficial echogenic line represents the reflection arising from the interface between the gallbladder wall and the liver.

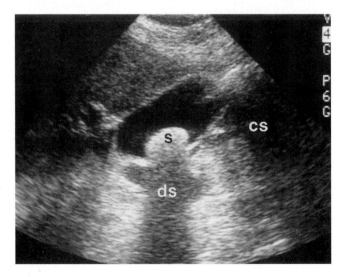

Fig. 2-11   Gallstone producing a relatively dirty shadow. Longitudinal view of the gallbladder demonstrates an intraluminal stone *(s)* that is producing a dirty shadow *(ds)* when compared to the cleaner shadow *(cs)* arising from an adjacent loop of gas-filled bowel.

nondependent aspect of the gallbladder even when the bile has not been altered (Fig. 2-14). This occurs when the specific gravity of bile is greater than the specific gravity of the stone and always indicates that the stones are cholesterol in nature.

SLUDGE

Sludge consists of calcium bilirubinate granules and cholesterol crystals in thick, viscous bile. It appears as

low- to high-level, nonshadowing reflectors in the gallbladder. Typically sludge localizes in the dependent portion of the gallbladder and forms a bile-sludge level (Fig. 2-13). In some cases the crystalline components of sludge float in the nondependent portion of the gallbladder lumen (Fig. 2-15). Sludge may completely fill the gallbladder lumen or it may form mass-like aggregates called sludge balls or tumefactive sludge (Fig. 2-16). In some cases sludge will have a very inhomogeneous appearance with prominent hypoechoic regions. It can also form echogenic bands that can be confused with sloughed membranes (Fig. 2-17). The lack of shadowing distinguishes the different forms of sludge from gallstones, and mobility distinguishes sludge from polyps and tumors. In rare cases, it will not be possible to demonstrate mobility of sludge. In such cases a follow-up examination several weeks later is often helpful to demonstrate mobility or a change in appearance and thus exclude gallbladder neoplasm. Color Doppler imaging is also potentially useful in isolated cases since detection of blood flow excludes tumefactive sludge from the differential diagnosis. Lack of detectable flow is not helpful because it can occur in hypovascular tumors in addition to tumefactive sludge.

The clinical significance of sludge is not entirely clear but it can probably be thought of as an asymptomatic dynamic equilibrium between crystal development and elimination in the majority of patients. Nonetheless, in a minority of patients it probably represents the early stage of gallstone formation.

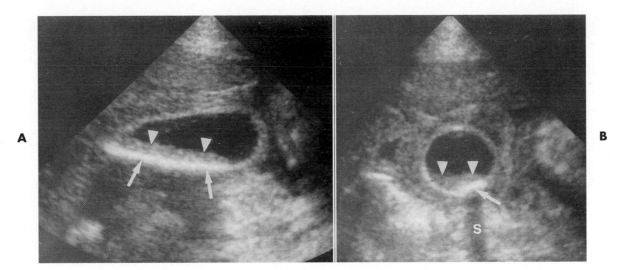

Fig. 2-13   Gallbladder sludge and multiple small gallstones layering in the dependent portion of the gallbladder. **A,** Longitudinal view of the gallbladder demonstrates sludge *(arrowheads)* in the dependent portion of the gallbladder lumen. The dependent wall of the gallbladder appears echogenic due to multiple small stones *(arrows)* layering on top of the wall. Posterior acoustic shadowing is present but difficult to appreciate. **B,** Transverse view of the gallbladder again demonstrates sludge *(arrowheads).* Note the lack of shadowing posterior to the sludge. The gallstones *(arrow)* and the acoustic shadow they produce *(s)* are more easily perceived than on the longitudinal view.

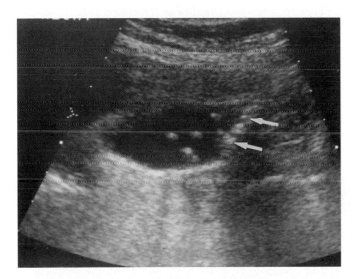

Fig. 2-14   Floating stones. Longitudinal view of the gallbladder obtained with the patient upright demonstrates multiple stones that have fallen to the dependent portion of the gallbladder *(arrows).* In addition however, there are multiple stones that are seen to float in the nondependent portion of the gallbladder lumen.

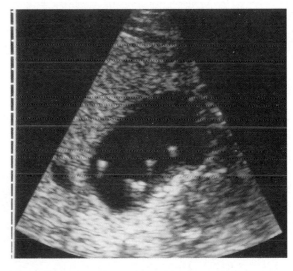

Fig. 2-15   Intraluminal cholesterol crystals. Longitudinal view of the gallbladder demonstrates multiple bright reflectors in the gallbladder lumen. The short comet tail artifacts and the lack of acoustic shadowing are characteristic of cholesterol crystals and distinguish them from floating stones.

ACUTE CHOLECYSTITIS

In the majority of cases, acute cholecystitis occurs from persistent obstruction of the cystic duct or gallbladder neck by an impacted gallstone. If the stone does not spontaneously disimpact or some form of therapy is not initiated, the gallbladder may become necrotic and perforate. In most cases the inflammatory process and the

patient's symptoms can be controlled by antibiotics and supportive care so that cholecystectomy can be performed electively in 2 to 4 days.

There are a number of sonographic findings that support the diagnosis of acute cholecystitis and of advanced acute cholecystitis (Boxes 2-1 and 2-2). They include (1) gallstones, (2) gallbladder wall thickening, (3) gallbladder enlargement, (4) pericholecystic fluid, and (5) focal ten-

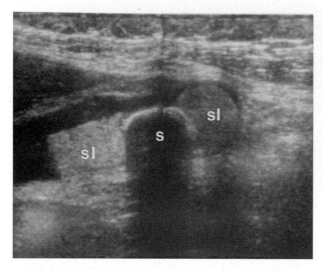

Fig. 2-16   Tumefactive sludge. Longitudinal view of the gall-bladder demonstrates a shadowing stone *(s)* and two adjacent non-shadowing intraluminal structures consistent with tumefactive sludge *(sl).*

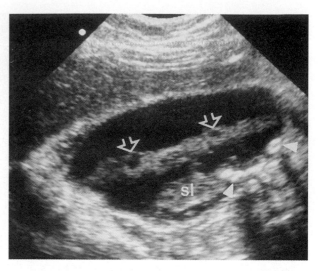

Fig. 2-17   Membranous-appearing sludge. Longitudinal view of the gallbladder demonstrates shadowing stones *(arrowheads)* and sludge *(sl)* in the dependent portion of the gallbladder. A linear membrane-like accumulation of nondependent sludge is also seen in the gallbladder lumen. Several focal hypoechoic areas *(open arrows)* are also seen in the sludge.

Box 2-1 Sonographic Signs of Acute Cholecystitis	
Gallstones	Pericholecystic fluid
Wall thickening (≥3 mm)	Sonographic Murphy's
Gallbladder enlargement	sign

Box 2-2   Sonographic Signs of Advanced Acute Cholecystitis
Pericholecystic fluid
Sloughed mucosal membranes
Irregular striated intramural sonolucencies
Wall disruption

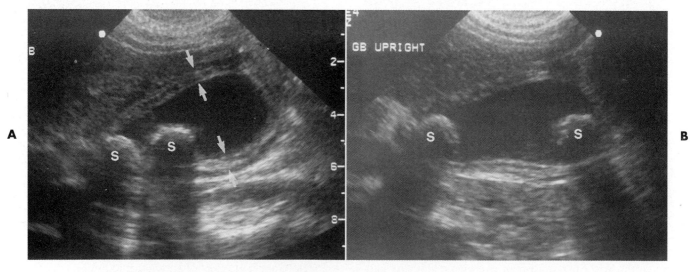

Fig. 2-18   Acute cholecystitis. **A,** Longitudinal view of the gallbladder with the patient supine demonstrates two shadowing stones *(s)* in the gallbladder lumen. The gallbladder wall *(arrows)* is diffusely thickened. **B,** Upright view of the gallbladder demonstrates that one stone has rolled into the dependent portion of the gallbladder, but the other stone is impacted in the gallbladder neck. This impacted stone was the cause of the acute cholecystitis in this patient.

derness directly over the gallbladder. By themselves, none of these findings are pathognomonic for acute cholecystitis, but the combination of several findings in the appropriate clinical setting is highly suggestive. The positive predictive value of gallstones and a positive sonographic Murphy's sign is 92%, whereas the negative predictive value is 95%.

Gallbladder wall thickening greater than or equal to 3 mm occurs in the majority of patients with acute cholecystitis (Fig. 2-18). Unfortunately there are many other causes of wall thickening and the sonographic appearance of the thickened gallbladder wall is not helpful in distinguishing cholecystitis from other abnormalities. However, in patients with acute cholecystitis, the finding of irregular, striated sonolucencies in the thickened wall is suggestive of necrosis and indicates a more advanced form of cholecystitis (Fig. 2-19). Another sonographic sign of gallbladder wall necrosis is sloughed mucosal membranes (Fig. 2-20), which is rarely seen, and as previously mentioned, can be simulated by sludge.

Pericholecystic fluid collections occur in approximately 20% of patients with acute cholecystitis and generally indicate perforation and/or abscess formation. Many of these collections occur in the gallbladder fossa between the gallbladder and the liver. Others are located in the gallbladder wall itself (Fig. 2-21) or are loculated in the peritoneal cavity (Fig. 2-20). Pericholecystic fluid is important to recognize since it usually indicates more advanced cholecystitis and the need for more urgent surgical intervention.

There continues to be debate about the use of sonography vs. hepatobiliary scintigraphy in patients with suspected acute cholecystitis. The reasons for starting with sonography are the following:

1. Approximately 70% of patients with clinically suspected acute cholecystitis will have some other

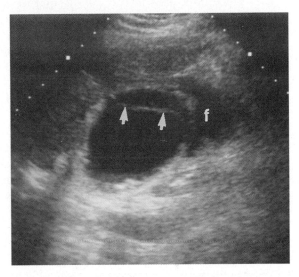

Fig. 2-20   Acute cholecystitis with sloughed membranes. Transverse view of the gallbladder demonstrates a linear intraluminal structure *(arrows)* secondary to sloughed mucosal membranes. In addition, a focal crescentic-shaped pericholecystic fluid collection *(f)* is seen adjacent to the medial gallbladder wall.

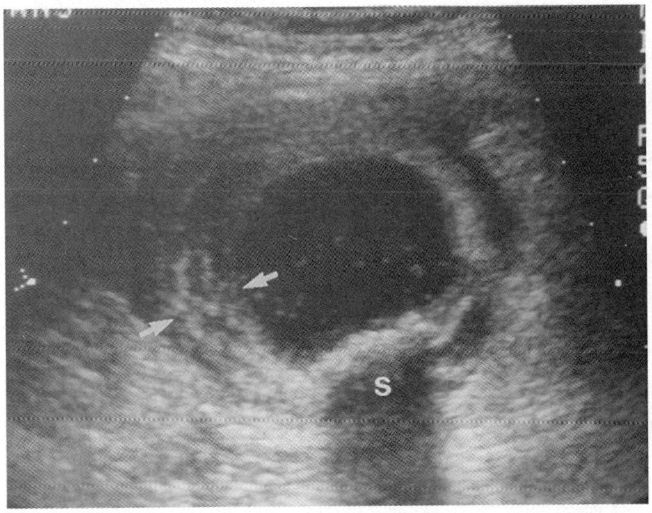

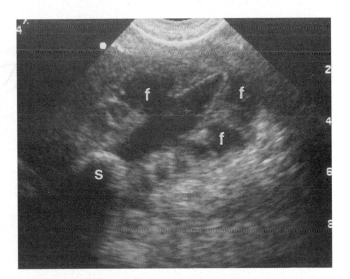

Fig. 2-19   Acute cholecystitis with gallbladder wall necrosis. Transverse view of the gallbladder demonstrates shadowing stones *(s)* and gallbladder wall thickening. Irregular intramural sonolucencies are seen along the lateral gallbladder wall *(arrows)*. Although these sonolucencies can be seen with many causes of gallbladder wall thickening, in the setting of acute cholecystitis, they are suggestive of gallbladder wall necrosis.

Fig. 2-21   Acute cholecystitis with intramural pericholecystic fluid. Longitudinal view of the gallbladder demonstrates a stone *(s)* impacted in the gallbladder neck. Multiple fluid collections *(f)* are seen in the thickened gallbladder wall. Communication between the gallbladder lumen and anterior fluid collection is apparent.

problem, and by showing a normal gallbladder, ultrasound can exclude cholecystitis in the majority of these patients. In addition, ultrasound is much more likely to identify a specific alternative diagnosis than is biliary scintigraphy (Fig. 2-22).

2. Ultrasound is a relatively inexpensive means of obtaining morphologic information about all the right upper quadrant organs. This is becoming particularly more important in the era of laparoscopic cholesystectomies since the surgeon has less capability of examining these organs during the operation. In addition, the size of the gallbladder, size of the largest stone, status of the gallbladder wall (Fig. 2-23), and presence of biliary dilatation are all important preoperative data that can be obtained with sonography but not with scintigraphy.

3. Most ultrasound exams that are considered false positive for acute cholecystitis occur in patients with gallstones and symptomatic chronic cholecystitis. Since these patients require cholecystectomy anyway, the impact of a preoperative diagnosis of acute cholecystitis is minimal.

Despite the advantages of sonography, the sonographic diagnosis remains in doubt in some patients. In these patients, hepatobiliary scintigraphy is extremely valuable as a problem-solving technique to exclude or establish the diagnosis of acute cholecystitis.

Approximately 5% of cases of acute cholecystitis occur in the absence of gallstones and are referred to as acalculous cholecystitis. The etiology is multifactorial and includes ischemia, gallbladder wall infection, chemical toxicity to the gallbladder wall, and cystic duct obstruction. Acalculous cholecystitis occurs predominantly in very sick patients, particularly following major surgery, extensive burns, major trauma, and prolonged total parenteral nutrition. Therefore the absence of stones is not a reliable means of excluding cholecystitis in this group of patients. Secondary signs must be relied upon to make the diagnosis (Fig. 2-24). Unfortunately, most very ill patients have many potential causes of secondary signs, such as gallbladder enlargement and wall thickening. It can also be difficult to assess for tenderness in a semiresponsive patient. Scintigraphy is probably more sensitive than sonography for acalculous cholecystitis, but it is also prone to false positive results.

Emphysematous cholecystitis is another unusual form and tends to occur in elderly men. Since it is caused by ischemia, it occurs more often in diabetics and is not often associated with gallstones. The gas that develops is because of infection with gas-forming organisms and can occur in the gallbladder wall and/or lumen. Perforation of

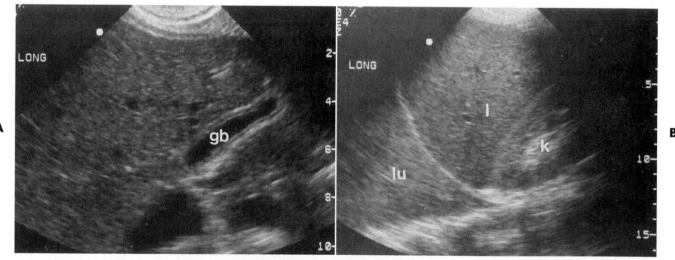

Fig. 2-22   Right lower lobe pneumonia masquerading as acute cholecystitis. **A,** Longitudinal view of the right upper quadrant in a patient presenting primarily with right upper quadrant pain shows a gallbladder *(gb)* that is contracted but free of stones or other abnormalities. Note the demarcation of the echogenic mucosa and the hypoechoic muscularis in this contracted gallbladder. **B,** Longitudinal view of the liver *(l)* and right kidney *(k)* demonstrates consolidation of the right lung base *(lu)* with equal echogenicity of the lung and liver. This is referred to as hepatization of the lung and is consistent with pneumonia. This diagnosis could not have been made with hepatobiliary scintigraphy and demonstrates one of the advantages of sonography in patients presenting with right upper quadrant symptoms.

the gallbladder is five times more likely with emphysematous cholecystitis than with gallstone-induced cholecystitis; therefore the distinction is clinically significant.

Sonographically, emphysematous cholecystitis usually manifests as very bright reflections from a nondependent portion of the gallbladder wall (Fig. 2-25). The associated acoustic shadow is usually dirty and in many cases has a demonstrable ring-down artifact that is a reliable sign of gas. Detection of gas in the bile ducts can be a helpful clue to the diagnosis since intraluminal gallbladder gas may pass through the cystic duct and into the intrahepatic or extrahepatic bile ducts.

CARCINOMA

Gallbladder cancer is the fifth most common GI malignancy. It probably occurs because of chronic irritation of the gallbladder wall by stones. Therefore the vast majority of gallbladder cancers are associated with gallstones and develop more commonly in women than in men. The 5-year survival rate for patients with gallbladder cancer is less than 20%, although the prognosis for patients with tumor confined to the gallbladder wall is much better. Unfortunately, up to 80% of these patients have direct tumor invasion of the liver or portal node involvement at the time of diagnosis.

The most common sonographic appearance for gallbladder cancer is a soft tissue mass centered in the gallbladder fossa that completely (Fig. 2-26) or partially obliterates the lumen (Fig. 2-27; Box 2-3). Identification of gallstones within the mass can help to confirm that the origin of the mass is the gallbladder rather than adjacent organs. Approximately 15% to 30% of gallbladder cancers appear as focal or diffuse gallbladder wall thicken-

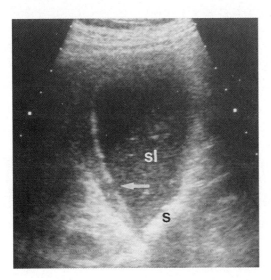

Fig. 2-23   Acute cholecystitis with disrupted gallbladder wall. Longitudinal view of the gallbladder demonstrates shadowing stones *(s)* and sludge *(sl)* in the lumen of the gallbladder. Focal disruption of the gallbladder wall *(arrow)* is also apparent. Successful laparoscopic cholecystectomy will be more difficult in this setting than with an intact gallbladder wall.

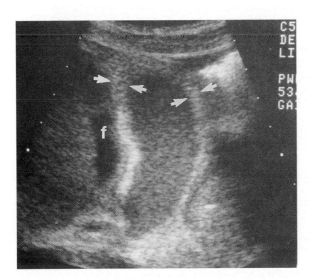

Fig. 2-24   Acalculous cholecystitis. Longitudinal view of the gallbladder demonstrates wall thickening *(arrows)*, intraluminal sludge, and pericholecystic fluid *(f)*. No stones were present. This gallbladder was drained percutaneously and cultures grew out *Staphylococcus aureus*.

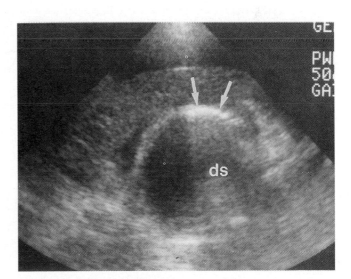

Fig. 2-25   Emphysematous cholecystitis. Transverse view of the gallbladder demonstrates a focal highly reflective region in the nondependent portion of the gallbladder wall *(arrows)*. Posterior to this portion of the gallbladder is a dirty shadow *(ds)*. These findings are suggestive of emphysematous cholecystitis and this diagnosis was confirmed with an abdominal radiograph.

ing. In the vast majority of these cases the thickening is irregular, asymmetric, and eccentric (Fig. 2-28). The least common form of gallbladder cancer is a polypoid intraluminal mass (Fig. 2-29). This form is usually larger than a centimeter, which helps in distinguishing it from gallbladder polyps. The differential diagnosis for gallbladder masses includes tumefactive sludge (Fig. 2-16), inflammatory wall thickening (Fig. 2-30), focal adenomyomatosis, and polyps (see Box 2-3). When the diagnosis is in doubt, detection of metastatic disease in the regional lymph nodes (Fig. 2-27, *B*), adjacent organs, or peritoneal cavity can be very useful.

CHOLESTEROLOSIS

Cholesterolosis is a condition where cholesterol is deposited within the lamina propia of the gallbladder. Al-

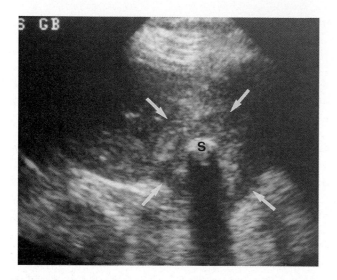

Fig. 2-26   Gallbladder carcinoma. Transverse view of the gallbladder demonstrates a soft tissue mass *(arrows)* in the expected region of the gallbladder fossa. A shadowing stone *(s)* is seen in the middle of this mass confirming that this is centered on the gallbladder. This is the most common appearance for gallbladder carcinoma.

Box 2-3   Sonographic Appearance of Gallbladder Cancer
Mass centered on gallbladder fossa with associated stones Eccentric irregular wall thickening Bulky intraluminal polypoid mass Infiltration of adjacent liver Periportal and/or peripancreatic lymphadenopathy Bile duct obstruction

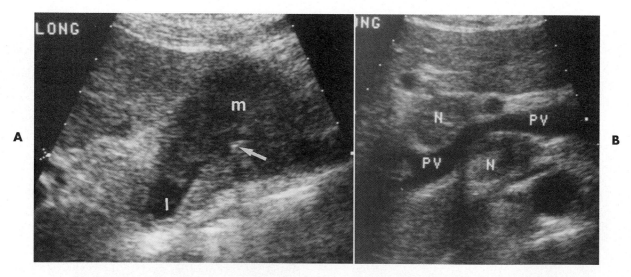

Fig. 2-27   Gallbladder carcinoma. **A,** Longitudinal view of the gallbladder demonstrates a hypoechoic soft tissue mass *(m)* in the region of the gallbladder fundus. A small shadowing stone *(arrow)* is seen imbedded in the mass. A small portion of residual gallbladder lumen *(l)* is seen in the region of the gallbladder neck. **B,** Longitudinal view through the porta hepatis demonstrates two enlarged lymph nodes *(N)* compressing and distorting the portal vein *(PV)*. The porta hepatis, the porto-caval space, and the area around the pancreatic head are typical sites for regional lymph node spread in gallbladder carcinoma.

though the cause is unknown, cholesterolosis does not appear to be related to serum lipid level, atherosclerosis, diabetes, cholesterol stones, or hyperconcentration of cholesterol in the bile. It is sometimes referred to as *strawberry gallbladder* because the mucosa bears a resemblance to a strawberry.

Most cases of cholesterolosis are of the planar variety and produce no detectable changes in the appearance or thickness of the gallbladder wall on ultrasound or other imaging tests. However, a minority of cases of cholesterolosis are of the polypoid variety and can be detected by imaging tests such as ultrasound (Fig. 2-31). Cholesterol polyps are by far the most comon type of gallbladder polyp. There are usually multiple polyps, although it is not uncommon to detect only the largest one sonographically. Cholesterol polyps are usually less than 5 mm in size and only rarely get bigger than 10 mm. They can be distinguished from gallbladder stones by their lack of a shadow

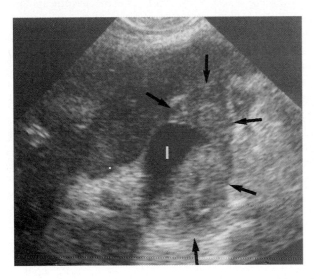

Fig. 2-28 Gallbladder carcinoma. Longitudinal view of the gallbladder demonstrates thickening of the gallbladder wall *(arrows)* along the wall opposite the liver. The gallbladder lumen *(l)* is preserved. Gallstones were identified on other images.

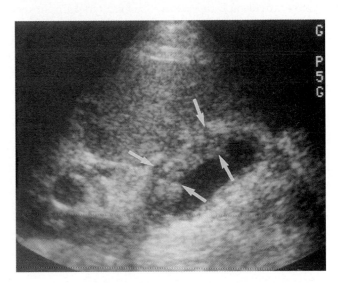

Fig. 2-30 Chronic cholecystitis mimicking gallbladder carcinoma. Longitudinal view of the gallbladder demonstrates focal eccentric gallbladder wall thickening *(arrows)*. Gallstones were seen on other views. This was considered highly suspicious for gallbladder carcinoma, but pathology of the resected specimen revealed only inflammatory changes.

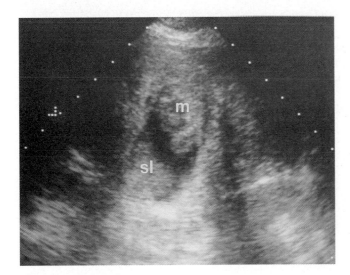

Fig. 2-29 Gallbladder carcinoma. Transverse view of the gallbladder demonstrates a polypoid intraluminal mass *(m)* arising from the fundus. Sludge *(sl)* is seen in the dependent portion of the gallbladder.

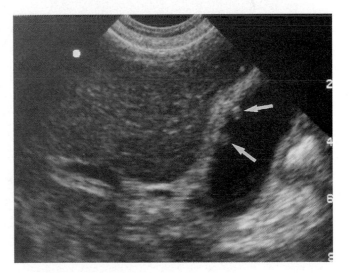

Fig. 2-31 Cholesterol polyps. Longitudinal view of the gallbladder demonstrates two <5 mm nonshadowing intraluminal soft tissue polyps *(arrows)* adjacent to the nondependent gallbladder wall. This is a classic appearance for cholesterol polyps. Several other small polyps were identified elsewhere in this gallbladder.

and nonmobile nature, and from sludge balls by their lack of mobility. Their small size and multiplicity help to distinguish them from true neoplasms of the gallbladder wall.

Metastatic disease to the gallbladder is very uncommon but can produce multiple polypoid lesions. Melanoma has the greatest tendency to spread to the gallbladder, therefore detection of gallbladder polyps should be viewed with a high level of suspicion in patients with a history of melanoma. Generally there will be further evidence of metastatic disease in the liver, lymph nodes, or bowel in these patients.

It has been well established that polypoid lesions of the gallbladder wall that are 5 mm or less require no further evaluation or therapy. Lesions that are between 5 and 10 mm should be monitored to ensure their stability, but if they are multiple, they are almost certainly cholesterol polyps and can be ignored (Fig. 2-32). Lesions that are larger than 10 mm should probably be removed because of the possibility of cancer.

ADENOMYOMATOSIS

Adenomyomatosis is one of two forms of hyperplastic cholecystoses (cholesterolosis is the other). Like choles-

terolosis, the etiology is unknown. Pathologically, adenomyomatosis is characterized by mucosal hyperplasia and thickening of the muscular layer of the gallbladder. Mucosal herniations into the muscular layer are called Rokitansky-Aschoff sinuses and they frequently contain cholesterol crystals. Adenomyomatosis is unrelated to gallstones and occurs equally in men and women.

Sonographically, the cholesterol crystals deposited in the Rokitansky-Aschoff sinuses result in bright reflections and short *comet-tail artifacts* arising from the gallbladder wall (Fig. 2-33). The comet-tail artifact is the most obvious finding in many cases of adenomyomatosis and is almost exclusively seen along the near wall of the gallbladder. This does not reflect focal disease, but instead occurs because the artifact is only visible when it is displayed in the anechoic background of the gallbladder lumen, not the echogenic background of the tissues deep to the gallbladder. Occasionally, large Rokitansky-Aschoff sinuses will be resolved as cystic or hypoechoic spaces in the gallbladder wall. Adenomyomatosis may also appear as diffuse wall thickening, focal segmental annular thickening (Fig. 2-34), or a fundal mass (Fig. 2-35; Box 2-4).

In many cases ultrasound will show such characteristic findings that the diagnosis is unequivocal. However, when the diagnosis of adenomyomatosis is in doubt as a result of the sonographic findings, an oral cholecys-

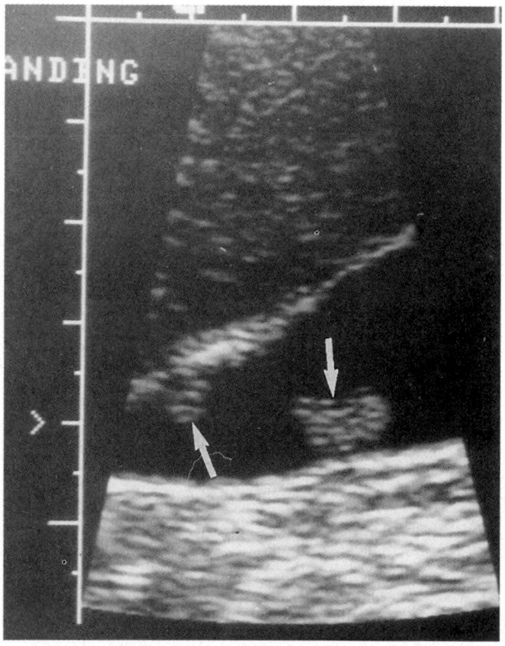

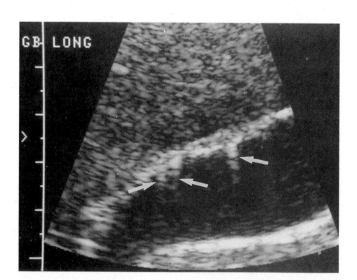

Fig. 2-32   Unusually large cholesterol polyp. Magnified longitudinal view of the gallbladder with the patient standing demonstrates two nondependent, nonmobile polyps *(arrows)*. The polyp arising from the posterior wall of the gallbladder is 9 mm in maximum dimension. However, because there were multiple lesions in this gallbladder, they are almost certainly all cholesterol polyps and require no further evaluation.

Fig. 2-33   Adenomyomatosis. Magnified longitudinal view of the gallbladder demonstrates three, short, comet-tail artifacts *(arrows)* arising from the anterior wall of the gallbladder. These result from cholesterol crystals that are deposited in Rokitansky-Aschoff sinuses that are otherwise too small to be resolved sonographically.

togram should be obtained since it can demonstrate the Rokitansky-Aschoff sinuses and establish the diagnosis more definitively.

GALLBLADDER WALL THICKENING

As mentioned previously, the normal upper limit for the gallbladder wall is 3 mm. A large number of processes can result in a thickened gallbladder wall (Box 2-5). In addition to acute cholecystitis, gallbladder cancer, and adenomyomatosis, other abnormalities related to the biliary tract that can thicken the gallbladder wall are AIDS cholangiopathy, and sclerosing cholangitis.

A large number of nonbiliary processes can also cause gallbladder wall thickening resulting from edema. Hypoproteinemia [from cirrhosis (Fig. 2-36), nephrotic syndrome, etc.], congestive heart failure (Fig. 2-37), venous congestion from portal hypertension, lymphatic obstruction from portal lymph node disease, and adjacent inflammatory processes like pancreatitis are all potential causes. Hepatitis is another cause of gallbladder wall thickening that is often overlooked despite the fact that it can cause marked thickening (Fig. 2-38). This may be due to the adjacent inflammation of the liver or excretion of the virus in the bile and direct infection of the gallbladder. Hepatitis is also often associated with a contracted gallbladder.

Box 2-4 **Causes of Gallbladder Masses**	
COMMON	**UNCOMMON**
Polyps	Metastases
Adenomyomatosis	Chronic cholecystitis
Gallbladder cancer	
Tumefactive sludge	

Box 2-5 **Causes of Gallbladder Wall Thickening**	
BILIARY	**NONBILIARY**
Cholecystitis	Hepatitis
Adenomyomatosis	Pancreatitis
Cancer	Heart failure
AIDS cholangiopathy	Hypoproteinemia
Sclerosing cholangitis	Cirrhosis
	Portal hypertension
	Lymphatic obstruction

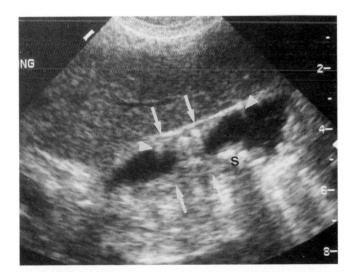

Fig. 2-34   Segmental adenomyomatosis. Longitudinal view of the gallbladder demonstrates a focal region of gallbladder wall thickening along the anterior and posterior wall *(arrows)* that has compartmentalized that gallbladder into a superior and inferior compartment. Several bright reflectors *(arrowheads)* with associated comet-tail artifacts are seen arising from the anterior wall consistent with cholesterol crystals deposited in Rokitansky-Aschoff sinuses. Gallstones *(s)* are present in the inferior compartment of the gallbladder.

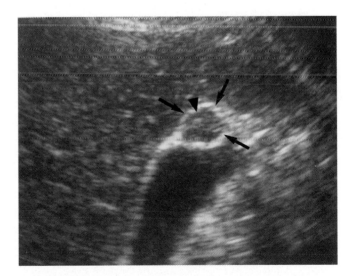

Fig. 2-35   Fundal adenomyomatosis. A small soft tissue mass *(arrows)* is seen arising from the gallbladder fundus. At least one small cystic space *(arrowhead)* is seen within this mass. This was pathologically proven to represent adenomyomatosis with several Rokitansky-Aschoff sinuses. It is unusual for these sinuses to be big enough to be resolved sonographically.

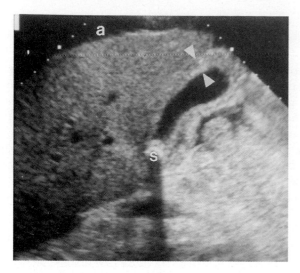

Fig. 2-36 Gallbladder wall thickening due to cirrhosis. Longitudinal view of the right upper quadrant demonstrates a thickened gallbladder wall *(arrowheads)* and a shadowing stone *(s)*. Ascites *(a)* is seen around the liver. The liver surface is slightly nodular, consistent with the patient's history of cirrhosis, and in this case there were no symptoms to suggest acute cholecystitis. The gallbladder wall thickening is due to cirrhosis and its associated hypoproteinemia. The presence of ascites is a good indication that the patient is suffering from some type of edema-forming state which can also affect the gallbladder wall.

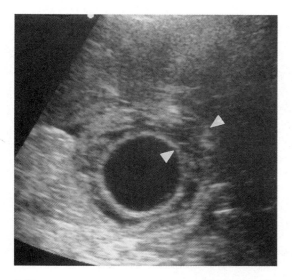

Fig. 2-37 Gallbladder wall thickening related to congestive heart failure. Transverse view of the gallbladder demonstrates gallbladder wall thickening *(arrowheads)* that exceeds 1 cm. Irregular intramural striations are present but no stones are visualized. This patient did complain of upper abdominal pain and acalculous cholecystitis was considered a possible cause of this patient's symptoms. However, hepatobiliary scintigraphy showed normal filling of the gallbladder and in this case, the marked gallbladder wall thickening was due to edema secondary to heart failure.

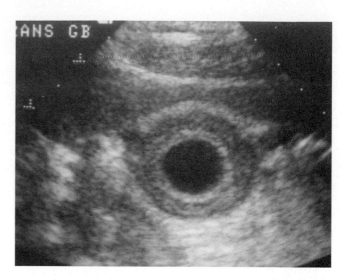

Fig. 2-38 Gallbladder wall thickening due to hepatitis. Transverse view of the gallbladder demonstrates diffuse concentric homogeneous thickening. No stones were identified and subsequent serologic studies confirmed that this patient had hepatitis.

Most nonbiliary causes of gallbladder wall thickening produce concentric thickening that may be uniform in echogenicity or may have a regular or irregular layered appearance with both hypoechoic and echogenic components. The actual sonographic appearance of the thickened wall is not helpful in distinguishing acute cholecystitis from nonbiliary thickening. However, in most cases the clinical setting and the presence or absence of a sonographic Murphy's sign can help to make the diagnosis. In some instances, associated sonographic signs can be very useful. For instance, heart failure often produces abnormally pulsatile portal venous flow, and cirrhosis produces secondary signs of portal hypertension and a nodular liver surface.

PORCELAIN GALLBLADDER

Extensive calcification of the gallbladder produces a brittle bluish wall that has led to the term *porcelain gallbladder.* It is associated with chronic gallbladder inflammation and 95% of the cases have gallstones. The clinical significance of porcelain gallbladder is the increased risk of gallbladder carcinoma. Estimates of this risk range from 13% to 61%. Since many uncomplicated and occult cases of porcelain gallbladder probably never come to clinical attention, the true incidence of carcinoma in this condition is probably overestimated in the literature. Nonetheless, most authorities would still recommend prophylactic cholecystectomy unless there are medical contraindications to surgery.

When the gallbladder wall is heavily calcified and the wall is diffusely involved, it will appear as an echogenic

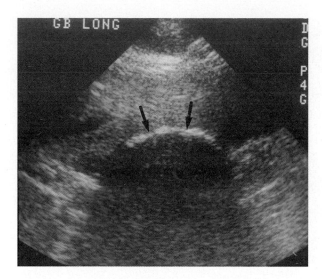

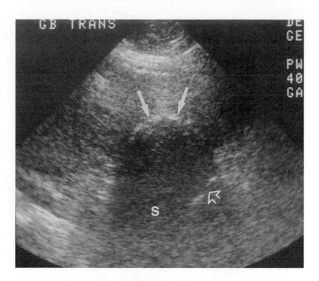

Fig. 2-39 Porcelain gallbladder. Longitudinal view of the right upper quadrant demonstrates a highly echogenic curvilinear reflector *(arrows)* with a dense posterior acoustic shadow. This sonographic appearance is most consistent with porcelain gallbladder, although a stone-filled gallbladder and emphysematous cholecystitis are other less likely possibilities. A CT scan in this case confirmed the presence of gallbladder wall calcification.

Fig. 2-40 Porcelain gallbladder. Transverse view of the gallbladder demonstrates an echogenic anterior wall *(arrows)* and a posterior acoustic shadow *(s)*. However, a small portion of the posterior gallbladder wall *(open arrow)* is still visualized. A stone-filled gallbladder would produce a more complete shadow, preventing visualization of the back wall of the gallbladder. Therefore, these findings are most consistent with gallbladder wall calcification. Emphysematous cholecystitis is a less likely possibility.

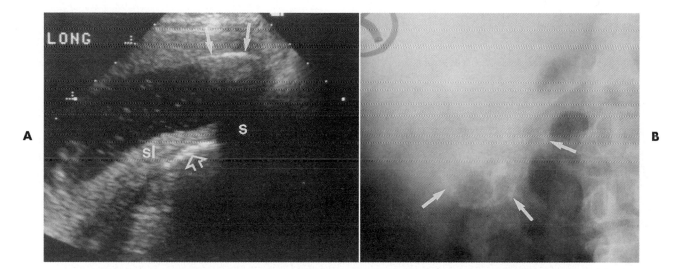

Fig. 2-41 Partial calcification of the gallbladder wall. **A,** Longitudinal view of the gallbladder demonstrates a focal area of increased echogenicity arising from the anterior fundal portion of the gallbladder wall *(arrows)* with a clean posterior acoustic shadow *(s)* obscuring the wall deep to this area. Stones *(open arrow)* and sludge *(sl)* are also seen in this gallbladder. Either calcium or gas in the wall of the gallbladder could produce these findings. The clean shadow favors calcification. **B,** Magnified view of an abdominal radiograph demonstrates flakelike calcification *(arrows)* in the right upper quadrant conforming to the shape of a gallbladder that is consistent with a porcelain gallbladder.

arc with dense posterior shadowing (Fig. 2-39). Less extensive calcification will produce only partial shadowing so that the back wall of the gallbladder remains visible (Fig. 2-40). In early cases, only segments of the gallbladder wall may be affected (Fig. 2-41). Given the increased risk of gallbladder carcinoma, whenever wall calcification is detected, a careful search should be made for evidence of malignancy (Fig. 2-42).

The major differential diagnosis for porcelain gallbladder is a gallbladder that is completely filled with stones

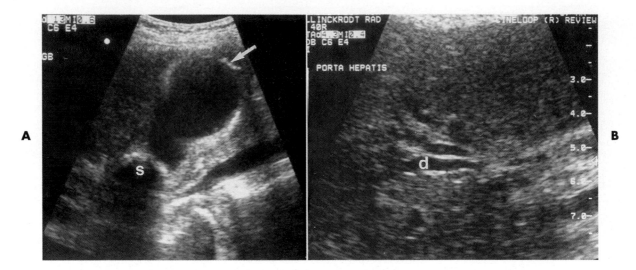

Fig. 2-42   Gallbladder wall calcification with associated gallbladder carcinoma. **A,** Longitudinal view of the gallbladder shows a stone *(s)* in the neck and a focal region of increased echogenicity in the fundus *(arrow)*. The remainder of the gallbladder was difficult to visualize but no obvious gall-bladder mass was seen on this view or other views. **B,** Longitudinal view of the liver hilum shows a dilated intrahepatic duct *(d)* that rapidly tapers in the region of the porta hepatis. This suggests a malignant process in the porta, and combined with gallbladder wall calcification, a gallbladder can-cer was considered likely. A subsequent CT scan confirmed gallbladder wall calcification as well as a mass arising from the lateral margin of the gallbladder that infiltrated the adjacent liver parenchy-ma and invaded the porta hepatis.

Table 2-3 Causes of shadowing from gallbladder fossa			
	Shadow	**WES**	**Back wall**
Gallbladder full of stones	Usually clean	Often	Not seen
Porcelain gallbladder	Variable	Rare	Occasionally seen
Intramural gas	Usually dirty	Rare	Occasionally seen

and emphysematous cholecystitis. If a wall-echo-shadow complex is seen, then it is almost certainly a stone-filled gallbladder. If the back wall of the gallbladder is visible, then a gallbladder filled with stones can be excluded. If ring-down artifact is detected, then emphysematous cholecystitis can be diagnosed. In cases where it is not possible to distinguish these three possibilities sono-graphically, abdominal radiographs and/or CT will be helpful. Table 2-3 summarizes the causes of shadowing from the gallbladder fossa.

Key Features

Gallstones appear as mobile, dependent, shadowing echogenic structures in the gallbladder lumen. Sonography is the most accurate means of detecting gallstones.

Sonography is the method of choice in the initial evaluation of patients with suspected acute cholecystitis. Findings include gallstones, wall thickening, gallbladder enlargement, pericholecystic fluid, and a sonographic Murphy's sign.

Gallbladder cancer typically presents late as a mass obliterating the gallbladder and engulfing gallstones. Wall thickening and intraluminal masses are less common findings.

Cholesterolosis is a benign, usually asymptomatic condition that may produce cholesterol polyps, which are usually small and represent the most common polypoid lesion of the gallbladder wall.

Adenomyomatosis is a benign, usually asymptomatic condition that may produce focal or diffuse wall thickening. Cholesterol crystals deposited in Rokitansky-Aschoff sinuses are a characteristic finding.

Gallbladder wall thickening is a nonspecific finding with a lengthy differential diagnosis.

Calcification of the gallbladder wall places a patient at a significantly increased risk of gallbladder cancer.

SUGGESTED READINGS

Berk RN, Armbuster RG, Saltzstein SL: Carcinoma in the porcelain gallbladder, *Radiology* 106:29-31, 1973.

Berk RN, van der Vegt JH, Lichtenstein JE: The hyperplastic cholecystoses: cholesterolosis and adenomyomatosis, *Radiology* 146:593-601, 1983.

Brandt DJ et al: Gallbladder disease in patients with primary sclerosing cholangitis, *AJR* 150:571-574, 1988.

Callen PW, Filly RA: Ultrasonographic localization of the gallbladder, *Radiology* 133:687-691, 1979.

Carroll BA: Gallbladder wall thickening secondary to focal lymphatic obstruction, *J Ultrasound Med* 2:89-91, 1983.

Carroll BA: Gallstones: in vitro comparison of physical, radiographic, and ultrasonic characteristics, *AJR* 131:223-226, 1978.

Cooperberg PL, Gibney RG: Imaging of the gallbladder, *Radiology* 163:605-613, 1987.

Cover KL, Slasky BS, Skolnick ML: Sonography of cholesterol in the biliary system, *J Ultrasound Med* 4:647-653, 1985.

Cover KL, Slasky BS, Skolnick ML: Sonography of cholesterol in the biliary system, *J Ultrasound Med* 4:647-653, 1985.

Eelkema HH, Hodgson JR, Stauffer MH: Fifteen year follow-up of polypoid lesions of the gallbladder diagnosed by cholecystography, *Gastroenterology* 42:144-147, 1962.

Filly RA et al: In vitro investigation of the origin of echoes within biliary sludge, *J Clin Ultrasound* 8:193-200, 1980.

Fiske CE, Laing FC, Brown TW: Ultrasonographic evidence of gallbladder wall thickening in association with hypoalbuminemia, *Radiology* 135:713-716, 1980.

Grieco RV, Bartone NF, Vasilas A: A study of fixed filling defects in the well opacified gallbladder and their evolution, *AJR* 90(4):844-853, 1963.

Jeanty P, Amman W, Cooperberg PL: Mobile intraluminal masses of the gallbladder, *J Ultrasound Med* 2:65-71, 1983.

Jivegord I, Thornell E, Svanvik J: Pathophysiology of acute obstructive cholecystitis: implications for nonoperative management, *Br J Surg* 74:1084-1086, 1987.

Jutras JA: Hyperplastic cholecystoses, *AJR* 83:795-827, 1960.

Juttner HU et al: Thickening of the gallbladder wall in acute hepatitis: ultrasound demonstration, *Radiology* 142:465-466, 1982.

Kane RA et al: Porcelain gallbladder ultrasound and CT appearance, *Radiology* 152:137-141, 1984.

Kidney M, Goiney R, Cooperberg PL: Adenomyomatosis of the gallbladder: a pictorial exhibit, *J Ultrasound Med* 5:331-333, 1986.

Koga A et al: Diagnosis and operative indications for polypoid lesions of the gallbladder, *Arch Surg* 123:26-29, 1988.

Lafortune M et al: The V-shaped artifact of the gallbladder wall, *AJR* 147:505-508, 1986.

Laing FC et al: Ultrasonic evaluation of patients with acute right upper quadrant pain, *Radiology* 140:449-455, 1981.

Laing FC: Diagnostic evaluation of patients with suspected acute cholecystitis, *Radiol Clin North Am* 21:477-493, 1983.

Lane J, Buck JL, Zeman RK: Primary carcinoma of the gallbladder: a pictorial essay, *Radiographics* 9:209-228, 1989.

Lee SP, Maher K, Nicholls JF: Origin and fate of biliary sludge, *Gastroenterology* 94:170-176, 1988.

Lee SP, Nicholls JF: Nature and composition of biliary sludge, *Gastroenterology* 90:677-686, 1986.

Lim JH, Ko YT, Kim SY: Ultrasound changes of the gallbladder wall in cholecystitis: sonographic-pathologic correlation, *Clin Radiol* 38:389-393, 1987.

MacDonald FR, Cooperberg PL, Cohen MM: The WES triad—a specific sonographic sign of gallstones in the contracted gallbladder. *Gastrointest Radiol* 6:39-41, 1981.

Matron KI, Doubilet P: How to study the gallbladder, *Ann Intern Med* 109:752-754, 1988.

Melson GL, Reiter F, Evens RG: Tumorous conditions of the gallbladder, *Sem Roentgenol* 11(4):269-282, 1976.

Mentzer RM et al: A comparative appraisal of emphysematous cholecystitis, *Am J Surg* 124:10-15, 1975.

Mirvis SE et al: The diagnosis of acute acalculous cholecystitis: a comparison of sonography, scintigraphy, and CT, *AJR* 147:1171-1175, 1986.

Nemcek AA et al: The effervescent gallbladder: a sonographic sign of emphysematous cholecystitis, *AJR* 150:575-577, 1988.

Ochsner SF: Solitary polypoid lesions of the gallbladder, *Radiol Clin North Am* 4:501-510, 1966.

Parulekar SG: Sonographic findings in acute emphysematous cholecystitis, *Radiology* 145:117-119, 1982.

Phillips G et al: Ultrasound patterns of metastatic tumors in the gallbladder, *J Clin Ultrasound* 10:379-383, 1982.

Price RJ et al: Sonography of polypoid cholesterolosis, *AJR* 139:1197-1198, 1982.

Raghavendra BN et al: Acute cholecystitis: sonographic-pathologic analysis, *AJR* 137:327-332, 1981.

Raghavendra BN et al: Sonography of adenomyomatosis of the gallbladder: radiologic-pathologic correlation, *Radiology* 146:747-752, 1983.

Ralls PW et al: Prospective evaluation of ^{99m}Tc-IDA cholescintigraphy and gray-scale ultrasound in the diagnosis of acute cholecystitis, *Radiology* 144:369-371, 1982.

Ralls PW et al: Real-time sonography in suspected acute cholecystitis. Prospective evaluation of primary and secondary signs, *Radiology* 155:767-771, 1985.

Ralls PW et al: Prospective evaluation of the sonographic Murphy sign in suspected acute cholecystitis, *J Clin Ultrasound* 10:113-115, 1982.

Rice J et al: Sonographic appearance of adenomyomatosis of the gallbladder, *J Clin Ultrasound* 9:336-337, 1981.

Romano AJ et al: Gallbladder and bile duct abnormalities in AIDS sonographic findings in eight patients, *AJR* 150:123-127, 1988.

Sharp KW: Acute cholecystitis, *Surg Clin North Am* 68(2): 269-279, 1988.

Shieh CJ, Dunn E, Standard JE: Primary carcinoma of the gallbladder: a review of a 16-year experience at the Waterbury Hospital Health Center, *Cancer* 47:996-1004, 1981.

Shlaer WJ, Leopold GR, Scheible FW: Sonography of the thickened gallbladder wall: a nonspecific finding, *AJR* 136:337-339, 1981.

Shuman WP et al: Evaluation of acute right upper quadrant pain: sonography and ^{99m}Tc-HIDA cholescintigraphy, *AJR* 139:61-64, 1982.

Shuman WP et al: Low sensitivity of sonography and cholescintigraphy in acalculous cholecystitis, *AJR* 142:531-534, 1984.

Sommer FG, Taylor KJW: Differentiation of acoustic shadowing due to calculi and gas collections, *Radiology* 135:399-403, 1980.

Teefey SA, Baron RA, Bigler SA: Sonography of the gallbladder: significance of striated (layered) thickening of the gallbladder wall, *AJR* 156:945-947, 1991.

Weiner SN et al: Sonography and computed tomography in the diagnosis of carcinoma of the gallbladder, *AJR* 142:735-739, 1984.

Yeh HC, Goodman J, Rabinowitz JG: Floating gallstones in bile without added contrast material, *AJR* 146:49-50, 1986.

CHAPTER 3

Bile Ducts

For a Key Features summary see p. 71.

ANATOMY

The bile ducts are generally divided into the intrahepatic and extrahepatic portions. The intrahepatic ducts run in the portal triads parallel to the portal veins and hepatic arteries. Although it was once thought that the intrahepatic ducts traveled anterior to the adjacent portal veins, it is now recognized that the relationship of the intrahepatic ducts with the portal veins and hepatic arteries is quite variable.

The extrahepatic portion includes the common hepatic duct, common bile duct, and a small portion of the distal right and left ducts. The common hepatic duct is the segment located above the cystic duct insertion and the common bile duct is the segment below (Fig. 3-1). In most cases the cystic duct is not seen, so it is not possible to distinguish the common hepatic from the common bile duct. Because of this, most people simply refer to the duct as the *common duct* and divide it subjectively into the proximal, mid, and distal segments. At the porta hepatis the proximal common duct runs anterior to the right and main portal vein and the right hepatic artery (Fig. 3-2). The midduct runs posterior to the duodenum. Inferiorly the distal common duct enters the head of the pancreas and travels along the posterior-most aspect of the pancreatic head (Fig. 3-3).

The hepatic artery arises from the celiac axis and travels in the hepatoduodenal ligament medial to the common duct. On transverse views of the porta hepatis this configuration produces the "Mickey Mouse" appearance (Fig. 3-4). The right hepatic artery passes between the common duct and the portal vein in approximately 85% of patients (see Fig. 3-2) and passes anterior to the common duct in approximately 15% (Fig. 3-5). The hepatic artery is relatively tortuous, so it is difficult to display more than 2 to 3 cm of its long axis in any plane. In addition, the hepatic artery remains relatively similar in caliber throughout its course. On the other hand, the common duct is relatively straight and its diameter varies. Therefore a tubular structure in front of the portal vein

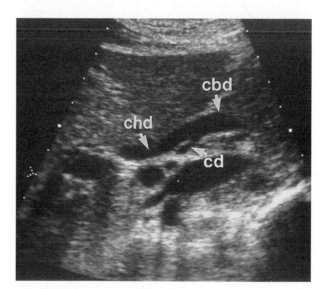

Fig. 3-1 Normal extrahepatic bile ducts. Longitudinal view of the porta hepatis demonstrates the cystic duct insertion *(cd)* into the extrahepatic duct. The common bile duct *(cbd)* is the segment below the cystic duct insertion and the common hepatic duct *(chd)* is the segment above the cystic duct insertion.

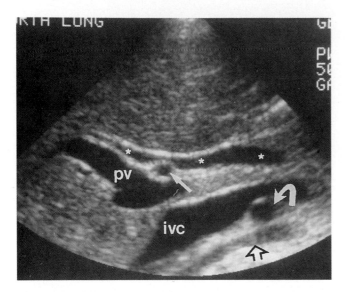

Fig. 3-2   Normal porta hepatis. Longitudinal view of the porta hepatis demonstrates the common duct (*) running anterior to the right hepatic artery *(arrow)* and the portal vein *(pv)*. Note that the common duct is seen along approximately 4 cm of its long axis and that it varies in caliber along its course. Also seen in this view are the inferior vena cava *(ivc)*, right renal artery *(curved arrow)*, and crus of the diaphragm *(open arrow)*.

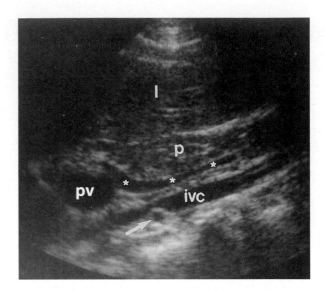

Fig. 3-3   Normal distal common bile duct. Longitudinal view through the pancreatic head *(p)* using the liver *(l)* as an acoustic window shows the distal intrapancreatic portion of the common bile duct (*) running through the posterior-most aspect of the pancreatic head. Note the close relationship of the distal common bile duct to the inferior vena cava *(ivc)*. Also seen in this view are the portal vein *(pv)* and right renal artery *(arrow)*.

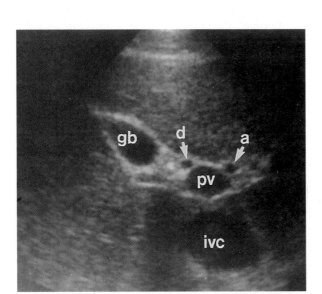

Fig. 3-4   Normal porta hepatis. Transverse view of the porta hepatis demonstrates the typical "Mickey Mouse" appearance. The portal vein *(pv)* forms the head, the hepatic artery *(a)* forms one ear, and the bile duct *(d)* forms the other ear. Also seen in this view are the gallbladder *(gb)* and the inferior vena cava *(ivc)*.

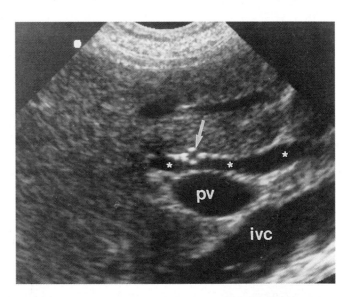

Fig. 3-5   Anomalous position of the right hepatic artery. Longitudinal view through the porta hepatis demonstrates the right hepatic artery *(arrow)* coursing anterior to the bile duct (*). This is a relatively common normal variant. Also seen in this view are the portal vein *(pv)* and inferior vena cava *(ivc)*.

that changes in diameter and can be shown in its long axis for 3 to 4 cm or more is almost certainly the common duct and not the hepatic artery (see Figs. 3-2 and 3-5; Table 3-1).

A replaced right hepatic artery arising from the superior mesenteric artery is a common normal variant, and this vessel runs between the inferior vena cava and the portal vein (Fig. 3-6, *A*) and is situated on the lateral aspect of the portal vein. It can be distinguished from the bile duct that usually occupies this location by following it to its origin or by Doppler analysis (Fig. 3-6, *B*). Another potentially confusing anatomic variant in this area is a cystic duct that inserts unusually low. In such cases it will appear as a tubular structure that parallels the distal common duct before joining it (Fig. 3-7). Occasionally a tortuous gallbladder neck simulates the appearance of the proximal common duct. Careful scanning in multiple obliquities usually reveals the continuity of a tortuous neck with the rest of the gallbladder. In addition, it is not possible for a tortuous gallbladder neck to elongate to the same extent as the common duct.

TECHNIQUE

The proximal common duct is usually best seen by placing the patient in a left lateral decubitus or left posterior oblique position and by scanning from a right anterior oblique approach during a deep inspiration. The distal common duct is best seen by visualizing the head of the pancreas. This is usually easiest from an anterior epigastric approach using the liver as an acoustic window. If

Table 3-1	Differentiation between common duct and hepatic artery	
Characteristics	**Duct**	**Artery**
Location	Anterior to right hepatic artery (85%)	Between duct and portal vein (85%)
	Posterior to right hepatic artery (15%)	Anterior to duct (15%)
	Lateral to hepatic artery	Medial to duct
Visible length	Long	Short
Diameter	Variable	Constant
Doppler signal	Absent	Present

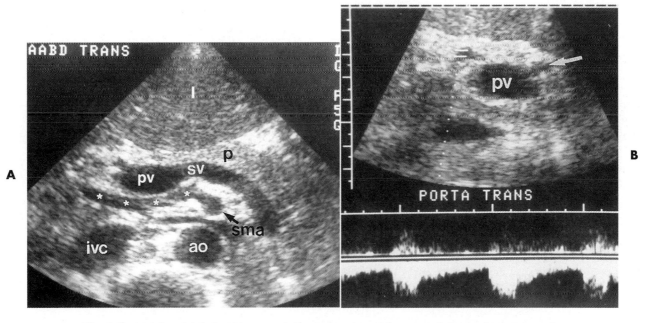

Fig. 3-6   Replaced right hepatic artery. **A,** Transverse view of the upper abdomen demonstrates the superior mesenteric artery *(sma)* anterior to the aorta *(ao)*. A replaced right hepatic artery (*) is seen arising from the superior mesenteric artery and coursing between the portal vein *(pv)* and the inferior vena cava *(ivc)*. Also seen in this image are the pancreas *(p)*, splenic vein *(sv)*, and left lobe of the liver *(l)*. **B,** Transverse view of the porta hepatis demonstrates the portal vein *(pv)* and the left hepatic artery *(arrow)*. The Doppler sample volume has been positioned in the expected location of the bile duct, yet the pulsed-Doppler waveform indicates that the structure seen is an artery. This represents the typical location of the replaced right hepatic artery. In this case the bile duct is small and not seen in this image.

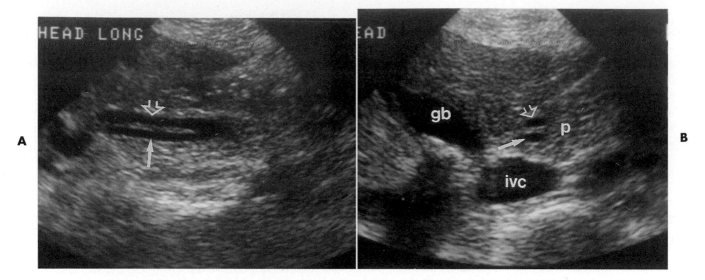

Fig. 3-7   Low-inserting cystic duct. **A,** Longitudinal view in the suprapancreatic region shows two parallel tubular structures that join inferiorly. The anterior structure is the common hepatic duct *(open arrow)* and the posterior structure is the low-inserting cystic duct *(arrow).* **B,** Transverse view through the superior portion of the pancreatic head demonstrates the common hepatic duct *(open arrow)* and the low-inserting cystic duct *(arrow)* within the pancreatic head *(p).* Also seen in this view are the gallbladder *(gb)* containing stones and the inferior vena cava *(ivc).*

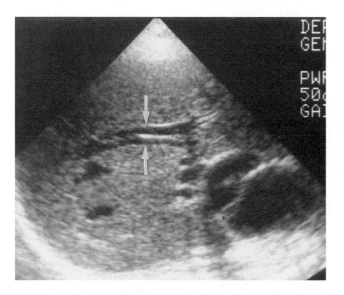

Fig. 3-8   Intrahepatic biliary ductal dilatation. Transverse view of the liver demonstrates parallel channels in the right lobe *(arrows).* The anterior channel in this case is the portal vein and the posterior channel is a dilated bile duct. Note that the bile duct is greater than 40% of the diameter of the adjacent portal vein.

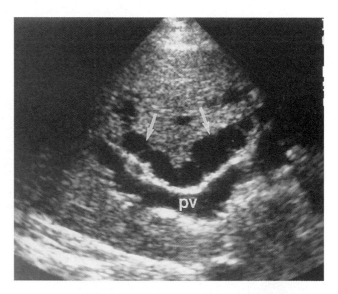

Fig. 3-9   Intrahepatic biliary ductal dilatation. Transverse view of the liver shows the bifurcation of the portal vein *(pv).* Anteriorly is the dilated left and right bile duct *(arrows).* Note the duct wall irregularity and tortuosity.

overlying bowel gas is a problem, pressure can be applied with the transducer to push the gas out of the way. In some cases it is necessary to have the patient drink water to displace gas out of the stomach and duodenum. Changing the patient from a supine to an upright position is also occasionally useful. When the anterior epigastric ap-

proach fails to allow visualization of the distal common duct, a right lateral approach with the patient in a left posterior oblique position frequently allows the distal common duct to be visualized in a semicoronal plane. Another useful technique is to position the patient (usually in a left posterior oblique or left lateral decubitus posi-

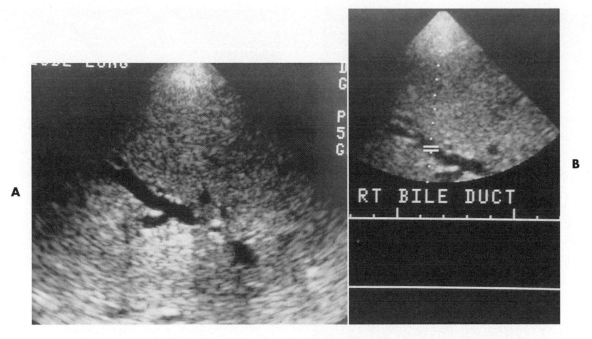

Fig. 3-10   Intrahepatic biliary ductal dilatation. **A,** Longitudinal view of the right lobe of the liver demonstrates a branching tubular structure, which in isolation could represent an intrahepatic portal vein. However, the amount of increased through-transmission behind this structure would be very unusual for a portal vein. **B,** Pulsed-Doppler analysis of this tubular structure demonstrates no detectable blood flow, confirming that this does not represent a branch of the portal vein.

tion) so that the gallbladder is directly over the head of the pancreas. This allows the gallbladder to be used as an acoustic window.

BILIARY OBSTRUCTION

Obstructed bile ducts are diagnosed sonographically by the finding of ductal dilatation. In the past, intrahepatic ductal dilatation was diagnosed whenever parallel channels were seen running adjacent to intrahepatic portal veins. With the advent of modern electronically focused transducers, resolution has been improved to the point that normal intrahepatic arteries or bile ducts, or both, can now be seen as parallel channels adjacent to portal veins. Revised criteria for diagnosing intrahepatic ductal dilatation states that the diameter of normal ducts should not be more than 40% of the diameter of the adjacent portal vein (Fig. 3-8). Dilated intrahepatic ducts can be distinguished from portal veins by their tortuosity or wall irregularity (Fig. 3-9), by the presence of increased through-transmission (Fig. 3-10), and by a stellate configuration centrally (Fig. 3-11). Doppler analysis is useful for confirmation and as an aid in equivocal cases (see Fig. 3-10). Doppler analysis is also helpful for distinguishing between an enlarged hepatic artery and a dilated duct. Confusion occurs most often in the setting of portal hypertension when hepatic arterial flow increases to com-

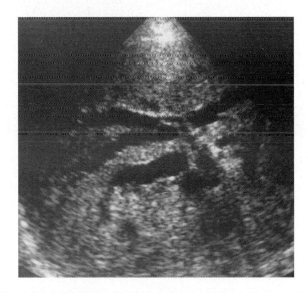

Fig. 3-11   Dilated intrahepatic bile ducts. Transverse view of the liver demonstrates multiple dilated tubular structures that form a stellate configuration radiating toward the porta hepatis. This is typical of markedly dilated intrahepatic bile ducts.

pensate for decreased portal venous flow (Fig. 3-12 [see also color insert, Plate 14]; Box 3-1).

Extrahepatic ductal dilatation is considered present when the maximum diameter of the common duct is 7 mm or greater, but this measurement is not universally ap-

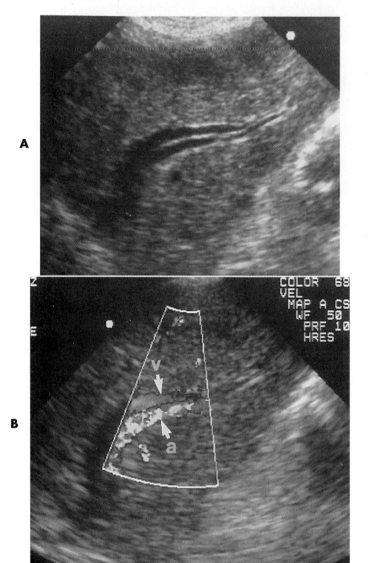

A

B

Fig. 3-12 Enlarged hepatic artery simulating a dilated bile duct. **A,** Longitudinal view of the liver demonstrates parallel tubular structures that simulate intrahepatic biliary ductal dilatation. **B,** Similar Doppler view shows that both of these structures are vascular. The enlarged hepatic artery *(a)* is seen posterior to the portal vein *(v)*. Flow is reversed in the portal vein secondary to severe portal hypertension (see color insert, Plate 14).

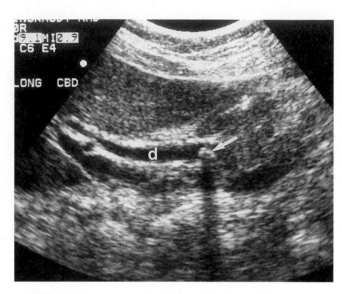

Fig. 3-13 Choledocholithiasis. Longitudinal view of the porta hepatis demonstrates a dilated bile duct *(d)* containing a shadowing intraluminal stone *(arrow)*.

Box 3-1	Criteria for Dilated Intrahepatic Ducts

>40% of diameter of adjacent portal vein
Increased through transmission
Irregular, tortuous walls
Stellate configuration centrally
Lack of Doppler signal

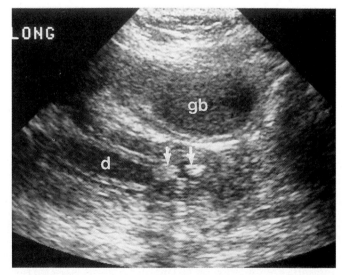

Fig. 3-14 Distal common bile duct stones seen using a gallbladder window. Longitudinal view of the distal common bile duct *(d)* demonstrates two weakly shadowing stones *(arrows)*. The gallbladder *(gb)* provided an adequate acoustic window for visualizing these distal stones that were not visualized from other approaches. Also notice the thickening of the common bile duct wall. Bile duct stones are one of the causes of bile duct wall thickening.

plicable in all situations. For instance, the common duct varies in diameter along its course: the diameter is generally greater in the midsegment and distal segment than it is in the proximal segment. In addition, the common duct enlarges with age. Finally, the common duct is larger in patients who have had cholecystectomies. Therefore, midduct diameters that exceed 7 mm may be normal in elderly patients, but proximal duct diameters that are less than 7 mm may be abnormal in younger patients.

Another complicating factor is that acute, intermittent, and partial obstruction may be present in the absence of ductal dilatation. Because sonography only displays morphology, the detection of an abnormality in such cases usually depends on actual identification of the obstructing process, such as an intermittently obstructing common duct stone or a partially obstructing pancreatic mass. Evaluation of the ductal response to a fatty meal can also be helpful. In normal patients a fatty meal will produce either no change or a decrease in the common duct diameter because fatty meals will cause the sphincter of Oddi to relax and bile to drain from unobstructed bile ducts. In patients with obstructed ducts, relaxation of the sphincter has no effect on biliary drainage, but the other effects of fatty meals—increased bile production and gallbladder contraction—cause the common duct diameter to increase by 1 mm or more.

In addition to distinguishing obstructive from nonobstructive jaundice, another major role of sonography is to determine the level and cause of obstruction. Findings from the most recent studies suggest that sonography can determine the level of obstruction in more than 90% of the patients and can identify the cause of obstruction in approximately 80%. In patients without obstruction other causes of jaundice should be sought.

CHOLEDOCHOLITHIASIS

Choledocholithiasis is one of the most common causes of biliary obstruction. As with gallbladder stones, ductal stones classically appear as hyperechoic, shadowing, intraductal structures (Fig. 3-13). Unlike gallbladder stones, in approximately 20% of the cases it is not possible to demonstrate an acoustic shadow behind a ductal stone. This likely is related to the lack of a significant amount of bile surrounding ductal stones. Most stones are located in the distal intrapancreatic portion of the duct. Methods for visualizing this segment include scanning after the oral administration of water, scanning with the patient in an upright or right posterior oblique position, and using the gallbladder as a window (Fig. 3-14).

The reported sensitivity of sonography for detecting ductal stones varies greatly. The best sensitivity that has been reported is approximately 75%. Most false-negative results are due to failure to visualize the distal common bile duct (Fig. 3-15). Although 25% or more of ductal stones may not be visualized sonographically, most of these patients will have dilated ducts and will eventually undergo some form of cholangiography to establish the cause of obstruction. False-positive results are less com-

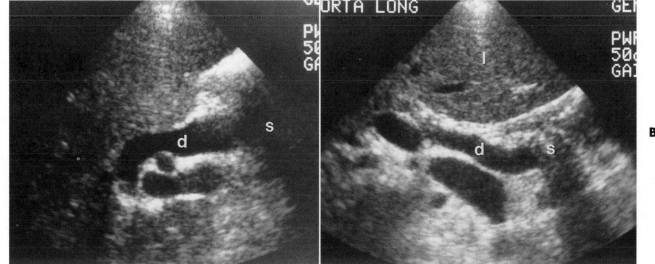

Fig. 3-15   False-negative sonographic findings in a patient with a distal common bile duct stone. **A,** Initial sonogram visualized the proximal common bile duct *(d)* and demonstrated ductal dilatation at this level. The distal common bile duct could not be visualized due to shadowing *(s)* from overlying bowel gas. **B,** Repeat examination later that day using a right coronal approach and the right lobe of the liver *(l)* as a sonographic window allowed for better visualization of the distal common bile duct *(d)* and showed a shadowing stone *(s)* in the distal-most segment.

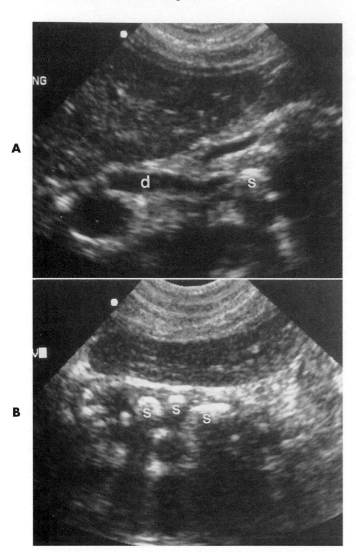

Fig. 3-16   Pancreatic calcifications simulating choledocholithiasis. **A,** Longitudinal view of the common duct *(d)* demonstrates ductal dilatation and an echogenic shadowing structure *(s)* adjacent to the distal duct at the level of obstruction. **B,** Transverse view of the pancreas demonstrates multiple echogenic shadowing structures *(s)* in the body of the pancreas. These are all pancreatic calcifications secondary to chronic calcific pancreatitis.

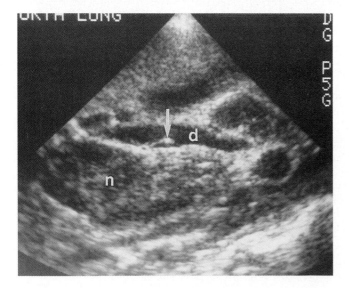

Fig. 3-17   Cystic duct insertion simulating a common bile duct stone. Longitudinal view of the common bile duct *(d)* demonstrates an echogenic nonshadowing focus *(arrow)* extending into the lumen of the duct. Note that there is a small septation extending from this focus to the wall of the duct superiorly. This represents the septation between the cystic duct and the common duct. An enlarged periportal lymph node *(n)* is seen posterior to the duct in this patient with lymphoma.

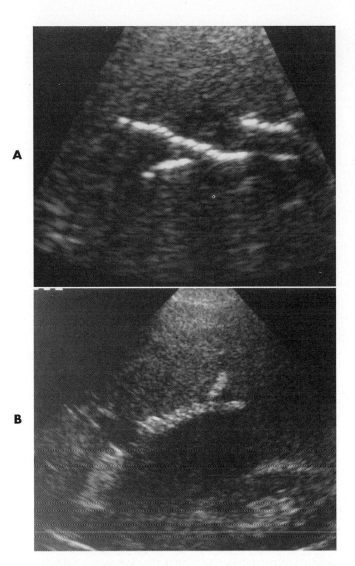

A

B

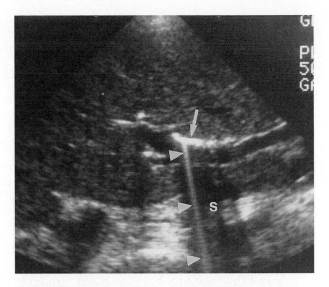

Fig. 3-19   Intrahepatic biliary gas with a ring-down artifact. Transverse view of the liver demonstrates a highly echogenic interface *(arrow)* anterior to the portal bifurcation. Shadowing *(s)* is seen posterior to this interface. In addition, a distinctive ring-down artifact *(arrowheads)* is seen. This artifact confirms that the bright reflection is arising from gas and not stones.

Fig. 3-18   Differentiation between intrahepatic gas and intrahepatic stones. **A,** Transverse view of the right lobe demonstrates a very echogenic branching structure with faint posterior acoustic shadowing consistent with intrahepatic biliary gas. **B,** Longitudinal view of the right lobe demonstrates a less echogenic branching structure with posterior acoustic shadowing due to intrahepatic biliary stones.

mon than false-negative results, but do occur. Calcifications in the hepatic artery and pancreatic head can sometimes be confused with ductal stones (Fig. 3-16). Gas in duodenal diverticula can also be misinterpreted to be choledocholithiasis. In all these instances transverse views of the duct are valuable for distinguishing between an intraductal and extraductal abnormality. In rare instances the cystic duct insertion can simulate a stone (Fig. 3-17). Recognition of the possibility of this pitfall is usually enough to avert misinterpretation. Intrabiliary gas is occasionally indistinguishable from stones. In most cases gas produces a brighter reflection (Fig. 3-18, *A*) and dirtier

shadow than do stones (Fig. 3-18, *B*). A ring-down artifact is only seen behind gas and, when found, is useful for establishing the diagnosis (Fig. 3-19).

CHOLANGIOCARCINOMA

Cancer of the bile ducts is slightly less common than gallbladder cancer. It occurs most commonly at the bifurcation of the common hepatic duct, with involvement of both the central left and right duct. Tumors at this location are referred to as *Klatskin tumors*. Bile duct cancer occurs less frequently in the distal and midcommon duct. Approximately 5% of cholangiocarcinomas are multicentric. In the most common pattern of growth, the tumor infiltrates the duct wall and occasionally the adjacent liver parenchyma and produces a focal stricture. Less commonly, cholangiocarcinomas grow either as an intraluminal polypoid mass or in a diffuse sclerosing pattern. The tumors in most patients are unresectable because of invasion of the liver or vascular structures or regional lymph node or distant metastatic spread.

In most cases cholangiocarcinomas appear as a dilated duct that abruptly terminates at the level of the tumor (Fig. 3-20 [for Fig. 3-20, *B*, see also color insert, Plate 15]). A mass may or may not be seen to explain the obstruction. When detected, the tumor itself is usually poorly marginated and may range from hypoechoic to hyperechoic (Fig. 3-21). Klatskin tumors classically appear as di-

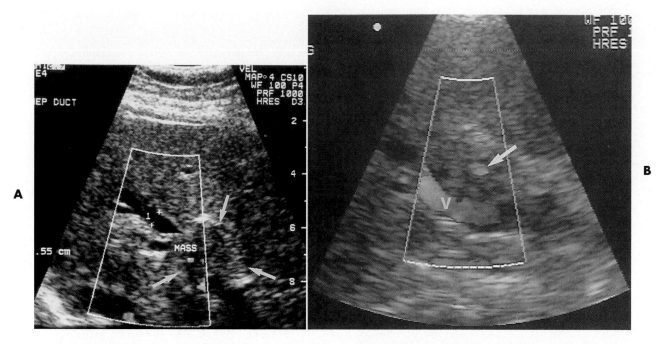

Fig. 3-20   Cholangiocarcinoma. **A,** Longitudinal view of the liver demonstrates a dilated left hepatic duct *(cursors)* that terminates abruptly centrally. There is a vaguely defined mass *(arrows)* that is isoechoic to the liver at the level of obstruction. **B,** Doppler view at the level of the mass demonstrates the hepatic artery *(arrow)* completely encased by this mass. This is generally regarded as a sign of nonresectability. The portal vein *(v)* is compressed by the mass (see color insert, Plate 15).

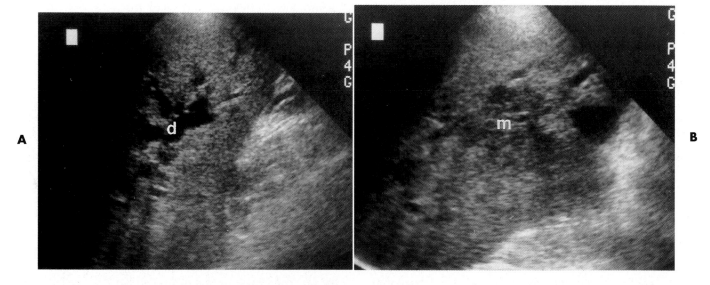

Fig. 3-21   Cholangiocarcinoma. **A,** Longitudinal view of the liver demonstrates multiple dilated central intrahepatic ducts *(d)*. **B,** Longitudinal view through the porta hepatis at the level of the biliary obstruction demonstrates an irregularly marginated hypoechoic mass *(m)* infiltrating the hepatic parenchyma.

lated intrahepatic ducts with no communication between the left and right duct (Fig. 3-22). Focal thickening of the bile duct wall without a mass is an uncommon but well-described sonographic appearance of cholangiocarcinoma (Fig. 3-23). Polypoid intraluminal masses are only rarely seen sonographically (Fig. 3-24). The differential diagnosis of cholangiocarcinoma depends on its location. Lesions at the ductal confluence can also be due to gallbladder carcinoma and hepatoma. Lesions in the distal duct can also be due to pancreatic or ampullary cancer.

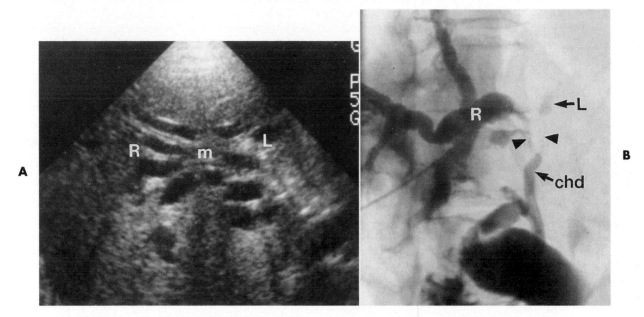

Fig. 3-22   Cholangiocarcinoma. **A,** Transverse view of the liver demonstrates dilated bile ducts in both the right *(R)* and left *(L)* lobes of the liver. There is no communication between these dilated ducts because of the presence of a central isoechoic mass *(m)*. **B,** Percutaneous transhepatic cholangiogram from the right side shows marked dilatation of the right hepatic ducts *(R)* due to a tight stricture *(arrowheads)* that involves both the right and left hepatic duct at their confluence with the common hepatic duct *(chd)*. There is minimal filling of the left hepatic duct *(L)* above the stricture. This is a classic cholangiographic appearance of a Klatskin tumor.

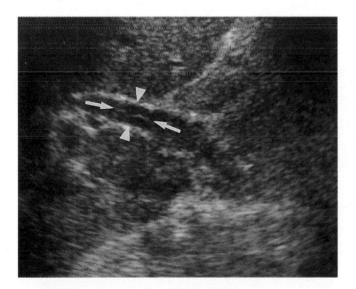

Fig. 3-23   Cholangiocarcinoma presenting as duct wall thickening. Longitudinal view of the porta hepatis demonstrates a common hepatic duct with a completely obliterated lumen. The reflection from the lumen is seen as a thin white line *(arrows)*. The space between the obliterated lumen and the outer duct walls *(arrowheads)* is due to the marked duct wall thickening.

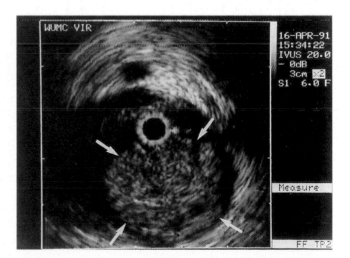

Fig. 3-24   Polypoid cholangiocarcinoma. Intraluminal ultrasound study using a miniaturized catheter-based transducer positioned in the lumen of the duct demonstrates an intraluminal polypoid mass *(arrows)* secondary to cholangiocarcinoma.

Metastatic disease to the duct or adjacent nodes can simulate cholangiocarcinoma at any level (Fig. 3-25).

Once the diagnosis is suspected, sonography can serve as a complementary tool to computed tomography and angiography in determining the resectability of the lesion. Hepatic metastases, invasion of the portal vein, and en-

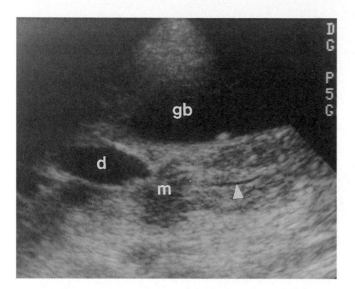

Fig. 3-25   Metastatic breast carcinoma simulating cholangiocarcinoma. Longitudinal view of the mid–common bile duct *(d)* demonstrates ductal dilatation to the level of a hypoechoic mass *(m)*. The distal duct *(arrowhead)* is almost completely decompressed. The gallbladder *(gb)* was used as an acoustic window to obtain this image. Brush biopsy specimens of this lesion revealed histologic findings identical to those of the patient's known breast carcinoma.

casement of the hepatic artery are all generally regarded as signs of nonresectability (see Fig. 3-20, *B*).

SCLEROSING CHOLANGITIS

Sclerosing cholangitis is characterized by fibrotic thickening of the bile ducts and adjacent fibrofatty tissues. Patients initially exhibit a cholestatic picture, and cirrhosis and its complications may then ensue. It most frequently affects young men and is strongly associated with inflammatory bowel disease, especially ulcerative colitis. It affects the intrahepatic and extrahepatic ducts in the majority of patients and occasionally involves the gallbladder and cystic duct.

The sonographic hallmark in the common duct is wall thickening that may appear smooth or irregular (Fig. 3-26). Multifocal strictures and beading develop in the intrahepatic ducts and these are optimally displayed by cholangiography but are seen occasionally sonographically (Fig. 3-27). Sonography more reliably detects intrahepatic disease when the strictures are associated with ductal dilatation (see Fig. 3-26, *B* and *C*).

Patients with sclerosing cholangitis are predisposed to the development of cholangiocarcinoma. It is generally not possible to detect coexistent sclerosing cholangitis and cholangiocarcinoma sonographically. However, cancer should be suspected whenever biliary centered or hepatic parenchymal mass lesions are detected in a patient with sclerosing cholangitis. Duct wall thickening greater than 5 mm and disproportionately dilated intrahepatic ducts should also raise the suspicion of cholangiocarci-

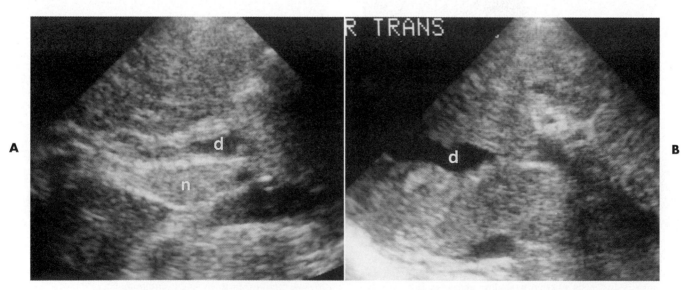

Fig. 3-26   Sclerosing cholangitis. **A,** Longitudinal view of the porta hepatis demonstrates a mildly dilated common duct *(d)* with slightly irregular wall thickening. Posterior to the duct is an enlarged reactive lymph node *(n)*. **B,** Transverse view of the liver demonstrates a dilated tubular structure *(d)* in the periphery of the right lobe.   *Continued.*

noma. It is not uncommon to see prominent nodes in the porta hepatis in patients with uncomplicated sclerosing cholangitis (see Fig. 3-26, *A*). This is therefore not a reliable sign of metastatic disease stemming from superimposed cholangiocarcinoma.

Other causes of bile duct wall thickening include choledocholithiasis (see Fig. 3-14), acquired immunodeficiency syndrome (AIDS) cholangiopathy (Fig. 3-28), pancreatitis, and oriental cholangiohepatitis. AIDS cholangiopathy is due to infection with cytomegalovirus or *Cryptosporidium* organisms. There are two forms—one that exactly mimics sclerosing cholangitis and one that produces isolated papillary stenosis. Oriental cholangiohepatitis is also known as *recurrent pyogenic cholangitis*. It appears to be caused by biliary flukes such as *Clonorchis sinensis* or *Ascaris lumbricoides*. Superimposed bacterial infection causes deconjugation of bilirubin diglucuronoside, and in 90% of patients this is associated with the formation of pigment stones in both the intrahepatic and extrahepatic ducts (Box 3-2).

CYSTIC DISEASE

Cystic lesions of the bile ducts are very unusual and occur more commonly in girls and women. They are be-

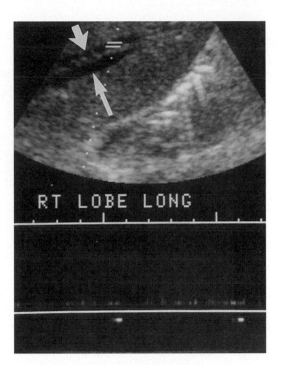

Fig. 3-27   Sclerosing cholangitis. Longitudinal magnified view of the right lobe of the liver demonstrates a dilated and slightly beaded intrahepatic bile duct *(short arrow)* adjacent to a normal intrahepatic portal vein *(long arrow)*. Pulsed-Doppler analysis of the duct confirms absence of flow and distinguishes it from a hepatic artery.

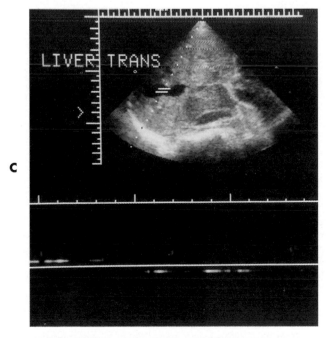

Fig. 3-26, cont'd.   **C,** Pulsed-Doppler analysis of this structure shows no detectable blood flow and confirms that this represents a dilated intrahepatic bile duct and not a vascular structure.

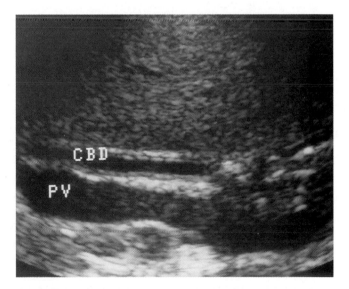

Fig. 3-28   AIDS cholangiopathy. Longitudinal view of the porta hepatis demonstrates the common bile duct *(CBD)* anterior to the portal vein *(PV)*. The bile duct exhibits a typical appearance of wall thickening with a hypoechoic submucosal layer.

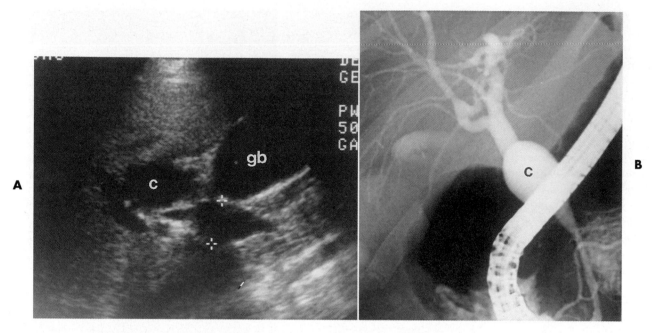

Fig. 3-29 Choledochal cyst. **A,** Longitudinal view of the porta hepatis demonstrates fusiform dilatation of the mid-common bile duct *(cursors)*. This represents a type 1 choledochal cyst. Also seen in this image is the gallbladder *(gb)* and an intrahepatic cyst *(c)* in the left lobe of the liver. **B,** Endoscopic retrograde cholangiopancreatography documenting the fusiform dilatation of the mid-common bile duct *(c)* consistent with a choledochal cyst.

Box 3-2 Causes of Bile Duct Wall Thickening	
Sclerosing cholangitis	AIDS cholangiopathy
Common bile duct stones	Cholangiocarcinoma
Pancreatitis	Oriental cholangiohepatitis
Ascending cholangitis	

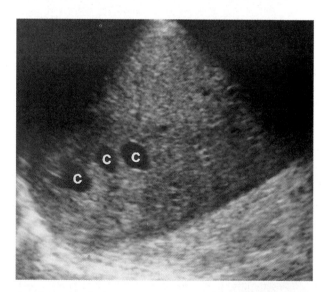

Fig. 3-30 Caroli's disease. Longitudinal view of the right lobe of the liver demonstrates three adjacent cystic lesions *(c)*. Communication between these three structures and the bile ducts was not evident sonographically, but was confirmed subsequently with hepatobiliary scintigraphy.

lieved to develop as the result of an anomalous connection of the common bile duct and pancreatic duct, such that pancreatic secretions can then reflux into the biliary tract. Classification schemes vary but all agree on the definitions of types 1 through 3. The most common is type 1, which is a fusiform dilatation of the extrahepatic duct (Fig. 3-29). Type 2 is a diverticular outpouching of the extrahepatic duct. Type 3 is a choledochocele, which is a dilatation of the distal intramural portion of the common bile duct that protrudes into the duodenum. Some authorities define type 4 as multifocal dilatations of the intrahepatic and extrahepatic bile ducts and type 5 as Caroli's disease.

The classic clinical triad of choledochal cysts comprises jaundice (occurring in approximately 80%), a palpable mass (occurring in approximately 50%), and abdominal pain (occurring in approximately 50%). Although choledochal cysts are typically thought of as pediatric le-

sions, it is not uncommon to first detect them during adulthood. The differential diagnosis includes cysts of the liver, right kidney, duodenum, mesentery, and omentum, as well as pancreatic pseudocysts and hepatic artery aneurysms (Box 3-3).

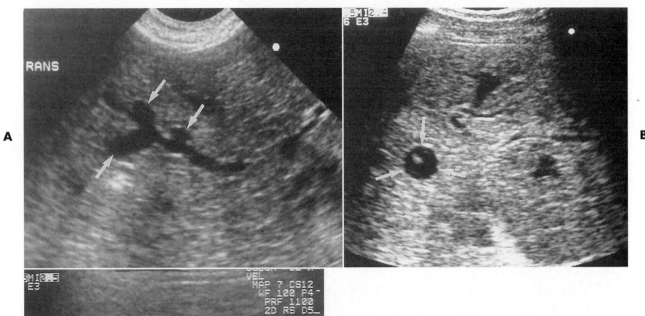

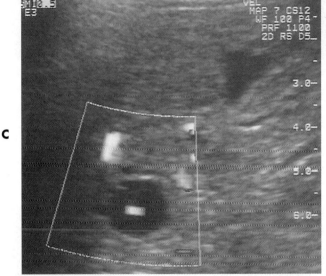

Fig. 3-31 Caroli's disease with associated hepatic fibrosis. **A,** Transverse view of the liver demonstrates an intrahepatic bile duct with several areas of saccular dilatation *(arrows)* at areas of branching. The underlying hepatic parenchyma is also coarsened due to hepatic fibrosis. **B,** Longitudinal view of the right lobe shows a dilated duct in cross-section *(arrows).* A central echogenic focus is present. This is the classic "central dot" sign. **C,** Doppler view similar to the previous image shows flow within the central dot, confirming its vascular nature (see color insert, Plate 16).

Continued.

Box 3-3   Differential Diagnosis of Choledochal Cysts

Duplication cyst of duodenum
Omental or mesenteric cyst
Pancreatic pseudocyst
Right renal cyst
Hepatic artery aneurysm

Caroli's disease is characterized by saccular dilatations of the intrahepatic bile ducts with sparing of the extrahepatic ducts. In its classic form, patients exhibit multiple complications of biliary stasis, including ductal stones and obstruction, cholangitis, and liver abscesses. More commonly it is associated with hepatic fibrosis, which leads to portal hypertension and variceal bleeding. Cystic disease of the kidney, especially medullary sponge disease

(tubular ectasia), is also strongly associated with Caroli's disease.

The sonographic features of Caroli's disease are predictable. Cystic intrahepatic lesions are the hallmark. In some cases it is difficult to document communication with the bile ducts (Fig. 3-30); in this event it is necessary to identify the secondary signs of portal hypertension (Fig. 3-31, *D*) or renal disease (Figs. 3-31, *E,* and 3-32, *B*) to suggest the diagnosis. Cholangiography or hepatobiliary scintigraphy can then be used to document the communication between the cysts and the bile ducts, but this can be documented sonographically in most cases (see Figs. 3-31 and 3-32). A very specific sonographic sign of Caroli's disease is the "central dot" sign, which occurs when the dilated segment of the bile duct surrounds the adjacent hepatic artery and portal vein so that these vascular structures produce a small focus in the middle of the dilated duct (see Fig. 3-31, *B* and *C* [for Fig. 3-31, *C,* see also color insert, Plate 16]).

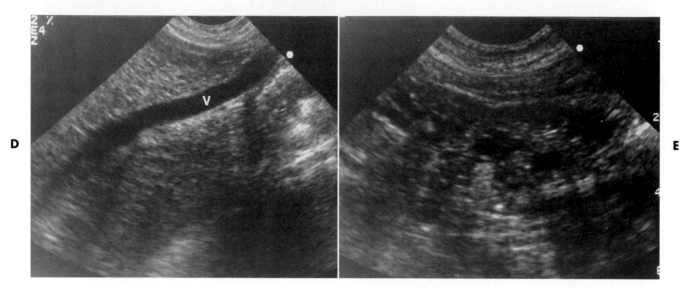

Fig. 3-31, cont'd.   **D,** Longitudinal view of the left lobe of the liver demonstrates an enlarged recanalized paraumbilical vein *(v)* exiting the inferior aspect of the liver. This provides evidence of underlying portal hypertension. **E,** Longitudinal view of the right kidney demonstrates distortion of the normal renal architecture by multiple small cystic lesions. This patient actually presented with progressive renal failure and was being evaluated in preparation for transplantation.

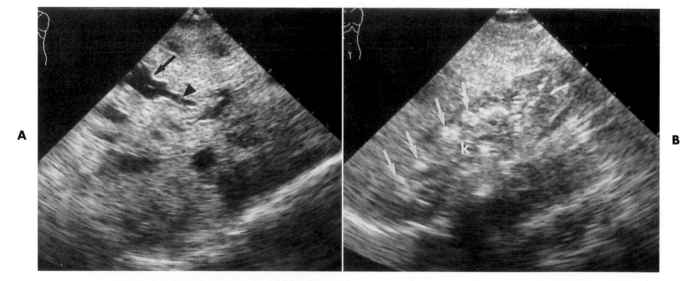

Fig. 3-32   Caroli's disease. **A,** Transverse view of the liver demonstrates a focal saccular region of biliary dilatation *(arrow)* peripherally, which communicates with a less-dilated bile duct centrally *(arrowhead).* **B,** Longitudinal view of the right kidney *(k)* demonstrates echogenic medullary pyramids *(arrows)* secondary to nephrocalcinosis related to underlying medullary sponge disease. Medullary sponge disease is the most frequent renal abnormality associated with Caroli's disease.

MIRIZZI'S SYNDROME

Mirizzi's syndrome is quite rare and is important more from an academic standpoint than from a clinical standpoint. It consists of a common duct obstruction caused by a gallstone in the cystic duct or, less commonly, in the gallbladder neck. For this to occur, usually the cystic duct must insert low and travel in a common sheath with the common duct. The obstruction may be caused by the actual mass effect of the stone or by an associated inflammatory reaction in the hepatoduodenal ligament. It is a particular problem for the surgeon because it may be difficult to distinguish the cystic duct from the common duct, resulting in inappropriate ligation of the common duct. Therefore preoperative knowledge of this condition is extremely valuable.

Sonographic findings can occasionally suggest the diagnosis in the setting of dilated ducts if an extrinsic mass effect from a shadowing structure is seen at the level of obstruction (Fig. 3-33). Often this is not possible, however, and the patient will need to undergo cholangiography for the diagnosis to be established. Cholangiography is also valuable for detecting the fistulas that often complicate the condition.

Key Features

The proximal common duct normally runs anterior to the portal vein and right hepatic artery.

Biliary obstruction is suspected when the bile ducts are dilated. The patient's age and the location of the diameter measurements are important factors in interpreting the significance of ductal size.

The detection of choledocholithiasis is improved by concentrating on the distal-most intrapancreatic portion of the common bile duct. At best, the sensitivity is 75%.

Cholangiocarcinoma should be suspected when there is abrupt termination of a dilated duct with little or no visible mass.

Sclerosing cholangitis is one of several conditions that cause bile duct wall thickening. It also produces multifocal intrahepatic duct strictures.

Choledochal cysts should be considered when cystic lesions are detected in the hepatoduodenal ligament. The most common appearance is focal fusiform dilatation of the common bile duct.

Caroli's disease produces a segmental saccular dilatation of the intrahepatic ducts and is usually associated with hepatic fibrosis and renal cystic disease.

Mirizzi's syndrome consists of a common bile duct obstruction resulting from a stone in the cystic duct or gallbladder neck.

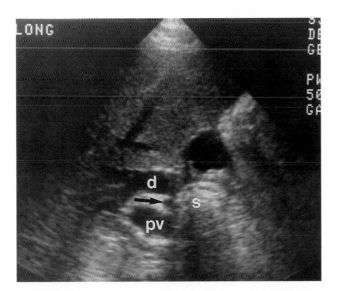

Fig. 3-33   Mirizzi's syndrome. Longitudinal view of the porta hepatis demonstrates a dilated common hepatic duct *(d)* that abruptly terminates at the level of an echogenic shadowing stone *(s)*. Although this could represent a large stone within the common duct itself, the presence of a wall-echo-shadow complex suggests that this actually resides within the gallbladder neck. The extrinsic nature of this obstructing stone was subsequently confirmed by cholangiography, and the diagnosis of Mirizzi's syndrome was established. Also seen in this view are the portal vein *(pv)* and the right hepatic artery *(arrow)*.

SUGGESTED READINGS

Babbit DP, Starshak RJ, Clemett AR: Choledochal cyst: a concept of etiology, *AJR* 119:57, 1973.

Becker CD, Hassler H, Terrier F: Preoperative diagnosis of Mirizzi syndrome: limitations of sonography and computed tomography, *AJR* 143:591, 1984.

Brandt DJ et al: Gallbladder disease in patients with primary sclerosing cholangitis, *AJR* 150:571, 1988.

Bressler EL, Rubin JM, McCracken S: Sonographic parallel channel sign: a reappraisal, *Radiology* 164:343, 1987.

Bret PM, deStempel JV, Atri M et al: Intrahepatic bile duct and portal vein anatomy revisited, *Radiology* 169:405, 1988.

Carroll BA, Oppenheimer DA: Sclerosing cholangitis: sonographic demonstration of bile duct wall thickening, *AJR* 139:1016, 1982.

Choi BI et al: Hilar cholangiocarcinoma: comparative study with sonography and CT, *Radiology* 172:689, 1989.

Choi BI, Yeon KM, Kim SH, Han MC: Caroli disease: central dot sign in CT, *Radiology* 174:161, 1990.

Coffey RJ, Wiesnet RH, Beaver SJ: Bile duct carcinoma: a late complication of end-stage primary sclerosing cholangitis, *Hepatology* 4:1056, 1984.

Darweesh R et al: Fatty-meal sonography for evaluating patients with suspected partial common duct obstruction, *AJR* 151:63, 1988.

Dolmatch BL et al: AIDS-related cholangitis: radiographic features in nine patients, *Radiology* 163:313, 1987.

Gibson RN et al: Bile duct obstruction: radiologic evaluation of level, cause, and tumor resectability, *Radiology* 160:43, 1986.

Hilger DJ, VerSteeg KR, Beaty PJ: Mirizzi syndrome with common septum: ultrasound and computed tomography findings, *J Ultrasound Med* 7:409, 1988.

Klatskin G: Adenocarcinoma of the hepatic duct at its bifurcation within the portal hepatis. An unusual tumor with distinctive clinical and pathological features, *Am J Med* 38: 241, 1965.

Laing FC et al: Biliary dilatation: defining the level and cause by real-time US, *Radiology* 160:39, 1986.

Laing FC, Jeffrey RB, Wing VW: Improved visualization of choledocholithiasis by sonography, *AJR* 143:949, 1984.

Laing FC, London LA, Filly RA: Ultrasonographic identification of dilated intrahepatic bile ducts and their differentiation from portal venous structures, *J Clin Ultrasound* 6:73, 1978.

Lim JH et al: Oriental cholangiohepatitis: sonographic findings in 48 cases, *AJR* 155:511, 1990.

Lim JH: Oriental cholangiohepatitis: pathologic, clinical, and radiologic features, *AJR* 157:1–8, 1991.

Li-Yeng C, Goldberg HI: Sclerosing cholangitis: broad spectrum of radiographic features, *Gastrointest Radiol* 9:39, 1984.

MacCarty RL et al: Cholangiocarcinoma complicating primary sclerosing cholangitis: cholangiographic appearances, *Radiology* 156:43, 1985.

Marchal GJ et al: Caroli disease: high-frequency US and pathologic findings, *Radiology* 158:507, 1986.

Meyer DG, Weinstein BJ: Klatskin tumors of the bile ducts: sonographic appearance, *Radiology* 148:803, 1983.

Miller DR, Egbert RM, Braunstein P: Comparison of ultrasound and hepatobiliary imaging in the early detection of acute total common bile duct obstruction, *Arch Surg* 119:1233, 1984.

Nagorney DM, McIlrath DC, Adson MA: Choledochal cysts in adults: clinical management, *Surgery* 96:656, 1984.

Nesbit GM et al: Cholangiocarcinoma: diagnosis and evaluation of resectability by CT and sonography as procedures complementary to cholangiography, *AJR* 151:933, 1988.

Ralls PW et al: The use of color Doppler sonography to distinguish dilated intrahepatic ducts from vascular structures, *AJR* 152:291, 1989.

Romano AJ et al: Gallbladder and bile duct abnormalities in AIDS: sonographic findings in eight patients, *AJR* 150:123, 1988.

Schulte SJ et al: CT of the extrahepatic bile ducts: wall thickness and contrast enhancement in normal and abnormal ducts, *AJR* 154:79, 1990.

Simeone JF et al: The bile ducts after a fatty meal: further sonographic observations, *Radiology* 154:763, 1985.

Subramanyam BR et al: Ultrasonic features of cholangiocarcinoma, *J Ultrasound Med* 3:405, 1984.

Takasan H et al: Clinicopathologic study of seventy patients with carcinoma of the biliary tract, *Surg Gynecol Obstet* 150: 721, 1980.

Teixidor HS, Godwin TA, Ramirez EA: Cryptosporidiosis of the biliary tract in AIDS, *Radiology* 180:51, 1991.

Todani T et al: Congenital bile duct cysts. Classification, operative procedures, and review of thirty-seven cases including cancer arising from choledochal cyst, *Am J Surg* 134:263, 1977.

Wiesner RH, LaRusso NF: Clinicopathologic features of the syndrome of primary sclerosing cholangitis, *Gastroenterology* 79:200, 1980.

Wu CC, Ho Y-H, Chen C-Y: Effect of aging on common bile duct diameter: a real-time ultrasonographic study, *J Clin Ultrasound* 12:473, 1984.

Yeung EYC et al: The ultrasonographic appearance of hilar cholangiocarcinoma (Klatskin tumours), *Br J Radiol* 61:991, 1988.

Kidney

For a Key Features summary see p. 119.

ANATOMY

Unlike the other solid abdominal organs, the kidneys have a very complex internal architecture that is responsible for producing a variety of internal echogenicities.

The central renal sinus is composed of fibrofatty tissue that appears echogenic on sonograms. The renal vessels and pelvis are occasionally seen as thin anechoic, fluid-containing structures located within the echogenic tissues of the renal sinus. The lymphatics also pass through the renal sinus, but cannot be resolved sonographically. Each kidney consists of multiple functional units called *lobes*. The archetypal lobe contains a calix, a medullary pyramid, cortical tissue, and vessels. In the adult there is an average of eleven pyramids and nine calices. This discrepancy is due to the presence of compound calices that drain more than one pyramid. Sonographically the pyramids are cone- or heart-shaped, hypoechoic structures (Fig. 4-1). The cortex is slightly more echogenic than the pyramids, although this distinction is not always apparent. The cortical echogenicity of the kidney should be equal or slightly less than that of the liver and substantially less than that of the spleen. The kidneys are slightly ovoid in cross-section, with the longest dimension directed from anteromedial to posterolateral. Therefore longitudinal views of the kidney will demonstrate a different shape depending on how the view was obtained (see Fig. 4-1).

The external contour of the kidney is generally smooth. A common normal variant, called the *junctional parenchymal defect* or the *interrenuncular junction,* produces a wedge-shaped hyperechoic defect in the anterior aspect of the kidney near the junction of the upper and middle thirds. It occurs because of incomplete embryologic fusion of the upper and lower poles. It can be distinguished from a scar or mass by its typical triangular shape and location. In addition, the junctional parenchymal defect communicates with the renal sinus medially (Fig. 4-2). Slight lobulation of the external contour of the kidney can also be seen as a result of persistent fetal lobation.

The size of the kidney varies with the age, sex, height, and weight of the person. In adults the average length of the kidney is approximately 10.5 to 11 cm. The lower and

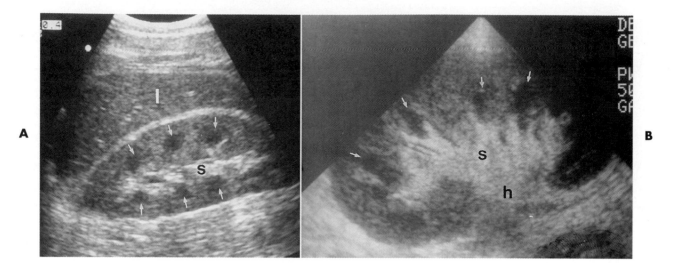

Fig. 4-1   Normal kidney. **A,** Longitudinal view of the kidney obtained from an anterior approach demonstrates the hyperechoic renal sinus *(s)* completely surrounded by renal parenchyma. The cortical echogenicity is equal to that of the overlying liver *(l)*. Several slightly hypoechoic renal pyramids *(arrows)* are seen at the junction of the renal cortex and renal sinus. The kidney has a relatively flattened appearance in this view. **B,** Longitudinal view obtained from a lateral approach demonstrates the renal sinus *(s)* extending to the renal hilum *(h)*. In this view the kidney appears bulbous rather than flattened. The pyramids again are visible as slightly hypoechoic structures *(arrows)*.

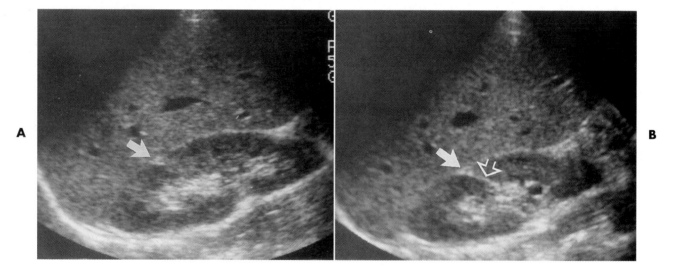

Fig. 4-2   Junctional parenchymal defect. **A,** Longitudinal view of the right kidney demonstrates a triangular, peripherally located hyperechoic area in the kidney at the junction of the upper pole and midpole *(arrow)*. **B,** Longitudinal view obtained slightly medial to **A** demonstrates the continuity of this triangular, hyperechoic region with the renal sinus fat via a thin bright line *(open arrow)*. These features are typical of the junctional parenchymal defect.

upper limits of normal are approximately 9 and 13 cm, respectively. The renal anteroposterior thickness and renal width can also be measured to calculate the renal volume based on the formula for an ellipsoid: volume = (length × thickness × width)/2. (See Table 4-1 for a summary of the characteristics of the normal kidney.)

A number of congenital anomalies of the kidneys can be detected sonographically. Agenesis is associated with an empty renal fossa and an elongated ipsilateral adrenal. The latter is much easier to detect in the neonatal period than later in life. Hypertrophy of the contralateral kidney is also usually present in cases of renal agenesis. Detec-

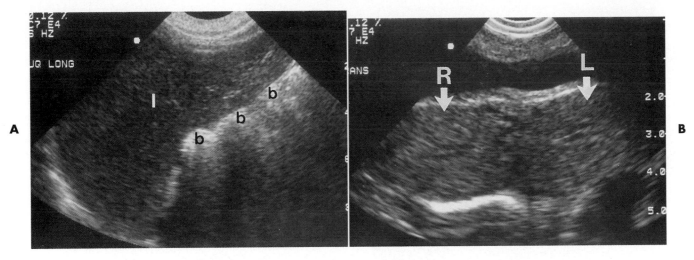

Fig. 4-3   Renal agenesis. **A,** Longitudinal view of the right upper quadrant demonstrates shadowing bowel gas *(b)* posterior to the liver *(l)* but no identifiable kidney within the right renal fossa. **B,** Transverse transvaginal scan of the uterus demonstrates two uterine horns and two separate endometrial stripes consistent with the right *(R)* and left *(L)* horns of a bicornuate uterus. Genitourinary anomalies often coexist, as they did in this patient.

Table 4-1 Characteristics of normal kidney	
Characteristic	**Appearance**
Size	Average, 11 cm (range, 9-13 cm)
Echogenicity	Right, ≤ liver; left, < spleen
Parenchyma	Inhomogeneous
Surface	Smooth

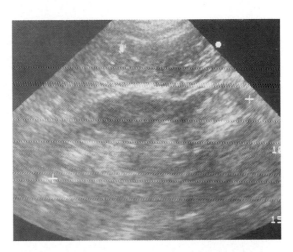

Fig. 4-4   Crossed, fused renal ectopia. Longitudinal view of the left upper quadrant demonstrates an elongated (15.45 cm) and distorted-appearing left kidney. No kidney was found in the right renal fossa and a subsequent intravenous urogram confirmed crossed, fused renal ectopia.

tion of renal agenesis should prompt a search for other anomalies in the genitourinary tract, such as duplication anomalies of the uterus (Fig. 4-3) and anomalies of the seminal vesicles and vas deferens. Ectopic kidneys can also appear as an empty renal fossa. Most ectopic kidneys are found inferior to the renal fossa, often in the pelvis. They have also been reported to occur in the thorax. Crossed, fused renal ectopy also occurs, and may appear as an unusually large kidney with a duplicated renal sinus or as a mass arising from the lower pole (Fig. 4-4). Fusion anomalies in general are relatively common (1 in 250). The most common fusion anomaly is the horseshoe kidney. This appears as renal tissue extending from both lower poles to connect anterior to the aorta (Fig. 4-5). It should be suspected when the axis of the kidney is distorted and the lower poles of the kidneys are hard to image sonographically.

TECHNIQUE

The native kidneys are best imaged with a 2- to 5-MHz transducer, depending on the patient's body habitus and the depth of the kidney. Higher frequencies can occasionally be used in renal transplants. Sector-type probes or curved arrays are generally best for imaging native kidneys, and linear arrays or curved arrays are best for imaging renal transplants.

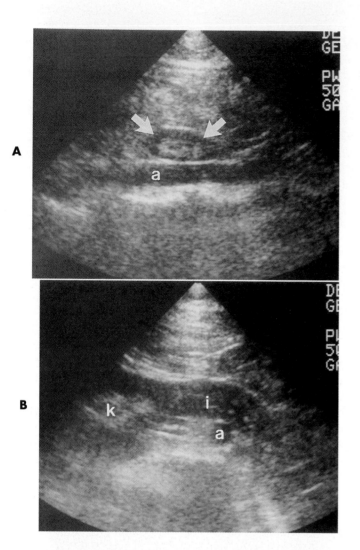

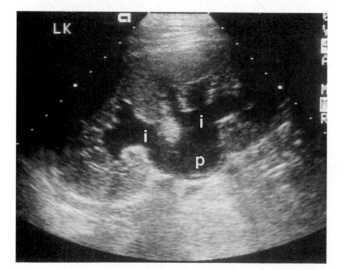

Fig. 4-5   Horseshoe kidney. **A,** Longitudinal view of the aorta *(a)* demonstrates an ovoid structure *(arrows)* resembling renal parenchyma and renal sinus fat anterior to the aorta. **B,** Transverse view of the aorta *(a)* demonstrates the lower pole of the right kidney *(k)* in continuity with this structure, which represents the isthmus *(i)* of a horseshoe kidney.

Fig. 4-6   Moderate hydronephrosis. Longitudinal view of the left kidney obtained from a lateral approach demonstrates dilated renal calices communicating with the central renal pelvis *(p)* via two distended infundibula *(i).*

The native kidneys can be viewed from a variety of approaches. The upper poles of each kidney are often seen best with the patient supine and by using a high posterior intercostal approach and the liver or spleen as a window. Failure to go high enough and posterior enough is the most common reason for inadequate visualization of the upper pole, especially on the left. The lower poles can be seen best using a subcostal approach, usually during a deep inspiration. The transducer location should be varied from anterior to lateral to posterior and the patient position should be varied from supine to decubitus until the best view is obtained. In some persons the lower pole of the left kidney can be seen best from an anterolateral approach with the patient in a right lateral decubitus position. This view seems to be especially advantageous in obese patients.

OBSTRUCTION

Approximately 5% of the patients with renal failure suffer from urinary obstruction. In most cases bilateral obstruction is required for renal insufficiency to develop. Early detection is important, as obstruction is easily treated and can lead to irreversible renal damage if untreated. The degree of long-term functional loss depends on both the degree and duration of obstruction. In dogs complete ureteral obstruction lasting 7 days results in an average long-term recovery of only 70% of function. If an obstructed kidney is also infected, permanent renal dam-

age can occur much more rapidly. Patients with signs of infection who are suspected to have renal obstruction should be treated as emergencies, with immediate renal sonography and urgent drainage performed if hydronephrosis is detected. In general, uninfected patients with suspected renal obstruction are not considered emergencies and are scanned as soon as is reasonable.

The likelihood of sonographic detection of hydronephrosis in patients with renal failure depends on the patient's history. In patients with no risk factors for urinary obstruction, only 1% will have hydronephrosis detected sonographically. In many of these patients, the ultrasound finding of hydronephrosis will prove to be falsely positive or the patient will receive no therapy despite the ultrasound results. On the other hand, approximately 30% of the patients affected by the following conditions or circumstances will have hydronephrosis: a known pelvic tumor, a palpable abdominal or pelvic mass, a history of renal stone disease, renal colic, sepsis, recent surgery, or history of bladder outlet obstruction.

The sonographic diagnosis of obstruction has traditionally relied on the detection of a dilated collecting system. This appears as anechoic spaces that conform to the expected location and shape of the renal calices and infundibula and generally communicate with a dilated renal pelvis (Fig. 4-6). Communication with the renal pelvis is best shown on coronal or semicoronal views (Fig. 4-7). *Marked hydronephrosis* refers to severe dilatation that is associated with cortical thinning. *Moderate hydroneph-*

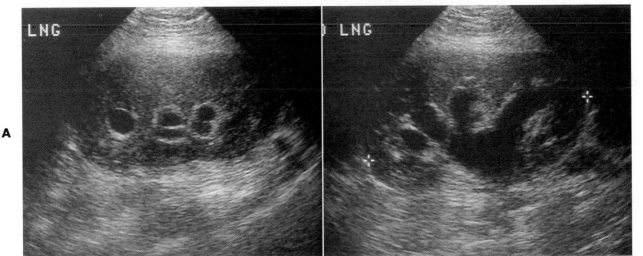

Fig. 4-7   Variation in the appearance of hydronephrosis depending on transducer position. **A,** Longitudinal view of the kidney from an anterior approach demonstrates several cystic structures that are surrounded by hyperechoic renal sinus fat. In this single view these could represent dilated renal calices or peripelvic cysts. **B,** Longitudinal view of the same kidney from a lateral approach demonstrates multiple dilated renal calices and infundibula connecting to a central renal pelvis, confirming that this is in fact a case of hydronephrosis and not peripelvic cysts.

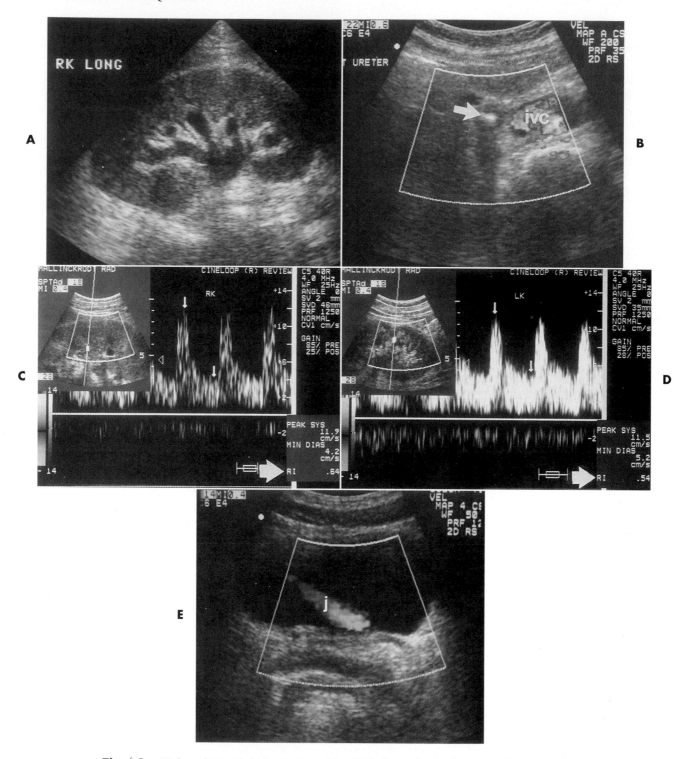

Fig. 4-8   High-grade ureteral obstruction with mild hydronephrosis. **A,** Longitudinal view of the right kidney demonstrates mild hydronephrosis. **B,** Transverse view of the midabdomen demonstrates a shadowing echogenic focus within the lumen of the right ureter *(arrow)*. The inferior vena cava *(ivc)* is also identified on this image. **C,** Intrarenal arterial waveform from the right kidney discloses a resistive index of 0.64 *(arrow)*. Taken by itself, this value would not be considered abnormal because it is less than 0.70. **D,** Intrarenal arterial waveform from the left kidney demonstrates a resistive index of 0.54 *(arrow)*. Because the right resistive index is 0.10 greater than the left, the value on the right should be considered abnormal and indicative of a high-grade obstruction. **E,** Transverse view of the bladder demonstrates a ureteral jet *(j)* arising from the left ureteral orifice and crossing the midline to the right. No ureteral jet is seen arising from the right ureteral orifice and no right ureteral jet was detected over 5 minutes despite multiple detectable left ureteral jets. This also provides evidence that there is a moderate to high-grade obstruction of the right ureter.

rosis refers to dilatation of the collecting system that is readily evident but not associated with cortical thinning (see Figs. 4-6 and 4-7). Neither moderate nor marked hydronephrosis is difficult to identify or interpret correctly on sonograms. *Mild hydronephrosis* refers to minimal amounts of urine producing slight distention of the collecting system (Fig. 4-8). Detecting the various grades of hydronephrosis is much less difficult than determining their significance. In general, the more distended the renal

collecting system, the more likely it is due to a clinically significant obstruction. However, recurrent or long-standing obstruction may cause a dilated, ectatic collecting system that persists even when obstruction is relieved (Fig. 4-9), and acute high-grade obstruction may produce minimal hydronephrosis (see Fig. 4-8) or may be imaged before any hydronephrosis develops. For this reason, comparison with old studies is extremely valuable. Mild hydronephrosis is much more likely to be due to ob-

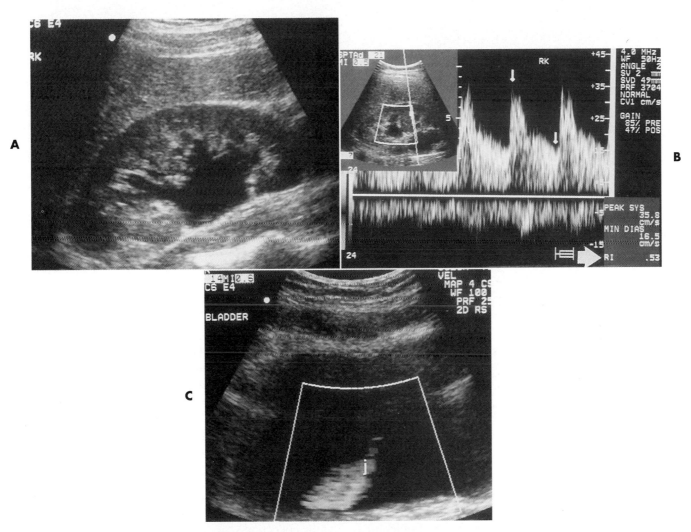

Fig. 4-9 Nonobstructive hydronephrosis. **A,** Longitudinal view of the right kidney demonstrates moderate right hydronephrosis. No obstructing stone or other abnormality was seen in the pelvis or along the expected course of the right ureter. **B,** Intraarterial Doppler waveform from the right kidney has a normal appearance and a measured resistive index of 0.53 *(arrow)*. This would argue against a high-grade obstruction. **C,** Transverse view of the bladder demonstrates a normal-appearing ureteral jet *(j)* arising from the right ureteral orifice and crossing the midline to the left. This provides further evidence against a moderate or high-grade obstruction. This patient had undergone endopyelotomy 2 years before for a ureteropelvic junction obstruction. After the procedure, there was no evidence of a urodynamically significant obstruction on retrograde pyelograms or renal scintigrams. The sonographic findings correlate with these other study findings and indicate a dilated but nonobstructed collecting system.

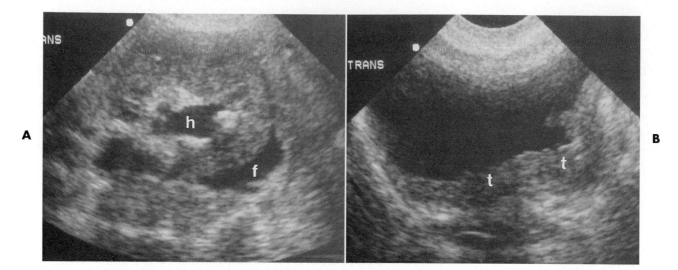

Fig. 4-10   Transitional cell carcinoma of the bladder producing hydronephrosis. **A,** Transverse view of the left kidney demonstrates a hydronephrotic collecting system *(h)* as well as a small amount of perinephric fluid *(f)*. Small perinephric fluid collections such as this are common in patients with urinary obstruction, especially acute obstruction. **B,** Transverse view of the bladder demonstrates extensive thickening *(t)* of the posterior and left lateral bladder wall. This case illustrates the value of obtaining views of the pelvis and bladder in patients with hydronephrosis or suspected urinary obstruction.

Box 4-1   Causes of Hydronephrosis

COMMON

Obstruction
Previous obstruction
Extrarenal pelvis
Distended bladder
Pregnancy

UNCOMMON

Active diuresis
Diabetes insipidus
Reflux nephropathy

---

struction if it is a new finding. On the other hand, even moderate hydronephrosis is less likely to be due to obstruction when it is a chronic unchanged finding.

In addition to obstruction, there are a number of processes that can cause a dilated renal collecting system (Box 4-1). They include very active physiologic diuresis, diuresis related to diabetes insipidus, overdistention of the urinary bladder, pregnancy, vesicoureteral reflux, and previous episodes of obstruction. The best way to determine if sonographically detected hydronephrosis is actually due to obstruction is to identify an obstructing lesion. Most obstructing lesions occur in the pelvis (Fig. 4-10). When the pelvis is normal, one should scan along the course of the ureters searching for masses, fluid collections, or stones

(see Fig. 4-8). In many cases the ureters themselves are not seen, even though the obstructing process is identified.

Doppler evaluation is useful when evaluating hydronephrosis or suspected renal obstruction. Prominent renal vessels (usually veins) mimic a dilated renal collecting system in up to 50% of the patients with apparent mild hydronephrosis. Doppler analysis can distinguish these patients from those with true renal pelvis dilatation (Fig. 4-11). In addition, resistance to renal arterial flow is increased in the setting of obstruction due to the release of vasoactive substances and to vasoconstriction. This produces an elevated resistive index (>0.7) or asymmetry between the ipsilateral and contralateral resistive index (a difference of 0.1 or more). Therefore a unilateral elevated resistive index suggests the presence of obstruction even when the hydronephrosis is mild (see Fig. 4-8) and also suggests obstruction in patients with an obstruction suspected on clinical grounds, even if there is no hydronephrosis. On the other hand, a normal resistive index in the setting of hydronephrosis suggests that the dilatation of the collecting system is not due to obstruction (see Fig. 4-9). Although the results of initial studies have indicated that intrarenal arterial waveforms and renal resistive indexes are both sensitive and specific in their ability to detect renal obstruction, the results have not been reproduced widely and the methods remain very controversial. One of the difficulties with intrarenal arterial resistive indexes is that they may not detect either acute or partial obstruction.

Analysis of ureteral jets is another way Doppler studies can assist in the evaluation of the potentially obstructed

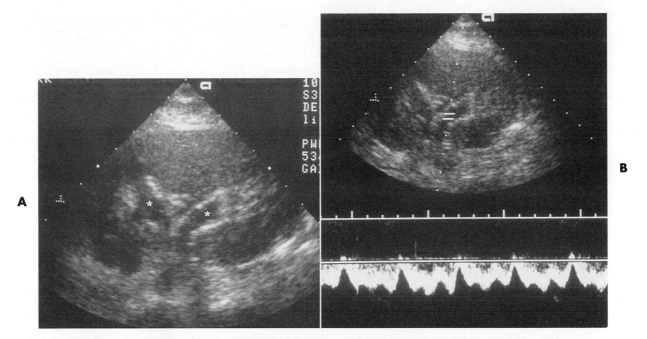

Fig. 4-11   Prominent renal veins simulating hydronephrosis. **A,** Longitudinal view of the right kidney demonstrates prominent hypoechoic structures in the central renal sinus (*) that could easily be mistaken for a distended renal collecting system. **B,** Pulsed-Doppler waveform analysis of these structures documents venous flow and confirms that this represents prominent renal veins rather than hydronephrosis.

kidney. In this method, the bladder is scanned in the region of the trigone using color-Doppler sonography to detect intermittent bursts of urine flow out of the ureteral orifices. Ureteral jets are absent in the presence of urinary obstruction (see Fig. 4-8) but are maintained in the presence of nonobstructive hydronephrosis. The advantage of this technique over intrarenal arterial analysis is that it can detect acute obstruction. However, as with renal resistive index measurements, a low-grade partial obstruction may not eliminate ureteral jets and thus may go undetected with this technique. The detection of ureteral jets depends on differences in density between urine in the bladder and urine exiting the ureters. Because the density of urine in the bladder is the average density of ureteral urine collected over long periods, it usually differs from the density of urine exiting the ureter at any point in time. This is not so after the patient has recently voided. Therefore patients should not be allowed to void completely before the examination as the fresh urine collecting in the bladder would then have the same density as the urine exiting the ureters.

The sensitivity of ultrasound studies in detecting obstruction is approximately 95%. Sources of false-negative findings include acute or partial obstruction, obstruction in a dehydrated patient, and lack of recognition of mild hydronephrosis. A number of abnormalities can be mistaken for hydronephrosis and lead to a false-positive diagnosis of obstruction. These include dilated renal vessels, peripelvic cysts, chronic reflux nephropathy, and severe papillary necrosis. In most cases, gray-scale sonography is capable of distinguishing these other abnormalities from hydronephrosis. Chronic reflux nephropathy affects the calices and produces cortical thinning, but spares the renal pelvis (Fig. 4-12). Severe papillary necrosis causes the papillae to be replaced with urine-filled sacs that simulate dilated calices, but again the renal pelvis and infundibula are spared (Fig. 4-13).

Pyonephrosis refers to an obstructed and infected collecting system. In some such cases echogenic pus can be seen filling the collecting system or layering in the dependent portion of the collecting system (Fig. 4-14). Unfortunately ultrasound analysis is neither sensitive nor specific in the detection of pyonephrosis, and the diagnosis should be suspected in any patient with hydronephrosis and clinical evidence of urinary tract infection.

CYSTIC DISEASES (Table 4-2)

Benign Cysts

Renal cysts are the most common renal mass. Their frequency increases with age and they are present in half the population above the age of 50. The etiology of renal cysts is not known, but it is possible that they form from the epithelial overgrowth of tubules or collecting ducts, with resulting distention of the nephron. This would explain why cysts enlarge over time, and the involvement

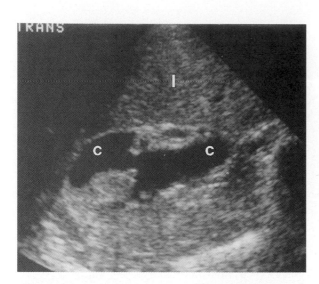

Fig. 4-12 Reflux nephropathy. Transverse view of the right kidney demonstrates dilated anterior calices *(c)*. The renal parenchyma overlying the abnormal calices is extremely thin and the echogenicity of the remainder of the renal cortex is increased compared with that of the overlying liver *(l)*. Despite the distention of the renal collecting system, this patient had no evidence of urinary obstruction and the findings just described are typical of reflux nephropathy.

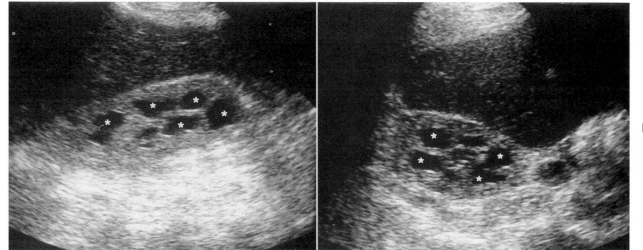

Fig. 4-13 Papillary necrosis. **A,** Longitudinal view of the right kidney in a patient with sickle cell anemia demonstrates multiple cystic structures (*) in the expected location of the renal pyramids. **B,** Transverse view of the same patient also demonstrates the cystic structures. On neither of these views is communication with a central renal pelvis evident. The renal cortex is also increased in echogenicity, reflecting the existence of underlying parenchymal disease. The sonographic findings and the patient's history of sickle cell disease are typical of severe papillary necrosis rather than hydronephrosis.

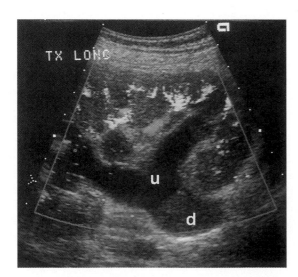

Fig. 4-14 Pyonephrosis. Longitudinal view of a renal transplant demonstrates mild hydronephrosis. A layer of slightly more echogenic debris *(d)* is seen in the renal pelvis, contrasting with the more anechoic urine *(u)* within the intrarenal collecting system. This appearance usually reflects either pus or blood within the collecting system.

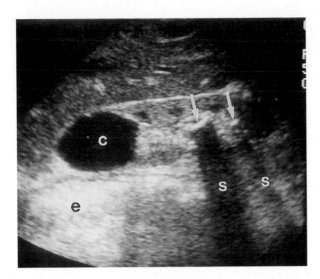

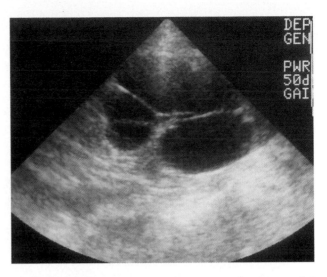

Fig. 4-15   Simple renal cyst. Longitudinal view of the kidney demonstrates an anechoic mass in the upper pole with well-defined walls consistent with a cyst *(c)*. The echogenicity of the tissues posterior to the cyst is increased secondary to acoustic enhancement *(e)*. Also seen in this kidney are two stones in the lower pole *(arrows)* with posterior acoustic shadowing *(s)* and increased cortical echogenicity.

Fig. 4-16   Multiseptated renal cyst. Longitudinal view of the lower pole of the kidney demonstrates a cystic mass with multiple internal septations. The septations coalesce centrally into a more solid-appearing component. Because of this, cystic renal cell carcinoma was considered a possibility. The lesion was resected and found to be a benign multiseptated cyst.

Table 4-2   Renal cystic disease

Disorder	Kidney size	Kidney tumors	Extrarenal cysts	Extrarenal tumors and other lesions
Autosomal dominant polycystic disease	Normal to large	None	Liver	Cerebral aneurysms
von Hippel–Lindau disease	Normal to large	RCCa	Pancreas	Pancreatic cystic neoplasms, CNS hemangioblastomas, retinal angiomas, pheochromocytomas
Acquired cystic disease	Small	RCCa	None	None
Tuberous sclerosis	Normal to large	AML	None	Cerebral hamartomas, periventricular nodules, subungual fibromas, cardiac rhabdomyomas, pulmonary lymphangiomyomatosis

RCCa, renal cell carcinoma; *CNS,* central nervous system; *AML,* angiomyolipoma.

of adjacent nephrons might explain why thin septations develop.

Sonography is the best way of initially evaluating cystic lesions in the kidney. To qualify as a simple cyst, the lesion should have the following characteristics.

1. Anechoic lumen
2. Well-defined back wall
3. Acoustic enhancement deep to the lesion
4. No measurable wall thickness

The image of the cyst shown in Fig. 4-15 satisfies all of the criteria for a simple cyst. However, not all features need to be evident on every view. Small cysts may have low-level artifactual internal echoes due to slice thickness limitations or to degradation of the ultrasound beam by overlying soft tissues such as fat. Small cysts may also not have demonstrable acoustic enhancement. All cysts, regardless of size, should have a well-defined back wall because of the acoustic impedance mismatch between fluid and the cyst wall.

A cyst can still be considered benign if it contains a limited number of thin internal septations, provided it satisfies the other criteria. Thick septations should be considered suspicious for a cystic neoplasm. They can be seen in the setting of cystic renal cell carcinoma, benign cystic neoplasms, and complicated cysts (Fig. 4-16). Overall, septations are seen in approximately 5% of benign renal cysts.

Cysts are complicated by intraluminal hemorrhage approximately 5% of the time. Hemorrhage may cause diffuse low-level internal echoes, fibrinous membranes, an echogenic clot, or a fluid-debris level (Fig. 4-17). Follow-up scans should show resolution of these findings in 2 to 3 months. The Doppler characteristics of hemorrhagic cysts overlap with those of infected renal cysts, and this distinction can only be made on the basis of clinical findings and the findings yielded by cyst aspiration (Fig. 4-18). A common clinical problem is a hyperdense mass seen on computed tomography (CT) usually due to hemorrhage or to a high protein content in the cyst fluid. Sonography is extremely useful in excluding the less likely possibility of a solid mass.

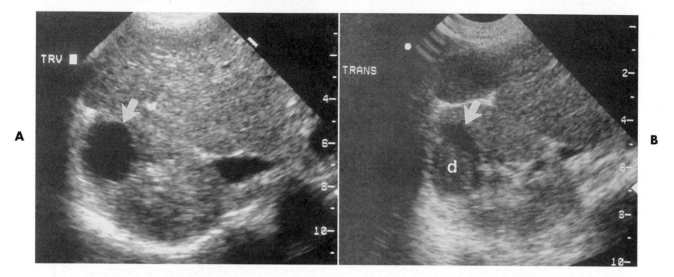

Fig. 4-17   Hemorrhagic renal cyst. **A,** Baseline transverse view of the upper pole of the right kidney demonstrates an uncomplicated-appearing renal cyst *(arrow)*. **B,** Similar view obtained 6 months later demonstrates a cyst *(arrow)* with debris *(d)* layering in the dependent aspect of the lumen. This is consistent with hemorrhage or pus. In this case hemorrhage was subsequently proved by the results of percutaneous aspiration.

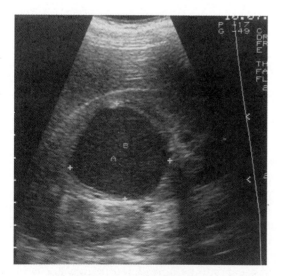

Fig. 4-18   Infected renal cyst. Longitudinal view of the kidney demonstrates a well-defined mass with increased through-transmission but low-level internal echoes. These findings are consistent with either an infected or hemorrhagic renal cyst. Results of percutaneous drainage confirmed that the low-level echoes were secondary to pus rather than blood.

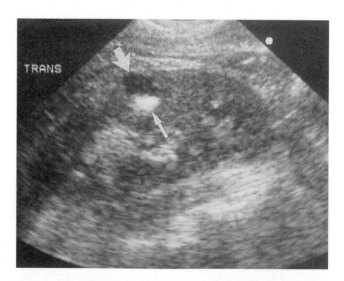

Fig. 4-19   Cyst with milk of calcium. Longitudinal view of the kidney demonstrates a cyst *(short arrow)* in the midpole. Echogenic material *(long arrow),* seen in the dependent aspect of the cyst, is casting a faint acoustic shadow consistent with milk of calcium.

Calcifications occur in 1% to 3% of cysts and usually result from prior hemorrhage, infection, or ischemia. Thin, curvilinear, peripheral calcifications should not raise the suspicion of carcinoma, but thick, globular calcification may indicate an underlying malignancy. Crystalline material can accumulate in cysts and produce shadowing, echogenic material that layers in the dependent aspect of the lumen (Fig. 4-19). In some cases crystals may form in cysts that are too small to resolve sonographically. In these cases the echogenic crystals are all that is detected.

The differential diagnosis of simple cysts includes caliceal diverticula, aneurysms and pseudoaneurysms (Fig. 4-20), arteriovenous malformations, papillary necrosis, obstructed upper pole duplications (Fig. 4-21), and lymphoma.

Cysts that form in the renal sinus fat are called *peripelvic cysts*. These cysts are probably lymphatic in origin and are located within the renal sinus. They are frequently bilateral and are important only because they can be confused with hydronephrosis (Fig. 4-22). However,

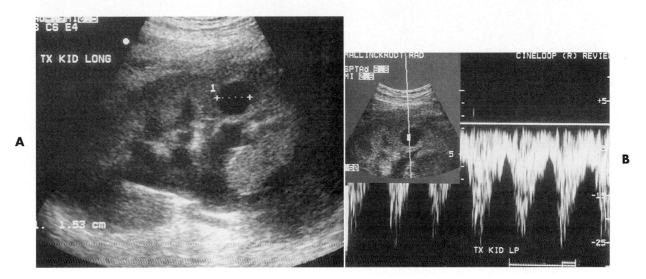

Fig. 4-20 Pseudoaneurysm simulating a renal cyst. **A,** Longitudinal view of a renal transplant demonstrates an anechoic cystic-appearing lesion *(cursors)* in the lower pole. Mild hydronephrosis is also present. **B,** Pulsed-Doppler waveform analysis of this apparent cyst confirms arterial flow within the lumen, consistent with a pseudoaneurysm.

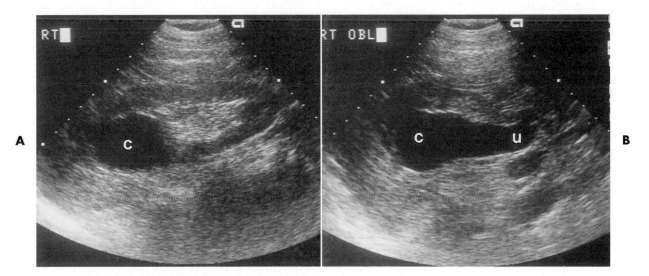

Fig. 4-21 Obstructed duplicated upper pole simulating a renal cyst. **A,** Longitudinal view of the right kidney demonstrates an anechoic mass with well-defined walls and increased through-transmission in the upper pole simulating a renal cyst *(c)*. **B,** Oblique view through the apparent cyst *(c)* shows continuity with a dilated upper pole ureter *(u)*, which could be traced inferiorly to the urinary bladder.

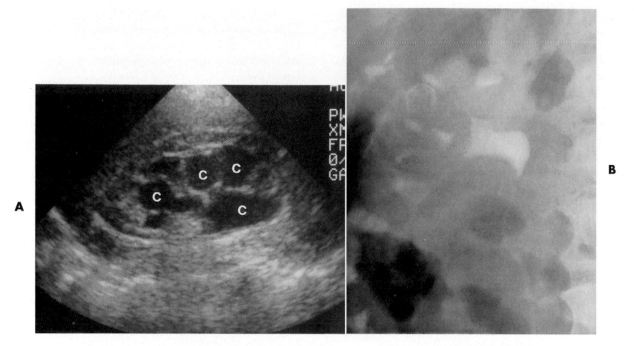

Fig. 4-22   Peripelvic cysts simulating hydronephrosis. **A,** Longitudinal view of the kidney demonstrates multiple centrally located adjacent cysts *(c)*. On no view was it possible to connect these cysts together or with a more central renal pelvis. Nevertheless, the possibility of hydronephrosis was entertained. **B,** Magnified view of the same kidney from an intravenous urogram demonstrates no evidence of hydronephrosis, but distortion and displacement of the renal collecting system and renal pelvis by the peripelvic cysts seen on sonography.

unlike hydronephrosis, they do not communicate with each other or with a dilated renal pelvis. In general it is more difficult to demonstrate the classic criteria of a cyst for peripelvic cysts than for cortically based cysts, possibly because of the renal sinus fat that surrounds the peripelvic cyst.

Autosomal Dominant Polycystic Disease

Autosomal dominant polycystic disease affects the kidney to a greater degree than any other organ. For this reason it is commonly referred to as *adult polycystic kidney disease.* However, the liver is involved in approximately 50% of the patients, the pancreas in 5% to 10% of the patients, and other organs in an even smaller percentage. Cerebral aneurysms occur in approximately 20% or more of the patients and are the cause of death in up to 10%. Despite the autosomal dominant pattern of inheritance, up to 50% of the patients have no family history of the disease. This is due to the variable expression of the disorder and the occurrence of spontaneous mutations. The disease generally becomes clinically apparent in the fourth or fifth decade, but it can cause renal failure in utero or may not become clinically evident until the eighth or ninth decade. The classic signs and symptoms of

the disease are hypertension and renal failure. Others include a palpable mass, abdominal pain, hematuria, renal infection, and polycythemia. It is unusual for affected patients to reach age 60 without renal failure.

The most conspicuous sonographic feature of autosomal dominant polycystic disease are multiple, variably sized cortical and medullary based cysts in the kidneys (Fig. 4-23). If cysts are not detected by age 30, it is very unlikely that the patient has the disease. The process affects the kidneys bilaterally in almost all instances, but it may be quite asymmetric. Early in the disease it is possible to detect normal renal parenchyma, but with time, the kidney becomes completely replaced by cysts and no normal parenchyma is identified. As the cysts become more numerous and enlarged, the kidney itself enlarges. Hemorrhage into the cyst is common and assumes the appearance of a solid-appearing mass (Fig. 4-24), a complex cyst, or a cyst with a fluid-debris level. Hemorrhagic cysts are much more common than neoplasms in patients with autosomal dominant polycystic disease, so a complex-appearing mass should be monitored rather than removed. Hemorrhagic cysts will resolve with time, but neoplasms will persist or enlarge, or both. The mass effect of the cyst can cause compression and partial obstruction of the collecting system. The resulting urinary stasis likely explains

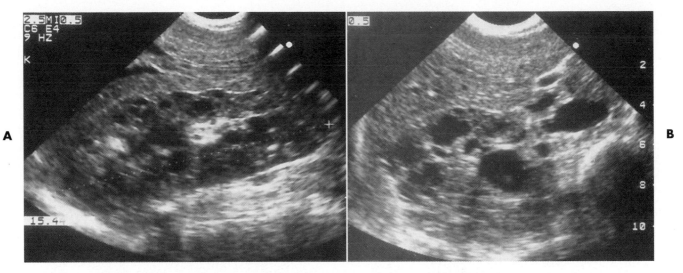

Fig. 4-23   Autosomal dominant polycystic disease. **A,** Longitudinal view of the right kidney demonstrates a distorted renal cortex secondary to the presence of multiple variously sized renal cysts. The kidney is also enlarged, measuring 15.44 cm in length. **B,** Transverse view of the same kidney also demonstrates distorted renal appearance due to the multiple variously sized renal cysts.

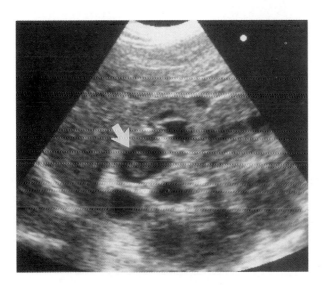

Fig. 4-24   Autosomal dominant polycystic disease with hemorrhagic cyst. Transverse view of the kidney demonstrates multiple cysts. One of the cysts *(arrow)* has a solid-appearing internal structure, which represented clotted blood.

the increase in stone formation in these patients. Detectable calcification may also be located in the walls of the cysts.

Acquired Cystic Disease

Multiple renal cysts develop in patients on long-term dialysis if they live long enough. This process is called *acquired cystic disease* and occurs in up to 90% of the patients who have been on dialysis for 3 years or more. Rarely it can occur in patients with chronic renal failure who are not receiving dialysis treatment. The etiology is unknown, although it seems likely that dialysis fails to clear renotropic substances that accumulate and promote

cyst formation. The cysts range in size and are usually seen in the setting of a small echogenic kidney. Occasionally the cysts become so numerous that the kidney is actually enlarged. Cyst hemorrhage is common and can result in complex-appearing masses. Follow-up scans obtained 2 to 3 months later should show clearing of hemorrhagic cysts, and thereby exclude the possibility of neoplasm. Major hemorrhage into the retroperitoneum is the most serious complication of acquired cystic disease.

Solid renal neoplasms occur in approximately 7% of patients with acquired cystic disease, but most are small (<3 cm) and exhibit benign behavior (Fig. 4-25). The risk of invasive or metastatic renal cell carcinoma is three to six times that for the general population, but it is not clear

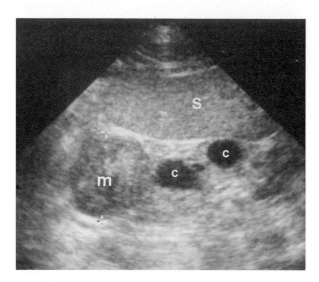

Fig. 4-25 Acquired cystic disease with associated renal cell carcinoma. Longitudinal view of the left kidney using the spleen *(s)* as a window shows two cysts *(c)* but little normal renal parenchyma, as is typical of acquired cystic disease. The solid mass *(m)* in the upper pole was proved surgically to be a renal cell carcinoma.

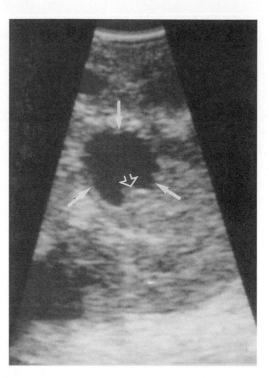

Fig. 4-26 von Hippel–Lindau disease. Intraoperative ultrasound scan demonstrates a small renal cyst *(arrows)* with slight wall irregularity. In addition, there is a solid mural nodule *(open arrow)*. This was resected and proved to be a renal cell carcinoma arising within the wall of a cyst.

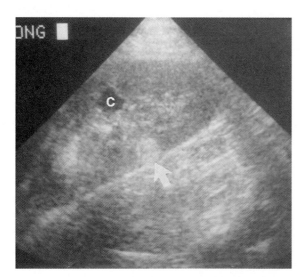

Fig. 4-27 von Hippel–Lindau disease. Longitudinal view of the lower pole of the left kidney demonstrates a small renal cyst *(c)*. Other renal cysts were also present bilaterally. Also seen is a small hyperechoic solid renal mass *(arrow)*. This was proved surgically to be a renal cell carcinoma.

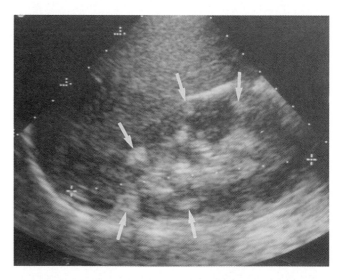

Fig. 4-28 Tuberous sclerosis with multiple angiomyolipomas. Longitudinal view of the right kidney demonstrates multiple small hyperechoic masses scattered throughout the renal cortex *(arrows)*. Similar findings were seen in the contralateral kidney and represent multiple angiomyolipomas in a patient with known tuberous sclerosis.

that sonographic screening for neoplasms is truly cost-effective.

von Hippel–Lindau Disease

von Hippel–Lindau disease is inherited as an autosomal dominant trait. It usually becomes clinically evident by the third to fifth decade of life. In affected patients neoplasms or cysts, or both, form in a variety of organs. Most commonly the presenting symptoms are those produced by cerebellar or spinal cord hemangioblastomas or retinal angiomas. Occasionally, abdominal manifestations arise before these other problems.

Approximately 30% to 70% of the patients with von Hippel–Lindau disease have renal involvement in the form of multiple renal cysts. Despite their multiplicity, the cysts do not cause renal failure or hypertension and do not generally cause renal enlargement. There is, however, an increased incidence of tumors developing in the cyst walls (Fig. 4-26). Therefore even benign-appearing cysts should be monitored.

Renal cell carcinoma occurs in up to 75% of the patients with von Hippel–Lindau disease whose kidneys are involved. These tumors are most often multiple and bilateral and they occur at a much earlier age than does the sporadic form of renal cell carcinoma. They may either develop in the walls of cysts or as separate solid tumors (Fig. 4-27).

The overall incidence of pheochromocytomas is increased in patients with von Hippel–Lindau disease and occurs in up to 20%, though most cases are isolated to certain kindreds in which the incidence is even higher. Pheochromocytomas produce symptoms less frequently in this population than do sporadic varieties, despite the fact that they are more frequently multiple and located in extraadrenal sites.

The pancreas is also affected, with an increased incidence of simple cysts that are generally asymptomatic. There is also, however, an increased risk of islet cell tumors and cystic pancreatic neoplasms in these patients.

Family members at risk of inheriting the disease should be evaluated in late adolescence for both genetic counseling and therapeutic reasons. The brain, spinal cord, orbit, and abdomen should all be imaged in some fashion to search for the major manifestations of the disease. CT is the best means of initially evaluating the abdomen, and is preferred for following the progress of the disease in affected patients. Sonography is valuable as a means of evaluating indeterminate masses in the kidney and pancreas. Intraoperative ultrasound examination is quite useful in patients undergoing partial nephrectomy for renal cell carcinoma (see Fig. 4-26). It is very sensitive for both detecting additional solid lesions and characterizing the nature of indeterminate lesions.

Tuberous Sclerosis

Tuberous sclerosis is another multisystem disorder that is associated with the formation of renal cysts and neoplasms. Its classic clinical triad consists of mental retardation, seizures, and cutaneous lesions. In addition to the renal abnormalities, central nervous system lesions (cortical hamartomas, periventricular subependymal glial nodules, subependymal giant cell astrocytomas, and retinal hamartomas), cardiovascular lesions (cardiac rhabdomyomas), pulmonary lesions (lymphangiomyomatosis), and skeletal lesions (sclerotic patches and cystic lesions) may develop.

The kidneys are affected in up to 95% of adult patients, with 50% to 80% having multiple bilateral angiomyolipomas. These are usually small (Fig. 4-28), but they can become quite large and eventually replace most of the renal parenchyma. Their sonographic characteristics are identical to those of sporadic isolated angiomyolipomas. Renal cysts occur in 20% to 40% of patients. Cysts are a more common renal manifestation in infancy and childhood.

RENAL MASSES

Renal Cell Carcinoma

Renal cell carcinoma constitutes approximately 90% of the primary renal malignancies and is the most common solid renal mass in adults. Each year 15,000 new cases are detected in the U.S. population. Risk factors include advanced age, smoking, von Hippel–Lindau disease, and long-term dialysis. The male-to-female ratio is approximately 2:1. Hematuria occurs in approximately 60% of the patients. Other signs and symptoms include weight loss, anemia, and fatigue. Paraneoplastic or hormonally related symptoms such as fever, erythrocytosis, and anorexia are also well described. One percent of the renal cell carcinomas are bilateral at presentation and 1% of the patients will be found to have a contralateral renal cell carcinoma on follow-up. Ten percent of the renal cell tumors are multifocal within the same kidney at the time of presentation. Histologically they can be described in terms of the cell type (clear cell or granular cytoplasm), cellular organization (papillary, tubular, or medullary), and cellular morphology (well differentiated, poorly differentiated, or undifferentiated).

Fifty percent of the renal cell carcinomas are hyperechoic compared with the normal adjacent renal parenchyma. Forty percent are only slightly more echogenic than the renal parenchyma (Fig. 4-29, *A*), but 12% are markedly hyperechoic to the point that they are similar to the echogenicity of the renal sinus (Fig. 4-29, *B*). This latter finding can potentially be confused with the appear-

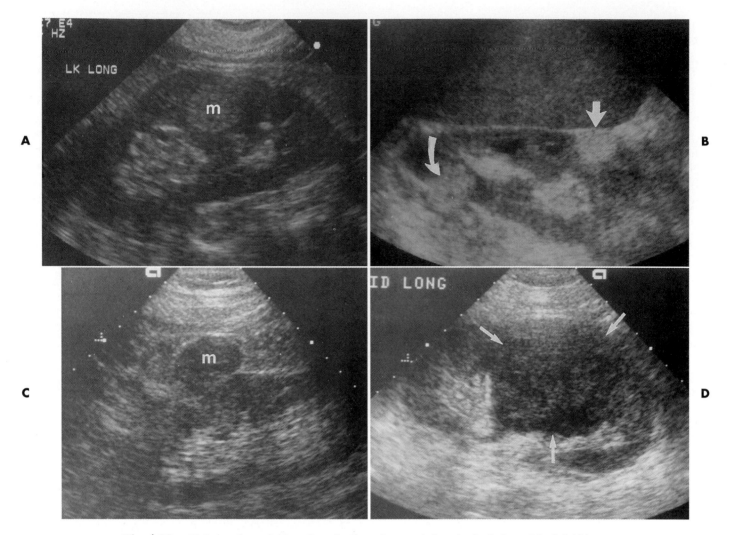

Fig. 4-29   Various echogenicities of renal cell carcinoma. **A,** Longitudinal view of the left kidney demonstrates a renal mass *(m)* that is more echogenic than the adjacent renal parenchyma but less echogenic than renal sinus fat. **B,** Longitudinal view of the left kidney demonstrates a markedly hyperechoic mass in the upper pole *(curved arrow)* that is similar in echogenicity to adjacent fatty tissues in the renal sinus and perinephric space. Biopsy findings proved this to be a renal cell carcinoma. In addition, another mass with a similar echogenicity is seen in the midpole *(straight arrow)*. This mass was found to contain fat on CT scans, which proves that it represents an angiomyolipoma. This case demonstrates the need to further evaluate hyperechoic renal masses. **C,** Longitudinal view of the left kidney demonstrates an isoechoic mass *(m)* projecting from the midpole of the kidney. Isoechoic masses such as these are seen when they are exophytic or distort the renal contour. **D,** Longitudinal view of the left kidney demonstrates a slightly hypoechoic renal mass *(arrows)* in the midpole.

ance of angiomyolipomas. Thirty percent of renal cell cancers are isoechoic to the renal parenchyma (Fig. 4-29, *C*) and 10% are hypoechoic (Fig. 4-29, *D*). Isoechoic tumors are detected when they are exophytic or when they distort the renal contour. Twenty to thirty percent of renal cell cancers contain identifiable calcification that may appear punctate, amorphous, or mottled (Fig. 4-30). It is very unusual for renal cell tumors to have peripheral rimlike calcification.

All solid renal masses in adults should be assumed to be renal cell carcinoma unless there is unequivocal evidence to contrary. For practical purposes the only way to prove that a solid mass is not a renal cancer is to document the presence of fat in the mass. This is best done with non–contrast-enhanced CT, using thin sections when necessary.

Although it is not uncommon for renal cell carcinoma to contain areas of necrosis or hemorrhage, predomi-

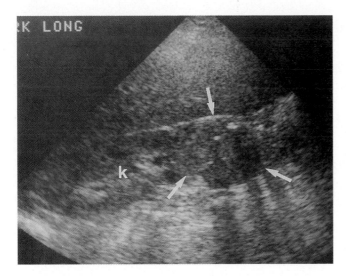

Fig. 4-30   Renal cell carcinoma with calcification. Longitudinal view of the right kidney *(k)* shows a slightly hyperechoic mass in the lower pole *(arrows).* Several bright shadowing foci are seen within the mass, consistent with calcification.

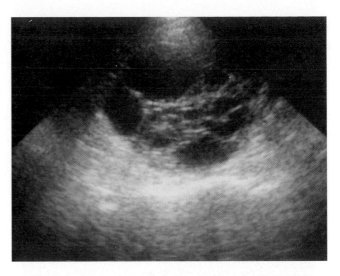

Fig. 4-31   Cystic renal cell carcinoma. Transverse view of the lower pole of the left kidney demonstrates a predominantly cystic but very complex mass containing thick septations and solid components. This was confirmed surgically to represent a cystic renal cell carcinoma.

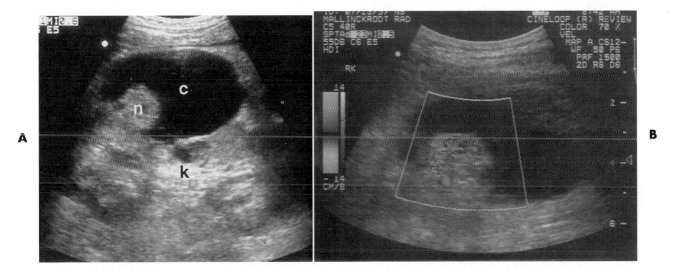

Fig. 4-32   Cystic renal cell carcinoma. **A,** Longitudinal view of the right kidney *(k)* demonstrates a large midpole cyst *(c).* A solid hyperechoic nodule *(n)* is seen adjacent to the cyst wall. The gray-scale appearance is consistent either with a tumor nodule growing in the cyst wall or a blood clot adjacent to the cyst wall. **B,** Longitudinal Doppler view of the same cyst demonstrates vascularity within the mural nodule. This rules out the possibility of an adherent blood clot. Renal cell carcinoma arising from the wall of the cyst was confirmed surgically in this patient (see color insert, Plate 17).

nantly cystic renal cell carcinomas are unusual and account for less than 5% of the total cases. They may assume the form of a cyst with multiple thick septations (Fig. 4-31), a thick or irregular wall or a cyst with a solid mural nodule (Fig. 4-32 [for Fig. 4-32, *B,* see also color insert, Plate 17]). In general the likelihood of malignancy increases with an increasing number and thickness of sep-

tations and with increased wall thickness or irregularity. Detection of blood flow within the substance of a complex cystic lesion should be taken as strong evidence of malignancy, as hemorrhage or otherwise complicated cysts should not contain internal vascularity (Fig. 4-32, *B*). Predominantly cystic lesions that are well seen sonographically and have features worrisome for malignancy should be considered potentially malignant regardless of the findings from other imaging studies such as CT or magnetic resonance imaging. On the other hand, the findings yielded by these other studies are very useful in excluding malignancy in lesions that are truly indeterminate or are poorly visualized sonographically.

In addition to detecting and characterizing tumors, sonography is also an excellent means of identifying inferior vena cava invasion (Fig. 4-33), and to a lesser degree renal vein invasion (Fig. 4-34). This not only provides useful staging information but also helps in planning surgical treatment (Fig. 4-35).

Occasionally, normal renal parenchyma can assume a masslike appearance and be confused with a renal cell carcinoma (Box 4-2). Hypertrophied columns of Bertin are common variants that appear as isoechoic cortical tissue protruding centrally into the renal sinus fat in the interpolar region. In some cases a renal pyramid is also seen (Fig. 4-36). Residual functioning renal parenchyma can also be confused with a solid mass when it is surrounded

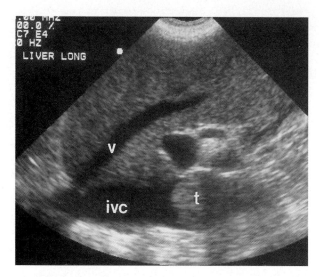

Fig. 4-33 Renal cell carcinoma with tumor thrombus involving the inferior vena cava. Longitudinal view of the liver and inferior vena cava *(ivc)* demonstrates a solid tumor thrombus *(t)* within the subhepatic portion of the inferior vena cava. The relationship of the tumor thrombus to the hepatic veins *(v)* is well demonstrated. This type of thrombus can be effectively removed during an isolated abdominal procedure.

Box 4-2 Differential Diagnosis of Solid Renal Masses

Renal cell carcinoma
Angiomyolipoma
Transitional cell carcinoma
Oncocytoma
Lymphoma
Metastasis
Juxtaglomerular cell tumor
Column of Bertin
Focal parenchymal hypertrophy
Focal pyelonephritis

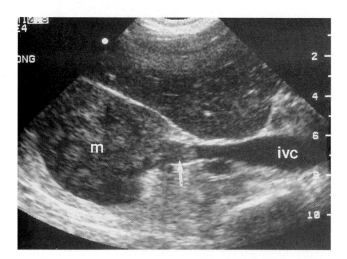

Fig. 4-34 Renal cell carcinoma with renal vein invasion. Transverse view of the right kidney demonstrates a mass *(m)* replacing most of the renal parenchyma. A tumor thrombus is seen extending into the right renal vein *(arrow)*. The inferior vena cava *(ivc)* is free of tumor.

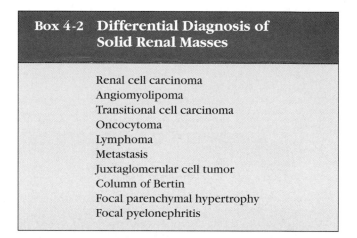

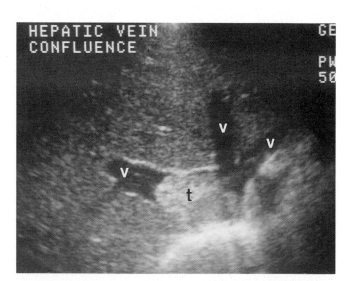

Fig. 4-35 Renal cell carcinoma with tumor thrombus in the intrahepatic portion of the inferior vena cava. Transverse view of the liver at the level of the hepatic vein confluence demonstrates solid tumor thrombus *(t)* extending to this level. All three hepatic veins *(v)* are patent. The tumor thrombus in this case extended above the diaphragm, and both an abdominal and thoracic procedure were required to remove it.

by atrophic renal parenchyma (Fig. 4-37). In most cases knowledge of these potential pitfalls is enough to allow for a confident diagnosis to be made. When there is doubt, renal scintigraphy is a useful tool for further evaluation (Fig. 4-37, *B*).

Angiomyolipoma

As the name implies, angiomyolipomas are tumors composed of vessels, muscles, and fat. They are the most common benign renal neoplasm and are second only to renal cell carcinoma in overall frequency. They have no malignant potential and rarely cause symptoms. Bleeding is the only serious complication, but it is rare. These tumors occur most frequently in middle-aged women.

The classic sonographic appearance, seen approximately 80% of the time, is a homogeneous, well-defined cortical mass that is as echogenic as renal fat (Fig. 4-38). Although this is very suggestive of angiomyolipoma, approximately 12% of renal cell carcinomas can also have this appearance (see Fig. 4-29, *B*). One distinguishing feature, seen in approximately 20% to 30% of the angiomyolipomas, is some degree of acoustic shadowing (Fig. 4-39). In the absence of calcification, this is not a feature of renal cell carcinoma. The shadowing associated with angiomyolipomas is probably due to attenuation of the sound beam by fatty elements of the tumor. Another useful feature to look for, as it is rare in angiomyolipomas but seen occasionally in hyperechoic renal cell cancers, are cystic components (Fig. 4-40). Hyperechoic renal masses that show no partial shadowing require further evaluation. If an an-

giomyolipoma is 1 cm or larger, thin-section CT should be able to detect fat. Volume-averaging effects make it difficult to detect fat in angiomyolipomas less than 1 cm, and it is reasonable to monitor such masses with periodic ultrasound studies at 6- to 12-month intervals. If fat is not de-

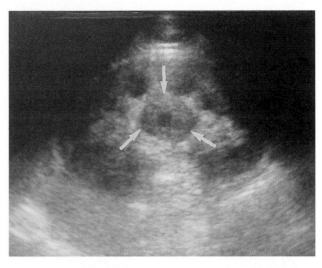

Fig. 4-36   Hypertrophied column of Bertin. Longitudinal view of the kidney obtained from a lateral approach demonstrates a rounded masslike structure protruding into the renal sinus *(arrows)*. This is isoechoic to the renal cortex, which is typical of a hypertrophied column of Bertin. In addition, a central hypoechoic region is also seen, consistent with a renal pyramid. Identification of renal pyramids such as this is unusual within columns of Bertin, but these are a very characteristic finding when seen.

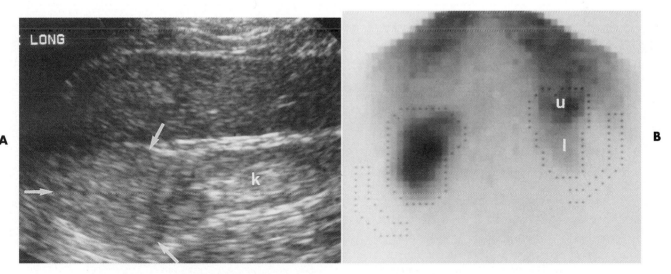

Fig. 4-37   Focal cortical hypertrophy simulating a renal mass. **A,** Longitudinal view of the right kidney demonstrates an isoechoic masslike lesion *(arrows)* arising from the upper pole of the kidney *(k)*. However, the kidney itself is atrophic and echogenic. The possibility of focal cortical hypertrophy in the upper pole was suggested, and renal scintigraphy was recommended for further evaluation. **B,** Posterior view of the renal scan demonstrates atrophy of the right lower pole *(l)* with decreased function. The upper pole *(u)* is enlarged and more normally functioning.

tected in a lesion larger than 1 cm, this indicates a renal cell carcinoma and it should be handled accordingly.

Transitional Cell Carcinoma

Transitional cell carcinoma accounts for more than 90% of the urothelium-based tumors. Most of the rest are squamous cell carcinomas. Transitional cell carcinoma of the intrarenal collecting system is five to ten times less frequent than renal cell carcinoma. Multiplicity and bilaterality are relatively common, and up to 10% of the patients have bilateral metachronous or synchronous primary tumors. The presence of a transitional cell carcinoma indicates that the entire urothelium is at risk, with the bladder at greatest risk followed by the renal pelvis and the ureter.

Most transitional cell carcinomas are too small to be detected by sonography. Intravenous urography and retrograde pyelography are the main methods used to detect this carcinoma in the kidney and ureter. Sonography can detect bulky upper urinary tract lesions but is much less sensitive in the detection of smaller lesions. The sonographic appearance of transitional cell carcinoma includes an intraluminal polypoid mass (Fig. 4-41, *A*), thickening of the urothelium (Fig. 4-41, *B*), and an otherwise nonspecific solid mass centered in the renal sinus (Fig. 4-41, *C*). Infiltration of the adjacent renal parenchyma can occur, and in such cases it is not possible to distinguish transitional cell carcinoma from renal cell carcinoma. Besides transitional cell carcinoma, other lesions that appear as intraluminal masses in the collecting system include blood clots, fungus balls, fibroepithelial polyps, malacoplakia, and calculi. Sonography is good at distinguishing stones in the collecting system from the other lesions, but cannot distinguish among the other lesions.

One potential pitfall is mistaking prominent renal papillae as a filling defect in the calices. This can occur in the setting of hydronephrosis (Fig. 4-42). The primary

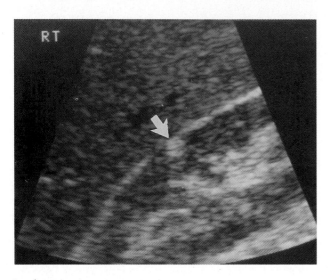

Fig. 4-38 Small angiomyolipoma. Magnified longitudinal view of the right kidney demonstrates a 5-mm, round hyperechoic mass along the anterior cortex *(arrow)*. The echogenicity of the mass is similar to that of renal sinus fat. This is consistent with an angiomyolipoma.

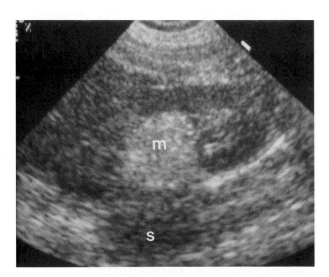

Fig. 4-39 Angiomyolipoma with partial acoustic shadowing. Longitudinal view of the left kidney demonstrates a hyperechoic mass *(m)* in the central portion of the kidney. There is partial acoustic shadowing *(s)* posterior to this lesion. Shadowing independent of calcification is seen only in angiomyolipomas.

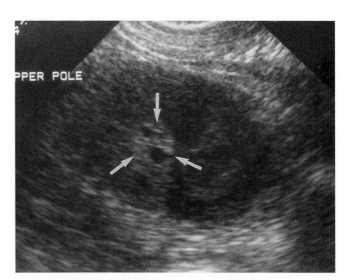

Fig. 4-40 Hyperechoic renal cell carcinoma with cystic components. Magnified transverse view of the upper pole of the kidney demonstrates a hyperechoic mass *(arrows)*. Two small cysts are seen within the substance of this mass, which was confirmed surgically to be a small renal cell carcinoma.

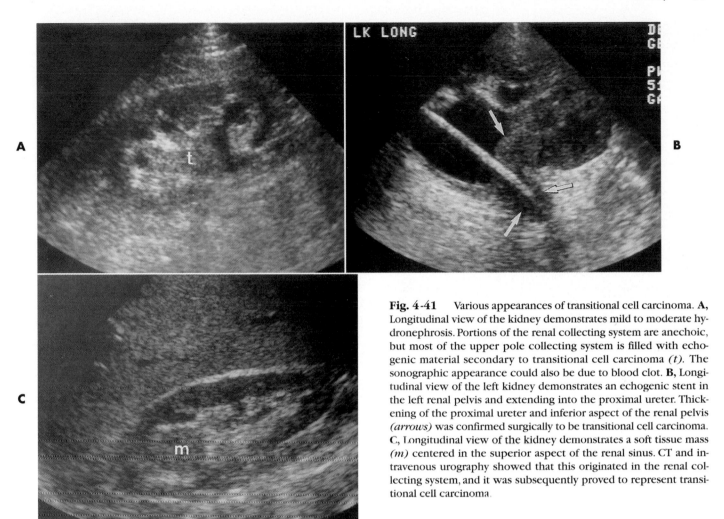

Fig. 4-41   Various appearances of transitional cell carcinoma. **A,** Longitudinal view of the kidney demonstrates mild to moderate hydronephrosis. Portions of the renal collecting system are anechoic, but most of the upper pole collecting system is filled with echogenic material secondary to transitional cell carcinoma *(t)*. The sonographic appearance could also be due to blood clot. **B,** Longitudinal view of the left kidney demonstrates an echogenic stent in the left renal pelvis and extending into the proximal ureter. Thickening of the proximal ureter and inferior aspect of the renal pelvis *(arrows)* was confirmed surgically to be transitional cell carcinoma. **C,** Longitudinal view of the kidney demonstrates a soft tissue mass *(m)* centered in the superior aspect of the renal sinus. CT and intravenous urography showed that this originated in the renal collecting system, and it was subsequently proved to represent transitional cell carcinoma.

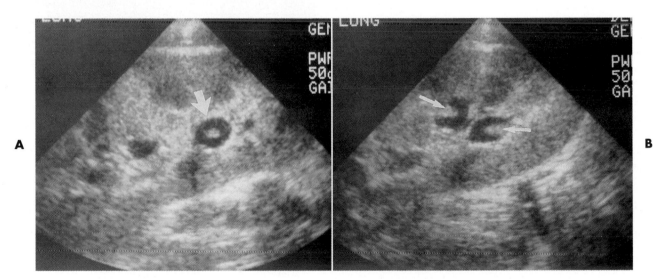

Fig. 4-42   Renal papillae simulating filling defects within the calices. **A,** Longitudinal view of the kidney demonstrates a distended renal calix *(arrow)*. An echogenic filling defect is seen in the middle of this calix. **B,** Oblique view through the same region demonstrates two distended calices, both of which contain prominent papillary tips *(arrows)* protruding into the caliceal lumen. These should not be confused with tumors, blood clots, or other abnormal filling defects.

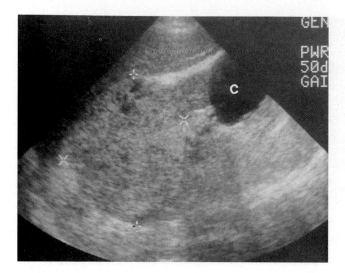

Fig. 4-43 Oncocytoma. Longitudinal view of the left kidney demonstrates a cyst *(c)* in the lower pole and a slightly hyperechoic and mildly nonhomogeneous solid mass in the upper pole *(cursors)*. The most likely diagnosis in this case is renal cell carcinoma, but this was proved pathologically to be an oncocytoma.

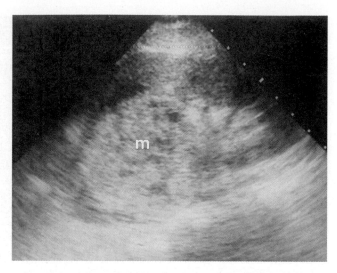

Fig. 4-44 Juxtaglomerular cell tumor. Longitudinal view of the left kidney demonstrates a hyperechoic nonhomogeneous mass *(m)* in the midpole to upper pole. This was a young patient with hypertension. A nephrectomy was performed and the mass was proved pathologically to be a juxtaglomerular cell tumor.

distinguishing feature of papillae is that they appear in all the calices, but other lesions such as transitional cell carcinoma appear only in one or a very limited number of calices.

Oncocytoma

Oncocytomas are a type of renal adenoma with large epithelial cells rich in granular eosinophilic cytoplasm. They account for approximately 5% of renal neoplasms. Their sonographic appearance is generally nonspecific (Fig. 4-43). A stellate hypoechoic central scar is a characteristic of oncocytomas, but it is not present in many lesions. Unfortunately, renal cell carcinomas can also have a central scar, so these lesions almost always must be surgically removed to determine if they are malignant. A partial nephrectomy occasionally can be substituted for radical nephrectomy if the preoperative diagnosis of oncocytoma is confirmed by frozen section findings.

Juxtaglomerular Cell Tumor

A juxtaglomerular cell tumor is a rare benign tumor that is also called a *reninoma* because it secretes renin. It occurs most often in young women, and patients typically initially exhibit signs and symptoms relating to severe hypertension. The sonographic characteristics of this lesion are variable, but they are most often hyperechoic (Fig. 4-44).

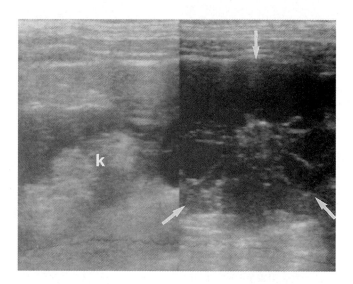

Fig. 4-45 Multilocular cystic nephroma. Longitudinal composite view of the left kidney *(k)* shows a large complex cystic mass *(arrows)* arising from the lower pole. Multiple septations are present. This sonographic appearance is consistent with either a cystic renal cell carcinoma or multilocular cystic nephroma. The latter was confirmed surgically.

Multilocular Cystic Nephroma

Multilocular cystic nephroma goes by a variety of names, and this has resulted in a certain amount of confusion about its characteristics. Most experts consider it to

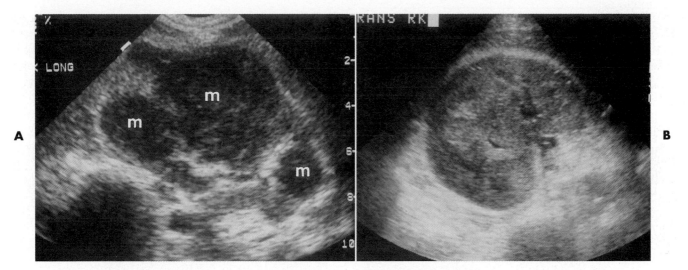

Fig. 4-46   Sonographic appearances of renal lymphoma. **A,** Longitudinal view of the left kidney demonstrates multiple hypoechoic masses *(m)* consistent with renal lymphoma in this patient with widely disseminated lymphoma elsewhere in the body. **B,** Transverse view of the right kidney in another patient demonstrates loss of normal renal echoarchitecture and swelling. This represented diffuse infiltration secondary to lymphoma.

be a benign renal neoplasm composed of multiple large, noncommunicating cystic spaces. It is an encapsulated lesion that contains no differentiated renal tissue and tends to afflict young boys and older women. Although a multilocular cystic mass is a characteristic sonographic appearance of multilocular cystic nephroma (Fig. 4-45), this finding is also exhibited by cystic renal cell carcinoma (see Fig. 4-31) and by cystic Wilms' tumors occurring in childhood (Box 4-3). For practical purposes, multilocular cystic-appearing masses must be removed surgically because of the possibility of malignancy. If the preoperative diagnosis of multilocular cystic nephroma is suggested radiographically, a partial nephrectomy may be performed rather than a radical nephrectomy.

Lymphoma

The vast majority of renal lymphomas occur in the setting of more widespread disease and are caused by hematogenous spread or by direct invasion from adjacent involved lymph nodes. It is most often bilateral and occurs much more commonly in patients with non-Hodgkins lymphomas than in those with Hodgkins disease. Renal involvement is found at autopsy in up to one third of the patients with lymphoma, but is not noted this frequently on imaging studies due to the small size of the nodules or occasionally to the diffusely infiltrating nature of the process. It is unusual for renal lymphoma to produce symptoms.

Box 4-3   Differential Diagnosis of Complex Cystic Masses

Hemorrhagic cyst
Infected cyst
Multiseptated cyst
Abscess
Hematoma
Cystic renal cell carcinoma
Multilocular cystic nephroma

The most common sonographic finding is multiple bilateral hypoechoic masses (Fig. 4-46, *A*). Unifocal, unilateral disease occurs but is unusual. Diffuse infiltration and smooth renal enlargement may also be seen (Fig. 4-46, *B*). One unusual but fairly characteristic pattern of growth is for the tumor to grow into the perinephric space so that it surrounds and encapsulates the kidney (Fig. 4-47).

Because lymphoma is a very homogeneous tumor with a monotonous histologic composition and little stromal tissue, there are very few internal reflectors. This can result in an anechoic appearance that simulates cysts in the kidney (Fig. 4-48) and elsewhere in the body. In most cases the lack of acoustic enhancement deep to the mass provides a clue that it is solid and not cystic. In rare instances a certain amount of acoustic enhancement can be seen despite the solid nature of the tumor.

Metastatic Disease

Metastatic disease to the kidney generally occurs in the setting of known metastases elsewhere in the body. The most common primary tumors that spread to the kidneys are lung, colon, breast, stomach, prostate, and pancreas carcinoma and melanoma. The incidence of renal metastases in cancer patients is as high as 20% in autopsy series. Detection with imaging studies such as ultrasound and CT has increased, and this has created a previously

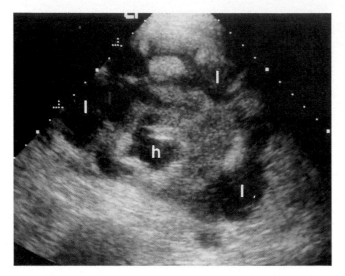

Fig. 4-47 Perirenal lymphoma. Transverse view of the left kidney demonstrates dilatation of the renal collecting system secondary to hydronephrosis *(h)*. In addition, there is extensive lymphomatous infiltration *(l)* surrounding the kidney. The sonographic appearance could also be secondary to perinephric fluid collections, but CT confirmed that this was solid tissue and showed other findings typical of extensive retroperitoneal lymphoma.

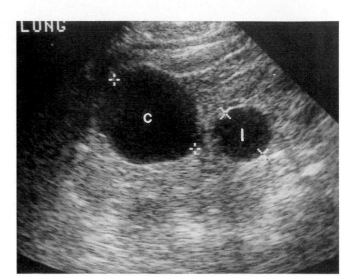

Fig. 4-48 Renal lymphoma simulating a renal cyst. Longitudinal view of the right kidney demonstrates two exophytic masses. The larger of the two represents a simple renal cyst *(c)*. The smaller one was shown to be solid on CT, and represents a lymphomatous mass *(l)* that has very similar sonographic characteristics to the adjacent cyst.

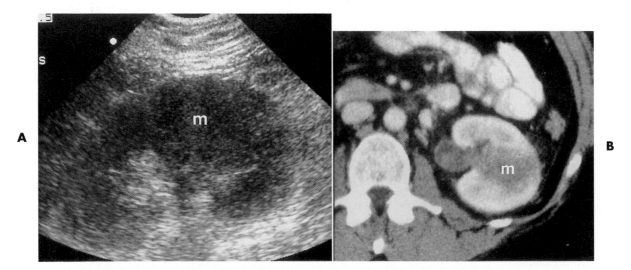

Fig. 4-49 Renal metastasis. **A,** Longitudinal view of the left kidney in a patient with squamous cell carcinoma of the head and neck demonstrates a slightly hypoechoic, poorly defined mass *(m)* in the midpole. **B,** Contrast-enhanced CT scan demonstrates a poorly defined region of decreased enhancement *(m)* in the midpole region. Percutaneous biopsy performed under ultrasound guidance yielded findings confirming squamous cell carcinoma.

unrecognized problem because it raises the question whether a new solid renal mass in a cancer patient is a renal metastasis or a primary renal cell carcinoma. It was originally thought that renal cell carcinoma was more likely by a ratio of 5 to 1. However, more recent data suggest just the opposite. The increased likelihood of a renal mass being metastatic disease in the setting of a known extrarenal carcinoma probably reflects the improved detection of smaller renal lesions with current state-of-the-art ultrasound and CT equipment. The sonographic characteristics of renal cell carcinoma and renal metastases overlap, and the diagnosis depends on biopsy findings (Fig. 4-49).

INFECTION

Pyelonephritis, as the name implies, refers to infection of the renal collecting system and renal parenchyma. It usually stems from the retrograde migration of bacteria up the ureter and into the kidney. This classically is associated with the reflux of urine from the bladder to the ureter, but in most adults and some children there is no evidence of vesicoureteral reflux and presumably bacteria ascend the ureter against the persistent antegrade flow of urine. Hematogenous transmission of infection to the kidneys also occurs generally in the setting of intravenous drug abuse or endocarditis, and occasionally originates from some other extraurinary site of infection.

As bacteria travel from the collecting system into the tubules, leukocytes migrate from the interstitium into the

affected tubules. The subsequent release of enzymes destroys tubular integrity and allows the bacteria to enter the interstitium. Casts of inflammatory cells in the tubules produce a focal microscopic obstruction that, when coupled with focal vasoconstriction, causes focal regions of decreased function and ischemia. Generally the process extends from the tip of the papilla to the periphery of the cortex and involves the kidney in a patchy manner. The demarcation between infected and normal parenchyma is usually sharp.

Clinically, patients present with flank pain, fever, leukocytosis, pyuria, bacteremia, and positive urine culture results. Uncomplicated cases of pyelonephritis treated with appropriate antibiotic therapy usually resolve within 72 hours. Chronic scarring may occur, particularly when there is associated vesicoureteral reflux. Severe forms of pyelonephritis may persist beyond 72 hours, and these are the patients who benefit from imaging studies such as ultrasound examination.

The ultrasound findings in most cases of uncomplicated pyelonephritis are normal. Occasionally the involvement of the collecting system produces urothelial thickening that is detectable on sonograms (Fig. 4-50). In the proper clinical setting this is a reliable sign of infection. However, it is nonspecific and can also be seen in association with calculi, after bouts of obstruction, with transitional cell carcinoma, and with renal transplant rejection and ischemia (Box 4-4).

More severe cases of pyelonephritis can alter the echogenicity of the renal parenchyma, producing areas of both increased and decreased echogenicity (Fig. 4-51). The overall renal size may increase or there may be focal areas of enlargement that can simulate a mass. In the past, focal masslike areas of renal inflammation have been referred to by a variety of names, including *acute focal bacterial nephritis, lobar nephronia, lobar nephritis,* and *preabscess.* These terms have appeared in the radiology literature, but are not recognized by most urologists or other clinicians and should probably be abandoned.

The primary role of sonography in evaluating patients with pyelonephritis is to exclude complications. These include hydronephrosis, renal abscess, or perinephric abscess. Renal abscesses appear as complex cystic masses

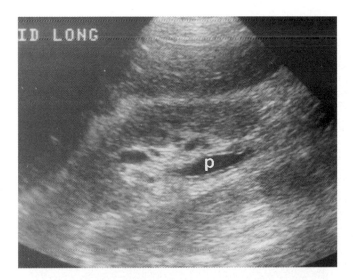

Fig. 4-50   Pyelonephritis with urothelial thickening. Longitudinal view of the kidney demonstrates thickening of the walls of the renal pelvis *(p)*. The walls of the collecting system should just appear as a thin bright stripe. In this case the mucosa appears bright and there is an external hypoechoic layer representing submucosal edema.

Box 4-4   Causes of Urothelial Thickening
Pyelonephritis
Ureteral calculi
Relieved obstruction
Transplant rejection
Transplant ischemia
Transitional cell carcinoma

(Fig. 4-52). The treatment of large and moderately sized renal abscesses generally consists of percutaneous drainage or occasionally surgery. However, small abscesses can be effectively treated with antibiotics. In such cases sonography can be valuable for monitoring the process of abscess healing and resolution (Fig. 4-53). Perinephric abscesses appear as complex perinephric fluid collec-

tions. Many patients with uncomplicated urinary obstruction have small anechoic perinephric fluid collections, and these should not be misinterpreted as abscesses. In addition, the perinephric fat can occasionally appear very hypoechoic and simulate perinephric fluid. This tends to occur in patients with renal atrophy and is bilateral in the vast majority of cases (Fig. 4-54). Identification of stones is also important, as they may form the nidus for persistent infection.

One unusual type of renal infection is xanthogranulomatous pyelonephritis. This is a chronic inflammatory process usually associated with long-standing urinary obstruction. The pathologic response to the infection is the formation of yellow inflammatory masses composed of lipid-laden macrophages. The most common organisms are *Proteus mirabilis* and *Escherichia coli.* More than 75% of patients will have a stone and most will be of the staghorn variety. The classic radiologic triad is a stone, renal enlargement, and lack of function. Sonographic findings include a shadowing stone in the renal pelvis together with dilated renal calices, perinephric fluid collection, and inflammatory tissue (Fig. 4-55).

Emphysematous pyelonephritis is a serious renal infection that typically occurs in diabetic women. It results from the formation of gas in the renal parenchyma stemming from high tissue glucose concentrations, vascular disease, and a necrotizing infection with a gas-forming organism such as *E. coli.* Nephrectomy is usually required for treatment. Emphysematous pyelitis is a less serious condition in which gas forms in the collecting system but not the renal parenchyma. The sonographic diagnosis de-

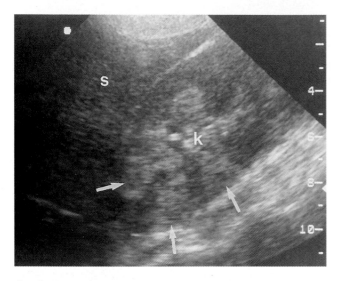

Fig. 4-51   Pyelonephritis. Longitudinal view of the left kidney *(k)* and spleen *(s)* demonstrates multiple wedge-shaped areas of increased echogenicity *(arrows)* extending from the central aspect of the kidney to the peripheral cortical rim. This reflects focal areas of pyelonephritis.

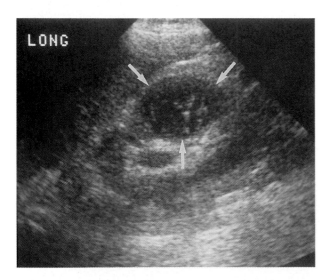

Fig. 4-52   Renal abscess. Longitudinal view of the kidney demonstrates a poorly marginated hypoechoic and anechoic mass *(arrows)* in the midpole. This was drained percutaneously and proved to be a renal abscess.

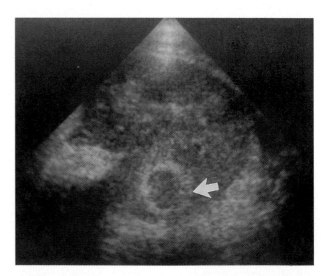

Fig. 4-53   Resolving renal abscess. Transverse view of the kidney demonstrates an isoechoic mass with a hyperechoic peripheral rim *(arrow)*. CT had previously shown a small renal abscess in this patient. She had been treated with antibiotics and was improving clinically at the time the ultrasound study was obtained.

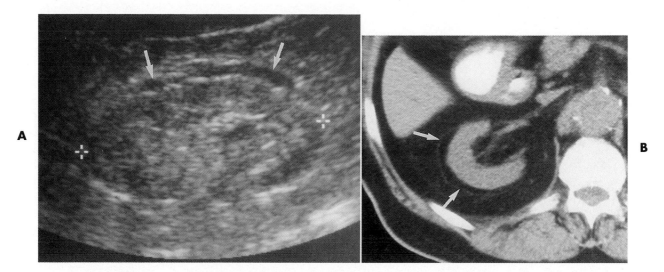

Fig. 4-54 Hypoechoic perinephric fat. **A,** Longitudinal view of the kidney *(cursors)* demonstrates a thin hypoechoic strip of material *(arrows)* anteriorly. This could be confused with perinephric fluid collections. However, a similar appearance was seen in the contralateral kidney, and this can occasionally be produced by perinephric fat. **B,** CT scan from the same patient demonstrates prominent perinephric fat within Gerota's fascia *(arrows)* but no evidence of perinephric fluid.

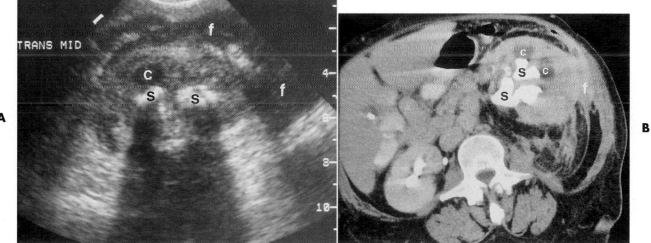

Fig. 4-55 Xanthogranulomatous pyelonephritis. **A,** Transverse view of the left kidney demonstrates shadowing stones *(s)* and a focally dilated renal calix *(c)*. In addition, there is hypoechoic perinephric tissue and fluid *(f)* surrounding the kidney. This appearance could be secondary to pyonephrosis and perinephric abscess or urinoma. However, xanthogranulomatous pyelonephritis should also be a consideration when these sonographic findings are encountered. **B,** CT scan from the same patient demonstrates an enlarged left kidney with a staghorn calculus *(s)* filling the renal pelvis and several infundibula. Two dilated calices *(c)* are seen and correspond to the dilated calix seen on sonography. In addition, a perinephric inflammatory process *(f)* is also present. Perinephric fluid was seen at other levels.

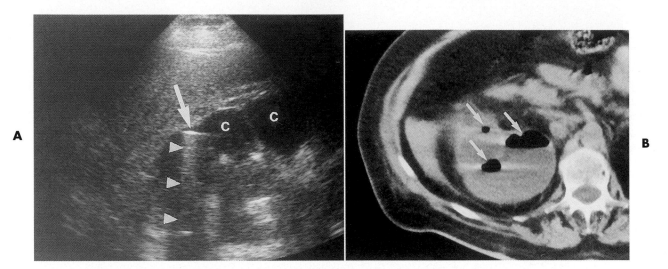

Fig. 4-56   Emphysematous pyelitis. **A,** Longitudinal view of the right kidney demonstrates little normal renal parenchyma and several markedly distended calices *(c).* A very bright reflector *(arrow)* is seen in the nondependent portion of one of these calices. The dirty posterior shadowing *(arrowheads)* suggests that this represents gas. **B,** Non–contrast-enhanced CT scan confirms multiple pockets of gas *(arrows)* within a markedly distended renal collecting system. No normal renal cortical tissue is identified.

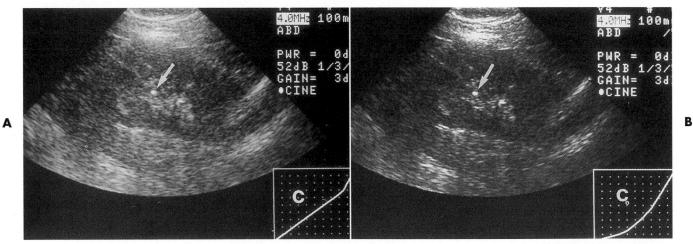

Fig. 4-57   Renal calculus. **A,** Longitudinal view of the kidney obtained using a standard postprocessing curve *(c)* demonstrates a bright reflector in the renal sinus *(arrow)* suspicious for a renal calculus. **B,** Identical view displayed with a different postprocessing curve *(c)* that accentuates differences in hyperechoic regions demonstrates decreased echogenicity of the renal sinus fat but a persistently bright reflection from the suspected stone. This increased contrast difference between the stone and the renal sinus fat allows for a more confident diagnosis of nephrolithiasis to be rendered in this case.

pends on the detection of bright reflectors with dirty shadows or ring-down artifacts (Fig. 4-56). It may be difficult to determine whether the gas is confined to the collecting system or involves the parenchyma. CT is helpful for making this distinction.

RENAL CALCULI

Urolithiasis is an extremely common problem, affecting 12% of the population by age 70. It affects men up to three times more often than women and is more common in whites than other racial groups. Risk factors include low fluid intake and diets high in animal protein. The latter factor may explain why stones are more common in affluent patients. Conditions that promote urinary stasis also predispose to the formation of stones; these include ureteropelvic junction obstruction, autosomal dominant polycystic disease, caliceal diverticula, tubular ectasia, and horseshoe kidneys. Stones can have a variety of compositions. Calcium-containing stones are most common (80% to 85%), and the calcium usually occurs in the form of calcium oxalate or calcium phosphate. Most calcium stones arise idiopathically in the absence of associated metabolic abnormalities. Uric acid stones account for approximately 5% to 10% of all calculi. They are commonly thought to be associated with gout, but only 25% of patients with gout have uric acid stones and only 25% of patients with uric acid stones have gout. Other conditions that predispose to the formation of uric acid stones include Crohn's disease and other small bowel abnormalities, as well as

myeloproliferative diseases that are being treated with chemotherapy. Pure uric acid stones are radiolucent. Cistine stones account for less than 5% of all renal calculi and are related to cistinuria, a rare metabolic disorder. They are relatively radiolucent. Approximately 10% of stones are associated with infection by urea-splitting bacteria such as *Proteus, Pseudomonas, Staphylococcus aureus,* and *Klebsiella.* These stones are composed of struvite (magnesium-ammonium-phosphate) or apatite (calcium phosphate), or both. They often develop into staghorn calculi.

As with gallstones, the sonographic appearance of renal stones depends on their size and not their composition. Stones of sufficient size produce an echogenic focus in the renal sinus with an associated acoustic shadow (see Fig. 4-16). Smaller stones may just appear as an echogenic focus without a shadow. These stones present a diagnostic problem, as the renal sinus itself is echogenic. Efforts should therefore be made to identify a shadow by using a high-frequency transducer that is focused at the appropriate depth and by viewing the stone from a variety of locations. If a shadow is not identified, it is possible to alter the postprocessing curve so that the gray-scale difference between the stones and renal sinus is accentuated (Fig. 4-57). This may increase diagnostic confidence that a stone is present even though there is no shadow. Another pitfall in the sonographic diagnosis of stones is refractive shadowing arising from the renal sinus. This occurs as the result of differences in the speed of sound between soft tissue, fluid, and fat. Because all three of these substances are present in the renal sinus, refractive shadowing is common. Therefore a shadow should not be taken as evidence of a stone unless it is arising from a definite echogenic focus. False-positive results can also occur in patients with renal arterial calcification, and should be suspected if the echogenic focus is elongated (Fig. 4-58).

The sensitivity of ultrasound studies in detecting renal calculi is superior to that of abdominal radiography and is only slightly less than that of the combined use of abdominal radiography and nephrotomography. However, sonography is not as accurate in determining stone size and in general should not be used to monitor the status of renal stones. Its sensitivity for detecting ureteral calculi is not as good as that for detecting renal calculi. Although stones can be seen in the proximal ureter and midureter (Fig. 4-59), they are considerably easier to detect in the distal ureter. Because most ureteral stones impact in the distal ureter near the ureterovesical junction, scans looking at the distal ureter through a moderately distended urinary bladder should always be obtained in someone suspected of passing a stone. In women, transvaginal sonography can visualize distal ureteral stones extremely well (Fig. 4-60). The exact role of sonography in evaluating patients with renal colic and suspected ureteral calculi is somewhat controversial. The combined use of gray-

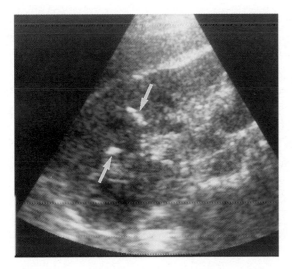

Fig. 4-58 Arterial calcification simulating nephrolithiasis. Longitudinal view of the kidney demonstrates two hyperechoic foci *(arrows)* in the upper pole of the kidney. The more anteriorly situated focus is linear and exhibits an appearance typical of arterial calcification. The posteriorly situated focus was also shown to be linear on other views.

scale sonography to detect the morphologic changes of hydronephrosis, perinephric fluid collections, and ureteral calculi, along with Doppler analysis of intrarenal resistive indexes and ureteral jets to estimate the degree of obstruction, is relatively effective and can provide adequate information to guide management in most cases. Nevertheless intravenous urography is easier to perform and probably more reliable, and should continue to be used in most patients, with sonography reserved for pregnant patients or those with allergies to contrast agents.

NEPHROCALCINOSIS

Nephrocalcinosis refers to calcification in the medullary pyramids rather than the renal collecting system. It is caused by a number of processes, but the three most

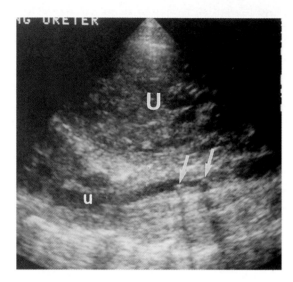

Fig. 4-59   Ureteral calculi. Longitudinal view of the ureter *(u)* in a pregnant patient demonstrates two small shadowing stones *(arrows)* in the midportion of the ureter. There is associated thickening of the ureteral wall, which is frequently seen with ureteral stones. In this case the lateral aspect of the uterus *(U)* was used as an acoustic window to visualize the midureter.

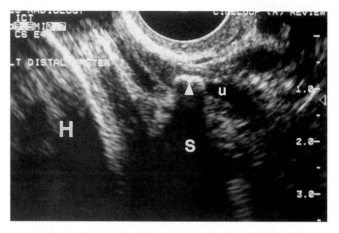

Fig. 4-60   Distal ureteral calculus seen from a transvaginal approach. Longitudinal view of the distal left ureter in another pregnant patient during her third trimester demonstrates a stone *(arrowhead)* with a well-defined posterior acoustic shadow *(s)*. A short segment of the distal left ureter *(u)* is seen leading to the stone. The fetal head *(H)* is seen superiorly.

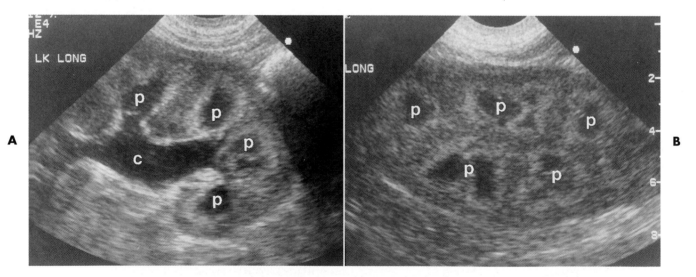

Fig. 4-61   Mild nephrocalcinosis. **A,** Longitudinal view of the left kidney from a lateral approach demonstrates mild dilatation of the collecting system *(c)*. The pyramids *(p)* are surrounded by a rim of increased echogenicity. **B,** Longitudinal view from an anterior approach shows multiple renal pyramids *(p)* with a peripheral hyperechoic rim. These should not be confused for dilated calices. This represents the earliest form of nephrocalcinosis and is seen sonographically before calcification is identifiable radiographically.

common ones are medullary sponge kidney (tubular ectasia), renal tubular acidosis, and hyperparathyroidism. In its early stages it causes increased medullary echogenicity at the periphery of the pyramids (Fig. 4-61) and eventually involves the entire pyramids (Fig. 4-62). With progressive calcification, shadowing begins to develop (Fig. 4-63).

Sonography is unusually sensitive in detecting this condition, and the sonographic changes predate any visible calcification on plain films and are generally more dramatic than the abnormalities seen on CT.

Parenchymal calcifications can be seen in the setting of conditions other than nephrocalcinosis. Multiple small punctate, cortical and medullary calcifications are occasionally seen in patients with the acquired immunodeficiency syndrome. These are usually due to disseminated *Pneumocystis* infection in patients being treated with aerosolized pentamidine (Fig. 4-64). Diffuse cortical calcification is rare and usually secondary to cortical necrosis and hyperoxaluria (Fig. 4-65).

RENAL PARENCHYMAL DISEASE

A large number of diseases affect the renal parenchyma and produce renal failure. The term "medical renal disease" is often used but is not truly appropriate because some of these patients will benefit from a surgical procedure, i.e., renal transplantation.

Increased parenchymal echogenicity is often seen in the setting of renal parenchymal disease. The degree of echogenicity correlates loosely with the severity of but not the type of histopathologic change. Therefore, although an underlying parenchymal abnormality is sug-

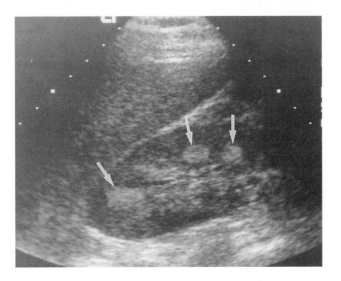

Fig. 4-62   Moderate nephrocalcinosis. Longitudinal view of the right kidney demonstrates several diffusely and uniformly hyperechoic medullary pyramids *(arrows).* This is the typical and classic appearance of nephrocalcinosis. No calcifications were apparent on this patient's abdominal radiographs, but the pyramids were slightly increased in attenuation on CT scans.

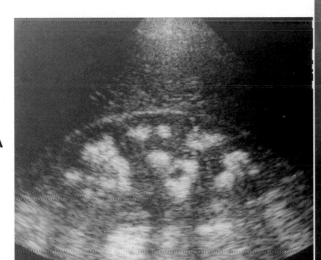

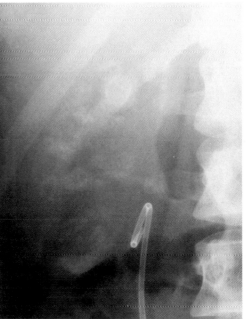

A

B

Fig. 4-63   Advanced nephrocalcinosis. **A,** Longitudinal view of the right kidney demonstrates renal pyramids that are diffusely increased in echogenicity. Most of these pyramids cast acoustic shadows. This is a finding typical of more advanced nephrocalcinosis. This view was obtained by angling the transducer just lateral to the renal sinus fat. **B,** Magnified view of an abdominal radiograph shows the radiographic findings typical of nephrocalcinosis involving all of the medullary pyramids.

gested by increased echogenicity, the cause cannot be determined (Fig. 4-66). Echogenicity is considered increased when the right kidney is more echogenic than the liver (Fig. 4-66) or when the echogenicity of the left kidney is equal or greater than that of the spleen. If images are not available to show the relative echogenicity of the kidneys and the liver or spleen, echogenicity is considered increased if the pyramids are unusually hypoechoic with respect to the renal cortex (Fig. 4-67). The main role of sonography in these patients is to exclude urinary obstruction and determine renal size. Renal biopsy of normal or enlarged kidneys may then be done to determine the underlying histologic diagnosis. Small kidneys usually indicate a chronic process with end-stage changes, and biopsy is often not indicated and the findings yielded are not helpful.

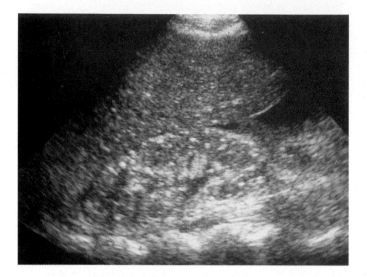

Fig. 4-64   Disseminated *Pneumocystis* infection of the kidney. Longitudinal view of the right kidney in a patient with AIDS demonstrates multiple small nonshadowing hyperechoic reflectors scattered throughout the kidney. Less numerous and less obvious findings are seen in the adjacent liver. The sonographic appearance is consistent with disseminated *Pneumocystis* infection in a patient with *Pneumocystis* pneumonia being treated with aerosolized pentamidine.

RENAL TRAUMA

Sonography is generally not recommended as a means of evaluating renal trauma, as contrast-enhanced CT is superior for detecting and determining the extent of posttraumatic abnormalities. Nevertheless, certain posttraumatic lesions are encountered frequently during the sonographic evaluations of other problems, so their sonographic appearance should be recognized. This is particularly true of renal hematomas. Acute hematomas appear echogenic or even hyperechoic, and can therefore mimic a solid renal mass (Fig. 4-68). With time, the echogenic clot retracts or lyses and the lesion assumes a more heterogeneous appearance, with echogenic, hypoechoic, and anechoic areas (Fig. 4-69). Eventually hematomas become completely anechoic. Subcapsular hematomas are particularly difficult to detect in the acute stages because they

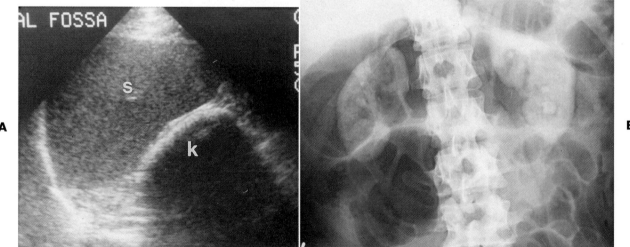

Fig. 4-65   Diffuse cortical calcification secondary to oxalosis. **A,** Longitudinal view of the left upper quadrant shows the spleen *(s)* and a shadowing hyperechoic structure in the expected location of the left kidney *(k)*. No normal renal tissue was identified elsewhere in the left upper quadrant. A similar shadowing structure was seen in the right upper quadrant. **B,** Abdominal radiograph of this patient obtained without any intravenous contrast material demonstrates diffuse cortical calcification of both kidneys as well as several discrete stones in the left kidney.

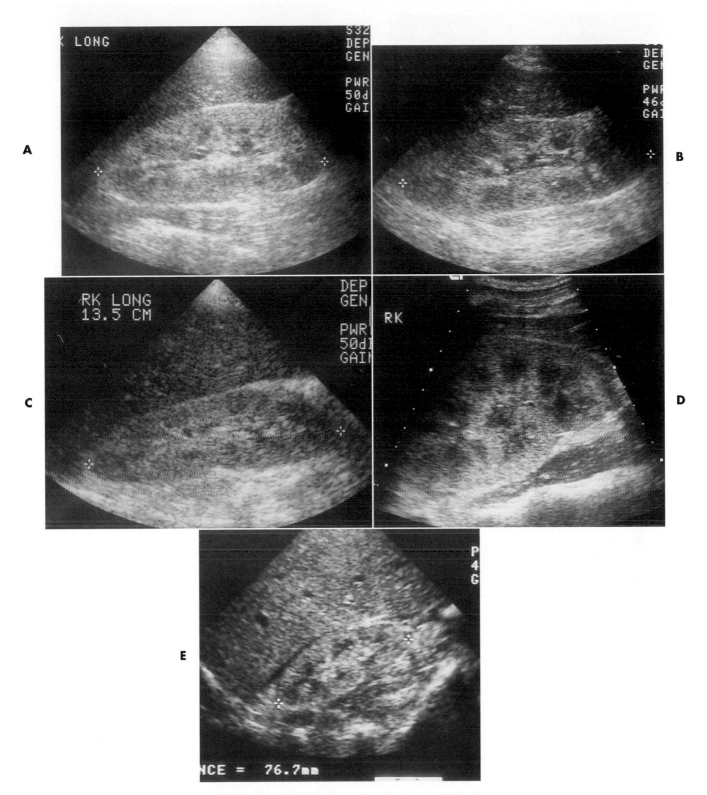

Fig. 4-66   Various renal parenchymal diseases manifesting as increased renal echogenicity. **A,** Acute glomerulonephritis. **B,** AIDS nephropathy. **C,** Amyloidosis. **D,** Heroin-induced nephropathy. **E,** End-stage hypertensive glomerulosclerosis. In all of these cases the kidneys are unusually echogenic versus the overlying liver. Percutaneous renal biopsy findings may be beneficial in the cases where the kidney is enlarged **(A, B, C,** and **D).**

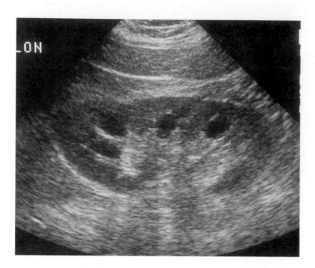

Fig. 4-67 Renal parenchymal disease. Longitudinal view of the left kidney obtained without adjacent splenic tissue for comparison. When liver or spleen are not imaged in the same view with the kidney, it is difficult to gauge renal echogenicity. In this case the renal pyramids are unusually hypoechoic. This does not reflect disease in the pyramids but rather disease in the renal cortex producing increased cortical echogenicity, and thus apparent decreased echogenicity of the pyramids.

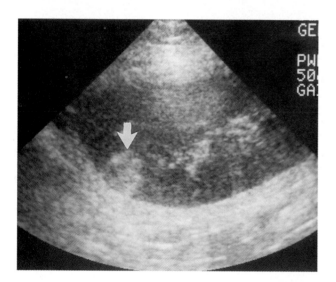

Fig. 4-68 Acute hematoma. Transverse view of the kidney demonstrates an echogenic cortical mass *(arrow)*. This was identified after a percutaneous renal biopsy and is an appearance consistent with acute cortical hematoma.

may be almost isoechoic to the kidney and they tend to distort the kidney so that the renal margins are difficult to discern (Fig. 4-70, *A*). When a subcapsular hematoma is suspected, follow-up scans can be very useful in documenting its presence (Fig. 4-70, *B*).

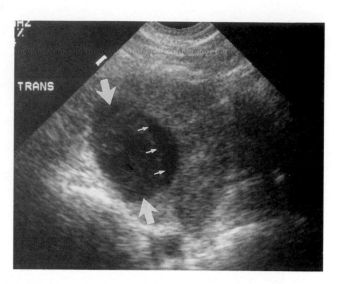

Fig. 4-69 Subacute hematoma. Transverse view of the kidney demonstrates a hypoechoic mass *(large arrows)*. More echogenic material is seen in the dependent aspect of the mass forming a fluid-debris level *(small arrows)*. This is consistent with a liquefying hematoma.

VASCULAR DISEASE

Normal Anatomic Characteristics and Hemodynamic Function

The kidneys are usually supplied by a single main renal artery that arises from the aorta just inferior to the origin of the superior mesenteric artery (Fig. 4-71 [see also color insert, Plate 18]). Accessory renal arteries occur in approximately 20% of the kidneys. The main renal arteries travel posterior to the corresponding vein and the right renal artery passes posterior to the inferior vena cava as well (Fig. 4-72 [see also color insert, Plate 19]). The renal arteries branch into multiple segmental arteries that travel from the renal hilum into the renal sinus. The segmental arteries subsequently branch into the interlobar arteries and arcuate arteries. The normal intrarenal arteries are rarely visible on gray-scale sonography but are routinely visible with color-Doppler analysis. The amount of detectable flow depends on the depth of the kidney and the type of Doppler technique and transducer used. With modern equipment using power-Doppler techniques, blood flow should be seen throughout the cortex to the capsular margin of the kidney in most superficial native kidneys and most renal transplants (Fig. 4-73). The difference in perfusion between the cortical tissues and the medullary pyramids is generally well displayed on color- and power-Doppler studies (Fig. 4-73, *B*). The pulsed-Doppler waveforms from the renal arteries show findings typical of a parenchymal organ with a low resistance pattern.

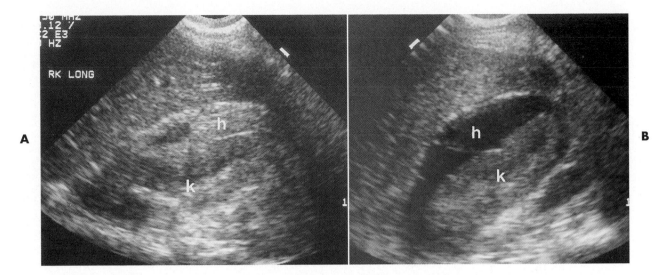

Fig. 4-70   Subcapsular hematoma. **A,** Longitudinal view of the right kidney *(k)* demonstrates a hyperechoic hematoma *(h)* anteriorly. Compression caused by this subcapsular hematoma causes marked distortion in the normal renal shape and morphology. **B,** Follow-up scan obtained 1 week later demonstrates near-complete liquefaction of the subcapsular hematoma *(h)*. The right kidney *(k)* remains somewhat distorted by the mass effect of the hematoma.

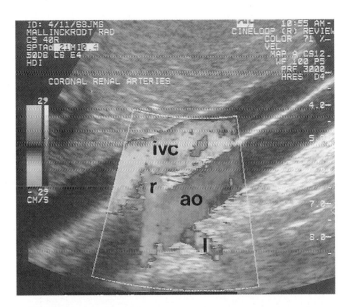

Fig. 4-71   Coronal view of the main renal arteries. Doppler image obtained from the right lateral aspect of the abdomen demonstrates the inferior vena cava *(ivc)* and the aorta *(ao)* traveling side-by-side. The origins of the right *(r)* and left *(l)* renal arteries are well demonstrated. Views of this clarity are difficult to obtain in most patients (see color insert, Plate 18).

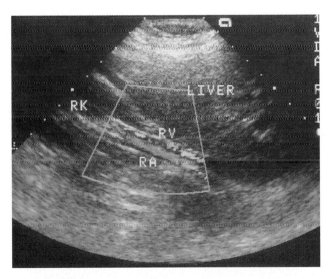

Fig. 4-72   Normal relationship of the renal vein and renal artery. Transverse Doppler view of the right upper quadrant shows the liver and right kidney *(RK)* as well as the main renal artery *(RA)* and renal vein *(RV)*. The renal artery travels posterior to the renal vein (see color insert, Plate 19).

The right renal vein is short and relatively constant in location and appearance. It is generally easily seen on both gray-scale and color-Doppler scans (Fig. 4-73 [see also color insert, Plate 20]). The left renal vein is approximately three times longer than the right and is consider-

ably more difficult to see along its entire length. It travels between the superior mesenteric artery and aorta in most subjects (Fig. 4-74). A retroaortic or circumaortic left renal vein is present in 3% and 17% of individuals, respectively (Fig. 4-75). The segment of left renal vein immediately to

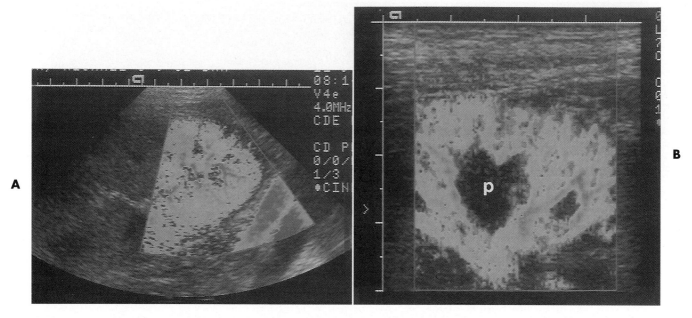

Fig. 4-73   Normal renal parenchymal blood flow. **A,** Longitudinal power-Doppler view of a renal transplant demonstrates normal perfusion throughout the renal parenchyma with vessels extending from the renal sinus to the capsular surface. The iliac vessels are seen on the inferior aspect of the transplant (see color insert, Plate 19). **B,** Transverse view of the superficial aspect of a renal transplant obtained with a 7.0-MHz linear array using power-Doppler imaging demonstrates a hypoechoic renal pyramid *(p)* exhibiting little detectable flow. There is readily detectable flow and multiple discrete identifiable vessels throughout the remainder of the cortex extending to the capsular surface of the transplant. This image graphically displays the difference in perfusion between the cortical tissue and the renal pyramids (see color insert, Plate 20).

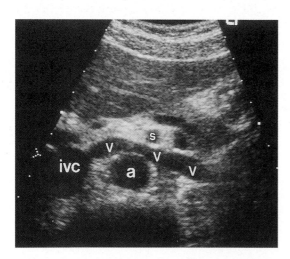

Fig. 4-74   Normal left renal vein. Transverse view of the upper abdomen demonstrates the aorta *(a)* and inferior vena cava *(ivc).* The left renal vein *(v)* travels between the aorta and superior mesenteric artery *(s)* before entering the vena cava.

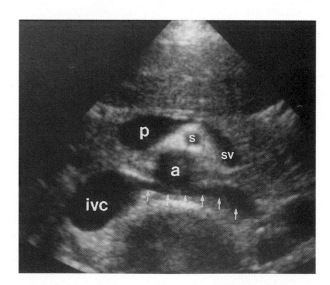

Fig. 4-75   Retroaortic left renal vein. Transverse view of the upper abdomen demonstrates an anomalous course of the left renal vein *(arrows)* behind the aorta *(a)* instead of between the aorta and the superior mesenteric artery *(s).* Also seen on this view are the inferior vena cava *(ivc),* portal vein *(p),* and splenic vein *(sv).*

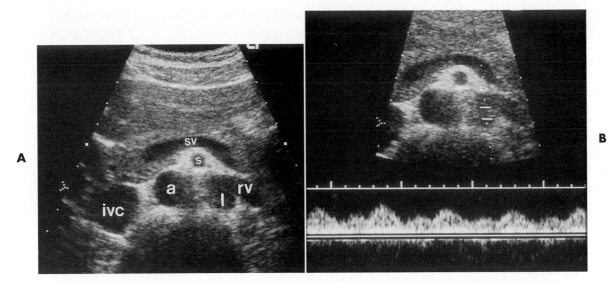

Fig. 4-76   Pseudomass produced by a prominent lumbar vein draining into the left renal vein. **A,** Transverse view of the upper abdomen demonstrates a prominent left renal vein *(rv)* as well as a prominent lumbar vein *(l)* that communicates with the renal vein. Also seen on this view are the aorta *(a)*, inferior vena cava *(ivc)*, superior mesenteric artery *(s)*, and splenic vein *(sv)*. **B,** Pulsed-Doppler waveform analysis of the pseudomass confirms venous flow directed toward the left renal vein.

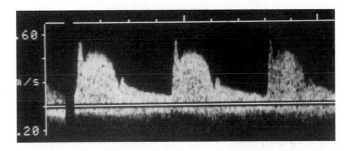

Fig. 4-77   Normal intrarenal arterial signal. Pulsed-Doppler waveform analysis of a normal intrarenal artery demonstrates a rapid systolic upstroke, which reflects normal early systolic acceleration. This should be contrasted with the slowed systolic acceleration seen secondary to renal artery stenosis in Fig. 4-78, *B*.

the left of the superior mesenteric artery and aorta is often relatively dilated and can simulate a periaortic mass. In addition, it may communicate with prominent lumbar veins that can also simulate a mass. Doppler techniques are effective in determining the nature of questionable lesions in this area (Fig. 4-76).

Renal Artery Stenosis

Hypertension affects up to 60 million people in the United States and is one of the most common diseases in the world. Three fourths of the cases are mild and controlled by diet and diuretics. Almost all of these patients have primary hypertension. Severe hypertension that is poorly controlled or controlled only with multiple medications is more likely to be caused by a secondary factor such as renal artery stenosis. Although renal artery stenosis accounts for only 5% of the total number of patients with hypertension, it is potentially curable. Therefore developing a noninvasive screening test that can identify patients with renal artery stenosis is important.

Doppler ultrasound examination is among the methods used to detect renal artery stenosis. Initial efforts were focused on the evaluation of the main renal arteries. Criteria advocated as useful for establishing renal artery stenosis included a peak renal artery velocity exceeding 100 cm/sec and a peak renal artery velocity-to-peak aortic velocity ratio of greater than 3.5. Results of initial studies evaluating these criteria were encouraging, but the results of subsequent studies have been quite disappointing. A number of difficulties with this approach exist. Perhaps the most significant is accessory renal arteries that may be stenotic and the cause of hypertension, but which are extremely difficult to detect and analyze with Doppler techniques. In addition, it often takes more than an hour to evaluate the main renal arteries.

More recently attention has been focused on the evaluation of the intrarenal arteries. Normally, intrarenal arterial waveforms show an extremely rapid early systolic acceleration that is reflected by an almost vertical early systolic upstroke (Fig. 4-77). Study findings have suggested that a marked stenosis of the main renal artery produces a slowed systolic upstroke and a delayed time to peak systole. This dampening of the distal arterial waveforms has been referred to as the *parvus-tardus effect.* In severe cases this effect is detectable subjectively (Fig. 4-78). In less severe cases, the effect can be detected quantitatively by measuring the early systolic acceleration. Values less than 300 cm/sec² are considered abnormal. The potential advantage of this method is that the intrarenal arteries are more easily and reproducibly imaged than the main renal arteries. Nevertheless, early studies evaluating this method have produced widely disparate results. Therefore it is difficult to make recommendations about this technique, other than to say that, in its current state of development, Doppler ultrasound evaluation of renal artery stenosis in native kidneys is only practical at facilities with highly trained personnel who have abundant experience.

Renal Vein Thrombosis

Bland renal vein thrombosis is a relatively rare event. It occurs in the settings of dehydration, coagulopathy, trauma, and certain renal parenchymal processes that cause the nephrotic syndrome such as membranous glomerulonephritis. It may also occur secondary to inferior vena cava thrombosis or ovarian vein thrombosis.

The imaging characteristics of renal vein thrombosis depend on the rapidity of onset and the completeness of occlusion. Totally occlusive acute renal vein thrombosis

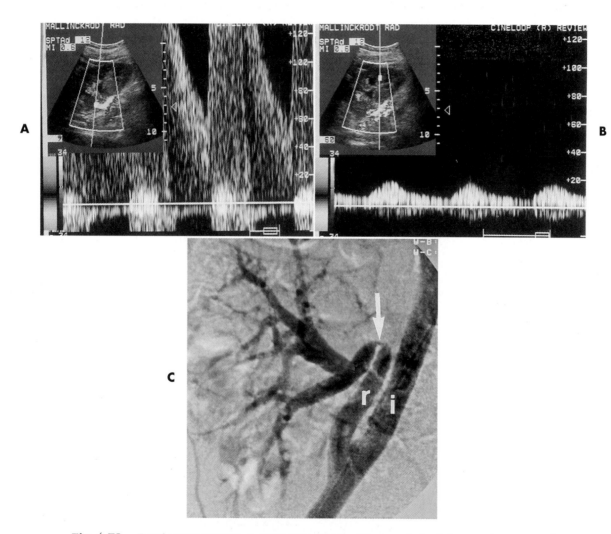

Fig. 4-78   Renal artery stenosis. **A,** Pulsed-Doppler waveform analysis of the superior aspect of the main renal artery in a renal transplant patient demonstrates markedly elevated flow velocities with extensive aliasing so that the systolic peak cannot be displayed on the highest possible Doppler scale. **B,** Pulsed-Doppler waveform analysis of an intrarenal artery demonstrates a dampened waveform with markedly decreased systolic acceleration. **C,** Angiogram demonstrates the renal artery *(r)* arising from the adjacent iliac artery *(i).* The renal artery is redundant, and this has produced a kink and resulting high-grade stenosis *(arrow)* in the superior aspect of the artery.

produces an enlarged kidney on gray-scale images. A defect in the renal vein may or may not be detected on gray-scale images, but no venous flow will be identified on pulsed- or color-Doppler studies. The venous outflow obstruction will result in diminished arterial inflow and cause a high-resistance arterial waveform. In some instances pandiastolic flow reversal occurs, and this should always raise a suspicion of underlying renal vein thrombosis (Fig. 4-79).

In most cases of native renal vein thrombosis, the clot develops slowly, which allows venous collaterals to form. In these cases the kidney remains normal in size and intrarenal arterial and venous flow is maintained. Because of this, the detection of venous flow in the kidney or renal hilum does not exclude renal vein thrombosis (Fig. 4-80 [for Fig. 4-80, *A*, see also color insert, Plate 20]). In fact, detection of venous flow in the vein itself does not exclude thrombosis because the thrombus is frequently nonocclusive (Fig. 4-81 [for Fig. 4-81, *C*, see also color insert, Plate 22]). The only way to establish the diagnosis in such cases is to identify the thrombus as a filling defect in the renal vein on either gray-scale or color-Doppler studies. In most cases it is possible to detect or exclude renal vein thrombosis on the right side because the vein is short and the liver provides an adequate acoustic win-

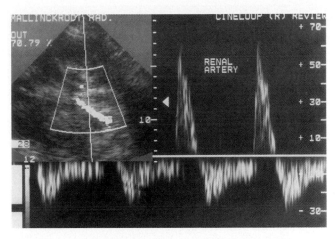

Fig. 4-79   Renal vein thrombosis. Pulsed-Doppler waveform analysis of the main renal artery of a renal transplant patient demonstrates markedly increased resistance to flow with reversal of flow throughout diastole. This type of pattern indicates that essentially all of the flow entering the kidney through the arterial system during systole rebounds out of the kidney through the arterial system during diastole. This reflects a lack of any effective renal perfusion. Renal vein thrombosis should always be considered whenever this type of arterial signal is encountered, and a careful evaluation of the renal vein should be performed. In this case, no renal venous flow was identified and thrombosis of the renal vein was subsequently confirmed surgically.

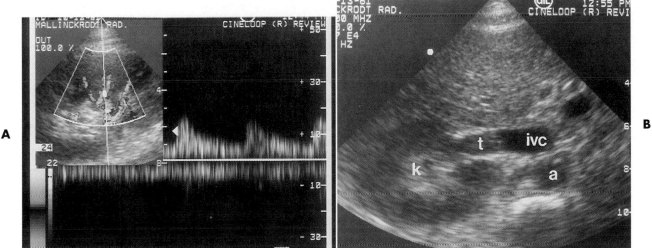

Fig. 4-80   Right renal vein thrombosis. **A,** Longitudinal Doppler image and pulsed-Doppler waveform analysis of the right kidney demonstrates normal-appearing intrarenal blood flow on the color-Doppler study and normal arterial and venous waveforms on pulsed-Doppler analysis (see color insert, Plate 21). **B,** Transverse gray-scale image of the right kidney *(k)* shows hypoechoic thrombus *(t)* in the right renal vein that is readily distinguished from the anechoic lumen of the inferior vena cava *(ivc)*. Also seen is the aorta *(a)*.   *Continued.*

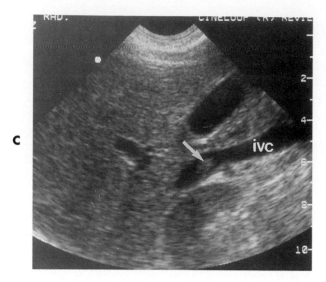

C

Fig. 4-80, cont'd.   **C,** Longitudinal view of the inferior vena cava *(ivc)* demonstrates that the right renal vein thrombus *(arrow)* is just barely extending into the lumen of the inferior vena cava. This case demonstrates why detection of normal arterial and venous flow within the renal parenchyma or hilum should not be used as a means of excluding renal vein thrombosis.

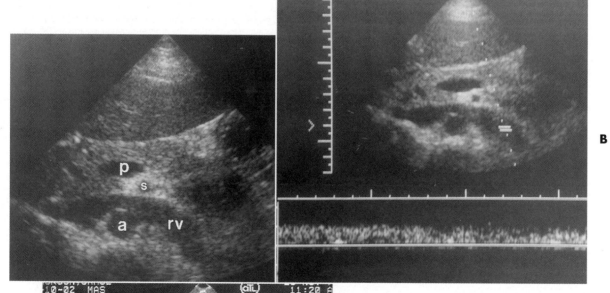

Fig. 4-81   Left renal vein thrombosis. **A,** Transverse gray-scale image of the upper abdomen demonstrates a prominent left renal vein *(rv).* Low-level echoes are seen within the lumen of the left renal vein, but similar echoes are seen within the lumen of the aorta *(a).* Also seen are the portal vein *(p)* and superior mesenteric artery *(s).* **B,** Transverse gray-scale image and pulsed-Doppler waveform analysis of the left renal vein confirm venous flow. This should not be mistaken as conclusive evidence against renal vein thrombosis. **C,** Transverse Doppler image confirms that there is some residual flow *(f)* within the posterior aspect of the left renal vein, but that there is nonocclusive thrombus *(t)* in the anterior aspect of the renal vein. This indicates the difficulty in relying just on gray-scale imaging and pulsed-Doppler waveform analysis for the diagnosis of renal vein thrombosis (see color insert, Plate 22).

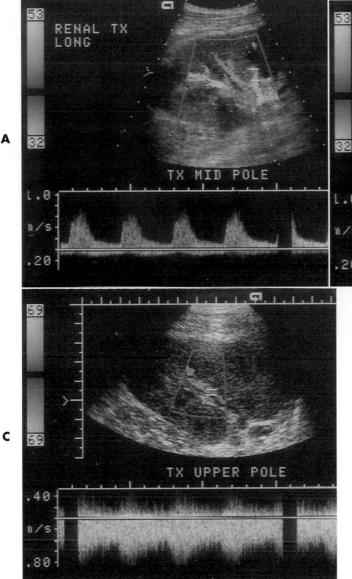

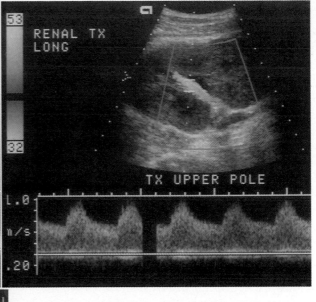

Fig. 4-82   Renal arteriovenous fistula (see color insert, Plate 23). **A,** Longitudinal Doppler image from the midpole of a renal transplant demonstrates several segmental vessels extending from the renal sinus into the renal parenchyma. The pulsed-Doppler sample volume is placed on a vessel in the midpole and the corresponding Doppler waveform shows slightly diminished diastolic flow but an otherwise normal appearance. **B,** Similar Doppler view, but in this case the pulsed-Doppler sample volume is placed on an artery leading to the upper pole. The corresponding waveform demonstrates increased flow velocities versus those in the vessel sampled in **A.** In addition, the diastolic flow is increased dramatically. These findings indicate a decreased resistance to flow in this vessel and are very suggestive of an arteriovenous fistula. **C,** Doppler view of the upper pole of the transplant demonstrates the pulsed-Doppler sample volume positioned over an upper pole draining vein. The waveform from this vein is arterialized. This provides conclusive evidence of an arteriovenous communication in the upper pole.

dow. As mentioned earlier, evaluation of the left renal vein is considerably more difficult because the vein is long and segments are often obscured by overlying bowel gas. Unless the entire left renal vein is seen and appears normal on both gray-scale and color-Doppler images, renal vein thrombosis cannot be excluded.

Arteriovenous Fistulas

Arteriovenous fistulas generally result from penetrating trauma, with percutaneous renal biopsy the most common cause. Small fistulas are probably fairly common after biopsies but they rarely cause symptoms. Occasion-ally, persistent bleeding occurs with or without associated urinary obstruction. Large fistulas are a rare cause of high-output cardiac failure, renal ischemia, and renal hypertension. Most renal arteriovenous fistulas resolve spontaneously without treatment.

In most cases there are no morphologic changes detectable with gray-scale sonography. Hemodynamic changes that can be detected with Doppler analysis include increased velocity and decreased resistance to flow in the supplying artery, increased velocity and arterialization of the draining vein, and perivascular soft tissue vibration in the region of the fistula (Fig. 4-82 [see also color insert, Plate 23]).

Pseudoaneurysms

Pseudoaneurysms are caused by trauma just as arteriovenous fistulas are. In fact, most pseudoaneurysms are associated with a fistula. They appear as cystic spaces on gray-scale images and can easily be mistaken for renal cysts. Ideally all renal cysts should undergo Doppler analysis to prove an absence of internal blood flow. Realistically this is not necessary in native kidneys because cysts are so common and pseudoaneurysms so rare. However, it is definitely necessary in renal transplants because then cysts are much less common and pseudoaneurysms are more frequent.

The color-Doppler characteristics of renal pseudoaneurysms are similar to those of pseudoaneurysms elsewhere in the body—a swirling pattern of internal blood flow (Fig. 4-83 [see also color insert, Plate 24]). However, because they are usually associated with an arteriovenous fistula, the flow usually progresses from the artery, to the pseudoaneurysm, and then to the vein. Therefore the characteristic "to-and-fro" flow pattern (seen in the neck of peripheral arterial pseudoaneurysms that communicate only with the artery via a single neck) is not present in most renal pseudoaneurysms.

RENAL TRANSPLANTS

The main role of sonography in the evaluation of renal transplants is to identify hydronephrosis and peritransplant fluid collections. Hydronephrosis has the same appearance in transplants as it does in native kidneys. However, because transplants are more superficially located and can be imaged with higher-resolution transducers, it is often possible to identify urine in the normal renal pelvis and even in the calices and infundibula. The findings revealed by this improved visualization of normal structures in the renal collecting system should not be confused with those of hydronephrosis. In addition, mild distention of the renal pelvis and intrarenal collecting system is common in transplants and should not be construed as functionally significant obstruction. It may stem from mild edema at the ureteroneocystostomy site in the early postoperative period and from a redundancy in the collecting system in the later postoperative period. Comparison with old studies is very helpful for eliminating doubt about the significance of mild collecting system dilatation. When old studies are not available, radionuclide scans can be used to determine the functional significance of the dilatation.

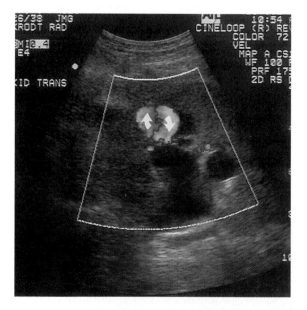

Fig. 4-83 Pseudoaneurysm. Transverse view of the upper pole of a renal transplant shows blood flow in the lumen of a rounded structure. The swirling pattern of flow, with half of the lumen exhibiting flow traveling toward the transducer and the other half showing flow away from the transducer *(curved arrows),* is characteristic of a pseudoaneurysm. Fig. 4-20 was also obtained from this patient (see color insert, Plate 24).

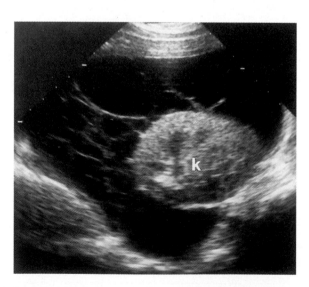

Fig. 4-84 Lymphocele. Transverse view of a renal transplant demonstrates an extensive septated fluid collection surrounding most of the kidney *(k).* This was drained surgically and shown to represent a lymphocele.

Peritransplant fluid collections are very common and readily visualized sonographically. Small hematomas are seen frequently in the early postoperative period and are of no importance. Larger hematomas may develop and become important if they compress the ureter and produce urinary obstruction. Compression of the renal parenchyma can also occur, especially with subcapsular hematomas, and this may cause a substantial reduction in renal blood flow. The sonographic appearance of peritransplant hematomas varies depending on their age, just as with hematomas elsewhere in the body. Acute hematomas are echogenic, but become hypoechoic and eventually anechoic as the clot retracts and lyses.

Lymphoceles are another common fluid collection encountered in transplant recipients. These typically arise 1 to 3 weeks postoperatively and are of concern only if they compress the ureter or cause local symptoms of pain and tenderness. They frequently appear as multiseptated fluid collections and can vary in size from a few centimeters to massive collections that surround the kidney (Fig. 4-84).

Urinomas typically occur as the result of a breakdown in the ureteral implantation into the bladder. Ureteric ischemia can be another cause. Urinomas tend to form in the first 2 postoperative weeks. They are due to urine extravasation and under most circumstances require surgical repair. Since they usually arise from the ureteral anastomosis, they generally occur in continuity with the bladder and often produce a mass effect on the bladder (Fig. 4-85). As they enlarge, they fill in the space between the lower pole of the transplant and the bladder. Their

sonographic characteristics are nonspecific and overlap with those of resolving hematomas and lymphoceles. Therefore diagnosis depends on the findings yielded by the aspiration and analysis of the fluid or the demonstration of urinary extravasation on renal scintigrams or contrast studies.

Abscesses may result from infection involving a pre-existing fluid collection or may develop de novo. They typically appear as complex fluid collections containing internal debris, just as they do elsewhere in the body. They are difficult to distinguish from other fluid collections, especially hematomas, so diagnosis depends on a high index of clinical suspicion coupled with the findings from analysis of the fluid aspirated.

Vascular complications of renal transplants include stenosis and thrombosis of the artery and vein, arteriovenous fistula, pseudoaneurysm, and segmental infarction. Most of these complications and their sonographic findings have been discussed already. The important difference with respect to transplants is that all of these vascular complications are easier to detect in them than in native kidneys. In particular, renal artery stenosis and renal vein thrombosis are much more reliably detected and excluded with sonography. Segmental infarcts have traditionally been difficult to detect with sonography, but with the development of color-Doppler sonography, moderate and large segmental infarcts can now be reliably documented (Fig. 4-86 [for Fig. 4-86, *C,* see also color insert, Plate 25]). Power-Doppler techniques will almost certainly further improve the detection of segmental infarcts.

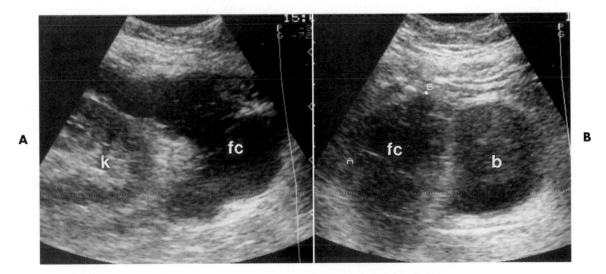

Fig. 4-85   Urinoma. **A,** Longitudinal view of a renal transplant demonstrates the lower pole of the kidney *(k)* with an adjacent associated fluid collection *(fc).* **B,** Transverse view of the urinary bladder *(b)* demonstrates that the fluid collection is in continuity with the right lateral aspect of the bladder and displaces the bladder to the left. This is a typical location and appearance for a urinoma, which in this case arose from an anastomotic leak between the ureter and bladder.

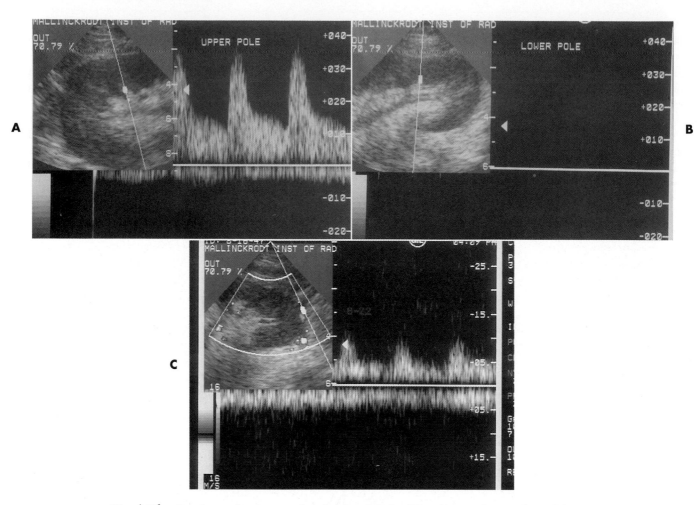

Fig. 4-86   Renal transplant lower pole infarction. **A,** Pulsed-Doppler waveform analysis of the upper pole of the transplant demonstrates normal arterial and venous flow. **B,** Pulsed-Doppler waveform analysis of the lower pole demonstrates no detectable arterial or venous flow. **C,** Doppler image from the lower pole confirms the absence of parenchymal flow but the presence of collateral flow around the renal capsule. Both arterial and venous capsular flow is identified on pulsed-Doppler waveform analysis (see color insert, Plate 25).

As with native kidneys, capsular collaterals form in areas of infarction and produce rim perfusion to the kidney.

Parenchymal processes affecting renal transplants are best diagnosed on the basis of the findings noted in specimens obtained by ultrasound-guided percutaneous biopsy. Sonography can often show gray-scale changes, but in most cases they are not specific enough to base management decisions on. Transplant rejection causes renal swelling that affects both the parenchyma and the urothelium (Fig. 4-87, *A*). It may also produce enlarged hypoechoic pyramids, cortical regions of decreased echogenicity, and decreased visibility of the renal sinus. The more of these abnormalities that are present, the more likely is the diagnosis of rejection. However, acute tubular necrosis, cyclosporin toxicity, and infection can also produce one or more of these abnormalities.

For some time there was great hope that Doppler waveform analysis of the intrarenal arteries could help in the effort to distinguish the different causes of transplant dysfunction. The belief was that rejection, particularly severe vascular rejection, affected the vasculature to a greater degree than did the other processes, and this would be reflected by a higher resistive index (Fig. 4-87, *B*). This has been shown to be statistically correct when large groups of patients with different diseases are compared, but there is a significant overlap in the resistive indexes obtained in the setting of the different parenchymal diseases that affect renal transplant recipients. Therefore it is probably best to use arterial waveform analysis in a manner similar to gray-scale changes, and to recognize that significantly elevated resistive indexes make rejection a more likely possibility but do not ensure the diagnosis.

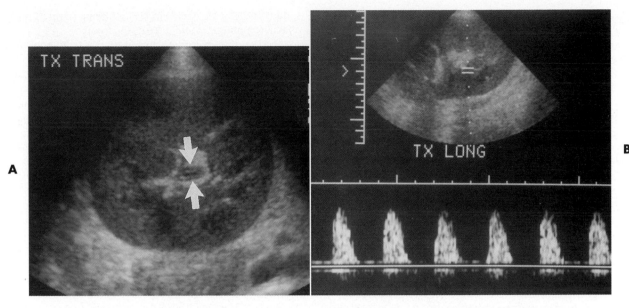

Fig. 4-87   Transplant rejection. **A,** Swelling of the renal transplant is manifested as a rounded appearance on this transverse view. In addition, there is thickening of the urothelium in the central renal collecting system *(arrows)* with a small amount of urine in the lumen. **B,** Pulsed-Doppler waveform analysis of an intrarenal artery demonstrates markedly increased vascular resistance with no diastolic flow. Although nonspecific, this type of a waveform pattern with absence of diastolic flow suggests rejection. Note that the minimal amount of noise seen on both sides of the waveform should not be confused with diastolic flow.

Key Features

The detection of urinary obstruction is one of the most common indications for abdominal sonography. Diagnosis relies on the detection of hydronephrosis and/or increased resistance to renal arterial flow and/or loss of ureteral jets.

Renal cysts are seen frequently. Patients with simple cysts require no further evaluation. Patients with complex cystic lesions require surgical treatment, evaluation with computed tomography, or periodic follow-up examinations.

Multiple renal cysts can occur in the settings of autosomal dominant polycystic disease, acquired cystic disease of dialysis, von Hippel–Lindau syndrome, and tuberous sclerosis.

Solid renal masses in adults should be considered renal cell carcinoma until proved otherwise. Small homogeneous hyperechoic masses are more likely to be angiomyolipomas, which can be confirmed with computed tomography or monitored sonographically, depending on size.

Pyelonephritis may cause focal areas of increased and decreased cortical echogenicity, renal enlargement, and urothelial thickening. However, sonographic findings are often normal in patients with pyelonephritis.

Sonography is a relatively effective means of detecting intrarenal calculi. Intravenous urography is an easier and more reliable means of detecting ureteral calculi. Sonography should be used to search for ureteral calculi in patients who are pregnant or patients who have allergies to contrast agents.

Nephrocalcinosis produces hyperechoic pyramids with or without shadowing.

Increased renal cortical echogenicity is a nonspecific finding that in general is associated with renal parenchymal diseases.

Renal artery stenosis can be detected with Doppler analysis on the basis of an elevated main renal artery-to-aortic velocity ratio or slowed segmental renal artery systolic acceleration. However, the use of sonography for this purpose remains controversial.

The detection and exclusion of renal vein thrombosis is relatively easy on the right side but relatively difficult on the left side.

In the evaluation of renal transplant dysfunction, sonography is most valuable in detecting the following surgical complications: urinary obstruction, postoperative fluid collections, and renal vascular thrombosis or stenosis.

SUGGESTED READINGS

al-Murrani B et al: Echogenic rings—an ultrasound sign of early nephrocalcinosis, *Clin Radiol* 44:49, 1991.

Banner MP et al: Multilocular renal cysts: radiologic-pathologic correlation, *AJR* 136:239, 1981.

Berland LL et al: Renal artery stenosis: prospective evaluation of diagnosis with color Doppler ultrasound compared with angiography, *Radiology* 174:421, 1990.

Bosniak MA et al: CT diagnosis of renal angiomyolipoma: the importance of detecting small amounts of fat, *AJR* 151:497, 1988.

Carter AR et al: The junctional parenchymal defect: a sonographic variant of renal anatomy, *Radiology* 154:499, 1985.

Charnsangavej C: Lymphoma of the genitourinary tract, *Radiol Clin North Am* 28:865, 1990.

Choyke PL et al: The natural history of renal lesions in von Hippel–Lindau disease: a serial CT study in 28 patients, *AJR* 159:1229, 1992.

Choyke PL et al: Renal metastases: clinicopathologic and radiologic correlation, *Radiology* 162:359, 1987.

Cronan JJ et al: Peripelvic cysts: an imposter of sonographic hydronephrosis, *J Ultrasound Med* 1:229, 1982.

Dalla Palma L, Stacul F, Bazzocchi M et al: Ultrasonography and plain film versus intravenous urography in ureteric colic, *Clin Radiol* 47:333, 1993.

Dillard JP, Talner LB, Pinckney L: Normal renal papillae simulating caliceal filling defects on sonography, *AJR* 148:895, 1987.

Dodd GD III, Tublin ME, Shah A, Zajko AB: Imaging of vascular complications associated with renal transplants, *AJR* 157:449, 1991.

Dunnick NR et al: The radiology of juxtaglomerular tumors, *Radiology* 147:321, 1983.

Forman HP, Middleton WD, Melson GL, McClennan BL: Increasing frequency of detection of hyperechoic renal cell carcinomas, *Radiology* 188:431, 1993.

Genkins SM, Sanfilippo FP, Carroll BA: Duplex Doppler sonography of renal transplants: lack of sensitivity and specificity in establishing pathologic diagnosis, *AJR* 152:535, 1989.

Glazer GM, Callen PW, Filly RA: Medullary nephrocalcinosis: sonographic evaluation, *AJR* 138:55, 1992.

Goiney RC et al: Renal oncocytoma: sonographic analysis of 14 cases, *AJR* 143:1001, 1984.

Goldman SM, Fishman EK: Upper urinary tract infection: the current role of CT, ultrasound, and MRI, *Semin Ultrasound CT MR* 12:355, 1991.

Grant DC et al: Sonography in transitional cell carcinoma of the renal pelvis, *Urol Radiol* 8:1, 1986.

Hartman DS et al: Renal lymphoma: radiologic-pathologic correlation of 21 cases, *Radiology* 144:759, 1982.

Hartman DS et al: Angiomyolipoma: ultrasonic-pathologic correlation, *Radiology* 139:451, 1981.

Hartman DS et al: Xanthogranulomatous pyelonephritis: sonographic-pathologic correlation of 16 cases, *J Ultrasound Med* 3:481, 1984.

Hayes WS, Hartman DS, Sesterhenn IA: From the archives of the AFIP. Xanthogranulomatous pyelonephritis, *Radiographics* 11:485, 1991.

Heiken JP, McClennan BL, Gold RP: Renal lymphoma, *Semin Ultrasound CT MR* 7:58, 1986.

Hoddick W, Filly RA, Backman U et al: Renal allograft rejection: US evaluation, *Radiology* 161:469, 1986.

Hricak H et al: Renal parenchymal disease: sonographic-histologic correlation, *Radiology* 144:141, 1982.

Jeffrey RB et al: Sensitivity of sonography in pyonephrosis: a re-evaluation, *AJR* 144:71, 1985.

Kliewer MA et al: Renal artery stenosis: analysis of Doppler waveform parameters and tardus-parvus pattern, *Radiology* 189:779, 1993.

Lafortune M et al: Sonography of the hypertrophied column of Bertin, *AJR* 146:53, 1986.

Letourneau JG, Day DL, Ascher NL, Castaneda-Zuniga WR: Imaging of renal transplants, *AJR* 150:833, 1988.

Levine E, Hartman DS, Smirniotopoulos JG: *Renal cystic disease associated with renal neoplasms.* In Pollack HM, editor: *Clinical urography,* Philadelphia, 1990, WB Saunders.

Levine E et al: Natural history of acquired renal cystic disease in dialysis patients: a prospective longitudinal CT study. *AJR* 156:501, 1991.

Madewell JE et al: Multilocular cystic nephroma: a radiographic-pathologic correlation of 58 patients, *Radiology* 146:309, 1983.

Middleton WD et al: Renal calculi: sensitivity for detection with US, *Radiology* 167:239, 1988.

Middleton WD et al: Postbiopsy renal transplant arteriovenous fistulas: color Doppler ultrasound characteristics, *Radiology* 171:253, 1989.

Middleton WD, Melson GL: Renal duplication artifact in ultrasound imaging, *Radiology* 173:427, 1989.

Nicolet V et al: Thickening of the renal collecting system: a nonspecific finding at ultrasound, *Radiology* 168:411, 1988.

Pagani JJ: Solid renal mass in the cancer patient: second primary renal cell carcinoma versus renal metastasis, *J Comput Assist Tomogr* 7:444, 1983.

Patriquin H, Robitaille P: Renal calcium deposition in children: sonographic demonstration of the Anderson-Carr progression, *AJR* 146:1253, 1986.

Piccirillo M, Rigsby CM, Rosenfield AT: Sonography of renal inflammatory disease, *Urol Radiol* 9:66, 1987.

Platt JF, Ellis JH, Rubin JM: Intrarenal arterial Doppler sonography in the detection of renal vein thrombosis of the native kidney, *AJR* 162:1367, 1994.

Platt JF et al: Duplex Doppler ultrasound of the kidney: differentiation of obstructive from nonobstructive dilatation, *Radiology* 171:515, 1989.

Pollack HM et al: The accuracy of gray-scale renal ultrasonography in differentiating cystic neoplasms from benign cysts, *Radiology* 143:741, 1982.

Pozniak MA et al: Extraneous factors affecting resistive index, *Invest Radiol* 23:899, 1988.

Quinn MJ et al: Renal oncocytoma: new observations, *Radiology* 153:49, 1984.

Radin DR et al: Visceral and nodal calcification in patients with AIDS-related *Pneumocystis carinii* infection, *AJR* 154:27, 1990.

Rifkin MD et al: Evaluation of renal transplant rejection by duplex Doppler examination: value of the resistive index, *AJR* 148:759, 1987.

Ritchie WW et al: Evaluation of azotemic patients: diagnostic yield of ultrasound examination, *Radiology* 167:245, 1988.

Rosenberg ER et al: The significance of septations in a renal cyst, *AJR* 144:593, 1985.

Rosenfield AT, Siegel NJ: Renal parenchymal disease: histopathologic-sonographic correlation, *AJR* 137:793, 1981.

Schwerk WB, Schwerk WN, Rodeck G: Venous renal tumor extension: a prospective ultrasound evaluation, *Radiology* 156:491, 1985.

Stavros AT et al: Segmental stenosis of the renal artery: pattern recognition of tardus and parvus abnormalities with duplex sonography, *Radiology* 184:487, 1992.

Taylor AJ et al: Renal imaging in long-term dialysis patients: a comparison of CT and sonography, *AJR* 153:765, 1989.

Taylor DC et al: Duplex ultrasound scanning in the diagnosis of renal artery stenosis: a prospective evaluation, *J Vasc Surg* 7:363, 1988.

Taylor KJW et al: Vascular complications in renal allografts: detection with duplex Doppler ultrasound, *Radiology* 162:31, 1987.

Vrtiska TJ et al: Role of ultrasound in medical management of patients with renal stone disease, *Urol Radiol* 14:131, 1992.

Warshauer DM et al: Unusual causes of increased vascular impedance in renal transplants: duplex Doppler evaluation, *Radiology* 169:367, 1988.

Wilson DA, Wenzl JE, Altshuler GP: Ultrasound demonstration of diffuse cortical nephrocalcinosis in a case of primary hyperoxaluria, *AJR* 132:659, 1979.

Wood BP et al: Tuberous sclerosis, *AJR* 158:750, 1992.

Yamashita Y et al: Small renal cell carcinoma: pathologic and radiologic correlation, *Radiology* 184:493, 1992.

Yousem DM et al: Synchronous and metachronous transitional cell carcinoma of the urinary tract: prevalence, incidence, and radiographic detection, *Radiology* 167:613, 1988.

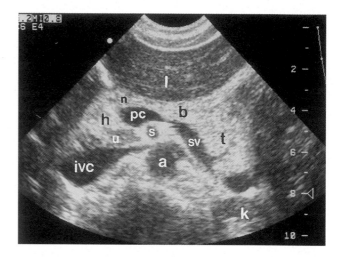

CHAPTER 5

Pancreas

Anatomy
Technique
Pancreatitis
Pancreatic Carcinoma
Islet Cell Tumors
Cystic Pancreatic Neoplasms
Rare Neoplasms

For a Key Features summary see p. 141.

ANATOMY

The pancreas is a retroperitoneal organ that develops from a large dorsal embryologic anlage and a smaller ventral anlage. The dorsal pancreatic anlage communicates by means of its central duct with the duodenum and the ventral anlage communicates with the biliary tract. During embryologic development these pancreatic anlagen rotate with the intestinal structures and ultimately fuse together so that the dorsal pancreas is located anterior and superior to the ventral pancreas. The associated pancreatic ductal structures rotate with the parenchymal structures so that the dorsal pancreatic duct empties into the duodenum several centimeters above the ventral duct. The ventral duct connects to the distal common bile duct at the ampulla. In 15% to 20% of persons these embryologic ductal anatomic characteristics persist, with a short ventral duct that drains the head of the pancreas by way of the major papilla and a long dorsal duct that drains the remainder of the pancreas via the minor papilla. This is referred to as *pancreas divisum.* In most persons the two ducts join and the minor papilla regresses so that the entire gland is drained via one duct that empties into the major papilla. Several other ductal patterns exist, but none are visible sonographically.

The pancreas is divided into a head, neck, body, tail, and uncinate process. The uncinate process extends inferiorly and medially from the head and is the only part of

Fig. 5-1 Normal pancreas. Transverse view of the pancreas demonstrates its relationship to adjacent structures. The head *(h)* and uncinate process *(u)* are immediately anterior to the inferior vena cava *(ivc).* The neck *(n),* body *(b),* and tail *(t)* are immediately anterior to the portosplenic confluence *(pc)* and the splenic vein *(sv).* The superior mesenteric artery *(s)* is surrounded by echogenic fibrofatty tissue that separates it from the pancreas. The splenic and superior mesenteric veins abut the pancreas and, unlike the superior mesenteric artery, do not have fatty tissue surrounding them and separating them from the pancreatic parenchyma. Note that the pancreas in this patient is quite echogenic compared with the overlying left lobe of the liver *(l).* Also seen are the aorta *(a)* and a portion of the left kidney *(k).*

the pancreas that is located posterior to the superior mesenteric vein. The head is located to the right of the mesenteric vessels, and the neck and body are located anterior to these vessels. The tail of the pancreas is located to the left of the mesenteric vessels and extends superiorly and posteriorly to the region of the splenic hilum (Fig. 5-1). In some references the tail of the pancreas is said to be that part that extends to the left of the vertebral column. Realistically though, the exact anatomic demar-

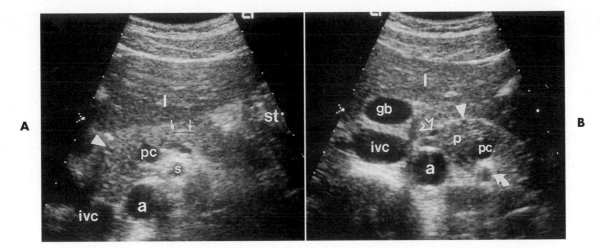

Fig. 5-2   Normal pancreas. **A,** Transverse view of the pancreas demonstrates the pancreatic head anterior to the inferior vena cava *(ivc)* and aorta *(a)*. The uncinate process of the pancreas is a small triangular extension of the pancreatic head that is positioned between the aorta and the portosplenic confluence *(pc)*. The superior mesenteric artery *(s)* is separated from the pancreas by a prominent rim of fibrofatty tissue. The pancreatic duct *(arrows)* is seen in the body of the pancreas and appears as a bright anterior and posterior wall with a thin internal lumen. Also seen are the left lobe of the liver *(l)*, the gastroduodenal artery *(arrowhead)*, and the stomach *(st)*. In this person the pancreas is just slightly hyperechoic to the liver. **B,** Transverse view of the pancreas obtained with the patient in a left lateral decubitus position and with the transducer positioned from a right anterolateral approach. The head of the pancreas *(p)* is seen, using the liver *(l)* as a window. Notice that the pancreatic head in this patient has shifted to the left so that it is anterior to the aorta *(a)* rather than the inferior vena cava *(ivc)*. This is brought about by the left lateral decubitus position. The relative location of the gastroduodenal artery *(arrowhead)* along the anterior aspect of the pancreatic head and of the common bile duct *(open arrow)* running through the posterior aspect of the head of the pancreas is well demonstrated on this view. Also seen are the gallbladder *(gb)*, portosplenic confluence *(pc)*, and the superior mesenteric artery *(curved arrow)*.   *Continued.*

cations between the different parts of the pancreas are poorly defined.

Because of its size, location, and echogenicity, the pancreas has always been one of the more difficult abdominal organs to image. For this reason adjacent vascular landmarks have been relied on heavily to help in the localization of the pancreas. The head of the pancreas is located immediately anterior to the inferior vena cava. However, when patients are in the left lateral decubitus or left posterior oblique position, the head of the pancreas may slide somewhat to the left so that it is located over the aorta. The body and tail of the pancreas are located immediately anterior to the splenic vein and the portal splenic confluence. The trifurcation of the celiac axis is located just superior to the pancreas, and the splenic artery generally runs near the superior aspect of the pancreas. The gastroduodenal artery arises from the common hepatic artery and travels inferiorly directly over the anterior and lateral aspects of the pancreatic head. The superior mesenteric vein is immediately adjacent to the posterior aspect of the pancreatic neck and body and to the medial aspect of the pancreatic head. There is no retroperitoneal fat between the superior mesenteric vein and the pan-

creas. There is, however, a prominent ring of retroperitoneal fat that separates the superior mesenteric artery from the pancreas (Fig. 5-2).

The pancreatic duct is seen segmentally in 85% of patients. It is most commonly seen in the body, where its walls are perpendicular to the sound beam. The portion of the pancreatic duct that travels through the head is more difficult to visualize sonographically. However, it is occasionally seen medial to the distal common bile duct and should not be confused with the bile duct or with a low-inserting cystic duct (Fig. 5-3). When the luminal diameter is very small, the pancreatic duct may appear as a single bright line. In most cases the diameter is sufficient to allow for resolution of both the anterior and posterior duct walls (see Fig. 5-2, *A*). The walls of the pancreatic duct should be smooth and parallel. Three millimeters is commonly used as the upper limit of normal for duct diameter in the body of the pancreas. However, the duct does enlarge with age, and this should be considered when scanning elderly patients.

Pancreatic echogenicity is variable, depending on the amount of fatty replacement. The normal pancreas is equal to, or more echogenic than, the normal liver. The

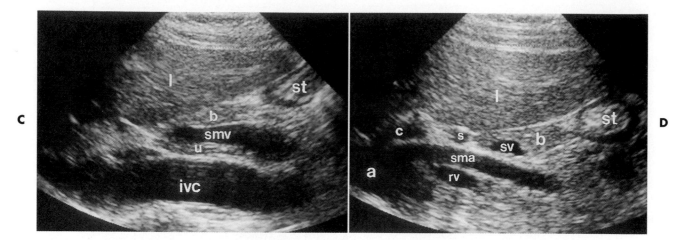

Fig. 5-2, cont'd.   C, Longitudinal view at the level of the superior mesenteric vein *(smv)* demonstrates the body of the pancreas *(b)* anterior to the vein. A small amount of pancreatic tissue is also seen posterior to the superior mesenteric vein, representing the uncinate process *(u)*. The pancreas is immediately anterior to the inferior vena cava *(ivc)*. Also seen are the left lobe of the liver *(l)* and the stomach *(st)*. Note the lack of fatty tissue between the superior mesenteric vein and the pancreas. **D,** Longitudinal view through the superior mesenteric artery *(sma)* demonstrates the splenic vein *(sv)* in cross-section immediately posterior to the body of the pancreas *(b)*. Note that the superior mesenteric artery is separated from the pancreas by fibrofatty tissue but that the splenic vein is immediately contiguous with the pancreas. Also seen are the aorta *(a)*, celiac axis *(c)*, left renal vein *(rv)*, splenic artery *(s)*, left lobe of the liver *(l)*, and stomach *(st)*.

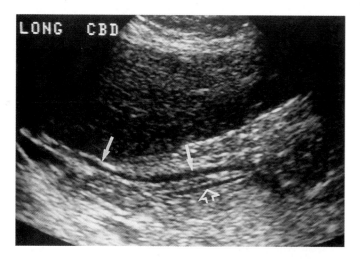

Fig. 5-3   Normal pancreatic duct and common bile duct. Coronal view of the pancreatic head obtained from a right lateral approach demonstrates the common bile duct *(arrows)* and the pancreatic duct *(open arrow)*. From this right coronal view, the lateral position of the common bile duct compared with the medial location of the pancreatic duct is apparent. Note that the two ducts begin to converge in the region of the major papilla.

pancreas may be hypoechoic, isoechoic, or hyperechoic with respect to the spleen (Fig. 5-4). With age, pancreatic echogenicity increases as the result of fatty replacement. In general the pancreas is homogeneous in echotexture. When the head is seen well, it is often possible to identify a focal area of decreased echogenicity in the posterior half of the pancreatic head. This is related to the lower fat content of the ventral embryologic anlage. This normal variant can be distinguished from pathologic processes that cause decreased pancreatic echogenicity (such as cancer and pancreatitis) by its straight border and lack of mass effect (Fig. 5-5).

The anteroposterior dimension of the pancreas varies throughout the gland, and the upper limit of normal for pancreatic measurements is not uniformly agreed upon. For practical purposes one can generally assume that the pancreas is abnormally enlarged when the thickness of the head, body, and tail is equal to or greater than 3.0, 2.5, and 2.0 cm, respectively. (See Table 5-1 for the normal characteristics of the pancreas.)

TECHNIQUE

The pancreas should be scanned with the patient in a fasting state to minimize the interference caused by overlying bowel gas. In most patients the body of the pancreas is well seen from an anterior subxiphoid approach using the left lobe of the liver as an acoustic window (see Figs. 5-1 and 5-2, *A*). This is generally aided by a deep inspiration. In some cases visualization of the body of the pancreas is improved by having the patient try to make a "beer belly." Portions of the head of the pancreas are usu-

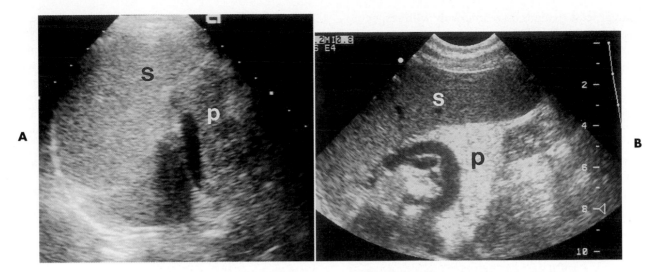

Fig. 5-4   Relative echogenicity of the pancreas and spleen. **A,** Coronal scan of the left upper quadrant in a normal volunteer demonstrates the spleen *(s)* and the pancreatic tail *(p)*. In this case the pancreas is less echogenic than the spleen. **B,** Similar view obtained in an older patient demonstrates increased pancreatic echogenicity compared with the adjacent spleen.

Table 5-1	Normal characteristics
Characteristic	**Normal finding**
Size	Head, <3 cm; body, <2.5 cm; tail, <2.0 cm
Echogenicity	> Liver, >/< spleen
Echotexture	Homogeneous
Surface	Smooth to slightly lobular

ally seen when the same anterior approach is employed as that used to see the body. However, it is often necessary to scan from a right subcostal approach with the transducer angled slightly medially to see the portions of the pancreatic head that are not well seen from an anterior approach (see Fig. 5-2, *B*). When this approach is used, the relationship of the pancreatic head to the adjacent structures will differ from that visualized by the more familiar anterior approach.

The tail of the pancreas is difficult to see in its entirety using the approach just described. To see the pancreatic tail well, it is usually necessary to have the patient drink water and to use the resulting fluid-filled stomach as a window. When this is not possible or is not helpful, the region of the pancreatic tail should be imaged by scanning from a left lateral intercostal approach and using the spleen as a window (see Fig. 5-4).

The uncinate process of the pancreas should be viewed in a manner similar to that used for the pancreatic head. It is important to remember that, because the

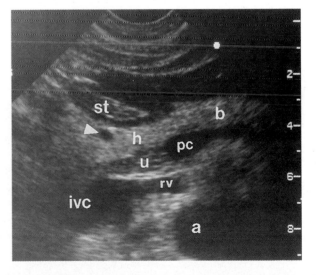

Fig. 5-5   Differential echogenicity of the pancreatic head and uncinate process. Transverse view of the pancreas shows the relative hyperechogenicity of the body *(b)* and head *(h)* of the pancreas with respect to the uncinate process *(u)*. The straight margin demarcating the uncinate process from the remainder of the pancreas is readily apparent. This is a normal variant that should not be confused with pathologic processes that can cause decreased pancreatic echogenicity. Also seen are the portosplenic confluence *(pc)*, inferior vena cava *(ivc)*, aorta *(a)*, left renal vein *(rv)*, gastroduodenal artery *(arrowhead)*, and antrum of the stomach *(st)*.

uncinate process extends quite inferiorly with respect to the pancreatic head and body, abnormalities in it can be easily overlooked if the scans are not extended inferiorly enough.

PANCREATITIS

Acute pancreatitis can be caused by a wide variety of abnormalities. The most common are alcohol abuse and gallstones. Less common causes include biliary sludge,

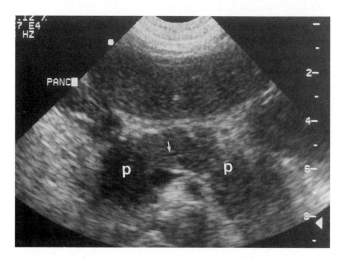

Fig. 5-6 Pancreatitis. Transverse view of the pancreas *(p)* demonstrates that it is enlarged and hypoechoic. No peripancreatic fluid collections are seen and the diameter of the pancreatic duct *(arrow)* is normal.

peptic ulcers, trauma, pregnancy, drugs, mumps, endoscopic retrograde cholangiopancreaticography (ERCP), tumors, hypercalcemia, hyperlipoproteinemia, and familial pancreatitis. The typical presenting features are upper abdominal and back pain and elevated levels of pancreatic enzymes in the blood or urine. The disease may be mild and respond well to supportive therapy, or it may progress to severe multisystem failure. Unfortunately, there are no pathognomonic clinical or laboratory findings that permit a definitive diagnosis of pancreatitis to be made.

One of the major roles of sonography in patients with pancreatitis is to evaluate the biliary tract for stone disease. This can not only identify the cause of the pancreatitis, but the findings can also be used to determine what the appropriate further management should be, such as cholecystectomy and, if necessary, preoperative ERCP. The detection of biliary obstruction is also quite important, as many of these patients have coexistent liver disease and the source of abnormal liver function test results may be difficult to sort out clinically. Obstruction of the bile ducts in patients with pancreatitis may be due to a stricture in the distal common bile duct or to compression of the common bile duct by either a pseudocyst or the inflammatory swelling of the pancreatic head.

The pancreas may appear normal in mild cases of acute pancreatitis, and sonography should therefore not be used to exclude the diagnosis. Nevertheless, when the pancreas does appear normal, other upper abdominal structures should be evaluated carefully to try and establish an alternative diagnosis such as cholecystitis, peptic ulcer disease, and hepatic abscess.

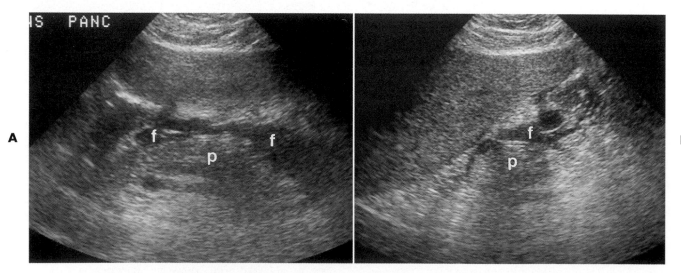

Fig. 5-7 Pancreatitis with a peripancreatic fluid collection. **A,** Transverse view of the pancreas *(p)* demonstrates a mantle of retroperitoneal fluid *(f)* anterior to the pancreas. **B,** Longitudinal view of the pancreas *(p)* also demonstrates this mantle of peripancreatic fluid *(f)* located superior, anterior, and inferior to the pancreas.

Pancreatic enlargement and decreased pancreatic echogenicity are the sonographic hallmarks of acute pancreatitis (Fig. 5-6). These changes are usually diffuse, but can, on occasion, be focal. Focal pancreatitis usually involves the pancreatic head.

The determination of pancreatic echogenicity relies on comparison with the echogenicity of the liver. When the liver is abnormally echogenic because of fatty infiltration, the pancreas may appear hypoechoic even though it is normal.

Alteration in the size and echogenicity of the pancreas is often subtle, and the diagnosis of pancreatitis is frequently based on the visualization of peripancreatic fluid collections in a patient with an appropriate clinical history. Using an anterior subxiphoid approach, sonography can visualize fluid collections around the body of the pancreas in many patients. Fluid may accumulate in a mantle anterior, superior, and inferior to the pancreas (Fig. 5-7). It may also dissect along the portal splenic confluence and the superior mesenteric vein. Using a left lateral approach and the spleen as a window, sonography can identify fluid in the left anterior pararenal space, the left perirenal space, and the interfascial plane (Fig. 5-8, *B*). Similar collections can be seen from a right lateral approach using the liver as a window (Fig. 5-9). Identifying fluid collections around the left and right kidneys and the duodenum

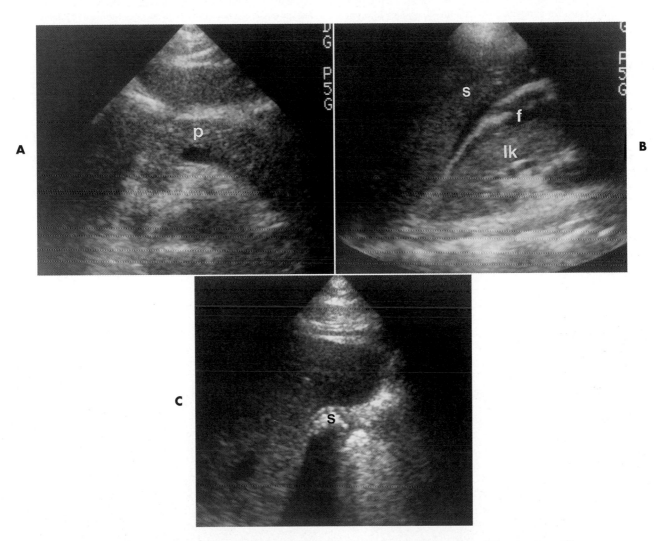

Fig. 5-8   Pancreatitis with normal-appearing pancreas. **A,** Transverse view of the pancreas *(p)* demonstrates normal size and echogenicity and no peripancreatic fluid collections. **B,** Coronal view of the left upper quadrant demonstrates the left kidney *(lk)* and the spleen *(s)*. A retroperitoneal fluid collection *(f)* is seen around the left kidney. This was the only sonographic evidence of pancreatitis in this patient with a well-established clinical diagnosis of pancreatitis. **C,** Transverse view of the right upper quadrant demonstrates a gallbladder filled with stones *(s)*. This establishes the cause of this patient's pancreatitis and indicates the need for cholecystectomy.

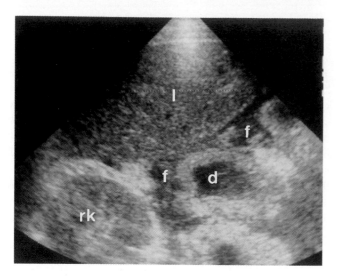

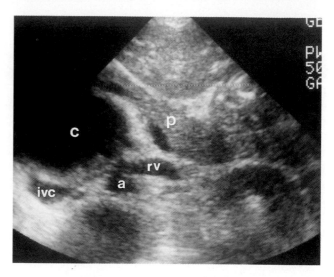

Fig. 5-9 Periduodenal fluid collection due to pancreatitis. Transverse view of the right upper quadrant obtained from a lateral approach demonstrates the fluid-filled duodenum *(d)* and an adjacent retroperitoneal fluid collection *(f)*. Also seen are the right kidney *(rk)* and the liver *(l)*. In this patient views of the pancreas could not be obtained because of overlying bowel gas, and the periduodenal and perirenal fluid collections on the right side were the only evidence of pancreatitis.

Fig. 5-10 Pancreatic pseudocyst. Transverse view of the upper abdomen demonstrates a large cystic structure *(c)* that is displacing the body and tail of the pancreas *(p)* anteriorly. This is a pseudocyst arising from the uncinate process of the pancreas. Its relationship to the aorta *(a)*, inferior vena cava *(ivc)*, and left renal vein *(rv)* is well demonstrated.

Box 5-1 Sonographic Signs of Acute Pancreatitis
Decreased pancreatic echogenicity
Pancreatic enlargement
Peripancreatic fluid collections
Perivascular fluid collections
Periduodenal fluid collections
Anterior pararenal fluid collections

Box 5-2 Complications of Pancreatitis
Pseudocyst formation
Bile duct obstruction
Pancreatic abscess
Pancreatic necrosis
Venous thrombosis
Pseudoaneurysm

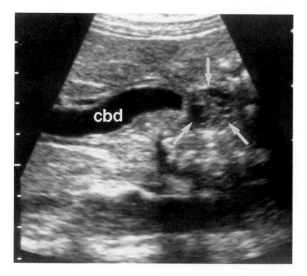

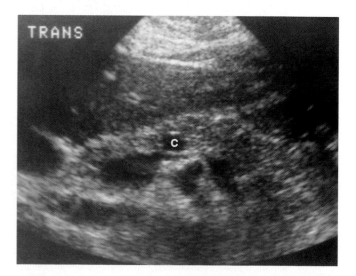

Fig. 5-11 Complex pseudocyst. Longitudinal view of a dilated common bile duct *(cbd)* demonstrates abrupt termination of the bile duct at the level of a complex-appearing, partially solid and partially cystic mass *(arrows)*. This was a hemorrhagic pseudocyst. Its cystic nature had been documented on previous scans.

Fig. 5-12 Pancreatic cyst in a patient with autosomal dominant polycystic disease. Transverse view of the pancreas demonstrates a small cyst *(c)* in the body of the pancreas. This is indistinguishable from an intrapancreatic pseudocyst. However, the presence of enlarged kidneys with multiple bilateral renal cysts and a positive family history of polycystic disease confirmed the diagnosis in this patient.

is extremely useful when visualization of the pancreas is limited or when the pancreas appears normal (see Fig. 5-8, *A*). Therefore these areas should be scanned carefully whenever pancreatitis is a consideration. (See Box 5-1 for a summary of the sonographic signs of acute pancreatitis.)

There are a number of complications that can occur in conjunction with acute pancreatitis (Box 5-2). One of

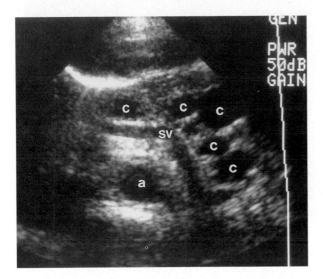

Fig. 5-13   Multiple pancreatic cysts in a patient with von Hippel–Lindau disease. Transverse view of the pancreas demonstrates multiple cystic lesions *(c)* scattered throughout the body and tail of the pancreas. The splenic vein *(sv)* is seen posterior to the pancreas. The aorta *(a)* is also identified.

the most common is pseudocyst formation. Pseudocysts are walled-off fluid collections that have a capsule composed of fibrous tissue but lacks true epithelial cells. They can form virtually anywhere, but most are located within or near the pancreas. Their sonographic appearance differs from that of other pancreatic fluid collections in that they have well-defined smooth margins and are loculated (Fig. 5-10). Their internal contents are usually anechoic, but the presence of debris can result in low-level internal echoes. Hemorrhage and infection can also produce complex internal echoes within a pseudocyst (Fig. 5-11).

The differential diagnosis of cystic pancreatic lesions is relatively broad. Besides pancreatitis, other causes of pancreatic cysts include cystic neoplasms, cysts related to autosomal dominant polycystic disease (Fig. 5-12), von Hippel–Lindau disease (Fig. 5-13), and cystic fibrosis. In addition, pancreatic cysts can be mimicked by a tortuous splenic artery (Fig. 5-14) or by a splenic artery aneurysm (Fig. 5-15 [for Fig. 5-15, *B*, see also color insert, Plate 26]) or pseudoaneurysm. Because of this, Doppler evaluation of suspected pancreatic cysts should always be performed, particularly if percutaneous drainage is being considered for treatment.

A number of vascular complications can occur in conjunction with pancreatitis. Thrombosis of the peripancreatic veins can arise as the result of compression and flow stasis. The splenic vein is involved most frequently, but the superior mesenteric vein may also be affected. Extension into the portal vein is also well described (Fig. 5-16). Splenic vein thrombosis should be suspected when-

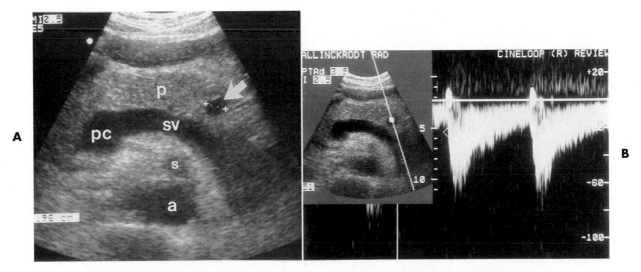

Fig. 5-14   Tortuous splenic artery simulating a pancreatic cyst. **A,** Transverse view of the pancreas *(p)* demonstrates a 1-cm, cystic-appearing structure *(arrow)* in the pancreatic tail. Also seen are the portosplenic confluence *(pc)*, splenic vein *(sv)*, superior mesenteric artery *(s)*, and aorta *(a)*. **B,** Pulsed-Doppler waveform analysis of the apparent cystic structure confirms arterial flow. On real-time color-Doppler scanning, this was shown to be a segment of a tortuous splenic artery that was viewed in cross-section.

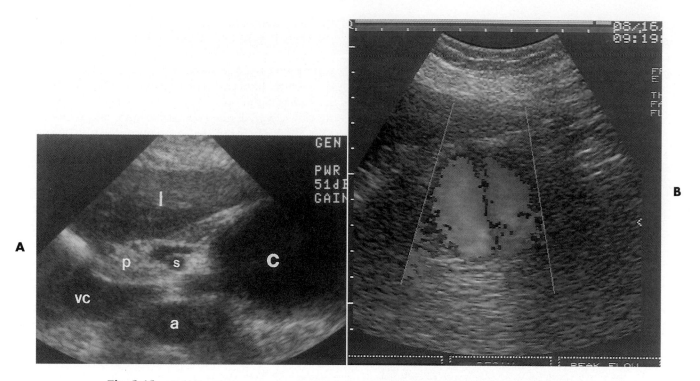

Fig. 5-15   Splenic artery aneurysm simulating a pancreatic cyst. **A,** Transverse view of the upper abdomen demonstrates a large cystic-appearing structure *(c)* in the left upper quadrant in the expected region of the pancreatic tail. The head of the pancreas *(p)* as well as the liver *(l)*, superior mesenteric artery *(s)*, aorta *(a)*, and inferior vena cava *(vc)* are also seen. **B,** Longitudinal Doppler view of the left upper quadrant demonstrates flow within the lumen of this cystic structure. The swirling pattern with flow both toward and away from the transducer is typical of flow within an aneurysm. Arteriography subsequently proved this was a large splenic artery aneurysm (see color insert, Plate 26).

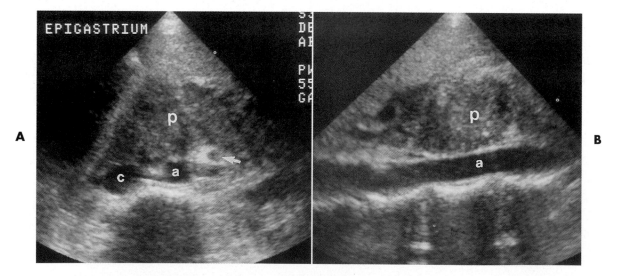

Fig. 5-16   Pancreatitis with associated venous thrombosis. **A,** Transverse view of the pancreas *(p)* demonstrates enlargement and decreased echogenicity. Despite the markedly abnormal gland, the fat plane between the pancreas and superior mesenteric artery *(arrow)* is maintained. Also seen are the aorta *(a)* and inferior vena cava *(c)*. **B,** Longitudinal view of the pancreatic head *(p)* again shows pancreatic enlargement and decreased pancreatic echogenicity. *a,* aorta

Continued.

ever gastric varices are seen in the absence of associated esophageal varices. This stems from the formation of collaterals that extend from the short gastric veins to the coronary vein and gastroepiploic veins. Pseudoaneurysms can also form as the result of erosion of the adjacent arteries produced by the proteolytic pancreatic enzymes. The splenic artery is involved most commonly, but any branch of the celiac axis can be affected. The gray-scale appearance of most pseudoaneurysms is indistinguishable from that of pseudocysts (Fig. 5-17). Detecting them sonographically requires a high level of suspicion combined with the Doppler evaluation of any cystic mass in or around the pancreas. Predominantly thrombosed pseudoaneurysms can be very difficult to diagnose correctly, as they can closely simulate the characteristics of solid pancreatic masses (Fig. 5-18). They should be suspected when a solid mass with a cystic component is identified.

Chronic pancreatitis is the permanent impairment of exocrine pancreatic function and permanent morphologic change in the gland as the result of persistent pan-

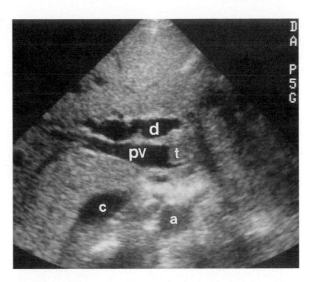

Fig. 5-16, cont'd.   **C,** Transverse view of the porta hepatis demonstrates a dilated common bile duct *(d)* and the portal vein *(pv)*. Thrombus *(t)* is seen in the extrahepatic portion of the portal vein. The aorta *(a)* and vena cava *(c)* are again seen.

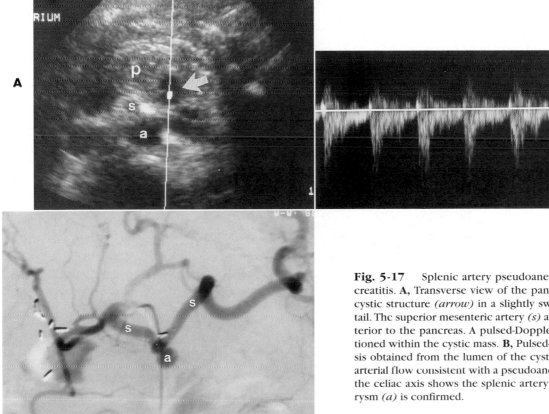

Fig. 5-17   Splenic artery pseudoaneurysm secondary to pancreatitis. **A,** Transverse view of the pancreas *(p)* demonstrates a cystic structure *(arrow)* in a slightly swollen pancreatic body or tail. The superior mesenteric artery *(s)* and aorta *(a)* are seen posterior to the pancreas. A pulsed-Doppler sample volume is positioned within the cystic mass. **B,** Pulsed-Doppler waveform analysis obtained from the lumen of the cystic mass confirms internal arterial flow consistent with a pseudoaneurysm. **C,** Arteriogram of the celiac axis shows the splenic artery *(s)*. A small pseudoaneurysm *(a)* is confirmed.

creatic inflammation. Pain may or may not be present and acute exacerbations may or may not occur.

The classic sonographic sign of chronic pancreatitis is pancreatic calcifications. These typically appear as multifocal punctate, hyperechoic foci in the pancreas (Fig. 5-19). Shadowing may or may not be present, depending on the size and extent of calcification (Fig. 5-20). Calcifications form as a consequence of increased pancreatic protein secretion and the subsequent calcification of intraductal protein plugs. Pancreatic calcifications occur commonly in the setting of alcoholic pancreatitis (20% to

40%) but rarely in the setting of gallstone pancreatitis (<2%). Although the pancreatic calcifications are intraductal, this is generally not apparent on ultrasound studies, which show them to be scattered in the pancreatic parenchyma. When calcifications erode from the small side branches into the main pancreatic duct, or form primarily in the main duct, they can cause pancreatic ductal obstruction and lead to persistent recurrent pancreatitis (Fig. 5-21).

Dilatation of the pancreatic duct is another sign of chronic pancreatitis. In many cases associated short stric-

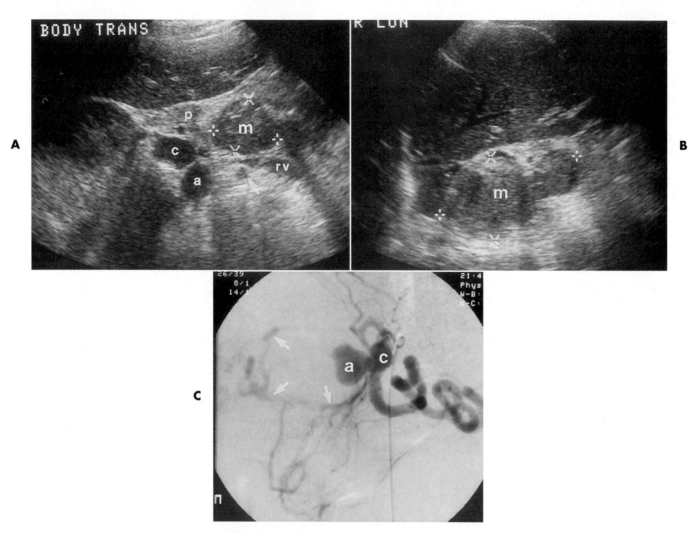

Fig. 5-18   Predominantly thrombosed pseudoaneurysm simulating a solid mass. **A,** Transverse view of the pancreas obtained from a right lateral approach demonstrates a solid-appearing mass *(m)* in the pancreatic body. The head of the pancreas *(p)* is seen to the right of the mass. Also identified are the aorta *(a)*, inferior vena cava *(c)*, superior mesenteric artery *(arrow)*, and left renal vein *(rv)*. **B,** Longitudinal view of the epigastric region demonstrates that the mass *(m)* has two components. The smaller component is centered over the body of the pancreas, but a larger component is seen extending into the suprapancreatic region. No cystic spaces were identified within this mass. **C,** Arteriogram of the celiac axis *(c)* demonstrates opacification of the lumen of a 1-cm pseudoaneurysm *(a)*. The thrombosed portion of the inferior component of the pseudoaneurysm is identified by an associated mass effect on the adjacent vessels *(arrows)*.

tures produce alternating areas of narrowing and dilatation that are referred to as a *chain of lakes.* Tortuosity of the pancreatic duct is also typical of chronic pancreatitis (Fig. 5-21). However, both of these patterns can be seen in patients with pancreatic carcinomas and associated ductal obstruction. Therefore a tortuous or beaded-appearing dilated duct should not be viewed as a pathognomonic sign of chronic pancreatitis.

As with acute pancreatitis, chronic pancreatitis can cause focal masses to develop that may be difficult to distinguish from cancers. The presence of calcifications is helpful in suggesting the diagnosis of focal pancreatitis, and an appropriate clinical history is also valuable (Fig. 5-22). Nevertheless, other diagnostic studies such as computed tomography (CT), ultrasound-guided biopsies, or ERCP are often required.

PANCREATIC CARCINOMA

Pancreatic carcinoma is adenocarcinoma arising from the ductal epithelium and constitutes more than 90% of all pancreatic tumors. Epithelial tumors arising from the acini are rare. Pancreatic carcinoma accounts for approximately 5% of all cancer deaths and is the fourth most common cause of cancer-related mortality, after lung, breast, and colon cancer. The 1-year survival is approximately 10%, with median survivals ranging from 3 to 8 months. Pancreatic carcinoma occurs primarily in elderly patients and is rare under the age of 40.

Most of the tumors arise in the pancreatic head and the typical presenting symptom in patients with tumors in this site is jaundice. Thirty percent of the tumors occur in the body and tail, and in this setting nonspecific symptoms such as weight loss and pain tend to be the presenting features. Tumors in the head may be detected when small because of the early biliary tract obstruction and jaundice that occur (Fig. 5-23). The strategic location of small tumors in the pancreatic head can cause early symptoms, and hence result in early detection and po-

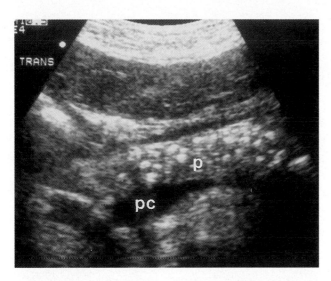

Fig. 5-19   Chronic calcific pancreatitis. Transverse view of the pancreas demonstrates multiple small hyperechoic foci scattered throughout the body of the pancreas *(p).* Note that there is minimal acoustic shadowing associated with these small calcific foci. The portosplenic confluence *(pc)* is seen posteriorly.

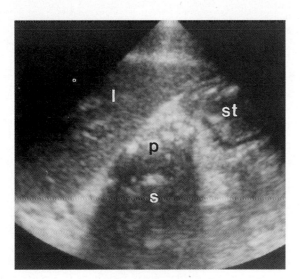

Fig. 5-20   Chronic calcific pancreatitis. Longitudinal view of the body of the pancreas *(p)* demonstrates multiple areas of increased echogenicity with a dense posterior shadow *(s)* from the entire substance of the gland. Also seen are the left lobe of the liver *(l)* and the stomach *(st).*

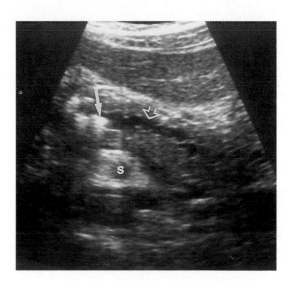

Fig. 5-21   Chronic pancreatitis with pancreatic duct calculus. Transverse view of the pancreas demonstrates a dilated and beaded pancreatic duct *(open arrow).* An echogenic shadowing stone *(arrow)* is seen in the duct, thereby accounting for the obstruction. The superior mesenteric artery *(s)* is seen posteriorly.

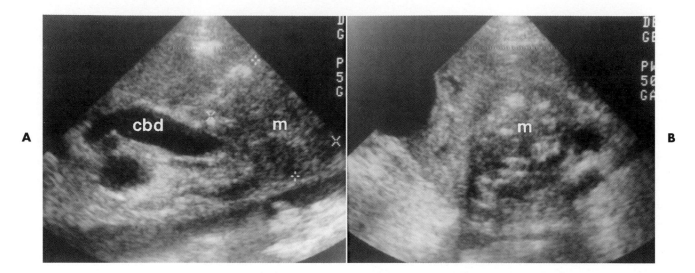

Fig. 5-22 Focal chronic pancreatitis. **A,** Longitudinal view of the right upper quadrant demonstrates a dilated common bile duct *(cbd)* that tapers to the level of an obstructing mass *(m)* in the pancreatic head. **B,** Transverse view of the mass *(m)* demonstrates multiple areas of increased echogenicity, some of which shadow partially. This makes chronic pancreatitis likely, and a clinical history of multiple past episodes of pancreatitis was obtained in this patient.

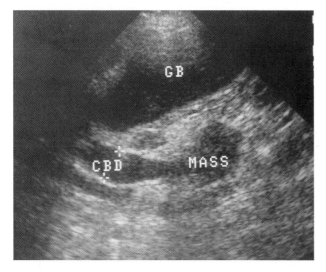

Fig. 5-23 Small pancreatic carcinoma. Longitudinal view of the right upper quadrant demonstrates a dilated common bile duct *(CBD)* that terminates at the level of a mass in the pancreatic head. In this patient the gallbladder *(GB)* was used as an acoustic window to visualize the distal common bile duct and mass. This mass measured 2 cm in diameter.

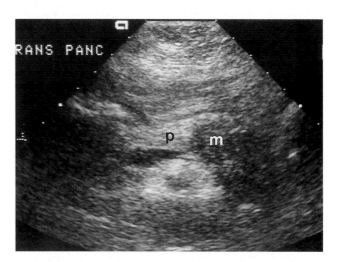

Fig. 5-24 Pancreatic carcinoma. Transverse view of the pancreas *(p)* demonstrates a hypoechoic mass *(m)* at the junction of the body and tail of the pancreas. This is the typical echogenicity of pancreatic carcinoma. The findings yielded by subsequent ultrasound-guided biopsy confirmed adenocarcinoma in this patient.

tential surgical cure. On the other hand, tumors in the body and tail tend to present as larger masses and are only rarely resectable.

Sonographically the vast majority of pancreatic cancers appear as hypoechoic masses when compared with the echogenicity of adjacent pancreatic parenchyma (Fig. 5-24). They may or may not distort the contour of the pan-

creas, depending on their size and location. Parenchymal atrophy may be present in the segment of pancreas distal to the tumor (Fig. 5-25). Obstruction of the pancreatic duct is a common finding in patients with pancreatic carcinoma. In general the duct appears less irregular and tortuous than does the ductal dilatation that is due to chronic pancreatitis (Fig. 5-25, *B*). However, there is over-

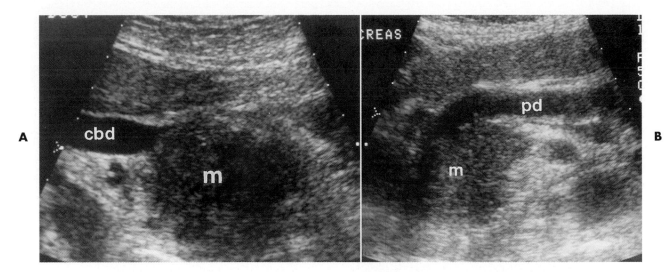

Fig. 5-25   Pancreatic carcinoma producing biliary and pancreatic ductal obstruction. **A,** Longitudinal view of the right upper quadrant demonstrates a dilated common bile duct *(cbd)* that terminates abruptly at the level of a mass *(m)* in the head of the pancreas. **B,** Transverse view of the pancreas again demonstrates the mass *(m)* in the region of the pancreatic head and uncinate process. A markedly dilated but smooth-walled pancreatic duct *(pd)* is identified in the pancreatic body. Note the marked atrophy of the pancreas, with essentially no normal pancreatic parenchyma seen surrounding the dilated pancreatic duct.

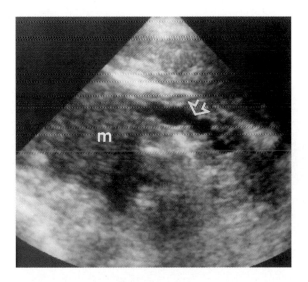

Fig. 5-26   Pancreatic carcinoma with pancreatic ductal dilatation. Transverse view of the pancreas demonstrates a hypoechoic mass *(m)* in the pancreatic head. A dilated tortuous pancreatic duct *(open arrow)* is seen in the pancreatic body and tail.

lap in the appearance of these diseases, and a careful search for a mass should be conducted in any patient with a dilated pancreatic duct (Fig. 5-26). Although sonography is similar to CT in its ability to identify cancer in those portions of the pancreas that can be well visualized sonographically, it cannot visualize the entire pancreas as

consistently as does CT. Therefore CT is the preferred imaging technique in patients with suspected pancreatic carcinoma. However, sonography is an extremely useful problem-solving tool in patients with equivocal CT results or in those with normal CT findings and a high suspicion of pancreatic carcinoma. ERCP is quite sensitive in detecting pancreatic cancer, but it is an invasive, costly procedure and can precipitate pancreatitis. In general it can be reserved for those patients whose CT and ultrasound findings are nondiagnostic or for patients requiring the placement of biliary or pancreatic duct stents.

In addition to detecting the primary tumor, sonography should be directed at identifying tumor spread. Although the criteria for determining resectability vary among surgeons, typical contraindications to surgery include the presence of hepatic or peritoneal metastases, the involvement of extrapancreatic vessels, invasion of adjacent organs other than the duodenum, and the presence of malignant ascites. Invasion of adjacent vessels generally takes the form of vascular encasement by hypoechoic soft tissue. This can be detected by gray-scale sonography supplemented by color-Doppler imaging (Fig. 5-27 [see also color insert, Plate 27]).

The differential diagnosis of hypoechoic pancreatic masses primarily includes pancreatic carcinoma and focal pancreatitis (Box 5-3). Focal pancreatitis can be excluded by the detection of metastases or vascular encasement. As mentioned earlier, the identification of scattered calcific foci in the hypoechoic mass makes focal chronic pancreatitis more likely. ERCP can provide useful information when the morphologic features revealed by ultrasound or CT studies overlap. Percutaneous biopsy findings are helpful when histologic analysis reveals malignancy, but normal biopsy findings do not exclude carcinoma. In addition to pancreatic carcinoma and focal pancreatitis, other uncommon lesions that produce pancreatic hypoechoic masses are other pancreatic tumors, metastases to the pancreas (Fig. 5-28), pancreatic lymphoma (Fig. 5-29), and peripancreatic lymph nodes.

ISLET CELL TUMORS

Endocrine tumors of the pancreas, referred to in the past as *APUD tumors* (*A*mine *P*recursor *U*ptake and *D*ecarboxylation), arise from the islets of Langerhans. They affect patients either because they are malignant and metastasize or because they produce excessive amounts of polypeptide hormones such as insulin, gastrin, glucagon, pancreatic polypeptide, and vasoactive intestinal peptide. Multiple islet cell tumors develop in patients with multiple endocrine neoplasm syndrome type I (MEN I).

Insulinomas account for 70% to 75% of islet cell tumors. They are usually small (<2 cm) and solitary, and 90% to 95% of them are benign. Patients exhibit symptoms related to hypoglycemia and are found to have elevated fasting levels of insulin. Like other islet cell tumors, insulinomas appear as hypoechoic solid masses. They can be located anywhere in the pancreas. The sensitivity of ultrasound studies varies widely, but in experienced hands they can detect up to 60% of insulinomas preoperatively. An intraoperative ultrasound study is the most sensitive

Box 5-3	Causes of Solid Hypoechoic Masses

Carcinoma
Focal pancreatitis
Lymphoma
Metastases
Islet cell tumors
Thrombosed aneurysms

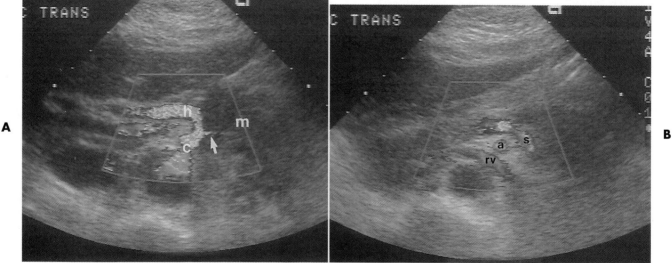

Fig. 5-27   Pancreatic carcinoma that involves the celiac axis but spares the superior mesenteric artery. **A,** Transverse Doppler view of the upper abdomen demonstrates the celiac axis *(c)* and hepatic artery *(h)*. A hypoechoic soft tissue mass *(m)* is seen obliterating the normal fat plane around these arteries. The soft tissue mass is also encasing and narrowing the origin of the splenic artery *(arrow)*. In this patient the primary mass arose at the junction of the body and tail of the pancreas and extended posteriorly to involve these vessels (see color insert, Plate 30). **B,** Transverse Doppler view slightly inferior to **A** shows the superior mesenteric artery *(a)* completely surrounded by echogenic fibrofatty tissue. At this level there is no evidence of arterial involvement. The splenic vein *(s)* and the left renal vein *(rv)* are also seen (see color insert, Plate 27).

means of imaging insulinomas, and can detect some tumors that are not palpable at surgery (Fig. 5-30).

Gastrinomas account for approximately 20% of islet cell tumors. Unlike insulinomas, most gastrinomas are malignant, with up to 40% of affected patients having metastatic disease at the time of diagnosis. Symptoms are due to excessive gastrin secretion, and include severe peptic ulcer disease and secretory diarrhea. Gastrinomas are small

tumors, and preoperative localization with sonography is limited. An intraoperative ultrasound study is useful for detecting lesions in the pancreas, but is significantly less sensitive in detecting extrapancreatic lesions that typically occur in the wall of the duodenum (Fig. 5-31).

Islet cell tumors that are nonfunctioning present as larger masses, usually with evidence of metastases at the time of diagnosis (Fig. 5-32). Approximately 20% of nonfunctioning islet cell tumors contain areas of calcification.

CYSTIC PANCREATIC NEOPLASMS

Cystic neoplasms of the pancreas account for less than 5% of pancreatic tumors. There are two types. Microcystic adenoma (serous cystadenoma and glycogen-rich cystadenoma) is a benign tumor seen predominantly in middle-aged and elderly women. It is a well-circumscribed and usually large mass (mean diameter, 10 cm) that contains multiple small cysts. A central stellate scar that may calcify is characteristic. Macrocystic adenoma (mucinous cystadenoma/cystadenocarcinoma) is either malignant or it is benign with a malignant potential. It occurs predominantly in middle-aged women, usually in the body or tail of the pancreas. It is typically made up of well-defined cysts containing thick mucinous fluid, internal septations, or mural nodules.

Because macrocystic tumors are malignant or premalignant, it is important to distinguish them from microcystic tumors. On sonograms macrocystic adenomas/adenocarcinomas generally appear as well-defined, pre-

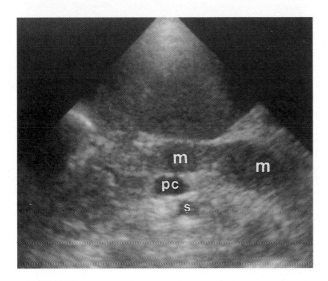

Fig. 5-28   Metastatic disease to the pancreas. Transverse view shows two hypoechoic masses *(m)* in the body of the pancreas. The primary tumor in this patient was renal cell carcinoma. *pc,* Portal splenic confluence; *s,* superior mesenteric artery.

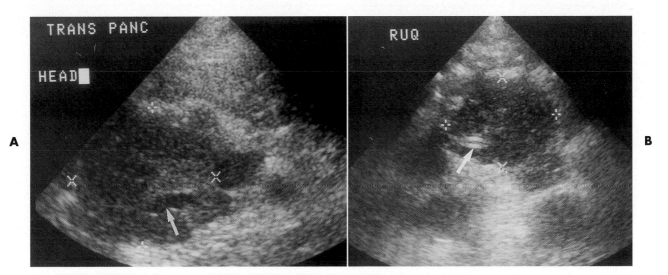

Fig. 5-29   Pancreatic lymphoma. **A,** Transverse view of the pancreatic head shows a large hypoechoic mass *(cursors)* in the pancreatic head. A dilated pancreatic duct *(arrow)* is seen. **B,** Longitudinal view of the pancreatic head shows the same mass *(cursors).* A stent *(arrows)* is in the common bile duct.

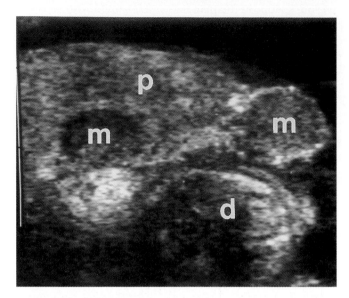

Fig. 5-30   Insulinomas. Longitudinal intraoperative scan shows the head of the pancreas *(p)* with two masses *(m)*. The inferior mass was palpable but the superior mass was not. Both were confirmed to be insulinomas on the basis of pathologic findings. The duodenum *(d)* is seen posteriorly.

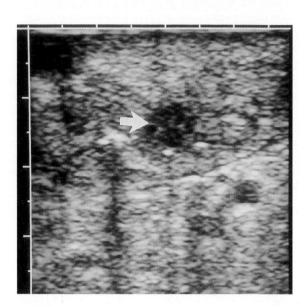

Fig. 5-31   Gastrinoma. Intraoperative scan of the duodenum shows a 6-mm mass *(arrow)* in the duodenal wall. This was resected and confirmed to be a gastrinoma on the basis of pathologic findings. No lesions were seen in the pancreas.

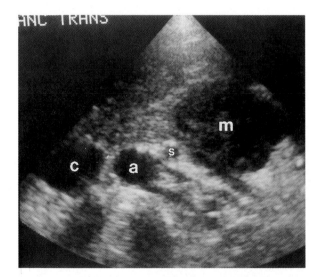

Fig. 5-32   Nonfunctioning islet cell tumor. Transverse view of the pancreas shows a large hypoechoic mass *(m)* in the junction of the body and tail. Also seen are the inferior vena cava *(c)*, aorta *(a)*, and superior mesenteric artery *(s)*.

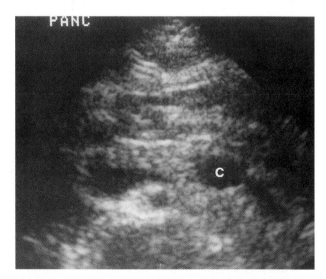

Fig. 5-33   Macrocystic adenoma. Transverse view of the pancreas shows a well-defined cyst *(c)* at the junction of the body and tail. This sonographic appearance is compatible with that of a pseudocyst, macrocystic adenoma, or a variety of other pancreatic cysts. The lack of a history of pancreatitis prompted surgery, at which this was proved to be a macrocystic adenoma. A distal pancreatectomy was performed because of the malignant potential of these lesions. The pathologic findings confirmed the diagnosis, and although atypical cells were seen, there was no evidence of malignancy.

dominantly cystic masses (Figs. 5-33 and 5-34). Internal septations are common but not uniformly present. Mural nodules and solid components may be seen, particularly in the frankly malignant lesions (Fig. 5-35). Peripheral calcification in the cyst wall is detected occasionally. The sonographic appearance of microcystic adenomas depends on the size of the cystic elements within the mass. When the internal cysts are very small, the mass itself will appear solid and may even be hyperechoic. When the internal cysts reach 5 to 10 mm in diameter, the mass itself appears multicystic (Fig. 5-36). Generally the individual

cysts are less than 2 cm in diameter and number more than six (Fig. 5-37). The central stellate scar seen on pathologic studies is generally difficult to identify sonographically.

Although sonography is relatively accurate in terms of the diagnosis and categorization of cystic pancreatic neoplasms, it is sometimes difficult to distinguish the neoplasms from one another or from pancreatic pseudocysts (Box 5-4). Necrotic pancreatic adenocarcinoma, adenocarcinomas with associated pseudocysts, solid and papillary epithelial neoplasm, and ductectatic carcinoma are also considerations. The clinical history is valuable in favoring a diagnosis of pseudocyst, as these patients frequently have a history of pancreatitis. Extrapancreatic signs of malignancy that are seen on imaging studies or are identified clinically are also useful because they would make the diagnosis of a macrocystic tumor much more likely (see Fig. 5-35, *B*).

Percutaneous biopsy and aspiration of pancreatic cystic tumors can be useful for diagnosis when mucin is detected either within the cells or in the fluid background of the tissue obtained. Because pancreatic pseudocysts often communicate with the ducts and cystic neoplasms rarely do so, ERCP can be useful in identifying these features.

RARE NEOPLASMS

Solid and papillary epithelial neoplasms of the pancreas are tumors that predominantly afflict young women. They are usually large tumors with a low-grade malignancy. They are solid lesions but characteristically have sizable cystic components that are due to hemor-

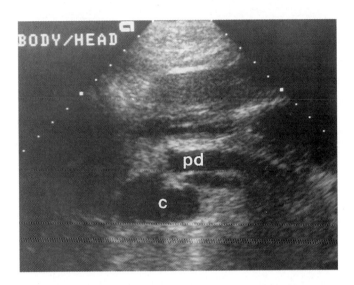

Fig. 5-34 Macrocystic mucinous adenocarcinoma. Transverse view of the pancreatic body and head shows a unilocular cystic mass *(c)* in the head. The pancreatic duct *(pd)* is dilated. This mass was resected and pathologic study revealed a well-differentiated mucinous cystadenocarcinoma.

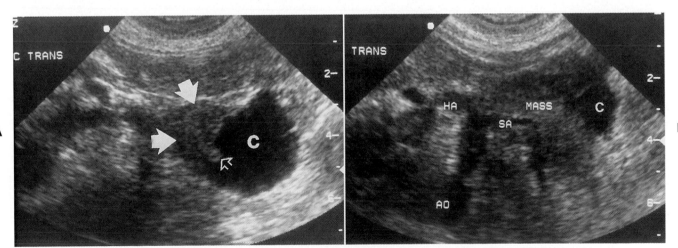

Fig. 5-35 Macrocystic mucinous adenocarcinoma. **A,** Transverse view of the pancreatic tail shows a large unilocular cyst *(c),* with a mural nodule *(open arrow)* and a solid component *(arrows).* **B,** Transverse view of the celiac axis shows the superior aspect of the cyst *(C)* and a soft tissue mass that encases the splenic artery *(SA).* Also seen are the aorta *(AO)* and the hepatic artery *(HA).*

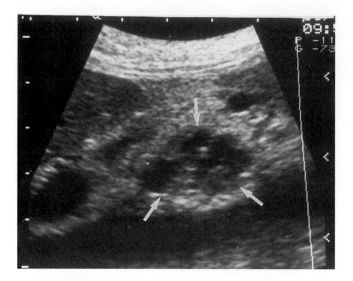

Fig. 5-36   Microcystic adenoma. Longitudinal view of the pancreatic head shows a hypoechoic mass *(arrows)* with some solid-appearing components and several small cystic components. This is a classic appearance of microcystic adenoma.

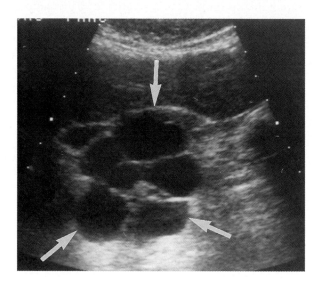

Fig. 5-37   Presumed microcystic adenoma. Transverse view through the region of the pancreatic head demonstrates a multicystic mass *(arrows)* with multiple variably sized internal cysts. This lesion has been monitored for many years. In that time it has shown minimal change and is presumed to be a microcystic adenoma. Further workup has not been attempted because there have been no symptoms and because of the patient's advanced age.

Box 5-4   Pancreatic Cystic Lesions

Pseudocyst
Macrocystic (mucinous) tumor
Microcystic (serous) tumors
Ductectatic carcinoma
Solid and papillary epithelial neoplasm
Autosomal dominant polycystic disease
von Hippel–Lindau disease
Cystic fibrosis
Aneurysm/pseudoaneurysm

rhage and necrosis. They should be considered whenever a complex solid and cystic mass is seen in a young woman who has no history of pancreatitis.

Ductectatic neoplasms are characterized by the massive mucinous distention of side branches of the pancreatic duct. The involved ductal epithelium is either hyperplastic and atypical or overtly malignant. They usually occur in the head and uncinate process of the pancreas. Unlike macrocystic neoplasms, there is no female predominance. They appear as nonspecific unilocular or multilocular cysts on sonography and CT. The ERCP findings can be diagnostic when mucinous material is seen draining from the pancreatic duct and dilated side branches are seen on a pancreatogram. When the tumor spreads into the main pancreatic duct or originally arises in the main duct, the main duct becomes dilated by the excess

Key Features

The echogenicity of the pancreas should be equal to or greater than that of the liver.

Pancreatitis is characterized by pancreatic enlargement, peripancreatic and retroperitoneal fluid collections, and decreased pancreatic echogenicity.

Complications of pancreatitis include biliary strictures, pseudocyst formation, splenic or portal vein thrombosis, splenic artery pseudoaneurysms, abscess, and pancreatic necrosis.

Chronic pancreatitis is characterized by pancreatic calcifications, ductal dilatation, and atrophy.

Pancreatic cancer and islet cell tumors are both typically hypoechoic.

mucin that is produced. This has been referred to as *mucin-hypersecreting carcinoma of the pancreas.*

SUGGESTED READINGS

Alpern MB, Sandler MA, Kellman GM, et al: Chronic pancreatitis: ultrasonic features, *Radiology* 155:215, 1985.

Bastid C, Sahel J, Sastre B, et al: Mucinous cystadenocarcinoma of the pancreas: ultrasonographic findings in 5 cases, *Acta Radiol* 30:45, 1989.

Bolondi L, LiBassi S, Saiani S, Barbara L: Sonography of chronic pancreatitis, *Radiol Clin North Am* 27:815, 1989.

Buck JL, Hayes WS: From the archives of the AFIP. Microcystic adenoma of the pancreas, *Radiographics* 10:313, 1990.

Campagno J, Oertel JE, Krezmar M: Solid and papillary epithelial neoplasm of the pancreas, probably of small duct origin: a clinicopathologic study of 52 cases [abstract], *Lab Invest* 40.248, 1979.

Campbell JP, Wilson SR: Pancreatic neoplasms: how useful is evaluation with US?, *Radiology* 167:341, 1988.

DelMaschio A, Vanzulli A, Sironi S, et al: Pancreatic cancer versus chronic pancreatitis: diagnosis with CA 19-9 assessment, US, CT and CT-guided fine-needle biopsy, *Radiology* 178:95, 1991.

Falkoff GE, Taylor KJW, Morse SS: Hepatic artery pseudoaneurysm: diagnosis with real-time and pulsed Doppler ultrasound, *Radiology* 58:55, 1986.

Freeny PC: Radiologic diagnosis and staging of pancreatic ductal adenocarcinoma, *Radiol Clin North Am* 27:121, 1989.

Friedman AC, Edmonds PR: Rare pancreatic malignancies, *Radiol Clin North Am* 27:15, 1989.

Friedman AC, Lichtenstein JE, Dachman AH: Cystic neoplasms of the pancreas. Radiological-pathologic correlation, *Radiology* 149:45, 1983.

Friedman AC, Lichtenstein JE, Fishman EK, et al: Solid and papillary epithelial neoplasm of the pancreas, *Radiology* 154:333, 1985.

Galiber AK, Reading CC, Charboneau JW, et al: Localization of pancreatic insulinoma: comparison of pre- and intraoperative US with CT and angiography, *Radiology* 166:405, 1988.

Glazer HS, Lee JKT, Balfe DM, et al: Non-Hodgkin lymphoma: computed tomographic demonstration of unusual extranodal involvement, *Radiology* 149:211, 1983.

Goekas MC: Etiology and pathogenesis of acute pancreatic inflammation: acute pancreatitis, *Ann Intern Med* 103:86, 1985.

Itai Y, Kokubo T, Atomi Y, et al: Mucin-hypersecreting carcinoma of the pancreas, *Radiology* 165:51, 1987.

Itai Y, Ohhashi K, Nagai H, et al: "Ductectatic" mucinous cystadenoma and cystadenocarcinoma of the pancreas, *Radiology* 161:697, 1986.

Jeffrey RB Jr: Sonography in acute pancreatitis, *Radiol Clin North Am* 27:5, 1989.

Jeffrey RB Jr, Laing FC, Wing VW: Extrapancreatic spread of acute pancreatitis: new observations with real-time US, *Radiology* 159:707, 1986.

Johnson CD, Stephens DH, Charboneau JW, et al: Cystic pancreatic tumors: CT and sonographic assessment, *AJR* 151:1133, 1988.

Jones SN, Lees WR, Frost RA: Diagnosis and grading of chronic pancreatitis by morphological criteria derived by ultrasound and pancreatography, *Clin Radiol* 39:43, 1988.

Mathieu D, Guigui B, Valette PJ, et al: Pancreatic cystic neoplasms, *Radiol Clin North Am* 27:163, 1989.

Norton JA, Cromack DT, Shawker TH: Intraoperative ultrasonographic localization of islet cell tumors, *Ann Surg* 207:160, 1988.

Ormson MJ, Charboneau JW, Stephens DH: Sonography in patients with a possible pancreatic mass shown on CT, *AJR* 148:551, 1987.

Ros PR, Hamrick-Turner JE, Chicchi MV, et al: Cystic masses of the pancreas, *Radiographics* 12:673, 1992.

Rossi P, Allison DJ, Bezzi M, et al: Endocrine tumors of the pancreas, *Radiol Clin North Am* 27:129, 1989.

Teefey SA, Stephens DH, Sheedy PF: CT appearance of primary pancreatic lymphoma, *Gastrointest Radiol* 11:41, 1987.

Warshaw AL, Compton CC, Lewandrowski K, et al: Cystic tumors of the pancreas. New clinical, radiologic, and pathologic observations in 67 patients, *Ann Surg* 212:432, 1990.

Warshaw AL, Swanson RS: Pancreatic cancer in 1988. Possibilities and probabilities, *Ann Surg* 208:541, 1988.

Wernecke K, Peters PE, Galanski M: Pancreatic metastases: ultrasound evaluation, *Radiology* 160:339, 1986.

White AF, Barum S, Buranasiri S: Aneurysms secondary to pancreatitis, *AJR* 127:393, 1976.

Wolfman NT, Ramquist NA, Karstaedt N, Hopkins MB: Cystic neoplasms of the pancreas: CT and sonography, *AJR* 138:37, 1992.

For a Key Features summary see p. 149.

ANATOMY

The spleen is an intraperitoneal organ that occupies the superior and lateral aspects of the left upper quadrant. It is normally in continuity with the diaphragm posteriorly, laterally, and superiorly. It contacts the kidney and splenic flexure inferiorly and the stomach and tail of the pancreas medially. The splenic artery arises from the celiac axis and travels along the posterior superior aspect of the pancreas toward the splenic hilum. It often becomes quite tortuous with aging. The splenic vein exits the spleen at the hilum and travels along the posterior aspect of the pancreas to form a confluence with the superior mesenteric vein and portal vein. The splenic vein is located slightly inferior to the splenic artery.

The splenic parenchyma appears very homogeneous on sonograms, and it is considerably more echogenic than the left kidney. It was thought that the spleen was equally echogenic to or less so than the liver, but it is now clear that the spleen is actually more echogenic than the liver.

The measurement of splenic size in the detection of splenomegaly has been the subject of much research, and a variety of methods have been proposed for doing this. In actual practice a length that exceeds 13 cm in a coronal plane is a reasonable cut-off between normal and enlarged. A thickness of 6 cm is also a useful cut-off when the length is borderline.

The shape of the spleen has a number of variations. The most common is a medial tubercle that extends as a tongue-shaped protrusion, usually positioned over the upper pole of the left kidney. On longitudinal scans this medial tubercle can occasionally be misconstrued to be a renal or adrenal mass. Splenules are also very common. They are supplied by branches of the splenic artery and usually arise immediately adjacent to the spleen, often near the splenic hilum. They tend to be round or ovoid and are isoechoic to the spleen (Fig. 6-1). They are more commonly seen in patients with splenomegaly. (See Table 6-1 for a summary of the normal characteristics of the spleen.)

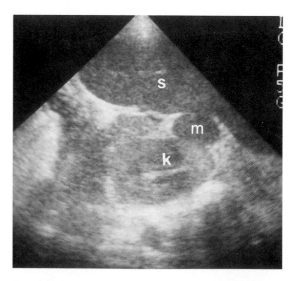

Fig. 6-1 Splenule. Transverse view of the left upper quadrant demonstrates an ovoid mass (*m*) positioned between the spleen (*s*) and left kidney (*k*). The mass is isoechoic to the spleen, and this appearance is consistent with that of a splenule. This should not be confused with an exophytic left renal mass. In this case the kidney is abnormally hyperechoic as the result of renal parenchymal disease.

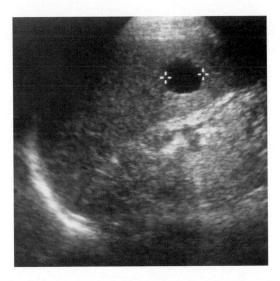

Fig. 6-2   Splenic cyst. Longitudinal view of the spleen demonstrates a well-defined anechoic mass *(cursors)* in the inferior aspect of the spleen. There are well-defined walls and good enhanced through-transmission.

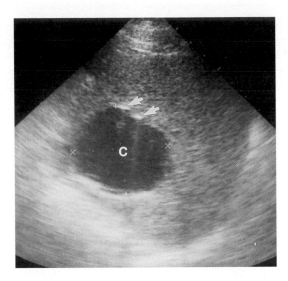

Fig. 6-3   Splenic cyst with wall calcification. Transverse view of the left upper quadrant demonstrates a cystic lesion *(c)* in the spleen. Note the highly echogenic foci *(arrows)* along the near wall of the cyst. These were shown by computed tomography to represent cyst wall calcifications.

TECHNIQUE

The spleen is generally best visualized from a high posterolateral intercostal approach with the patient supine. Failure to position the transducer superior and posterior enough is a common problem when sonographers and sonologists are inexperienced. In some patients the spleen is seen well from an anterolateral subcostal approach with the patient in a right lateral decubitus or right posterior oblique position. When scanning from a subcostal approach, a deep inspiration is often helpful in bringing the spleen further into the field of view. The right lateral decubitus and right posterior oblique positions should generally not be used when scanning from an intercostal approach as this causes the spleen to fall away from the chest and abdominal wall and causes aerated lung to migrate inferiorly and obscure an otherwise acceptable acoustic window.

CYSTS

Most splenic cysts result from trauma. They actually represent hematomas that have evolved into seromas and formed a pseudocapsule. Their appearance is similar to that of cysts in other organs, and this consists of the following characteristics: an anechoic lumen, well-defined walls, and increased through-transmission (Fig. 6-2). Cyst wall calcification is occasionally encountered, but if

Table 6-1   Normal characteristics

Characteristic	Normal finding
Size	≤13 cm long, ≤6 cm thick
Echogenicity	> Left kidney, > liver, >/< pancreas
Echotexture	Homogeneous
Surface	Smooth
Shape	Crescentic

found, this does not imply an increased risk of neoplasm (Fig. 6-3). True epithelial-lined cysts of the spleen are rare and are probably congenital. They are also referred to as *epidermoid cysts* because the wall generally contains squamous cells. Parasitic cysts can occur as the result of hydatid disease. These are an important consideration in persons living in endemic parts of the world, but are rare in residents of North America.

Pseudocysts of the pancreas can erode into the spleen and simulate the appearance of splenic cysts. As in any parenchymal organ, aneurysms, pseudoaneurysms, and vascular malformations can also mimic splenic cysts. Perisplenic cysts can arise from a variety of organs adjacent to the spleen. The most common are exophytic renal cysts and pancreatic pseudocysts (Fig. 6-4). Peritoneal-based cystic lesions such as endometriomas (Fig. 6-5) and metastatic ovarian carcinoma can also arise next to the spleen.

TUMORS

Primary splenic tumors are rare. Hemangiomas of the spleen occur but are much less common than they are in the liver. They are typically hyperechoic and homogeneous (Fig. 6-6) but are more variable in appearance than they are in the liver. Hemangiosarcomas are primary splenic malignancies that are extremely rare. They tend to be inhomogeneous in that they exhibit hyperechoic and hypoechoic areas. Splenic lymphangiomas are composed of multiple cystic spaces that vary in size. When the cysts are large enough, they will be seen as anechoic spaces, but collections of very small cysts will appear solid.

Lymphoma commonly involves the spleen in a unifocal (Fig. 6-7), multifocal (Fig. 6-8), or diffuse manner. Focal lesions are usually hypoechoic. Diffuse involvement of the spleen produces splenomegaly. Sonography is insen-

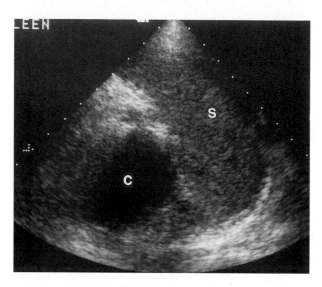

Fig. 6-4 Perisplenic pancreatic pseudocyst. Transverse view of the left upper quadrant demonstrates the spleen *(s)* and a poorly marginated cystic lesion *(c)* in the region of the splenic hilum. This represented an evolving pseudocyst in a patient with pancreatitis.

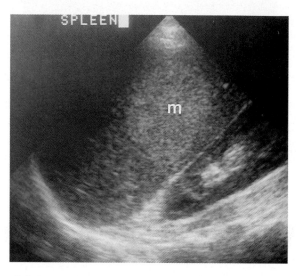

Fig. 6-6 Splenic hemangioma. Longitudinal view of the spleen demonstrates a homogeneous hyperechoic mass *(m)*. This mass was found to be stable over many years, and this behavior is most consistent with a hemangioma.

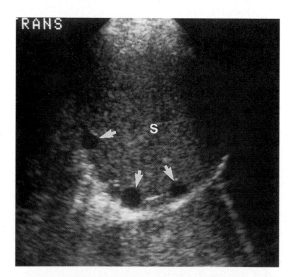

Fig. 6-5 Perisplenic endometriosis. Transverse view of the left upper quadrant demonstrates the superior aspect of the spleen *(s)* and multiple small cystic lesions *(arrows)* between the spleen and the diaphragm. Laparoscopic findings confirmed the diagnosis of endometriosis.

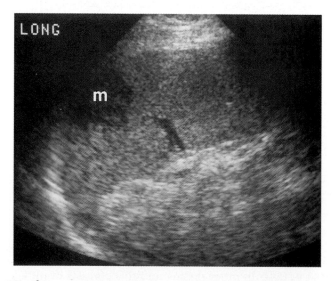

Fig. 6-7 Splenic lymphoma. Longitudinal view of the spleen demonstrates a hypoechoic mass *(m)* in the superior aspect of the spleen. This patient had biopsy-proven large cell lymphoma.

sitive in its ability to detect splenic lymphoma, but the detection of focal hypoechoic lesions is a relatively specific sign of splenic involvement in patients with known lymphoma.

Metastatic disease to the spleen is much less common than that to the liver. Overall the spleen is the tenth most common organ involved by metastatic spread. Generally, splenic metastases are believed to arise from hematoge-

nous routes. Melanoma is the primary tumor most likely to spread to the spleen, although the more common tumors such as lung, breast, and colon account for the majority of splenic metastases. In most cases splenic metastases occur in the setting of widespread metastases elsewhere in the body. The sonographic appearance of splenic metastases is quite variable, and all of the patterns exhibited by hepatic metastases are also exhibited by splenic metastases.

Besides tumors, other causes of multiple splenic masses include abscesses, sarcoidosis (Fig. 6-9), and extramedullary hematopoiesis. Due to the concave nature of the splenic hilum, partial volume effects can occasionally cause the higher-amplitude echoes from the hilum to appear intrasplenic and simulate the characteristics of a mass (Fig. 6-10). This potential pitfall can be averted by correlating longitudinal and transverse images. (See Box 6-1 for a listing of solid spleen lesions.)

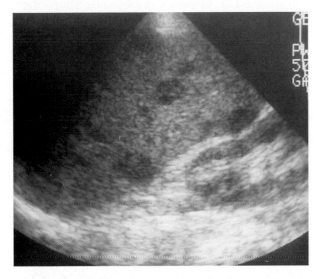

Fig. 6-8   Splenic lymphoma. Longitudinal view of the left upper quadrant demonstrates multiple hypoechoic lesions in the spleen. This patient also had hepatic masses. Findings from biopsy of the hepatic lesions revealed lymphoma.

Box 6-1 Solid Spleen Lesions	
Hemangiomas	Infarcts
Hemangiosarcomas	Abscesses
Lymphomas	Sarcoidosis
Metastases	Extramedullary hematopoiesis

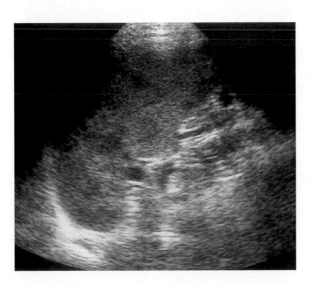

Fig. 6-9   Splenic sarcoid. Longitudinal view of the spleen demonstrates multiple poorly defined, hypoechoic lesions. This patient also had diffuse hepatic involvement as well as typical pulmonary sarcoidosis, which was proved by biopsy findings.

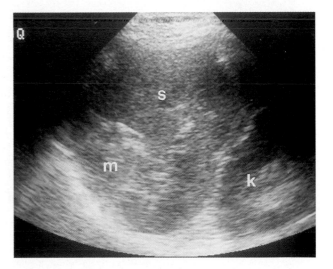

Fig. 6-10   Splenic pseudolesion. Longitudinal view of the left upper quadrant demonstrates the spleen *(s)* and upper pole of the left kidney *(k)*. An apparent hyperechoic mass *(m)* is seen in the spleen. The findings from real-time evaluation as well as transverse imaging confirmed that this represented fibrofatty tissue in the splenic hilum that appeared as an intrasplenic lesion on this longitudinal view because of the effects of volume averaging.

SPLENOMEGALY

A large number of processes can result in spleno-megaly, and a partial list of them is given in Box 6-2. In most cases it is not possible to determine the cause of splenic enlargement on the basis of the findings from the sonographic analysis of the spleen itself (Fig. 6-11 [see color insert, Plate 28]). Analysis of associated findings may, however, provide clues to the cause of spleno-megaly.

Box 6-2 Causes of Splenomegaly	
COMMON	**UNCOMMON**
Heart failure	Glycogen storage disease
Portal hypertension	Malaria
Leukemia	Myelofibrosis
Lymphoma	
Hepatitis	
Mononucleosis	
Hemolytic anemias	

INFECTIONS

Splenic abscesses are uncommon and probably due to the efficient phagocytic activity of its reticuloen-dothelial system leukocytes. However, these defenses may be insufficient in the settings of bacterial endo-carditis, septicemia, immunologic deficiencies, intra-venous drug abuse, and splenic trauma. Splenic abscesses tend to appear on sonograms as complex fluid-filled le-sions. However, they can also appear as hypoechoic solid lesions (Fig. 6-12). As with abscesses elsewhere, the dif-ferential diagnosis primarily includes hematoma and necrotic tumor.

Fungal abscesses of the spleen have an appearance similar to that of fungal abscesses in the liver. They are typically small and may appear as a target lesion (Fig. 6-13). Granulomatous infection of the spleen can occur in the settings of tuberculosis and histoplasmosis. In both situations multiple small punctate areas of increased echogenicity are seen and these represent calcifications.

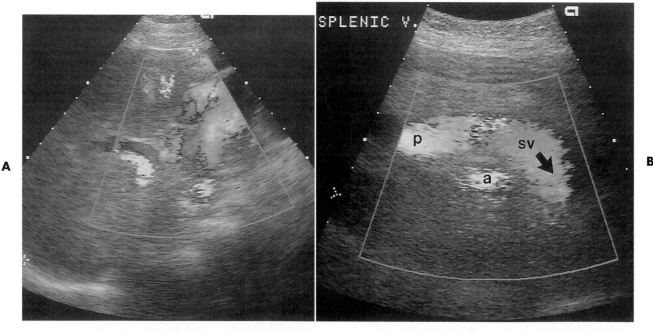

Fig. 6-11   Splenomegaly. **A,** Longitudinal view of the left upper quadrant demonstrates mild spleno-megaly with a splenic length of 14 cm. There are also prominent vessels in the splenic hilum dis-played on a color-Doppler study. Based on the findings in this image, the splenomegaly could be due to a number of factors. The prominent hilar vascularity suggests portal hypertension, but spleno-megaly stemming from other causes can also result in increased splenic blood flow and enlargement of the splenic hilar vessels (see also color insert, Plate 28). **B,** Transverse view of the epigastrium dem-onstrates the splenic vein *(sv)* and portosplenic confluence *(p)*. Blood flow in the splenic vein is re-versed *(arrow)* and traveling away from the portosplenic confluence. This is convincing evidence of portal hypertension with the development of splenic vein-to-systemic vein collaterals. A splenorenal shunt was subsequently identified in this patient. Also seen is the superior mesenteric artery *(a)*.

TRAUMA

The spleen is the most commonly involved organ in victims of upper abdominal trauma. Splenic disruption can occur with or without capsular laceration. If the capsule remains intact, an intraparenchymal or subcapsular hematoma may develop. Laceration of the splenic capsule can result in hemoperitoneum as well as splenic hematomas. In a trauma patient, the finding of localized fluid around the spleen suggests splenic laceration regardless of the sonographic appearance of the spleen.

Splenic hematomas, subcapsular hematomas, and perisplenic hematomas all vary in their sonographic appearance, depending on their age. In the acute phase they appear complex and hypoechoic. With clot formation they appear more echogenic and may be isoechoic to the splenic parenchyma. With time the clot lyses and liquefies and becomes more hypoechoic to anechoic. Although sonography is relatively sensitive in its ability to detect splenic lacerations and ruptures, it is significantly less accurate than computed tomography in its ability to determine the extent of an abnormality. In addition, it is more difficult to assess the other upper abdominal organs with sonography than with contrast-enhanced computed tomography. Therefore sonography has not been used extensively in North America to evaluate patients with suspected trauma to the abdomen.

One important pitfall to be aware of is the elongated left hepatic lobe that crosses the midline and insinuates itself between the spleen and the diaphragm. Because the liver is less echogenic than the spleen, this anatomic variant can give the false impression of a perisplenic or splenic subcapsular fluid collection (Fig. 6-14). In general, knowledge of this pitfall is sufficient to avert a diagnostic error. In addition, the detection of vascular structures running through the hepatic parenchyma can help in distinguishing it from perisplenic fluid.

A condition that may develop after splenic trauma is splenosis, and this consists of the implantation of splenic tissue onto intraperitoneal surfaces, with subsequent vascularization and growth. The end-result is the development of macroscopic nodules of splenic tissue. Like the spleen itself, these nodules are very homogeneous in their echogenicity and are usually round or ovoid (Fig. 6-15). The differential diagnosis includes other intraperitoneal masses. If there is a history of splenic trauma or splenic surgery, splenosis should be considered likely. Tagged damaged red blood cell scans can be used for confirmation in confusing cases.

INFARCTION

Splenic infarctions stem from an embolic phenomenon as well as from thrombosis of the splenic artery,

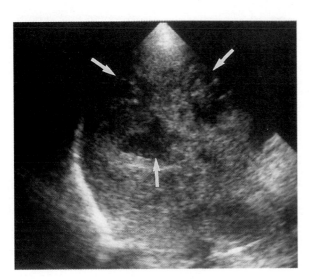

Fig. 6-12   Splenic abscess. Longitudinal view of the left upper quadrant demonstrates an inhomogeneous but predominantly hypoechoic mass *(arrows)* in the spleen. This patient was an intravenous drug abuser who had sustained several left rib fractures secondary to a recent motor vehicle accident.

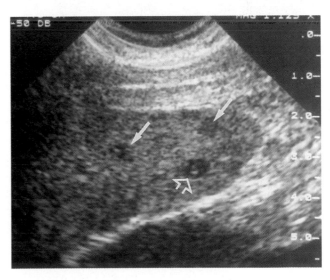

Fig. 6-13   Fungal abscess. Longitudinal view of the inferior aspect of the spleen demonstrates several lesions less than 1 cm in diameter *(arrows)*. The most prominent of these *(open arrow)* contains a central echogenic focus. This appearance is typical of *Candida* abscesses in the spleen and liver.

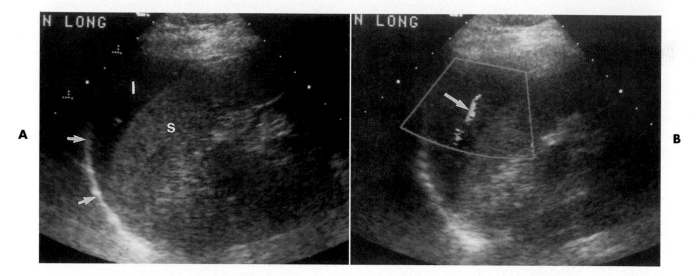

Fig. 6-14   Pseudo–perisplenic fluid. **A,** Longitudinal view of the left upper quadrant demonstrates the spleen *(s)* and an elongated left hepatic lobe *(l)* insinuating itself between the spleen and the diaphragm *(arrows).* The markedly decreased echogenicity of the liver versus that of the spleen could result in this anatomic variant being misinterpreted as perisplenic fluid. **B,** Gray-scale reproduction of a color-Doppler image demonstrates a portal vein *(arrow)* within the hepatic parenchyma. This confirms that this is liver and not a perisplenic fluid collection.

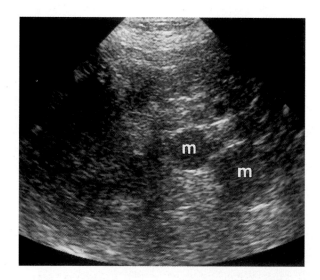

Fig. 6-15   Splenosis. Transverse view of the left upper quadrant demonstrates two adjacent hypoechoic masses *(m).* No spleen was identified, and it was later discovered that the patient had undergone a splenectomy many years ago because of splenic trauma. The two masses identified are consistent with the appearance of splenosis, and in retrospect were noted to be present and unchanged on old computed tomographic scans.

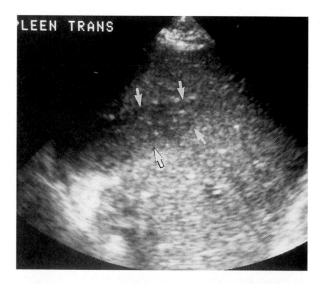

Fig. 6-16   Focal splenic infarction. Transverse view of the spleen demonstrates a wedge-shaped hypoechoic region that extends to the periphery of the spleen. This patient had bacterial endocarditis, and the sonographic finding is most consistent with the appearance of a splenic infarction.

splenic vein, and their branches. They are one of the most common causes of focal splenic lesions seen on cross-sectional images. Infarcts appear hypoechoic in the acute phase. With time scar formation causes them to become hyperechoic. When a wedge-shaped, peripherally located splenic lesion is identified, an infarct should be considered (Fig. 6-16). Complete infarction of the spleen can be more difficult to detect sonographically. However, as with focal infarcts, an alteration in splenic echogenicity can be a clue to an underlying infarct (Fig. 6-17).

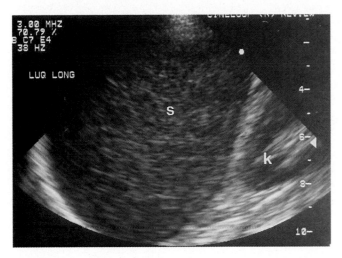

Fig. 6-17   Complete splenic infarction. Longitudinal view of the left upper quadrant demonstrates the spleen *(s)* and upper pole of the left kidney *(k)*. Note that the spleen is isoechoic to the renal cortex. In addition to the decreased splenic echogenicity, the splenic echotexture is also coarsened. Subsequent computed tomography demonstrated completely absent enhancement of the spleen due to splenic artery thrombosis.

Key Features

The spleen is normally more echogenic than the liver.
Splenic cysts are most frequently the result of prior episodes of trauma and hematoma formation.
Focal splenic masses have a variety of sonographic appearances, none of which is specific.
Ultrasound is an effective means of detecting splenomegaly, but in the absence of associated findings, it is not capable of distinguishing among the many potential causes.
Splenic abscesses share the sonographic characteristics of abscesses elsewhere in the body, ranging in appearance from solid-appearing masses to markedly or minimally complex fluid collections.
Splenic infarcts are common, and range from being hypoechoic in the acute stage to hyperechoic in the chronic phase. They may or may not appear wedge shaped.

SUGGESTED READINGS

Costello P, Kane RA, Oster J, et al: Focal splenic disease demonstrated by ultrasound and computed tomography, *J Can Assoc Radiol* 36:22, 1985.

Crivello MS, Peterson IM, Austin RM: Left lobe of the liver mimicking perisplenic collections, *J Clin Ultrasound* 14:697, 1986.

Dodds WJ, Taylor AJ, Erickson SJ et al: Radiologic imaging of splenic anomalies, *AJR* 155:805, 1990.

Goerg C, Schwerk WB: Splenic infarction: sonographic patterns, diagnosis, follow-up, and complications, *Radiology* 174:803, 1990.

Georg C, Schwerk WB, Goerg K: Splenic lesions: sonographic patterns, follow-up, differential diagnosis, *Eur J Radiol* 13:59, 1991.

Goerg C, Schwerk WB, Goerg K. Sonography of focal lesions of the spleen, *AJR* 156:949, 1991.

Li DK, Cooperberg PL, Graham MF, Callen P: Pseudo perisplenic "fluid collections": a clue to normal liver and spleen echogenic texture, *J Ultrasound Med* 5:397, 1986.

Maillard JC, Menu Y, Scherrer A, et al: Intraperitoneal splenosis: diagnosis by ultrasound and computed tomography, *Gastrointest Radiol* 14:179, 1989.

Maresca G, Mirk P, DeGaetano AM, et al: Sonographic patterns in splenic infarction, *J Clin Ultrasound* 14:23, 1986.

Pastakia B, Shawker TH, Thalar M, et al: Hepatosplenic candidiasis: wheels within wheels, *Radiology* 166:417, 1988.

Ross PR, Moser RP, Dackman AH, et al: Hemangioma of the spleen: radiologic-pathologic correlation in ten cases, *AJR* 162:73, 1987.

OBSTETRICS

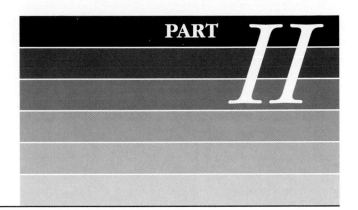

PART

II

CHAPTER 7

Guidelines to Obstetrical Examination and Appropriate Measurements

Equipment
Documentation
Guidelines for First-Trimester Sonography
Guidelines for Second- and Third-Trimester Sonography

Obstetric ultrasound examinations are performed by sonographers and sonologists (radiologists and obstetricians) who possess varied experience and use different equipment. An attempt to standardize the obstetric ultrasound study took place in 1985 when the American College of Radiology (ACR) and the American Institute of Ultrasound in Medicine (AIUM) approved examination guidelines. These guidelines have recently been updated, with some modifications. Although technical notes have been issued by the American College of Obstetrics and Gynecology, there has been no formal acknowledgment or endorsement of these guidelines.

Although it is not possible for sonography to detect all in utero problems, most of the significant abnormalities can be detected with a systematic approach. A uniform approach is necessary in all pregnant women, regardless of clinical history, as most of those with an abnormal fetus have no predisposing risk factors.

It had originally been suggested that the obstetric examination could be divided into two levels of study. In this concept, which was first developed in 1977 in conjunction with maternal serum alpha-fetoprotein (MSAFP) screening programs, level 1 sonography was to be used to detect obstetric problems resulting in elevated MSAFP levels (twins, incorrect dates, and fetal demise), with level 2 sonography reserved for identification of the fetal anomalies causing the elevated levels of MSAFP (open neural tube defects and abdominal wall defects). Many practitioners unfortunately misinterpreted the difference between level 1 and level 2 examinations as connoting a difference in skill and ability, in that, although it might be acceptable to have a level 1 study performed by someone with little expertise and inferior equipment, a level 2 study needed more operator experience and better machinery. To make matters more complicated, some practitioners dealing with complex cases declared themselves "level 3" examiners, a designation with no defined meaning. The concept of levels was therefore never properly applied and has further lost its validity. It is therefore recommended that this terminology be discarded.

Using the ACR/AIUM guidelines as a framework, the routine ultrasound obstetric examination in its updated version is described here. The standard anatomic views and their importance are stressed, and routine fetal biometry is also described, with measurement tables included.

EQUIPMENT

Studies should be performed with real-time scanners, using a transabdominal or transvaginal approach, or both. A transducer of appropriate frequency ($\geq$3 MHz for transabdominal examination or $\geq$5 MHz for transvaginal studies) should be used. The choice of frequency is a trade-off between beam penetration (better at lower frequencies) and resolution (better at higher frequencies). In general the highest frequency that still affords adequate penetration should be selected. The lowest ultrasound exposure settings should be used to gain necessary diagnostic information.

DOCUMENTATION

Adequate documentation is essential for ensuring appropriate patient care. A permanent record of the ultrasound images must be established that includes the measurements and anatomic findings of these guidelines. Images should be labeled with the examination date, patient's name or identification number, and image orientation, if needed. A written report of the ultrasound findings should be prepared and included in the patient's medical record.

GUIDELINES FOR FIRST-TRIMESTER SONOGRAPHY

1. The location of the gestational sac should be documented, the embryo identified, and the crown-rump length recorded.

In obstetric ultrasound examinations, the gestational age is equivalent to the fetal and menstrual age, all starting from the day of onset of the woman's last normal menstrual period. The gestational sac can routinely be identified transabdominally at 5 weeks' gestation and 1 to 2 weeks earlier transvaginally. Gestational age can be determined from measurement of the sac (Table 7-1). If the sac is round, only one measurement is needed, obtained from the inner-to-inner edge of the hyperechoic rim (Fig. 7-1). If the sac is ovoid, as is often the case, usually due to a mass effect from the distended bladder, three orthogonal measurements are averaged (Fig. 7-2). Although not as extensively studied as the characteristics of the embryo, the average sac diameter has been shown to have the same accuracy, ± 5 to 7 days. The smallest gestational sacs and their gestational ages have not been fully worked out. Although one of the earliest studies established a 10-mm sac diameter at 5 weeks' gestation, others have shown the gestational sac to be smaller at 5 weeks, even as small as 2 mm (Table 7-2).

To analyze the embryo, its long axis or crown-rump length is measured and compared to the gestational age (Fig. 7-3). A reanalysis has not led to a significant change from these earlier results (Table 7-3). This is discussed more completely in Chapter 9.

2. Presence or absence of fetal life should be reported.

Fetal life can be detected by the real-time observation of heart activity. Further documentation is not necessary, although M-mode cardiac ultrasound can be recorded. Cardiac activity should be evident in all embryos with a crown-rump length of 9 mm or more transabdominally and of 5 mm transvaginally, equivalent to 6.9 and 6.2 weeks, respectively. At 5 to 6 weeks, the heart rate should be 100 beats/min, rising to between 140 to 160 beats/min by 8 weeks. This rate is maintained throughout the rest of the first trimester and should not be less than 90 beats/min at 5 to 6 weeks or less than 120 beats/min by 8 weeks.

3. Fetal numbers should be documented.

Multiple gestations can be determined accurately through a careful analysis of the number of embryos and

Text continued on p. 158.

Table 7-1 Gestational sac measurement

Mean predicted gestational sac (mm)	Gestational age* (wks)
10	5.0
11	5.2
12	5.3
13	5.5
14	5.6
15	5.8
16	5.9
17	6.0
18	6.2
19	6.3
20	6.5
21	6.6
22	6.8
23	6.9
24	7.0
25	7.2
26	7.3
27	7.5
28	7.6
29	7.8
30	7.9
31	8.0
32	8.2
33	8.3
34	8.5
35	8.6
36	8.8
37	8.9
38	9.0
39	9.2
40	9.3
41	9.5
42	9.6
43	9.7
44	9.9
45	10.0
46	10.2
47	10.3
48	10.5
49	10.6
50	10.7
51	10.9
52	11.0
53	11.2
54	11.3
55	11.5
56	11.6
57	11.7
58	11.9
59	12.0
60	12.2

*Gestational age (wks) = (Gestational sac [mm] + 25.43)/7.02. (This formula was expressed in centimeters in its original form.)
From Hellman LM et al: Growth and development of the human fetus prior to the 20th week of gestation, *Am J Obstet Gynecol* 103:789-800, 1969.

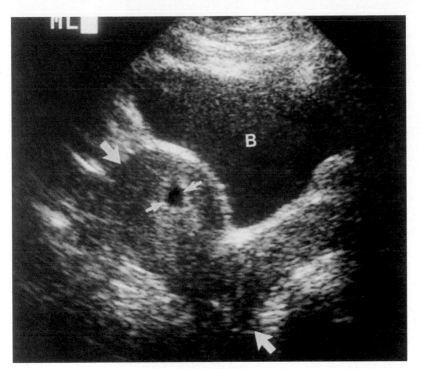

Fig. 7-1   Normal round early gestational sac, imaged transabdominally at less than 5 weeks. The uterus *(large arrows)* is shown in this sagittal view with the gestational sac normally positioned high in the body. The sac is anechoic and has a hyperechoic rim. Only one measurement of a round sac is needed, and this is taken in the anechoic space *(small arrows). B,* urinary bladder.

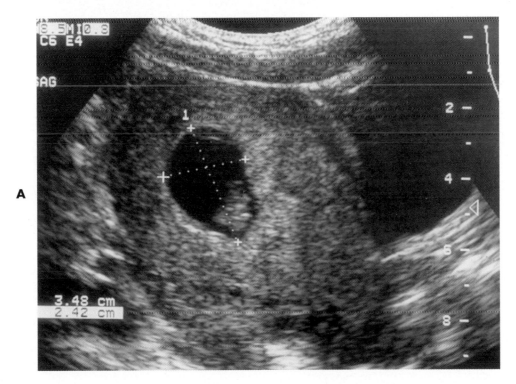

Fig. 7-2   Normal ovoid gestational sac, imaged transabdominally at 8 weeks' gestation. **A,** Sagittal view.   *Continued.*

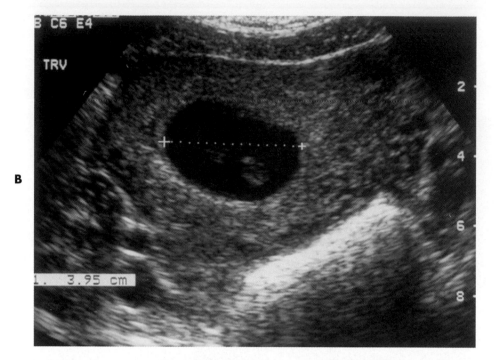

Fig. 7-2, cont'd. **B,** Transaxial view. Both views demonstrate the three orthogonal measurements (+) that should be averaged to obtain the mean diameter of the gestational sac.

Table 7-2   Mean diameter of gestational sac and corresponding estimates of gestational age*

Mean sac diameter (mm)	Mean gestational age (wk)	Gestational age (days)	
		Mean	95% confidence interval
2	5.0	34.9	34.3-35.5
3	5.1	35.8	35.2-36.3
4	5.2	36.6	36.1-37.2
5	5.4	37.5	37.0-38.0
6	5.5	38.4	37.9-38.9
7	5.6	39.3	38.9-39.7
8	5.7	40.2	39.8-40.6
9	5.9	41.1	40.7-41.4
10	6.0	41.9	41.6-42.3
11	6.1	42.8	42.5-43.2
12	6.2	43.7	43.4-44.0
13	6.4	44.6	44.3-44.9
14	6.5	45.5	45.2-45.8
15	6.6	46.3	46.0-46.6
16	6.7	47.2	46.9-47.5
17	6.9	48.1	47.8-48.4
18	7.0	49.0	48.6-49.4
19	7.1	49.9	49.5-50.3
20	7.3	50.8	50.3-51.2
21	7.4	51.6	51.2-52.1
22	7.5	52.5	52.0-53.0
23	7.6	53.4	52.9-53.9
24	7.8	54.3	53.7-54.8
25	7.9	55.2	54.6-55.7
26	8.0	56.0	55.4-56.7
27	8.1	56.9	56.3-57.6
28	8.3	57.8	57.1-58.5
29	8.4	58.7	58.0-59.4
30	8.5	59.6	58.8-60.4

*The mean gestational age was calculated from a regression equation.

From Daya S et al: Early pregnancy assessment with transvaginal ultrasound scanning, *Can Med Assoc J* 144:441-445, 1991.

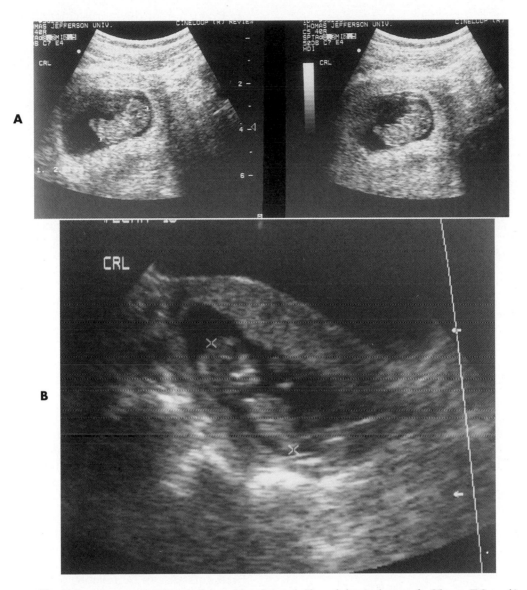

Fig. 7-3   Crown-rump length, denoted by pluses. **A,** Transabdominal scan of a 25-mm (7.2-week) embryo with normal heart motion. **B,** Transabdominal scan of a 57-mm (11.7-week) fetus. Note the better evaluation of the anatomic characteristics by the end of the first trimester.

Table 7-3 Predicted menstrual age from crown-rump length measurements from 5.7 to 12 weeks*

Crown-rump length (mm)	Menstrual age (wk)
2	5.7
3	5.9
4	6.1
5	6.2
6	6.4
7	6.6
8	6.7
9	6.9
10	7.1
11	7.2
12	7.4
13	7.5
14	7.7
15	7.9
16	8.0
17	8.1
18	8.3
19	8.4
20	8.6
21	8.7
22	8.9
23	9.0
24	9.1
25	9.2
26	9.4
27	9.5
28	9.6
29	9.7
30	9.9
31	10.0
32	10.1
33	10.2
34	10.3
35	10.4
36	10.5
37	10.6
38	10.7
39	10.8
40	10.9
41	11.0
42	11.1
43	11.2
44	11.2
45	11.3
46	11.4
47	11.5
48	11.6
49	11.7
50	11.7
51	11.8
52	11.9
53	12.0
54	12.0

*The 95% confidence interval is ±8% of the predicted age.
From Hadlock FP et al: Fetal crown-rump length: reevaluation of relation to menstrual age (5-8 weeks) with hi-res real-time ultrasound, *Radiology* 182:501-505, 1992.

the number of gestational sacs. Overestimations may occur if fluid in the endometrial cavity or the normal separation of the amnion and chorion is misinterpreted as a sac. Underestimation may also occur, particularly if there are more than two closely situated gestations on transabdominal images. In these cases transvaginal scanning will often be of diagnostic value.

4. Evaluation of the uterus (including the cervix) and adnexal structures should be performed.

The size and location of fibroids need to be noted and monitored, as they tend to enlarge during pregnancy. In the first trimester they are most likely to cause gestational sac malposition and miscarriage.

The most common adnexal mass, the corpus luteum cyst, tends to be less than 3 cm in diameter, is sonographically cystic in appearance, and tends to resolve by the mid–second trimester (Fig. 7-4). Noncystic adnexal masses should be evaluated for echogenicity and size. Surgical removal during pregnancy, usually in the second trimester, may be necessary in the event of a solid or complex mass (if there is a possible malignant potential) or of a large cul-de-sac mass (if there is a possibility of birth canal obstruction at term).

GUIDELINES FOR SECOND- AND THIRD-TRIMESTER SONOGRAPHY

1. Fetal life, number, and presentation should be documented.

As with first-trimester pregnancies, fetal life can be documented by the real-time observation of heart motion. M-mode ultrasound studies can be used, but this is not required. However, when an abnormal heart rate or rhythm is noted, it should probably be documented with M-mode studies. The sustained normal heart rate should be 140 to 160 beats/min throughout the second and third trimester. A rate of more than 180 or less than 120 beats/min should be considered potentially problematic at any time. However, mild transient episodes of bradycardia are usually normal.

Fetal number can be reliably documented. The amnionicity and chorionicity of multiple gestations is important information because it helps to assess the potential risk of complications associated with monoamniotic or monochorionic-diamniotic pregnancies. This is discussed in depth in Chapter 16. The comparison of fetal sizes as described in the guidelines is discussed later under item 4.

The fetal lie (presentation) should be recorded. The most common is cephalic (vertex) and is the most favorable one for a normal vaginal delivery. Breech and transverse lies are not uncommon early in pregnancy, but at

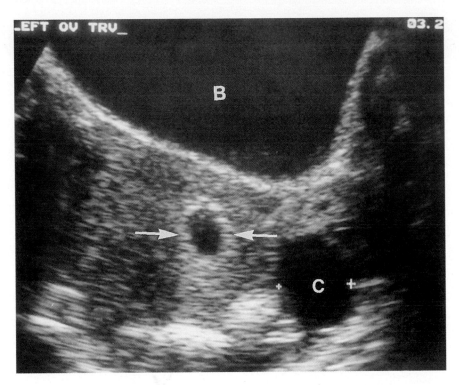

Fig. 7-4   Corpus luteum cyst of pregnancy *(C)*. Transaxial image shows an early intrauterine gestational sac *(arrows)* and a simple 2.2-cm cyst within the left ovary. *B*, urinary bladder.

term decrease in incidence to 3% to 4% and 0.25% to 0.5%, respectively. At term the fetal lie can have significant implications for the obstetric management, as it may determine the mode of delivery and whether fetal repositioning should be attempted.

2. An estimate of the amount of amniotic fluid (increased, decreased, or normal) should be reported.

Estimation of the amount of amniotic fluid is important, as either an excess or decreased amount is associated with increased perinatal morbidity and mortality. This estimate can be accurately performed both qualitatively (subjectively) and quantitatively (by measurement). This is discussed in Chapter 8.

3. The placenta location and appearance and its relationship to the internal cervical os should be recorded.

The placenta has a uniform hyperechoic echogenicity with a thin, very hyperechoic chorionic plate separating it from the amniotic fluid. The relationship of the placenta to the internal cervical os should be documented. If the placenta is not seen to extend to or cover the internal os on the initial transabdominal views (usually performed through a full or partially full urinary bladder), then a previa is excluded. If, however, the placenta is low-lying or

appears to cover the os, the patient should completely void because a distended bladder may have falsely elongated the lower uterine segment, giving the impression that the placenta covers the internal os. The study should be repeated transabdominally (through the amniotic fluid), transvaginally, or translabially. If a previa is still present, it should be deemed partial if it goes up to and only slightly covers the os or complete if it fully covers the os. A complete previa rarely changes position during pregnancy. However, a partial previa seen early in the second trimester may resolve, perhaps due to differential growth of the lower uterine segment.

The cervix should also be evaluated during routine imaging of the lower uterine segment to determine whether there is foreshortening or widening of the internal os, both signs of cervical incompetence. Precise measurements that identify incompetency are not available, however. Although not specifically mentioned in the guidelines, the placenta should also be carefully examined for evidence of abruption, which is the premature separation of the placenta from its myometrial attachment.

4. Gestational age should be assessed using a combination of biparietal diameter (or head circumference) and femur length. Fetal growth and weight (as opposed to age) should be assessed in the third trimester and should include abdominal

Table 7-4 Composite biparietal diameter table

Biparietal diameter (mm)	Gestational age (wk)		Biparietal diameter (mm)	Gestational age (wk)	
	Mean*	Range 90% variation†		Mean*	Range 90% variation†
20	12.0	12.0	61	24.2	22.6 to 25.8
21	12.0	12.0	62	24.6	23.1 to 26.1
22	12.7	12.2 to 13.2	63	24.9	23.4 to 26.4
23	13.0	12.4 to 13.6	64	25.3	23.8 to 26.8
24	13.2	12.6 to 13.8	65	25.6	24.1 to 27.1
25	13.5	12.9 to 14.1			
			66	26.0	24.5 to 27.5
26	13.7	13.1 to 14.3	67	26.4	25.0 to 27.8
27	14.0	13.4 to 14.6	68	26.7	25.3 to 28.1
28	14.3	13.6 to 15.0	69	27.1	25.8 to 28.4
29	14.5	13.9 to 15.2	70	27.5	26.3 to 28.7
30	14.8	14.1 to 15.5			
			71	27.9	26.7 to 29.1
31	15.1	14.3 to 15.9	72	28.3	27.2 to 29.4
32	15.3	14.5 to 16.1	73	28.7	27.6 to 29.8
33	15.6	14.7 to 16.5	74	29.1	28.1 to 30.1
34	15.9	15.0 to 16.8	75	29.5	28.5 to 30.5
35	16.2	15.2 to 17.2			
			76	30.0	29.0 to 31.0
36	16.4	15.4 to 17.4	77	30.3	29.2 to 31.4
37	16.7	15.6 to 17.8	78	30.8	29.6 to 32.0
38	17.0	15.9 to 18.1	79	31.1	29.9 to 32.5
39	17.3	16.1 to 18.5	80	31.6	30.2 to 33.0
40	17.6	16.4 to 18.8			
			81	32.1	30.7 to 33.5
41	17.9	16.5 to 19.3	82	32.6	31.2 to 34.0
42	18.1	16.6 to 19.8	83	33.0	31.5 to 34.5
43	18.4	16.8 to 20.2	84	33.4	31.9 to 35.1
44	18.8	16.9 to 20.7	85	34.0	32.3 to 35.7
45	19.1	17.0 to 21.2			
			86	34.3	32.8 to 36.2
46	19.4	17.4 to 21.4	87	35.0	33.4 to 36.6
47	19.7	17.8 to 21.6	88	35.4	33.9 to 37.1
48	20.0	18.2 to 21.8	89	36.1	34.6 to 37.6
49	20.3	18.6 to 22.0	90	36.6	35.1 to 38.1
50	20.6	19.0 to 22.2			
			91	37.2	35.9 to 38.5
51	20.9	19.3 to 22.5	92	37.8	36.7 to 38.9
52	21.2	19.5 to 22.9	93	38.8	37.3 to 39.3
53	21.5	19.8 to 23.2	94	39.0	37.9 to 40.1
54	21.9	20.1 to 23.7	95	39.7	38.5 to 40.9
55	22.2	20.4 to 24.0			
			96	40.6	39.1 to 41.5
56	22.5	20.7 to 24.3	97	41.0	39.9 to 42.1
57	22.8	21.1 to 24.5	98	41.8	40.5 to 43.1
58	23.2	21.5 to 24.9			
59	23.5	21.9 to 25.1			
60	23.8	22.3 to 25.5			

*Weighted least mean square fit equation: biparietal diameter (mm) = 34.5701 + 5.0157GA – 0.00441GA^2 (*GA*, mean gestational age).
†For each biparietal diameter, 90% of gestational age data points fell within this range.
From Kurtz AB et al: Analysis of biparietal diameter as an accurate indicator of gestational age, *J Clin Ultrasound* 8:319-326, 1980.

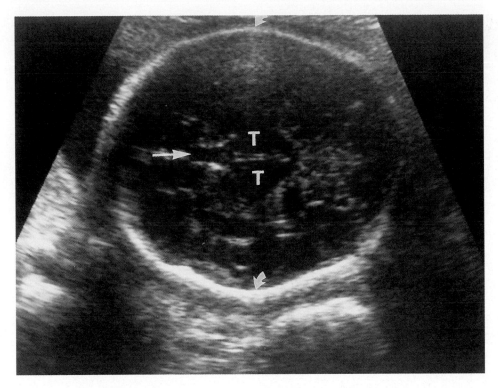

Fig. 7-5   Biparietal diameter. Transaxial image of the fetal head in the late second trimester, at the level of the thalami *(T)*. The biparietal diameter is measured from the leading edge to the leading edge *(curved arrows)*. The cavum septum pellucidum is also seen *(straight arrow)*.

diameters or circumferences. If previous studies have been performed, an estimate of the appropriateness of the interval change should be made.

a. Biparietal diameter at a standard reference level (which should include the cavum septum pellucidum and the thalamus) should be measured and recorded.

b. Head circumference is measured at the same level as the biparietal diameter.

c. Femur length should be measured routinely and recorded after 14 weeks' gestation.

d. Abdominal circumference should be determined at the level of the junction of the umbilical vein and portal sinus.

The gestational age assessment in the second and third trimesters (assuming no first-trimester study has been done) is primarily achieved by the measurement of the biparietal diameter (BPD). The BPD is obtained in a transaxial view, measured from the leading edge to the leading edge or from the outer edge of the closer temporoparietal bone to the inner edge of the farther temporoparietal bone (Fig. 7-5). The BPD is then compared to the gestational age and a mean age and a range around this mean are determined (Table 7-4).

The accuracy of the BPD is based on a normal head shape. If the fetal head is unusually rounded (brachycephalic) or elongated (dolichocephalic), the BPD will ei-

ther cause the gestational age to be overestimated or underestimated, respectively. To correct this inaccuracy, a second linear measurement is obtained from the same image as the BPD—the frontooccipital diameter (FOD). Using both measurements, a cephalic index (CI) (Fig. 7-6) is calculated by the formula: $CI = (BPD/FOD) \times 100$. The mean CI is 78.3 and the normal range is 70 to 86 at 2 standard deviations. For the purposes of this correction, both the BPD and FOD should ideally be obtained from outer edge to outer edge. In actuality the BPD is usually not remeasured but is kept as an outer-to-inner edge measurement.

If the CI as computed is at or beyond the limits of 70 and 86, the guidelines suggest one of two corrections: (1) an area-corrected BPD to correct the BPD measurement to an ideal head shape using the formula: $BPD_a = [(BPD \times FOD/1.265)]^{1/2}$ or (2) a head circumference (HC), obtained by tracing the perimeter of the calvarium with a digitizer (map reader) (Fig. 7-7) using the formula for the circumference of a circle: $\pi(BPD + FOD)/2 = (BPD + FOD) \times 1.57$. Both HC techniques have an equal technical accuracy and come within approximately 2% of the actual measurement. Reference can then be made to any standard table of HCs (Table 7-5).

The BPD measurement in the second trimester (up to 24 weeks) is accurate to ±5 to 7 days, the same as that of the first-trimester crown-rump length. By the third

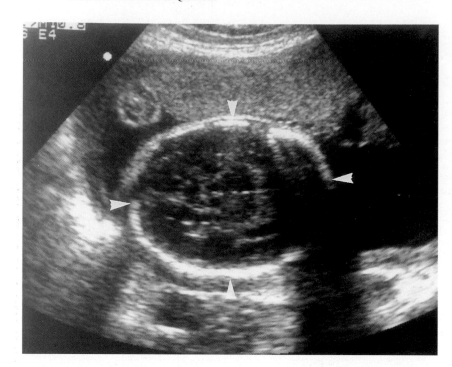

Fig. 7-6   Cephalic index *(CI)*. In the same transthalamic plane as the biparietal diameter, arrowheads denote the position of the outer-to-outer edge of the calvarium, where the biparietal and frontooccipital diameters are measured.

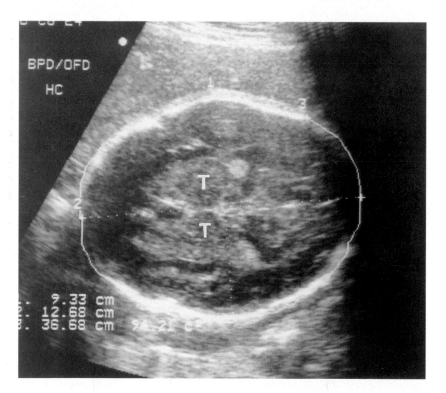

Fig. 7-7   Head circumference. Transaxial image of the fetal head in the late third trimester, at the level of the thalami *(T)*. The circumference is traced around the outer margin of the calvarium.

trimester, particularly after 30 weeks, the accuracy of the BPD decreases to ±2 weeks and new approaches ±4 weeks by term. When the HC is used, its accuracy is equivalent to that of the corrected BPD.

The femur length is an indicator of skeletal growth and can also be used to establish gestational age. The femur

is a linear structure and it is measured along its ossified shaft (diaphysis), disregarding the epiphyseal cartilages (Fig. 7-8). It is preferably obtained using a linear or phased-array transducer to eliminate the potential distortion that can be caused by some mechanical sector scanners as they age. The normal diaphysis has a straight lateral and

Table 7-5 Head circumference measurement

Head circumference (mm)	Gestational age (wk) Predicted mean values	Head circumference (mm)	Gestational age (wk) Predicted mean values
80	13.4	230	24.9
85	13.7	235	25.4
90	14.0	240	25.9
95	14.3	245	26.4
100	14.6	250	26.9
105	15.0	255	27.5
110	15.3	260	28.0
115	15.6	265	28.1
120	15.9	270	29.2
125	16.3	275	29.8
130	16.6	280	30.3
135	17.0	285	31.0
140	17.3	290	31.6
145	17.7	295	32.2
150	18.1	300	32.8
155	18.4	305	33.5
160	18.8	310	34.2
165	19.2	315	34.9
170	19.6	320	35.5
175	20.0	325	36.3
180	20.4	330	37.0
185	20.8	335	37.7
190	21.2	340	38.5
195	21.6	345	39.2
200	22.1	350	40.0
205	22.5	355	40.8
210	23.0	360	41.6
215	23.4		
220	23.9		
225	24.4		

Gestational age (wk)	Variability (wk) at 95% confidence limits
12 to 18	± 1.3
18 to 24	± 1.6
24 to 30	± 2.3
30 to 36	± 2.7
36 to 42	± 3.4

From Hadlock FP et al: Fetal head circumference: relation to menstrual age. *AJR* 138:649-653, 1982.

curved medial border. If measured medially, a straight measurement is still obtained that disregards the curvature. The femur length is considered to be as accurate as the BPD after 26 weeks, and can therefore be substituted for it when the BPD is considered unreliable for technical or pathologic reasons (Table 7-6). A more common use of the femur length is to analyze its proportionality to the

BPD, which can detect skeletal dysplasias and growth disturbances (Table 7-7).

The fetal abdomen is measured transaxially at the level of the fetal liver, using as a landmark the umbilical portion of the left portal vein at its junction with the portal sinus (Fig. 7-9). This vein should be imaged entirely within the liver and equidistant from the sides of the ab-

Text continued on p. 168.

Table 7-6   Femur and humerus measurement

Bone length (mm)	Gestational age (wk)			
	Femur		Humerus	
	Predicted mean value	Range from 5th to 95th percentile	Predicted mean value	Range from 5th to 95th percentile
10	12.6	10.4 to 14.9	12.6	9.9 to 15.3
11	12.9	10.7 to 15.1	12.9	10.1 to 15.6
12	13.3	11.1 to 15.6	13.1	10.4 to 15.9
13	13.6	11.4 to 15.9	13.6	10.9 to 16.1
14	13.9	11.7 to 16.1	13.9	11.1 to 16.6
15	14.1	12.0 to 16.4	14.1	11.4 to 16.9
16	14.6	12.4 to 16.9	14.6	11.9 to 17.3
17	14.9	12.7 to 17.1	14.9	12.1 to 17.6
18	15.1	13.0 to 17.4	15.1	12.6 to 18.0
19	15.6	13.4 to 17.9	15.6	12.9 to 18.3
20	15.9	13.7 to 18.1	15.9	13.1 to 18.7
21	16.3	14.1 to 18.6	16.3	13.6 to 19.1
22	16.6	14.4 to 18.9	16.7	13.9 to 19.4
23	16.9	14.7 to 19.1	17.1	14.3 to 19.9
24	17.3	15.1 to 19.6	17.4	14.7 to 20.1
25	17.6	15.4 to 19.9	17.9	15.1 to 20.6
26	18.0	15.9 to 20.1	18.1	15.6 to 21.0
27	18.3	16.1 to 20.6	18.6	15.9 to 21.4
28	18.7	16.6 go 20.9	19.0	16.3 to 21.9
29	19.0	16.9 to 21.1	19.4	16.7 to 22.1
30	19.4	17.1 to 21.6	19.9	17.1 to 22.6
31	19.9	17.6 to 22.0	20.3	17.6 to 23.0
32	20.1	17.9 to 22.3	20.7	18.0 to 23.6
33	20.6	18.3 to 22.7	21.1	18.4 to 23.9
34	20.9	18.7 to 23.1	21.6	18.9 to 24.3
35	21.1	19.0 to 23.4	22.0	19.3 to 24.9
36	21.6	19.4 to 23.9	22.6	19.7 to 25.1
37	22.0	19.9 to 24.1	22.9	20.1 to 25.7
38	22.4	20.1 to 24.6	23.4	20.6 to 26.1
39	22.7	20.6 to 24.9	23.9	21.1 to 26.6
40	23.1	20.9 to 25.3	24.3	21.6 to 27.1
41	23.6	21.3 to 25.7	24.9	22.0 to 27.6
42	23.9	21.7 to 26.1	25.3	22.6 to 28.0
43	24.3	22.1 to 26.6	25.7	23.0 to 28.6
44	24.7	22.6 to 26.9	26.1	23.6 to 29.0
45	25.0	22.9 to 27.1	26.7	24.0 to 29.6

From Jeanty P et al: Estimation of gestational age from measurements of fetal long bones, *J Ultrasound Med* 3:75-79, 1984.

Table 7-6	Femur and humerus measurement—cont'd

| | Gestational age (wk) | | | |
| | Femur | | Humerus | |
Bone length (mm)	Predicted mean value	Range from 5th to 95th percentile	Predicted mean value	Range from 5th to 95th percentile
46	25.4	23.1 to 27.6	27.1	24.6 to 30.0
47	25.9	23.6 to 28.0	27.7	25.0 to 30.6
48	26.1	24.0 to 28.4	28.1	25.6 to 31.0
49	26.6	24.4 to 28.9	28.9	26.0 to 31.6
50	27.0	24.9 to 29.1	29.3	26.6 to 32.0
51	27.4	25.1 to 29.6	29.9	27.1 to 32.6
52	27.9	25.6 to 30.0	30.3	27.6 to 33.1
53	28.1	26.0 to 30.4	30.9	28.1 to 33.6
54	28.6	26.4 to 30.9	31.4	28.7 to 34.1
55	29.1	26.9 to 31.3	32.0	29.1 to 34.7
56	29.6	27.2 to 31.7	32.6	29.9 to 35.3
57	29.9	27.7 to 32.1	33.1	30.3 to 35.9
58	30.3	28.1 to 32.6	33.6	30.9 to 36.4
59	30.7	28.6 to 32.9	34.1	31.4 to 36.9
60	31.1	28.9 to 33.3	34.9	32.0 to 37.6
61	31.6	29.4 to 33.9	35.3	32.6 to 38.1
62	32.0	29.9 to 34.1	35.9	33.1 to 38.7
63	32.4	30.1 to 34.6	36.6	33.9 to 39.3
64	32.9	30.7 to 35.1	37.1	34.4 to 39.9
65	33.4	31.1 to 35.6	37.7	35.0 to 40.6
66	33.7	31.6 to 35.9	38.3	35.6 to 41.1
67	34.1	32.0 to 36.4	38.9	36.1 to 41.7
68	34.6	32.4 to 36.9	39.6	36.9 to 42.3
69	35.0	32.6 to 37.1	40.1	37.4 to 42.9
70	35.6	33.3 to 37.7	—	—
71	35.9	33.7 to 38.1	—	—
72	36.4	34.1 to 38.6	—	—
73	36.9	34.6 to 39.0	—	—
74	37.3	35.1 to 39.6	—	—
75	37.7	35.6 to 39.9	—	—
76	38.1	36.0 to 40.4	—	—
77	38.6	36.4 to 40.9	—	—
78	39.1	36.9 to 41.3	—	—
79	39.6	37.3 to 41.7	—	—
80	40.0	37.9 to 42.1	—	—

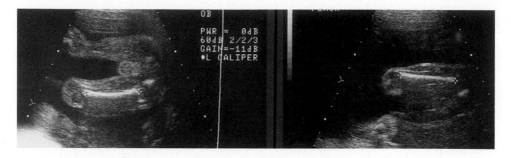

Fig. 7-8 Femur lengths. The end-points of the ossified diaphyseal shaft are shown (+). The right image is of the straight lateral margin and the left is of the curved inner margin of a femur. Both are measured linearly, disregarding any curvature.

Table 7-7   Fetal long bone measurement

| | True mean and range from 5th to 95th percentile (mm) (2 standard deviation) | | | | | |
| | Biparietal diameter | | Femur | | Humerus | |
Gestational age (wk)	True mean	2 Standard deviations	True mean	2 Standard deviations	True mean	2 Standard deviations
13	23	20 to 26	11	9 to 13	10	8 to 12
14	27	24 to 30	13	11 to 15	12	10 to 14
15	30	29 to 31	15	13 to 17	14	12 to 16
16	33	31 to 35	19	16 to 22	17	15 to 19
17	37	34 to 40	22	19 to 25	20	16 to24
18	42	37 to 47	25	22 to 28	23	20 to 26
19	44	40 to 48	28	25 to 31	26	23 to 29
20	47	43 to 51	31	28 to 34	29	26 to 32
21	50	45 to 55	35	31 to 39	32	28 to 36
22	55	50 to 60	36	33 to 39	33	30 to 36
23	58	53 to 63	40	36 to 44	37	34 to 40
24	61	56 to 66	42	39 to 45	38	34 to 42
25	64	59 to 69	46	43 to 49	42	38 to 46
26	68	63 to 73	48	44 to 52	43	40 to 46
27	70	67 to 73	49	46 to 52	45	43 to 47
28	73	68 to 78	53	48 to 58	47	43 to 51
29	76	71 to 81	53	48 to 58	48	44 to 52
30	77	71 to 83	56	53 to 59	50	45 to 55
31	82	75 to 89	60	54 to 66	53	49 to 57
32	85	79 to 91	61	55 to 68	54	50 to 58
33	86	82 to 90	64	59 to 69	56	51 to 61
34	89	84 to 94	66	60 to 72	58	53 to 63
35	89	82 to 96	67	61 to 73	59	53 to 65
36	91	84 to 98	70	63 to 77	60	54 to 66
37	93	84 to 102	72	68 to 76	61	57 to 65
38	95	89 to 101	74	68 to 80	64	61 to 67
39	95	89 to 101	76	68 to 84	65	59 to 71
40	99	92 to 107	77	73 to 81	66	62 to 70
41	97	91 to 103	77	73 to 81	66	62 to 70
42	100	95 to 105	78	71 to 83	68	61 to 75

From Merz E, Kim-Kern M, Pehl S: Ultrasonic mensuration of fetal limb bones in the second and third trimester, *J Clin Ultrasound* 15:175-183, 1987.

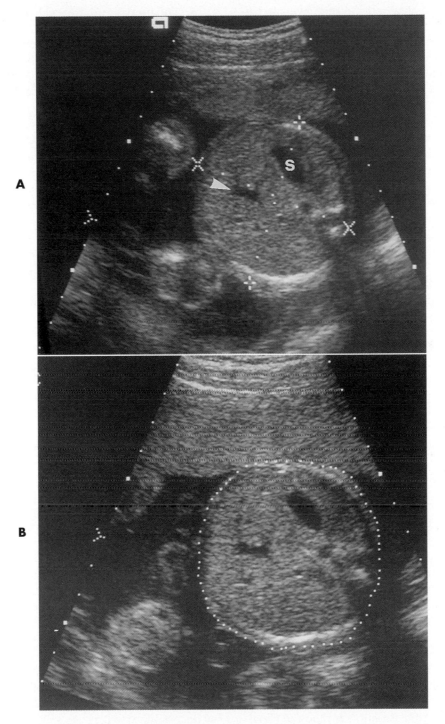

Fig. 7-9   Abdominal diameter/circumference. Transaxial view of the upper abdomen at 25 weeks. **A,** The umbilical portion of the left portal vein *(arrowhead)* is equidistant from the sides of the abdomen. The outer-to-outer edge measurement of the abdominal diameter is shown (+ and *x*). *s,* stomach. **B,** The abdominal circumference can be calculated or traced (as in this case) along its outer margin *(dotted circle)*.

domen, with the abdominal diameter measured from outer edge to outer edge. If the abdomen is round, one measurement will suffice; if it is ovoid, two orthogonal measurements should be obtained and then averaged. If necessary, the abdominal circumference can then be computed either by tracing the abdomen with a map reader (digitizer) or by using the same equation for the circumference of a circle. Abdominal measurements have not been shown to be as accurate as head and femur measurements from the standpoint of establishing gestational age. Their value lies instead in the determination of normal proportionality with the head so that growth disturbances can be identified by the head-to-abdominal circumference ratio (Table 7-8). Alternatively the proportionality of the BPD to the abdominal diameter can also be evaluated, and is normal if the values are within 5 mm of each other until at least 34 weeks (Table 7-9). With either method the head is normally larger than the body in the second and early third trimesters, with reversal near term.

The guidelines recommend that, whenever possible, gestational age should initially be determined in either the first or second trimester. If one or more studies are performed, the gestational age should not be reestablished at each examination, particularly in the third trimester. Instead, the current fetal age is the initial fetal age established by the first examination plus the number of weeks that have elapsed. For example, if a fetus with a crown-rump length equivalent to 7 weeks' gestation is restudied 20 weeks later, the gestational age is 27 weeks (7 weeks + 20 weeks) on the second study, regardless of the new fetal measurements.

In all follow-up studies, interval growth should be assessed so that macrosomia or intrauterine growth retardation (IUGR) is not missed. The BPD is the best-studied measurement available, as it was developed from longitudinal data (Table 7-10). However, abdominal growth should be even more helpful, particularly in the event of asymmetric IUGR in which the abdomen is considerably more affected and affected earlier. Unfortunately, findings from a longitudinal study of abdominal growth are not yet available. For now, cross-sectional studies have to suffice in the assessment of the abdomen.

The guidelines also suggest that fetal weight be assessed in the third trimester. These weights can be calculated from tables that incorporate head, body, and femur measurements (Tables 7-11 and 7-12). The utility of fetal weights is limited by a sizable variation around the mean weight (at least ±12%), an inability to predict asymmetric IUGR, and an uncertainty about the significance of the calculated weight unless an accurate fetal age has been established. If the fetal age is known, the calculated weight can be compared with the expected weight of a fetus for that age (Table 7-13).

In the setting of multiple gestations, particularly twins, gestational age and growth are similar to those of single-ton pregnancies and the same measurement tables can be used. This is described at length in Chapter 16.

5. The uterus and adnexal structure should be evaluated.

There should be a careful search for fibroids and adnexal masses. After 20 weeks the analysis is performed primarily to detect fibroids, particularly those in the lower uterine segment that could cause dystocia at delivery.

6. The study should include, but not necessarily be limited to, the following fetal anatomic characteristics: cerebral ventricles, four-chamber view of the heart (including its position within the thorax), spine, stomach, urinary bladder, umbilical cord insertion site on the anterior abdominal wall, and renal region.

A careful analysis of fetal structures is part of the guidelines. Although not all anomalies can be identified, the more important ones that affect the major organs can be. These anatomic areas are more completely discussed in the respective chapters on these topics.

In the head, the atria of the lateral ventricles are imaged by tilting the transducer slightly caudally from the standard transaxial view. The atrial measurement is easily reproducible and essentially constant from 14 to 38 weeks: 7.6 mm in the transverse dimension, with 10 to 12 mm usually considered the upper limit of normal. In addition, the hyperechoic choroid plexus normally take up at least 60% of the atria.

Although not now part of these guidelines, it seems certain that imaging of the posterior fossa will be a routine part of any future update. In the transaxial plane, the cerebellum and cisterna magna can be imaged by tilting the transducer slightly more posteriorly toward the occiput.

Careful analysis of the spine is important to detect neural tube defects, both meningoceles and myelomeningoceles. There are three ossification centers at each vertebral level: one anterior center (centrum), which forms the vertebral body, and two posterior centers, which form the neural arches. A complete examination requires visualization of all vertebral levels, evaluating the posterior centers and overlying soft tissues. The transverse view of the spine can visualize both the osseous and soft tissue and may be the only projection necessary if all segments are imaged adequately. If this is suboptimal, midline sagittal images can visualize the soft tissues and vertebral centrum, and coronal images can visualize the posterior ossification centers.

The lumbosacral region of the spine is the most important area to image because most of the defects occur there. Although the spine can be identified clearly by 16 weeks, the fifth lumbar vertebral body is the most caudal vertebral body that is reliably ossified at this time. After 16 weeks ossification proceeds in a cephalocaudal direc-

Table 7-8 Head-to-abdominal circumference ratio

Gestational age (wk)	Ratio of head circumference/abdominal circumference		
	5th Percentile	Mean	95th Percentile
13-14	1.14	1.23	1.31
15-16	1.05	1.22	1.39
17-18	1.07	1.18	1.29
19-20	1.09	1.18	1.29
21-22	1.06	1.15	1.25
23-24	1.05	1.13	1.21
25-26	1.04	1.13	1.22
27-28	1.05	1.13	1.22
29-30	0.99	1.10	1.21
31-32	0.96	1.07	1.17
33-34	0.96	1.04	1.11
35-36	0.93	1.02	1.11
37-38	0.92	0.98	1.05
39-40	0.87	0.97	1.06
41-42	0.93	0.96	1.00

From Campbell S, Thoms A: Ultrasound measurement of the fetal head to abdomen circumference in the assessment of growth retardation, *Br J Obstet Gynaecol* 84:165-174, 1977.

tion from L5 to S5, each additional vertebral level ossifying every 2 to 3 weeks.

The revised 1991 guidelines now recommend a four-chamber view of the heart. This view is obtained transaxially and can identify both ventricles and their interventricular septum, both atria and their foramen ovale, and the atrioventricular valves. From 18 weeks to term, a satisfactory view can be obtained in 95% of the fetuses. During the analysis, the position of the heart within the chest should be determined. It is normal if the heart is on the left side with the apex pointing toward the left anterior chest wall at an approximately 45-degree angle and the chamber closest to the chest wall is the right ventricle.

The fetal stomach is an anechoic structure in the left upper quadrant of the abdomen and is first visualized at approximately 11 menstrual weeks. By 16 weeks the stomach should routinely be identified during a standard obstetric examination. There is, however, a wide variation in stomach size, and in a small percentage of normal fetuses, nonvisualization of the stomach may require a follow-up scan in several hours or even days. However, when the stomach has not been seen from 19 weeks onward, with scanning performed for up to 60 minutes, all such fetuses have been found to be abnormal.

The kidneys can be identified by their paraspinal location, seen on a transaxial view just below the level of the liver. The kidneys may be recognized as early as 12 to 14 weeks, and by 17 weeks may be seen in up to 90% of fetuses. It may be difficult, however, to distinguish the kidneys from the surrounding perinephric tissues in the second trimester; after 26 weeks, the perinephric fat and renal sinus become more hyperechoic and the relatively hypoechoic renal parenchyma is identified more easily. Exact renal measurements are not obtained routinely, although ta-

bles of renal length, anteroposterior dimension, and width are available. Of note is the constant ratio of the renal-to-abdominal circumference or their anteroposterior lengths at 0.27 to 0.30 throughout the second and third trimesters. When the normal renal sinus is separated by an anechoic space, pyelectasis is likely present. This may also be a normal finding. On a transaxial image, the anteroposterior dimension of this anechoic space should be measured. In the third trimester moderate dilatation of up to 7 mm (and occasionally 10 mm) usually represents physiologic in utero reflux and not an obstructive uropathy. When it measures more than 7 mm, however, a follow-up examination is usually desirable, frequently postnatally. Significant pyelectasis is usually accompanied by caliectasis, often requiring postnatal surgical management. In the second trimester a mild dilatation of 4 mm or more is unusual.

The urinary bladder is a round or ovoid anechoic structure. It can be observed to fill and empty in cycles varying from 50 to 155 minutes. If the normal bladder is not seen initially, it will almost always appear if sequential scanning is performed at 10- to 15-minute intervals. Visualization of the bladder is usually all that is necessary. However, changeability over time should be documented in cases in which a urinary tract abnormality is suspected. When assessing the renal system, the amount of amniotic fluid should also be evaluated, as oligohydramnios is almost always associated with a significant impairment.

Finally, the insertion site of the umbilical cord into the fetal abdominal wall should be identified. This is done to exclude ventral abdominal wall defects, particularly omphalocele, which occur at the base of the cord. Gastroschisis, a defect usually seen in the right lower quadrant, can also commonly be excluded by a more thorough imaging of the anterior abdominal wall.

Text continued on p. 179.

Table 7-9   Abdominal diameter measurement

Gestational age (wk)	Predicted mean biparietal diameter (mm)	Average abdominal diameter (mm)	
		Predicted mean	Range from 5th to 95th percentile
13	25.6	22.7	18.2 to 27.2
14	28.5	26.4	21.7 to 31.1
15	31.5	30.1	25.3 to 34.9
16	34.6	33.7	28.6 to 38.8
17	37.7	37.3	32.0 to 42.7
18	40.9	40.9	35.4 to 46.5
19	44.1	44.5	38.7 to 50.3
20	47.4	48.0	41.9 to 54.0
21	50.6	51.4	45.2 to 57.7
22	53.9	54.9	48.3 to 61.5
23	57.1	58.3	51.4 to 65.2
24	60.4	61.7	54.5 to 68.9
25	63.5	65.0	57.5 to 72.6
26	66.6	68.4	60.5 to 76.2
27	70.0	71.7	63.4 to 79.9
28	72.6	74.9	66.3 to 83.6
29	75.4	78.2	69.1 to 87.2
30	78.1	81.4	71.9 to 90.9
31	80.7	84.6	74.6 to 94.5
32	83.1	87.7	77.2 to 98.2
33	85.4	90.8	79.8 to 101.8
34	87.5	93.9	82.4 to 105.5
35	89.4	97.0	84.8 to 109.2
36	91.1	100.1	87.3 to 112.9
37	92.6	103.1	89.5 to 116.5
38	93.8	106.1	91.9 to 120.3
39	94.8	109.0	94.1 to 124.0
40	95.5	112.0	96.2 to 127.8

From Eriksen PS, Sechor NJ, Weis-Bentzon M: Normal growth of the fetal biparietal diameter and the abdominal diameter in a longitudinal study, *Acta Obstet Gynecol Scand* 64:65-70, 1985.

Table 7-10   Biparietal diameter growth rate

Gestational age (wk)	Mean biparietal diameter (mm)	Predicted interval growth (mm/wk)				
		Percentiles				
		10%	20%	50%	80%	90%
15	32	—	—	3.88	—	—
16	36	—	—	3.20	—	—
17	39	—	2.86	3.20	3.44	—
18	41	—	2.85	3.05	3.85	—
19	44	—	2.80	3.25	3.90	—
20	48	2.56	2.69	3.15	3.33	3.63
21	50	2.56	2.70	3.10	3.70	3.89
22	54	2.50	2.78	3.09	3.43	3.90
23	57	2.31	2.58	2.85	3.31	3.49
24	59	2.32	2.56	2.85	3.20	3.47
25	63	2.41	2.55	2.74	3.06	3.36
26	66	2.26	2.34	2.58	3.01	3.21
27	68	2.16	2.33	2.57	2.97	3.22
28	71	2.12	2.25	2.47	2.76	3.06
29	75	2.06	2.17	2.42	2.68	2.93
30	78	1.86	2.00	2.30	2.64	2.90
31	80	1.69	1.87	2.16	2.42	2.68
32	82	1.56	1.78	2.02	2.37	2.61
33	84	1.17	1.45	1.92	2.32	2.56
34	85	1.15	1.39	1.85	2.23	2.60
35	87	0.95	1.21	1.67	1.95	2.25
36	89	0.90	1.10	1.56	1.95	2.44
37	90	0.76	0.91	1.40	1.91	2.25
38	92	0.69	0.89	1.45	1.92	2.36
39	93	0.43	0.85	1.38	1.94	2.88
40	94	0.57	0.87	1.38	2.35	2.91
41	94	0.63	0.87	1.57	2.86	2.93
42	95	0.62	0.87	1.38	1.91	1.95
43	95	—	—	—	—	—

From Levi S, Smets P: Intrauterine fetal growth studied by ultrasonic biparietal measurements, *Acta Obset Gynecol Scand* 52:193-198, 1973.

Table 7-11 Estimated fetal weight (g) based on biparietal diameter and abdominal circumference*

Biparietal diameter (mm)	Abdominal circumference (mm)												
	155	160	165	170	175	180	185	190	195	200	205	210	215
31	224	234	244	255	267	279	291	304	318	332	346	362	378
32	231	241	251	263	274	286	299	312	326	340	355	371	388
33	237	248	259	270	282	294	307	321	335	349	365	381	397
34	244	255	266	278	290	302	316	329	344	359	374	391	408
35	251	262	274	285	298	311	324	338	353	368	384	401	418
36	259	270	281	294	306	319	333	347	362	378	394	411	429
37	266	278	290	302	315	328	342	357	372	388	404	422	440
38	274	286	298	310	324	337	352	366	382	398	415	432	451
39	282	294	306	319	333	347	361	376	392	409	426	444	462
40	290	303	315	328	342	356	371	386	403	419	437	455	474
41	299	311	324	338	352	366	381	397	413	430	448	467	486
42	308	320	333	347	361	376	392	408	424	442	460	479	498
43	317	330	343	357	371	387	402	419	436	453	472	491	511
44	326	339	353	367	382	397	413	430	447	465	484	504	524
45	335	349	363	377	393	408	425	442	459	478	497	517	538
46	345	359	373	386	404	420	436	454	472	490	510	530	551
47	355	369	384	399	415	431	448	466	484	503	524	544	565
48	366	380	395	410	426	443	460	478	497	517	537	558	580
49	376	391	406	422	438	455	473	491	510	530	551	572	594
50	387	402	418	434	451	468	486	505	524	544	565	587	610
51	399	414	430	446	463	481	499	518	538	559	580	602	625
52	410	426	442	459	476	494	513	532	552	573	595	618	641
53	422	438	455	472	489	508	527	547	567	589	611	634	657
54	435	451	468	485	503	522	541	561	582	604	627	650	674
55	447	464	481	499	517	536	556	577	598	620	643	667	691
56	461	477	495	513	532	551	571	592	614	636	660	684	709
57	474	491	509	527	547	566	587	608	630	653	677	701	727
58	488	505	524	542	562	582	603	625	647	670	695	719	745
59	502	520	539	558	578	598	619	642	664	688	713	738	764
60	517	535	554	573	594	615	636	659	682	706	731	757	784
61	532	550	570	590	610	632	654	677	700	725	750	777	804
62	547	566	586	606	627	649	672	695	719	744	770	797	824
63	563	583	603	624	645	667	690	714	738	764	790	817	845
64	580	600	620	641	663	686	709	733	758	784	811	838	867
65	597	617	638	659	682	705	728	753	778	805	832	860	889
66	614	635	656	678	701	724	748	773	799	826	853	882	911
67	632	653	675	697	720	744	769	794	820	848	876	905	935
68	651	672	694	717	740	765	790	816	842	870	898	928	958
69	670	691	714	737	761	786	811	838	865	893	922	952	983
70	689	711	734	758	782	807	833	860	888	916	946	976	1008
71	709	732	755	779	804	830	856	883	912	941	971	1002	1033
72	730	763	777	801	827	853	880	907	936	965	996	1027	1060
73	751	775	799	824	850	876	904	932	961	991	1022	1054	1087
74	773	797	822	847	874	901	928	957	987	1017	1049	1081	1114
75	796	820	845	871	898	925	954	983	1013	1044	1076	1109	1143
76	819	844	870	896	923	951	980	1009	1040	1072	1104	1137	1172
77	843	868	894	921	949	977	1007	1037	1068	1100	1133	1167	1202
78	868	894	920	947	975	1004	1034	1065	1096	1129	1162	1197	1232
79	893	919	946	974	1003	1032	1062	1094	1126	1159	1193	1228	1264
80	919	946	973	1002	1031	1061	1091	1123	1156	1189	1224	1259	1296
81	946	973	1001	1030	1060	1090	1121	1153	1187	1221	1256	1292	1329
82	974	1001	1030	1059	1089	1120	1152	1185	1218	1253	1288	1325	1363
83	1002	1030	1059	1089	1120	1151	1183	1217	1251	1286	1322	1359	1397
84	1032	1060	1090	1120	1151	1183	1216	1249	1284	1320	1356	1394	1433
85	1062	1091	1121	1151	1183	1216	1249	1283	1318	1355	1392	1430	1469
86	1093	1122	1153	1184	1216	1249	1283	1318	1354	1390	1428	1467	1507
87	1125	1155	1186	1218	1250	1284	1318	1353	1390	1427	1465	1505	1545
88	1157	1188	1220	1252	1285	1319	1354	1390	1427	1465	1504	1543	1584
89	1191	1222	1253	1287	1321	1356	1391	1428	1465	1503	1543	1583	1625
90	1226	1258	1290	1324	1358	1393	1429	1456	1504	1543	1583	1624	1666
91	1262	1294	1327	1361	1396	1432	1468	1506	1544	1584	1624	1666	1708
92	1299	1332	1365	1400	1435	1471	1508	1546	1586	1626	1667	1709	1752
93	1337	1370	1404	1439	1475	1512	1550	1588	1628	1668	1710	1753	1796
94	1376	1410	1444	1480	1516	1554	1592	1631	1671	1712	1755	1798	1842
95	1416	1450	1486	1522	1559	1597	1635	1675	1716	1758	1800	1844	1889
96	1457	1492	1528	1565	1602	1641	1680	1720	1762	1804	1847	1892	1937
97	1500	1535	1572	1609	1547	1686	1726	1767	1809	1852	1895	1940	1986
98	1544	1580	1617	1654	1693	1733	1773	1815	1857	1900	1945	1990	2037
99	1589	1625	1663	1701	1740	1781	1822	1864	1907	1951	1996	2042	2089
100	1635	1672	1710	1749	1789	1830	1871	1914	1958	2002	2048	2094	2142

*Estimated fetal weights: Log (birth weight) = −1.7492 + 0.166 (biparietal diameter) + 0.046 (abdominal circumference) − 0.00264 (abdominal circumference × biparietal diameter).

From Shepard MJ et al: An evaluation of two equations for predicted fetal weight by ultrasound, *Am J Obstet Gynecol* 147:47-54, 1982.

Abdominal circumference (mm)

220	225	230	235	240	245	250	255	260	265	270	275	280
395	412	431	450	470	491	513	536	559	584	610	638	666
405	423	441	461	481	502	525	548	572	597	624	651	680
415	433	452	472	493	514	537	560	585	611	638	666	693
425	444	463	483	504	526	549	573	598	624	652	680	710
436	455	475	495	517	539	562	587	612	638	666	695	725
447	466	486	507	529	552	575	600	626	653	681	710	740
458	478	498	519	542	565	589	614	640	667	696	725	756
470	490	510	532	554	578	602	628	654	682	711	741	772
482	502	523	545	568	592	616	642	669	697	727	757	789
494	514	536	558	581	606	631	657	684	713	743	773	806
506	527	549	572	595	620	645	672	700	729	759	790	828
519	540	562	585	609	634	660	688	716	745	776	807	841
532	554	576	600	624	649	676	703	732	762	793	825	859
545	567	590	614	639	665	692	719	749	779	810	843	877
559	581	605	629	654	680	708	736	765	796	828	861	896
573	596	620	644	670	696	724	753	783	814	846	880	915
588	611	635	660	686	713	741	770	801	832	865	899	934
602	626	650	676	702	730	758	788	819	851	884	919	954
617	641	666	692	719	747	776	806	837	870	903	938	975
633	657	683	709	736	765	794	824	856	889	923	959	996
649	674	699	726	754	783	812	843	876	909	944	980	1017
665	690	717	744	772	801	831	863	895	929	964	1001	1039
682	708	734	762	790	820	851	883	916	950	986	1023	1061
699	725	752	780	809	839	870	903	936	971	1007	1045	1084
717	743	771	799	828	859	891	924	958	993	1030	1068	1107
735	762	789	818	848	879	911	945	979	1015	1052	1091	1131
753	780	809	838	869	900	933	966	1001	1038	1075	1114	1155
772	800	829	858	889	921	954	989	1024	1061	1099	1139	1180
792	820	849	879	911	943	977	1011	1047	1085	1123	1163	1205
811	840	870	900	932	965	999	1035	1071	1109	1148	1189	1231
832	861	891	922	955	988	1023	1058	1095	1134	1173	1214	1257
853	882	913	945	977	1011	1046	1083	1120	1159	1199	1241	1284
874	904	935	967	1001	1035	1071	1107	1145	1185	1226	1268	1311
896	927	958	991	1025	1059	1096	1133	1171	1211	1253	1295	1339
919	950	982	1015	1049	1084	1121	1159	1198	1238	1280	1323	1368
942	973	1006	1039	1074	1110	1147	1185	1225	1266	1308	1352	1397
965	997	1030	1065	1100	1136	1174	1213	1253	1294	1337	1381	1427
990	1022	1056	1090	1126	1163	1201	1241	1281	1323	1367	1411	1458
1015	1048	1082	1117	1153	1190	1229	1269	1310	1353	1397	1442	1489
1040	1074	1108	1144	1181	1219	1258	1298	1340	1383	1427	1473	1521
1066	1100	1135	1171	1209	1247	1287	1328	1370	1414	1459	1505	1553
1093	1128	1163	1200	1238	1277	1317	1358	1401	1445	1491	1538	1586
1121	1156	1192	1229	1267	1307	1548	1390	1433	1478	1524	1571	1620
1149	1184	1221	1259	1297	1338	1379	1421	1465	1511	1557	1605	1655
1178	1214	1251	1289	1328	1369	1411	1454	1499	1544	1592	1640	1690
1207	1244	1281	1320	1360	1401	1444	1487	1533	1579	1627	1676	1727
1238	1275	1313	1352	1393	1434	1477	1522	1567	1614	1663	1712	1764
1269	1306	1345	1385	1426	1468	1512	1557	1603	1650	1699	1749	1801
1301	1339	1378	1418	1460	1503	1547	1492	1639	1687	1737	1787	1840
1333	1372	1412	1453	1495	1538	1583	1629	1676	1725	1775	1826	1879
1367	1406	1446	1488	1531	1575	1620	1666	1714	1763	1814	1866	1919
1401	1441	1482	1524	1567	1612	1657	1704	1753	1803	1854	1906	1960
1436	1477	1518	1561	1605	1650	1696	1744	1793	1843	1895	1948	2002
1473	1513	1555	1599	1643	1689	1735	1784	1825	1884	1936	1990	2045
1510	1551	1594	1637	1682	1728	1776	1825	1875	1926	1979	2033	2089
1548	1589	1633	1677	1722	1769	1817	1866	1917	1969	2022	2077	2134
1586	1629	1673	1717	1764	1811	1859	1909	1960	2013	2067	2122	2179
1626	1669	1714	1759	1806	1854	1903	1953	2005	2058	2113	2169	2226
1667	1711	1756	1802	1849	1897	1947	1998	2050	2104	2159	2216	2274
1709	1753	1799	1845	1893	1942	1992	2044	2097	2151	2207	2264	2322
1752	1797	1843	1890	1938	1988	2039	2091	2144	2199	2255	2313	2372
1796	1841	1888	1936	1984	2035	2086	2139	2193	2248	2305	2363	2423
1841	1887	1934	1982	2032	2083	2135	2188	2242	2298	2356	2414	2475
1887	1934	1982	2030	2080	2132	2184	2238	2293	2350	2407	2467	2527
1935	1982	2030	2080	2130	2182	2235	2289	2345	2402	2460	2520	2582
1984	2031	2080	2130	2181	2233	2287	2342	2398	2456	2515	2575	2637
2033	2082	2131	2181	2233	2286	2340	2396	2452	2510	2570	2631	2693
2085	2133	2183	2234	2286	2340	2395	2451	2508	2567	2627	2688	2751
2137	2186	2237	2288	2341	2395	2450	2507	2565	2624	2684	2746	2810
2191	2241	2292	2344	2397	2452	2507	2564	2623	2682	2743	2806	2870

Continued.

Biparietal diameter (mm)	Abdominal circumference (mm)											
	285	290	295	300	305	310	315	320	325	330	335	340
31	696	726	759	793	828	865	903	943	985	1029	1075	1123
32	710	742	774	809	844	882	921	961	1004	1048	1094	1143
33	725	757	790	825	861	899	938	979	1022	1067	1114	1163
34	740	773	806	841	878	916	956	998	1041	1087	1134	1183
35	756	789	823	858	896	934	975	1017	1061	1107	1154	1204
36	772	805	840	876	913	953	993	1036	1080	1127	1175	1226
37	788	822	857	893	931	971	1012	1056	1101	1147	1196	1247
38	805	839	874	911	950	990	1032	1076	1121	1168	1218	1269
39	822	856	892	930	969	1009	1052	1096	1142	1190	1240	1292
40	839	874	911	949	988	1029	1072	1117	1163	1212	1262	1315
41	857	892	929	968	1008	1049	1093	1138	1185	1234	1285	1338
42	875	911	948	987	1028	1070	1114	1159	1207	1256	1308	1361
43	893	930	968	1007	1048	1091	1135	1181	1229	1279	1331	1385
44	912	949	987	1027	1069	1112	1157	1204	1252	1303	1355	1410
45	932	969	1008	1048	1090	1134	1179	1226	1275	1326	1380	1435
46	951	989	1028	1069	1112	1156	1202	1249	1299	1351	1404	1406
47	971	1010	1049	1091	1134	1178	1225	1273	1323	1375	1430	1486
48	992	1031	1071	1113	1156	1201	1248	1297	1348	1401	1455	1512
49	1013	1052	1093	1135	1179	1225	1272	1322	1373	1426	1482	1539
50	1034	1074	1115	1158	1203	1249	1297	1347	1399	1452	1508	1566
51	1056	1096	1138	1181	1226	1273	1322	1372	1425	1479	1535	1594
52	1078	1119	1161	1205	1251	1298	1347	1398	1451	1506	1563	1622
53	1101	1142	1185	1229	1276	1323	1373	1425	1478	1533	1591	1651
54	1124	1166	1209	1254	1301	1349	1399	1452	1506	1562	1620	1680
55	1148	1190	1234	1279	1327	1376	1426	1479	1534	1590	1649	1710
56	1172	1215	1259	1305	1353	1402	1454	1507	1562	1619	1678	1740
57	1197	1240	1285	1332	1380	1430	1482	1535	1591	1649	1709	1770
58	1222	1266	1311	1358	1407	1458	1510	1564	1621	1679	1739	1802
59	1248	1292	1338	1386	1435	1486	1539	1594	1651	1710	1770	1834
60	1274	1319	1366	1414	1464	1515	1569	1624	1682	1741	1802	1866
61	1301	1346	1393	1442	1493	1545	1599	1655	1713	1773	1835	1899
62	1328	1374	1422	1471	1522	1575	1630	1686	1745	1805	1868	1932
63	1356	1403	1451	1501	1552	1606	1661	1718	1777	1838	1901	1967
64	1385	1432	1481	1531	1583	1637	1693	1751	1810	1872	1935	2001
65	1414	1462	1511	1562	1615	1669	1725	1784	1844	1906	1970	2037
66	1444	1492	1542	1594	1647	1702	1759	1817	1878	1941	2006	2073
67	1474	1523	1574	1626	1679	1735	1792	1852	1913	1976	2042	2109
68	1505	1555	1606	1658	1713	1769	1827	1887	1949	2012	2078	2147
69	1537	1587	1639	1692	1747	1803	1862	1922	1985	2049	2116	2184
70	1570	1620	1672	1726	1781	1839	1898	1959	2022	2087	2154	2223
71	1603	1654	1706	1761	1817	1875	1934	1996	2059	2125	2193	2262
72	1636	1688	1741	1796	1853	1911	1971	2044	2098	2164	2232	2302
73	1671	1723	1777	1832	1890	1948	2009	2072	2137	2203	2272	2343
74	1706	1759	1813	1869	1927	1987	2048	2111	2176	2244	2313	2384
75	1742	1795	1850	1907	1965	2025	2087	2151	2217	2265	2354	2426
76	1779	1833	1888	1945	2004	2065	2127	2192	2258	2326	2397	2469
77	1816	1871	1927	1985	2044	2105	2168	2233	2300	2369	2440	2513
78	1855	1910	1966	2025	2085	2146	2210	2275	2343	2412	2484	2557
79	1894	1949	2006	2065	2126	2188	2252	2318	2386	2456	2528	2603
80	1934	1990	2048	2107	2168	2231	2296	2362	2431	2501	2574	2649
81	1975	2031	2089	2149	2211	2275	2340	2407	2476	2547	2620	2695
82	2016	2073	2132	2193	2255	2319	2385	2462	2522	2594	2667	2743
83	2059	2116	2176	2237	2300	2364	2431	2499	2569	2641	2715	2791
84	2102	2160	2220	2282	2345	2410	2477	2546	2617	2689	2764	2841
85	2146	2205	2266	2328	2392	2457	2525	2594	2665	2739	2814	2891
86	2192	2251	2312	2375	2439	2505	2573	2643	2715	2789	2864	2942
87	2238	2298	2359	2423	2488	2554	2623	2693	2765	2840	2916	2994
88	2285	2346	2408	2472	2537	2604	2673	2744	2817	2892	2968	3047
89	2333	2394	2457	2521	2587	2655	2725	2796	2869	2944	3021	3101
90	2382	2444	2507	2572	2639	2707	2777	2849	2923	2998	3076	3155
91	2433	2495	2559	2624	2691	2760	2830	2903	2977	3053	3131	3211
92	2484	2547	2611	2677	2744	2814	2885	2958	3032	3109	3187	3268
93	2536	2599	2664	2731	2799	2869	2940	3014	3089	3166	3245	3326
94	2590	2653	2719	2786	2854	2925	2997	3070	3146	3224	3303	3384
95	2644	2709	2774	2842	2911	2982	3054	3129	3205	3283	3362	3444
96	2700	2765	2831	2899	2969	3040	3113	3188	3264	3343	3423	3505
97	2757	2822	2889	2958	3028	3099	3173	3248	3325	3404	3484	3567
98	2815	2881	2948	3017	3088	3160	3234	3309	3387	3466	3547	3630
99	2874	2941	3009	3078	3149	3222	3296	3372	3450	3529	3611	3694
100	2935	3002	3070	3140	3211	3285	3359	3436	3514	3594	3676	3759

*Estimated fetal weights: Log (birth weight) = −1.7492 + 0.166 (biparietal diameter) + 0.046 (abdominal circumference) − 0.00264 (abdominal circumference × biparietal diameter).

From Shepard MJ et al: An evaluation of two equations for predicting fetal weight by ultrasound, *Am J Obstet Gynecol* 147:47-54, 1982.

Abdominal circumference (mm)

345	350	355	360	365	370	375	380	385	390	395	400
1173	1225	1279	1336	1396	1458	1523	1591	1661	1735	1812	1893
1193	1246	1301	1358	1418	1481	1546	1615	1686	1761	1838	1920
1214	1267	1323	1381	1441	1504	1570	1639	1711	1786	1865	1946
1235	1289	1345	1403	1464	1528	1595	1664	1737	1812	1891	1973
1256	1311	1367	1426	1488	1552	1619	1689	1762	1839	1918	2001
1278	1333	1390	1450	1512	1577	1645	1715	1789	1865	1945	2029
1300	1356	1413	1474	1536	1602	1670	1741	1815	1893	1973	2057
1323	1379	1437	1498	1561	1627	1696	1768	1842	1920	2001	2086
1346	1402	1461	1523	1586	1653	1722	1794	1870	1948	2030	2115
1369	1426	1486	1548	1612	1679	1749	1822	1898	1977	2059	2145
1393	1451	1511	1573	1638	1706	1776	1849	1926	2005	2088	2174
1417	1475	1536	1599	1664	1733	1804	1878	1954	2035	2118	2205
1442	1500	1562	1625	1691	1760	1832	1906	1984	2064	2148	2236
1467	1526	1588	1652	1718	1788	1860	1935	2013	2094	2179	2267
1492	1552	1614	1679	1746	1816	1889	1964	2043	2125	2210	2298
1518	1579	1641	1706	1774	1845	1918	1994	2073	2156	2241	2330
1545	1605	1669	1734	1803	1874	1948	2024	2104	2187	2273	2363
1571	1633	1697	1763	1832	1904	1976	2055	2136	2219	2306	2396
1599	1661	1725	1792	1861	1934	2009	2086	2167	2251	2339	2429
1626	1689	1754	1821	1891	1964	2040	2118	2200	2284	2372	2463
1655	1718	1783	1851	1922	1995	2071	2150	2232	2317	2406	2498
1683	1747	1813	1882	1953	2027	2103	2183	2266	2351	2440	2532
1713	1777	1843	1913	1984	2059	2136	2216	2299	2386	2475	2568
1742	1807	1874	1944	2016	2091	2169	2250	2333	2420	2510	2604
1773	1838	1906	1976	2049	2124	2203	2284	2368	2456	2546	2640
1803	1869	1938	2008	2082	2158	2237	2319	2403	2491	2582	2677
1835	1901	1970	2041	2115	2192	2272	2354	2439	2528	2619	2714
1866	1934	2003	2075	2150	2227	2307	2390	2475	2564	2657	2752
1899	1966	2037	2109	2184	2262	2342	2426	2512	2602	2694	2790
1932	2000	2071	2144	2219	2298	2379	2463	2550	2640	2733	2829
1965	2034	2105	2179	2255	2334	2416	2500	2588	2678	2772	2869
1999	2069	2140	2215	2291	2371	2453	2538	2626	2717	2811	2909
2034	2104	2176	2251	2328	2408	2491	2577	2665	2757	2851	2949
2069	2140	2213	2288	2366	2446	2530	2616	2705	2797	2892	2991
2105	2176	2250	2326	2404	2485	2569	2656	2745	2838	2933	3032
2142	2213	2287	2364	2443	2524	2609	2696	2786	2879	2975	3075
2179	2251	2326	2403	2482	2564	2649	2737	2827	2921	3018	3117
2217	2290	2365	2442	2522	2604	2690	2778	2869	2964	3061	3161
2255	2329	2404	2482	2563	2646	2732	2821	2912	3007	3104	3205
2295	2368	2444	2523	2604	2688	2774	2863	2955	3050	3149	3250
2334	2409	2485	2564	2646	2730	2817	2907	2999	3095	3193	3295
2375	2450	2527	2607	2689	2773	2861	2951	3044	3140	3239	3341
2416	2491	2569	2649	2732	2817	2905	2996	3089	3186	3285	3386
2458	2534	2612	2693	2776	2862	2950	3041	3135	3232	3332	3435
2501	2577	2656	2737	2821	2907	2996	3088	3182	3279	3380	3483
2544	2621	2700	2782	2866	2953	3042	3134	3229	3327	3428	3531
2588	2666	2746	2828	2912	3000	3090	3182	3277	3376	3477	3581
2633	2711	2792	2874	2959	3047	3137	3230	3326	3425	3526	3631
2679	2757	2838	2921	3007	3095	3186	3279	3376	3475	3576	3681
2725	2804	2886	2969	3056	3144	3235	3329	3426	3525	3627	3733
2773	2852	2934	3018	3105	3194	3286	3380	3477	3577	3679	3785
2821	2901	2983	3068	3155	3244	3336	3431	3529	3629	3732	3838
2870	2950	3033	3118	3206	3296	3388	3483	3581	3682	3785	3891
2920	3001	3084	3169	3257	3348	3441	3536	3634	3735	3839	3945
2970	3052	3135	3221	3310	3401	3494	3590	3688	3790	3894	4000
3022	3104	3188	3274	3363	3454	3548	3644	3743	3845	3949	4056
3074	3157	3241	3328	3417	3509	3603	3700	3799	3901	4005	4113
3128	3210	3295	3383	3472	3565	3659	3756	3855	3958	4063	4170
3182	3265	3351	3438	3528	3621	3716	3813	3913	4015	4120	4228
3237	3321	3407	3495	3585	3678	3773	3871	3971	4074	4179	4287
3293	3377	3464	3552	3643	3736	3832	3930	4030	4133	4239	4347
3350	3435	3522	3611	3702	3795	3891	3989	4090	4193	4299	4408
3409	3494	3581	3670	3761	3855	3951	4050	4151	4254	4361	4469
3468	3553	3641	3738	3822	3916	4013	4111	4213	4316	4423	4532
3528	3614	3701	3791	3884	3978	4075	4174	4275	4379	4486	4595
3589	3675	3763	3854	3946	4041	4138	4237	4339	4443	4550	4659
3651	3738	3826	3917	4010	4105	4202	4302	4404	4508	4615	4724
3715	3802	3890	3981	4074	4170	4267	4367	4469	4573	4680	4790
3779	3866	3956	4047	4140	4236	4333	4433	4536	4640	4747	4857
3845	3932	4022	4113	4207	4303	4400	4501	4603	4708	4815	4924

Table 7-12   Estimated fetal weight (g) based on abdominal circumference and femur length*

Femur length (mm)	Ratio of head circumference/abdominal circumference																			
	200	205	210	215	220	225	230	235	240	245	250	255	260	265	270	275	280	285	290	295
40	663	691	720	751	783	816	851	887	925	964	1006	1048	1093	1139	1188	1239	1291	1346	1403	1463
41	680	709	738	769	802	836	871	907	946	986	1027	1070	1115	1162	1211	1262	1315	1371	1429	1489
42	697	726	757	788	821	855	891	928	967	1007	1049	1093	1138	1186	1235	1287	1340	1396	1454	1515
43	715	745	776	808	841	875	912	949	988	1029	1071	1116	1162	1209	1259	1311	1365	1422	1480	1541
44	734	764	795	827	861	896	933	971	1010	1051	1094	1139	1185	1234	1284	1336	1391	1448	1509	1568
45	753	783	815	847	882	917	954	993	1033	1074	1118	1163	1210	1259	1309	1362	1417	1474	1534	1596
46	772	803	835	868	903	939	976	1015	1056	1098	1142	1187	1235	1284	1335	1388	1444	1501	1561	1623
47	792	823	856	889	924	961	999	1038	1079	1122	1166	1212	1260	1310	1316	1415	1471	1529	1589	1652
48	812	844	877	911	947	984	1022	1062	1103	1146	1191	1237	1286	1336	1388	1442	1498	1557	1618	1681
49	833	865	899	933	969	1007	1046	1086	1128	1171	1216	1263	1312	1363	1415	1470	1527	1585	1647	1710
50	855	887	921	956	993	1031	1070	1111	1153	1197	1243	1290	1339	1390	1443	1498	1555	1615	1676	1740
51	877	910	944	980	1016	1055	1095	1136	1179	1223	1269	1317	1367	1418	1471	1527	1584	1644	1706	1770
52	899	933	967	1004	1041	1080	1120	1162	1205	1250	1296	1344	1395	1447	1500	1556	1614	1647	1737	1801
53	922	956	992	1028	1066	1105	1146	1188	1232	1277	1324	1373	1423	1476	1530	1586	1645	1705	1768	1833
54	946	981	1016	1053	1091	1131	1172	1215	1259	1305	1352	1401	1452	1505	1560	1617	1675	1736	1799	1865
55	971	1005	1041	1079	1118	1158	1199	1242	1287	1333	1318	1431	1482	1535	1591	1648	1707	1768	1832	1897
56	995	1031	1067	1105	1144	1185	1227	1271	1316	1362	1411	1461	1513	1566	1622	1679	1739	1801	1864	1931
57	1021	1057	1094	1132	1172	1213	1255	1299	1345	1392	1441	1491	1544	1598	1654	1712	1772	1834	1898	1964
58	1047	1084	1121	1160	1200	1242	1285	1329	1375	1422	1472	1523	1575	1630	1686	1744	1805	1867	1932	1999
59	1074	1111	1149	1188	1229	1271	1314	1359	1406	1454	1503	1555	1608	1663	1719	1778	1839	1902	1966	2034
60	1102	1139	1178	1217	1258	1301	1345	1309	1437	1485	1535	1587	1641	1696	1753	1812	1873	1936	2002	2069
61	1130	1168	1207	1247	1289	1331	1376	1421	1469	1518	1568	1620	1674	1730	1788	1847	1908	1972	2038	2105
62	1160	1198	1237	1278	1319	1363	1408	1454	1501	1551	1602	1654	1709	1765	1823	1882	1944	2008	2074	2142
63	1189	1228	1268	1309	1351	1395	1440	1487	1535	1585	1636	1689	1744	1800	1858	1919	1981	2045	2111	2180
64	1220	1259	1299	1341	1384	1428	1473	1520	1569	1619	1671	1724	1779	1836	1895	1956	2018	2082	2149	2218
65	1251	1291	1332	1373	1417	1461	1507	1555	1604	1655	1707	1760	1816	1873	1932	1993	2056	2121	2188	2256
66	1284	1324	1365	1407	1451	1496	1542	1590	1640	1691	1743	1797	1853	1911	1970	2031	2094	2160	2227	2296
67	1317	1357	1399	1441	1486	1531	1578	1626	1676	1728	1780	1835	1891	1949	2009	2070	2134	2199	2267	2336
68	1351	1391	1433	1477	1521	1567	1615	1663	1713	1765	1819	1873	1930	1988	2048	2110	2174	2240	2307	2377
69	1385	1427	1469	1513	1558	1604	1652	1701	1752	1804	1857	1913	1970	2028	2089	2151	2215	2281	2348	2418
70	1421	1463	1506	1550	1595	1642	1690	1740	1791	1843	1897	1953	2010	2069	2130	2192	2256	2322	2391	2461
71	1458	1500	1543	1588	1633	1681	1729	1779	1830	1883	1938	1994	2051	2110	2171	2234	2299	2365	2433	2504
72	1495	1538	1581	1626	1673	1720	1769	1819	1871	1924	1979	2035	2093	2153	2214	2277	2342	2408	2477	2547
73	1534	1577	1621	1666	1713	1761	1810	1861	1913	1966	2021	2078	2136	2196	2258	2321	2386	2453	2521	2592
74	1573	1616	1661	1707	1754	1802	1852	1903	1955	2009	2065	2122	2180	2240	2302	2365	2431	2498	2566	2637
75	1614	1657	1702	1749	1796	1845	1895	1946	1999	2053	2109	2166	2225	2285	2347	2411	2476	2543	2612	2683
76	1655	1699	1745	1791	1839	1888	1939	1990	2043	2098	2154	2211	2270	2331	2393	2457	2523	2590	2659	2730
77	1698	1742	1788	1835	1883	1933	1983	2035	2089	2144	2200	2258	2317	2378	2440	2504	2570	2638	2707	2778
78	1741	1786	1833	1880	1928	1978	2029	2082	2135	2191	2247	2305	2365	2426	2488	2553	2618	2686	2755	2827
79	1786	1832	1878	1926	1975	2025	2076	2129	2183	2238	2295	2353	2413	2474	2537	2602	2668	2735	2805	2876
80	1832	1878	1925	1973	2022	2073	2124	2177	2232	2287	2344	2403	2463	2524	2587	2652	2718	2785	2855	2926
81	1879	1926	1973	2021	2071	2121	2173	2227	2281	2337	2394	2453	2513	2575	2638	2702	2769	2837	2906	2977
82	1928	1974	2022	2070	2120	2171	2224	2277	2332	2388	2446	2504	2565	2626	2690	2754	2821	2889	2958	3029
83	1978	2024	2072	2121	2171	2223	2275	2329	2384	2440	2498	2557	2617	2679	2743	2807	2874	2942	3011	3082

*Based on regression model: Log_{10} body weight = 1.3598 + 0.051 (abdominal circumference) + 0.1844 (femur length) − 0.0037 (abdominal circumference × femur length).

From Hadlock FP et al: Sonographic estimation of fetal weight, *Radiology* 150:535-540, 1984.

Ratio of head circumference/abdominal circumference

300	305	310	315	320	325	330	335	340	345	350	355	360	365	370	375	380	385	390	395	400
1525	1590	1658	1729	1802	1879	1959	2042	2129	2220	2314	2413	2515	2622	2734	2850	2972	3098	3230	3367	3511
1551	1617	1685	1756	1830	1907	1987	2071	2158	2249	2344	2442	2545	2652	2764	2880	3002	3128	3260	3397	3540
1578	1644	1712	1783	1858	1935	2016	2100	2187	2279	2373	2472	2575	2683	2794	2911	3032	3159	3290	3427	3570
1605	1671	1740	1812	1886	1964	2054	2129	2217	2308	2404	2503	2606	2713	2825	2942	3063	3189	3321	3458	3600
1632	1699	1768	1840	1915	1993	2075	2159	2247	2339	2434	2533	2637	2744	2856	2973	3094	3220	3352	3488	3630
1660	1727	1797	1869	1944	2023	2105	2189	2278	2370	2465	2565	2668	2776	2888	3004	3125	3251	3383	3519	3661
1688	1756	1826	1898	1974	2053	2135	2220	2309	2401	2497	2596	2700	2807	2919	3036	3157	3283	3414	3550	3692
1717	1785	1855	1928	2004	2084	2166	2251	2340	2432	2528	2628	2732	2840	2952	3068	3189	3315	3446	3582	3723
1746	1814	1885	1959	2035	2115	2197	2283	2372	2464	2560	2660	2764	2872	2984	3100	3221	3347	3478	3613	3754
1776	1845	1916	1990	2066	2146	2229	2315	2404	2497	2593	2693	2797	2905	3017	3133	3254	3380	3510	3645	3786
1806	1875	1947	2021	2098	2178	2261	2347	2437	2530	2626	2726	2830	2938	3050	3166	3287	3412	3542	3677	3818
1837	1906	1978	2053	2130	2210	2294	2380	2470	2563	2659	2760	2864	2972	3084	3200	3320	3445	3575	3710	3850
1868	1938	2010	2085	2163	2243	2327	2413	2503	2597	2693	2794	2898	3006	3117	3234	3354	3479	3608	3743	3882
1900	1970	2043	2118	2196	2277	2360	2447	2537	2631	2728	2828	2932	3040	3152	3268	3388	3513	3642	3776	3915
1933	2003	2076	2151	2229	2311	2395	2482	2572	2665	2762	2863	2967	3075	3186	3302	3422	3547	3676	3809	3948
1966	2036	2109	2185	2264	2345	2429	2516	2607	2700	2797	2898	3002	3110	3221	3337	3457	3581	3710	3843	3981
1999	2070	2143	2220	2298	2380	2464	2552	2642	2736	2833	2933	3038	3145	3257	3372	3492	3616	3744	3877	4015
2033	2104	2178	2254	2333	2415	2500	2587	2678	2772	2869	2970	3074	3181	3293	3408	3572	3651	3779	3911	4048
2068	2139	2213	2290	2369	2451	2536	2624	2714	2808	2905	3006	3110	3218	3329	3444	3563	3686	3814	3946	4082
2103	2174	2249	2326	2405	2488	2573	2660	2751	2845	2942	3043	3147	3254	3366	3480	3599	3722	3849	3981	4117
2139	2211	2286	2363	2442	2525	2610	2698	2789	2883	2980	3080	3184	3292	3403	3517	3636	3758	3885	4016	4151
2175	2248	2323	2400	2480	2562	2647	2736	2827	2921	3018	3118	3222	3329	3440	3554	3673	3795	3921	4052	4186
2212	2285	2360	2438	2518	2600	2686	2774	2865	2959	3056	3157	3260	3367	3478	3592	3710	3832	3957	4087	4222
2250	2323	2398	2476	2556	2639	2725	2813	2904	2998	3095	3195	3299	3406	3516	3630	3747	3869	3994	4124	4257
2289	2362	2437	2515	2595	2678	2764	2852	2943	3037	3134	3235	3338	3445	3555	3668	3785	3906	4031	4160	4293
2328	2401	2477	2555	2635	2718	2804	2892	2983	3077	3174	3274	3378	3484	3594	3707	3824	3944	4069	4197	4329
2367	2441	2517	2595	2675	2759	2844	2933	3024	3118	3215	3315	3418	3524	3633	3746	3863	3983	4106	4234	4366
2408	2481	2557	2636	2716	2800	2885	2974	3065	3159	3256	3355	3458	3564	3673	3786	3902	4021	4144	4271	4402
2449	2523	2599	2677	2758	2841	2927	3016	3107	3200	3297	3397	3499	3605	3714	3862	3941	4060	4183	4309	4439
2490	2564	2641	2719	2800	2884	2969	3058	3149	3242	3339	3438	3541	3646	3754	3866	3981	4100	4222	4347	4477
2533	2607	2683	2762	2843	2927	3012	3101	3192	3285	3381	3481	3583	3688	3796	3907	4022	4140	4261	4386	4514
2576	2650	2727	2806	2887	2970	3056	3144	3235	3328	3424	3523	3625	3730	3838	3948	4062	4180	4300	4425	4552
2620	2694	2771	2850	2931	3014	3100	3188	3279	3372	3468	3567	3668	3772	3880	3990	4104	4220	4340	4464	4591
2665	2739	2816	2895	2976	3059	3145	3233	3323	3416	3512	3610	3712	3816	3922	4032	4145	4261	4381	4503	4629
2710	2785	2861	2940	3021	3105	3190	3278	3369	3461	3557	3655	3756	3859	3966	4075	4187	4303	4421	4543	4668
2756	2831	2908	2987	3068	3151	3236	3324	3414	3507	3602	3700	3800	3903	4009	4118	4230	4344	4462	4583	4708
2803	2878	2955	3034	3115	3198	3283	3371	3461	3553	3648	3745	3845	3948	4053	4161	4272	4387	4504	4624	4747
2851	2926	3003	3081	3162	3245	3331	3418	3508	3600	4694	3791	3891	3993	4098	4205	4316	4429	4545	4665	4787
2899	2974	3051	3130	3211	3294	3379	3466	3555	3647	3741	3838	3937	4039	4143	4250	4360	4472	4588	4706	4827
2949	3024	3100	3179	3260	3343	3427	3514	3604	3695	3789	3885	3984	4085	4188	4295	4404	4515	4630	4748	4868
2999	3074	3151	3229	3310	3392	3477	3564	3653	3744	3837	3933	4031	4131	4234	4340	4448	4559	4673	4790	4909
3050	3125	3202	3280	3360	3443	3527	3614	3702	3793	3886	3981	4079	4179	4281	4386	4493	4604	4716	4832	4950
3102	3177	3253	3332	3412	3494	3578	3664	3752	3843	3935	4030	4127	4226	4328	4432	4539	4648	4760	4875	4992
3155	3230	3306	3384	2464	3546	3630	3716	3803	3893	3985	4080	4176	4275	4376	4479	4585	4693	4804	4918	5034

Table 7-13   Predicted fetal weight percentiles throughout pregnancy

Gestational age (menstrual weeks)	Smoothed percentiles				
	10	25	50	75	90
8	—	—	6	—	—
9	—	—	7	—	—
10	—	—	8	—	—
11	—	—	12	—	—
12	—	11	21	34	—
13	—	23	35	55	—
14	—	35	51	77	—
15	—	51	77	108	—
16	—	80	117	151	—
17	—	125	166	212	—
18	—	172	220	298	—
19	—	217	283	394	—
20	—	255	325	460	—
21	280	330	410	570	860
22	320	410	480	630	920
23	370	460	550	690	990
24	420	530	640	780	1080
25	490	630	740	890	1180
26	570	730	860	1020	1320
27	660	840	990	1160	1470
28	770	980	1150	1350	1660
29	890	1100	1310	1530	1890
30	1030	1260	1460	1710	2100
31	1180	1410	1630	1880	2290
32	1310	1570	1810	2090	2500
33	1480	1720	2010	2280	2690
34	1670	1910	2220	2510	2880
35	1870	2130	2430	2730	3090
36	2190	2470	2650	2950	3290
37	2310	2580	2870	3160	3470
38	2510	2770	3030	3320	3610
39	2680	2910	3170	3470	3750
40	2750	3010	3280	3590	3870
41	2800	3070	3360	3680	3980
42	2830	3110	3410	3740	4060
43	2840	3110	3420	3780	4100
44	2790	3050	3390	3770	4110

From Brenner WE, Edelman D, Hendricks CH: A standard of fetal growth for the USA, *Am J Obstet Gynecol* 126:555-564, 1976.

SUGGESTED READINGS

AIUM Guidelines, *J Ultrasound Med* 10:576, 1991.

Arger PH et al: Routine fetal genitourinary tract screening, *Radiology* 156:485, 1985.

Barss VA, Benacerraf BR, Frigoletto FD Jr: Ultrasonographic determination of chorion type in twin gestation, *Obstet Gynecol* 66:779, 1985.

Benson CB, Doubilet PM: Sonographic prediction of gestational age: accuracy of second- and third-trimester fetal measurements, *AJR* 157:1275, 1991.

Bowie JD et al: The changing sonographic appearance of fetal kidneys during pregnancy, *J Ultrasound Med* 2:505, 1983.

Bromley B et al: Fetal echocardiography: accuracy and limitations in a population at high and low risk for heart defects, *Am J Obstet Gynecol* 166:1473, 1992.

Budorick NE et al: Ossification of the fetal spine, *Radiology* 181:561, 1991.

Campbell S, Wladimiroff JW, Dewhurst CJ: The antenatal measurement of fetal urine production, *Br J Obstet Gynaecol* 80:680, 1973.

Cardoza JD, Goldstein BB, Filly RA: Exclusion of fetal ventriculomegaly with a single measurement: the width of the lateral ventricular atrium, *Radiology* 169:711, 1988.

Copel JA et al: Fetal echocardiographic screening for congenital heart disease: the importance of the four-chamber view, *Am J Obstet Gynecol* 157:648, 1987.

Doubilet PM, Greenes RA: Improved prediction of gestational age from fetal head measurements, *AJR* 142:797, 1984.

Filly RA: Level 1, level 2, level 3 obstetric sonography: I'll see your level and raise you one, *Radiology* 172:312, 1989.

Goldstein RB, Filly RA: Sonographic estimation of amniotic fluid volume. Subjective assessment versus pocket measurements, *J Ultrasound Med* 7:363, 1988.

Grannum P et al: Assessment of fetal kidney size in normal gestation by comparison of ratio of kidney circumference to abdominal circumference, *Am J Obstet Gynecol* 136:249, 1980.

Grumbach K et al: Twin and singleton growth patterns compared using ultrasound, *Radiology* 158:237, 1986.

Hadlock FP et al: Estimating fetal age: effect of head shape on BPD, *AJR* 137:83, 1981.

Hadlock FP et al: Fetal abdominal circumference as a predictor of menstrual age, *AJR* 139:369, 1982.

Hertzberg BS et al. Diagnosis of placenta previa during the third trimester: role of transperineal sonography, *AJR* 159:83, 1992.

Levi CS et al: Endovaginal US: demonstration of cardiac activity in embryos of less than 5.0 mm in crown-rump length, *Radiology* 176:71, 1990.

Mahony BS, Filly RA, Callen PW: Amnionicity and chorionicity in twin pregnancies: prediction using ultrasound, *Radiology* 155:205, 1985.

McGahan JP: Sonography of the fetal heart: findings on the four-chamber view, *AJR* 156:547, 1991.

Michaels WH et al: Ultrasound differentiation of the competent from the incompetent cervix. Prevention of preterm delivery, *Am J Obstet Gynecol* 154:537, 1986.

Pennell RG et al: Prospective comparison of vaginal and abdominal sonography in normal early pregnancy, *J Ultrasound Med* 10:63, 1991.

Pilu et al: Sonographic evaluation of the normal developmental anatomy of the fetal cerebral ventricles: II. The atria, *Obstet Gynecol* 783:250, 1989.

Pretorius DH et al: Sonographic evaluation of the fetal stomach: significance of non-visualization, *AJR* 151:987, 1988.

CHAPTER 8

Fetal Well-Being: Growth Retardation, Doppler Waveform Analysis, Biophysical Profile, and Macrosoma

Intrauterine Growth Retardation
  Ultrasound Characteristics
  Doppler Velocity Waveform Analysis
  Biophysical Profile
  Summary
Macrosomia

For a Key Features summary see p. 189.

For a Key Features summary see p. 189.

Improved equipment and increased ultrasound so-phistication have permitted the examiner to go beyond a routine evaluation of the fetal structure. Particularly in the third trimester, fetal function and measurements, separately or in combination with the clinical findings, have been used to analyze fetal well-being, thereby helping to predict fetuses that are either too small or too large. This approach has allowed increased accuracy in the detection of the compromised fetus and in some cases determination of the timing of delivery.

INTRAUTERINE GROWTH RETARDATION

Intrauterine growth retardation (IUGR) is a complex problem not always detected in utero. By definition, at birth a child with a low birth weight is deemed small for gestational age; the baby with IUGR is pathologically smaller than its expected gestational age, whereas the small but otherwise normal baby is constitutionally small.

Most studies use a weight cutoff for these growth-re-tarded babies of the lower 10th percentile or less, with increased specificity when the lower 5th or 3rd per-centile is used. The incidence of IUGR cited in different studies varies, but is typically between 3% and 10% of all births. On average, 1 in every 20 babies (5%) is growth re-tarded, with this approaching 1 in 10 babies in certain high-risk groups (10%).

The ideal fetal characteristics needed to predict growth retardation are age and weight. If these can be precisely determined, then the size of the fetus for its ges-tational age can be known. Unfortunately, the prenatal de-termination of age and weight is not sufficiently accurate. Using 2 standard deviations (2 SD, or 95%) in a large group of women, an optimal menstrual history can only predict fetal age to within ±2.5 weeks; when the dates are uncertain, this accuracy decreases to ±4 weeks or more. The first-trimester crown-rump length and second-trimester biparietal diameter (BPD) are more accurate up to 24 weeks, at ±1 week. However, in the third trimester, the overall accuracy of the BPD and head circumference is closer to ±3 to 4 weeks. Although the ultrasound-de-termined age is therefore better than that determined by the menstrual history, there is still a wide variation in its accuracy, particularly in the third trimester. Additionally, fetal weight is only accurate to at best ±10% to 15%. In the third trimester the 2-SD range can be as great as 1 kg!

To further complicate this analysis, there are numer-ous causes of IUGR and two types of growth retardation. The causes can be segregated into maternal, fetal, and pla-cental problems. High blood pressure, collagen vascular diseases, insulin-dependent diabetes, smoking, and certain drugs, including alcohol and cocaine, have adverse effects on fetal growth. Other maternal factors range from a young maternal age to a state of chronic hypoxia. Fetal risk factors include a previously growth-retarded fetus, structural and chromosomal abnormalities, and in utero infections (e.g., the TORCH viruses [*t*oxoplasmosis, *o*ther, *r*ubella, *c*ytomegalovirus, and *h*erpes simplex]). Placental problems include infarction, abnormal umbilical cord insertion, placenta previa, and abruption. Premature pla-cental aging (dysmaturity), vascular problems (anticardi-olipin antibodies and hypercoagulable states), and pla-cental tumors also adversely affect the fetus. Although not understood, women with persistently elevated α-fetoprotein levels (without structural fetal causes) have a higher incidence of growth-retarded fetuses.

Abnormally low growth can stem from two distinct mechanisms: fetal malnutrition and diminished cellular growth. These manifest themselves as two different types of IUGR, asymmetric and symmetric. Though separate entities, there is some degree of overlap. Asymmetric IUGR (malnutrition) constitutes 90% of the cases of growth retardation. It almost always is detected in the third trimester and rarely earlier. Placental and maternal problems predominate, with the fetus receiving a less-than-adequate blood supply and nourishment. Because asymmetric IUGR is a form of starvation, initially there is a loss of subcutaneous tissue and liver glycogen stores, and thus an initial decrease in abdominal size. The head and femur are also affected, but to a lesser extent. As starvation persists, however, the entire fetus becomes equally affected and the fetus assumes a "symmetric" appearance. This signifies severe growth retardation. Fetal malnutrition is infrequently accompanied by oligohydramnios. The differentiation in the third trimester between this severe form of asymmetric growth retardation and the truly symmetric growth retardation (described in the next paragraph) must often rely on history and, if present, on the finding of decreased amniotic fluid. The prognosis depends on the severity of the perinatal and immediate neonatal problems. If the problems are successfully resolved, this type of child will go on to experience normal development.

The symmetric type of IUGR (diminished cellular growth) makes up the other 10% and occurs early in pregnancy, usually in the first trimester. In it the fetus is considerably stunted as the result of an insult primarily to the fetus or its mother. The head and body (and femur) are equally affected and the fetus remains symmetric. The volume of amniotic fluid is typically normal. Because this form of IUGR occurs early when the central nervous system is forming, there are usually persistent neurologic problems after birth.

Normal growth of the fetal head and body is usually linear or mildly curvilinear. It is faster in the second trimester, becoming progressively slower until term. In asymmetric IUGR the fetus grows normally into the third trimester, with decreased growth (usually marked) in the third trimester. In symmetric IUGR the fetus grows slowly from the time of the insult onward. The small fetus with IUGR grows differently (slower) than a normal fetus of similar size.

The overall detection rate for in utero IUGR is 70%, commonly with asymmetric growth retardation more readily detected. When incorporated with the clinical evaluation, ultrasound can be used to accomplish different tasks in the detection and management of suspected growth abnormalities: to suggest that a low-risk fetus is smaller than expected, to determine if a fetus at high risk is too small, to find out if the ultrasound findings are compatible with the clinical impression of a small fetus, and to monitor the pregnancy when the diagnosis of a small fetus is made.

The accuracy of ultrasound is different in these different circumstances. For example, a small abdominal circumference detected during an examination performed solely to establish fetal age is less likely to be due to IUGR than it is in the fetus of a woman with hypertension. In a "screening" group, there is a larger proportion of constitutionally small fetuses than of those with IUGR, and consequently there is a higher false-positive rate and a lower positive predictive value for this group than those for a group of higher-risk women with hypertension (preeclampsia). Therefore, if only abnormal measurements are found, it is more prudent to initially call the fetus small for gestational age rather than growth retarded and request a follow-up study.

Ultrasound Characteristics

Because the precise fetal weight and age cannot be determined, ultrasound relies on more indirect characteristics of the fetus, amniotic fluid, and placenta to make the diagnosis of IUGR. The fetus should therefore be evaluated carefully to determine structural normalcy, as fetal anomalies may cause growth retardation. Even when the fetus appears grossly normal, however, chromosomal anomalies or in utero infection may still be present.

Aside from structure, almost all the fetal information can be obtained from measurements of the head and body, and occasionally of the femur. All standard ultrasound projections and measurements are performed according to the obstetric guidelines (see Chapter 7). The gestational age is ideally established by a first-trimester crown rump length (see Chapter 7, Table 7-3) or a second-trimester BPD (see Chapter 7, Table 7-4). In follow-up studies the fetal age is the initial ultrasound age plus the number of intervening weeks. The fetal head measurement, obtained in the transaxial plane at the level of the thalami or midbrain, yields the BPD and head circumference. The body measurement, obtained from the transaxial image of the liver where the umbilical portion of the left portal vein is detected, yields the average body diameter and abdominal circumference. The femur length is obtained from the diaphyseal shaft.

The calculated fetal weight, determined using a combination of measurements of the head, body, and femur (the latter representing fetal length), has shown value in the prediction of IUGR (see Chapter 7, Tables 7-11 and 7-12). Similarly, so has the measured abdominal circumference. Both are useful primarily when the fetal age is known. The *calculated* fetal weight and the *measured* abdominal circumference can then be compared with the *expected* weight and abdominal circumference for that fetal age. Percentile tables are available for both, using the

Table 8-1   Fetal abdominal circumference (mm)

Weeks of gestation	Percentile								
	2.5	5	10	25	50	75	80	95	97.5
18	98	103	109	119	131	142	145	159	164
19	111	116	123	133	144	156	159	172	178
20	121	126	133	143	154	166	169	182	188
21	137	142	148	159	170	181	184	198	203
22	147	152	158	169	180	191	194	208	213
23	160	165	171	182	193	204	207	221	226
24	172	177	183	194	205	216	219	233	238
25	180	185	191	202	213	224	227	241	246
26	188	193	199	210	221	232	235	249	254
27	204	209	215	226	237	248	251	265	270
28	220	225	231	242	253	264	267	281	286
29	236	241	247	258	269	280	283	297	302
30	241	246	252	263	274	285	288	302	307
31	247	252	258	269	280	291	294	308	313
32	254	259	265	276	287	298	301	315	320
33	257	262	268	279	290	301	304	318	323
34	268	273	279	290	301	312	315	329	334
35	289	294	300	311	322	333	336	350	355
36	300	305	311	322	333	344	347	361	366
37	311	316	322	333	344	355	358	372	377
38	324	329	335	346	357	368	371	385	390
39	326	331	337	348	359	370	373	387	392
40	328	333	339	350	361	372	375	389	394
41	338	343	349	360	371	382	385	399	404

From Tamura RK, Sabbagha RE: Percentile ranks of fetal sonar abdominal circumference measurements, *Am J Obstet Gynecol,* 138:475, 1980.

10th percentile as the cutoff (Table 8-1; see Chapter 7, Table 7-13). It is important to remember that, although fetuses who are small for gestational age are detected, neither low weight nor abdominal circumference can differentiate symmetric from asymmetric IUGR.

Ratios of these three characteristics have been used with variable success in predicting the presence of asymmetric IUGR. In asymmetric IUGR, because the abdomen is typically initially affected more severely than either the head or femur, the head-to-abdominal circumference ratio has a high sensitivity. A table of the normal head-to-abdominal circumference ratios from 13 to 42 weeks' gestation shows the head to be normally larger in the second trimester (ratio, >1), with reversal near term (ratio, <1) (see Chapter 7, Table 7-8). A comparison of the BPD to the average body diameter yields similar results (see Chapter 7, Table 7-9). If the ratio is normal, however, fetal malnutrition is not excluded. The femur length–to–abdominal circumference ratio is an age-independent ratio for use from 22 weeks to term (normal between 18 and

24). Although initially shown to be elevated in the setting of asymmetric IUGR (small body) and decreased in the setting of macrosomia (large body), subsequent studies have shown this ratio to have a poor sensitivity and poor positive predictive value for both conditions. Additionally, it is not as sensitive as the head-to-abdominal circumference ratio. In symmetric IUGR all fetal size characteristics are affected equally and ratios have no diagnostic value.

Interval growth is a way of identifying both types of growth retardation. To effectively analyze this growth, longitudinal growth tables are needed based on data from the measurement of the same fetuses multiple times throughout pregnancy. True growth can then be established with both an accurate mean and SD range. Unfortunately, most studies are cross-sectional and involve evaluating a single fetus only once at random gestational ages; only the mean gestational age is accurate. At present, accurate longitudinal growth tables are only available for the BPD (see Chapter 7, Table 7-10). The same concept (described in the next paragraph) will also apply for body and femur growth when good longitudinal studies become available.

Two fetal examinations are needed, separated by an interval of no less than 3 weeks in the third trimester. Three weeks is the necessary interval because there is a potential measurement error on any study of no less than 1 mm, with a combined error of at least 2 mm for two studies. If an interval growth taken from 1 week to the next were only 2 mm, it is possible that all the presumed growth could actually represent a 2-mm error. Enough expected true growth is therefore needed to render the potential 2-mm error inconsequential. BPD growth in the early second trimester is approximately 3.5 mm/wk, so that 2 weeks (7 mm of growth) is needed between studies. Near term the normal BPD growth is only 1.5 mm/wk, with a minimum of 3 weeks ideally needed between studies (4.5 mm of growth). Because asymmetric IUGR is primarily diagnosed late in the third trimester, there is often little time to make the diagnosis, and studies performed less than 3 weeks apart may be necessary. Although interval growth can still be determined, it will be less accurate.

It is anticipated that normal fetal growth should be above the 10th percentile. Although 10% of normal fetuses will grow slower, so will almost all fetuses with IUGR. It is also expected that most fetuses will maintain predetermined growth percentiles throughout fetal life.

For example, a fetus growing at the 10th or 50th percentile early in pregnancy will typically remain at that same percentile until term. Using these two pieces of information, most growth above the 10th percentile should be normal and most growth below it should be abnormal. Four types of growth patterns have been described. Growth consistently above the 10th percentile and growth spurts from below to above the 10th percentile are almost always normal. Continued slow growth (below the 10th percentile) or a growth slowdown from above to below the 10th percentile is likely to be abnormal.

In asymmetric IUGR caused by fetal starvation, the loss of fetal subcutaneous fat could have diagnostic value. Unfortunately, at present no measurement has proved predictive.

The calculated fetal weight has been successfully combined with the clinical severity of hypertension and the ultrasound-determined amount of amniotic fluid in an attempt to predict IUGR. A table using these features has been developed. A fetus is considered relatively unlikely to have growth retardation if it weighs more than a certain amount. As hypertension or oligohydramnios, or both, become more severe, the fetal weight must be higher to rule out IUGR.

Amniotic fluid   The entire uterus must be examined to determine the volume of amniotic fluid. The amniotic fluid volume can be analyzed either qualitatively (subjec-

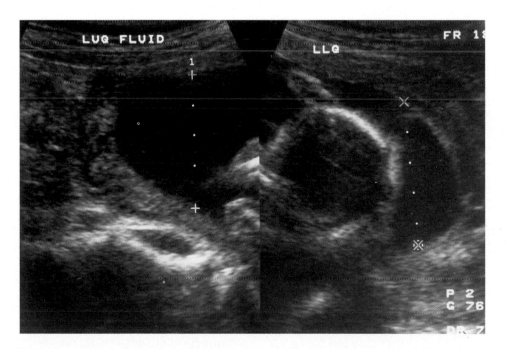

Fig. 8-1   Amniotic fluid index *(AFI)*. In this normal case sagittal images of the left upper quadrant *(LUQ)* and left lower quadrant *(LLQ)* were obtained. The largest amniotic fluid pockets were measured for the LUQ (+ and *dotted lines)* and the LLQ (x and *dotted lines)*. Additionally, the largest pockets in the right upper and lower quadrants are added to these measurements to obtain the AFI. All pockets are measured strictly from anterior to posterior and may contain umbilical cord or extremities.

tively) or quantitatively (by measurement). With real-time ultrasound only single pockets of fluid can be imaged at any one time. When the results of measurement techniques are compared with the findings from the subjective analysis of amniotic fluid, the subjective impression has been shown to be as accurate as the objective (quantitative) one, with excellent intraobserver and interobserver agreement.

Nevertheless, quantitative analysis can be performed and the findings obtained are at times helpful. The easiest method is to measure the largest single fluid pocket, with the measurement usually done in the anteroposterior dimension and avoiding a pocket of fluid containing mostly umbilical cord. This method is limited by its failure to analyze fluid in additional smaller pockets. To avert this pitfall, the amniotic fluid index is now used. In it the largest anteroposterior fluid pocket is imaged and measured in each of the four uterine quadrants (either in a sagittal or transaxial projection), and the four measurements are then totaled (Fig. 8-1). Although there are week-to-week fluctuations, the amniotic fluid index should usually be between 7 and 25 cm (Table 8-2).

It must be reemphasized that the subjective analysis of the amniotic fluid volume is equal in value to the amniotic fluid index. This is particularly true in borderline cases in which the index may be misleading. If, for example, the index is in the low normal range but subjectively the fluid appears decreased in volume, it is recommended that the examiner rely on the subjective interpretation and diagnose oligohydramnios. The result of the four-quadrant analysis should not be discarded, however, for it compels the examiner to examine the entire uterus.

The placenta   Asymmetric IUGR is caused by a placenta that does not supply adequate blood and nutrition to the fetus. Although there are no absolute criteria for identifying a dysfunctioning placenta, three placental properties have been analyzed: its thickness, its echogenicity, and its Doppler velocity waveform. The first two are discussed in Chapter 15 and the Doppler velocity waveform is described later in this chapter.

Grade 3 changes occur in only 15% of pregnancies. When detected, they are normally expected at 34 weeks and later. Although data from prospective studies are not available, a composite of data from case reports has shown that the incidence of asymmetric IUGR approaches 50% in fetuses younger than 34 weeks with grade 3 changes. Further work is needed, however, before the early appearance of grade changes can be considered a risk factor for IUGR.

Possible future characteristics   Two other ultrasound findings may be of value in diagnosing IUGR: the length of the liver and the epiphyseal centers, particularly at the distal end of the femur and the proximal end of the tibia. Although both need further evaluation in large prospective studies, they both hold promise in the detection of growth retardation.

The principle that underlies the use of the epiphyseal centers is that they are expected to develop at certain antenatal and postnatal ages. The distal femoral epiphysis has been shown to be 5 mm or more in its longest length by 32 weeks, with the proximal tibial epiphysis also growing to 5 mm or more by 36 weeks. If these lengths are found and yet the fetus is otherwise too small (by at least 2 weeks), this might suggest growth retardation. The overall length of the liver (the long axis of the right lobe) has proved of value for diagnosing normal and enlarged livers (fetal hydrops). Conversely, when the liver is smaller than expected, initial work has shown that this finding holds promise in the diagnosis of asymmetric IUGR. These findings are discussed more completely in Chapters 12 and 14.

The transverse cerebellar diameter increases normally as the fetus grows. Findings from initial studies of asymmetric growth retardation have suggested that this di-

Table 8-2	Amniotic fluid index values (cm) in normal pregnancy		
	Amniotic fluid index percentile values		
Week	**5th**	**50th**	**95th**
16	7.9	12.1	18.5
17	8.3	12.7	19.4
18	8.7	13.3	20.2
19	9.0	13.7	20.7
20	9.3	14.1	21.2
21	9.5	14.3	21.4
22	9.7	14.5	21.6
23	9.8	14.6	21.8
24	9.8	14.7	21.9
25	9.7	14.7	22.1
26	9.7	14.7	22.3
27	9.5	14.6	22.6
28	9.4	14.6	22.8
29	9.2	14.5	23.1
30	9.0	14.5	23.4
31	8.8	14.4	23.8
32	8.6	14.4	24.2
33	8.3	14.3	24.5
34	8.1	14.2	24.8
35	7.9	14.0	24.9
36	7.7	13.8	24.9
37	7.5	13.5	24.4
38	7.3	13.2	23.9
39	7.2	12.7	22.6
40	7.1	12.3	21.4
41	7.0	11.6	19.4
42	6.9	11.0	17.5

From Moore TR, Cayle JE: The amniotic fluid index in normal human pregnancy, *Am J Obstet Gynecol* 162:1168, 1990.

ameter would remain unaffected even when all other growth characteristics have shown a slowdown. More recently, however, the cerebellum has been shown to be equally affected by growth retardation.

Doppler Velocity Waveform Analysis

Placental circulation is composed of two parallel low-resistance, high-flow circulations. From the maternal side, approximately 100 spiral arteries feed the placenta through the uterine artery. From the fetal side, usually two but sometimes one umbilical artery flows to and one umbilical vein flows away from the placenta. The capillary vessels are long, tortuous, and dilated. This creates slow flow and a large surface area so that a maximum exchange of nutrients and waste products can take place. The low resistance ensures continuous blood flow throughout the fetal and maternal cardiac cycles.

The uterine and umbilical artery Doppler signals can be differentiated by their anatomic position: the uterine artery waveforms are obtained from either the basilar plate (between the placenta and myometrium) or lateral uterine wall, and the umbilical artery waveforms are obtained from the umbilical cord, usually in its middle. The heart rates also differ: the normal maternal heart rate is usually 80 beats/min, and the normal fetal heart rate is approximately 140 to 160 beats/min.

Obstetric Doppler examinations evaluate the flow of blood in the uterine spiral arteries and in the umbilical arteries. It is important to remember that this is a measurement of velocity of the arterial blood, and not true flow. To obtain true flow, an accurate blood vessel cross-sectional area and vessel angle would have to be computed simultaneously with the Doppler shift. These cannot be performed on routine ultrasound machines, and currently true flow has an error of 30% to 100%! Instead the arterial velocity waveform is analyzed by comparing peak systole (A) to end-diastole (B) in the same cycle as an A/B ratio. For maximum consistency, sampling should be repeated from at least three different waveforms and averaged. If variations in the ratio exist, some observers have suggested averaging as many as six consecutive A/B ratios. Because this is a comparison of the height of systole to end-diastole, the angle is not important.

Most studies have examined the uterine artery Doppler waveform in the third trimester and have found the A/B ratio to be fairly constant. The end-diastolic flow is always high (low resistance) and the mean A/B ratio is 2.0 at 28 weeks, decreasing slightly to 1.7 at term. It should not exceed 3.0 at any time. It is important to obtain the Doppler waveform from within the uterus, either from the basilar plate or within the uterine wall (Fig. 8-2). If a vessel outside the uterus exhibits a high-resistance signal, it may instead be a branch of the internal iliac artery (hypogastric artery) that is not feeding the uterus.

When Doppler waveform analysis is used on the umbilical cord, both the artery and vein signals are commonly identified: the typical pulsatile arterial flow of the

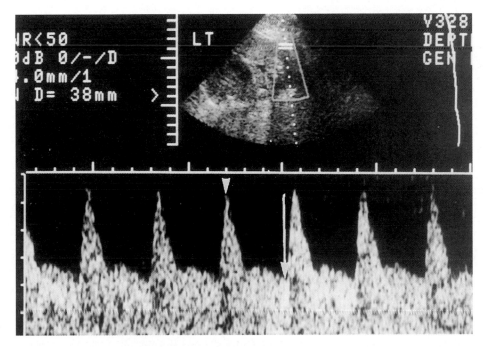

Fig. 8-2   Normal pulsed-Doppler evaluation of the uterine artery waveform, taken at the left lateral margin of the uterine wall. Peak systole, or A *(arrowhead)*, and end-diastole, or B *(arrow)*, are taken from the same waveform to obtain an A/B ratio.

umbilical artery on one side of the baseline and the nonpulsatile venous flow pattern of the umbilical vein on the other. The A/B ratio of the umbilical artery normally decreases throughout the second and third trimesters, from mean values of 4.25 at 16 weeks to 2.51 by term, with an abnormal ratio set at greater than the 90th percentile (Fig. 8-3; Table 8-3). The normal decrease in the ratio is caused by increasing diastolic flow. Because the ratio changes, knowledge of the fetal age is important. A top normal ratio at 28 weeks, for example, would be above the 90th percentile (abnormal) at 34 weeks.

If an abnormal Doppler signal is present, it may occur in the uterine artery, the umbilical artery, or both. Because many of the abnormal Doppler signals are encountered in women with vascular problems, usually essential or pregnancy-induced hypertension, it would be expected that the uterine artery waveform would initially become abnormal. Surprisingly, this is not always the case. Because the umbilical artery Doppler waveform analysis is more specific in identifying fetal problems, some have advocated using only the umbilical artery waveform.

Decreased blood flow to the fetus is usually caused by increased vascular resistance within the placental vascular bed, in the vessels supplying the placenta, or from the fetus. Less commonly it stems from maternal cardiovascular problems. As the resistance increases in any of these conditions, the diastolic flow decreases initially toward the baseline value, with reversal in more severe cases

(Fig. 8-4). If a further increase in resistance occurs, the systolic component becomes blunted and decreased in height.

An abnormal A/B ratio indicates an underlying fetal problem. However, once detected, can this abnormal ratio routinely be equated with fetal distress or demise? The

Table 8-3	Umbilical artery peak systolic–to–end-diastolic ratio		

Gestational age	Percentile		
	10th	50th	90th
16	3.01	4.25	6.07
20	3.16	4.04	5.24
24	2.70	3.50	4.75
28	2.41	3.02	3.97
30	2.43	3.04	3.80
32	2.27	2.73	3.57
34	2.08	2.52	3.41
36	1.96	2.35	3.15
38	1.89	2.24	3.10
40	1.88	2.22	2.68
41	1.93	2.21	2.55
42	1.91	2.51	3.21

From Fogarty P et al: Continuous wave Doppler flow velocity waveforms from the umbilical artery in normal pregnancy, *J Perinat Med* 18:51, 1990.

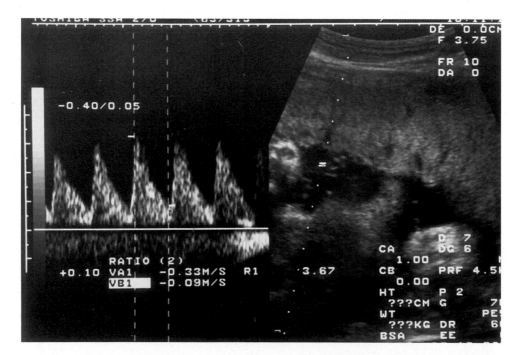

Fig. 8-3   Normal pulsed-Doppler evaluation of the umbilical artery waveform, taken in the midcord position, in a 32-week fetus. Peak systole and end-diastole, both denoted by a dash, are shown from the same waveform.

answer to this question is at present "no." Although the abnormal Doppler signal, particularly when other variables such as fetal biometric measurements are abnormal, elevates the fetus to an increased risk level, there is, nevertheless, not an absolute correlation between this and severe fetal compromise. In most pregnancies, close observation, not intervention, is considered the correct approach unless the fetus is mature enough to be delivered. As a general rule, however, the earlier an abnormal ratio is detected, the worse the prognosis.

Of additional importance, abnormal Doppler signals are not encountered in all cases of growth retardation. The indications for performing Doppler ultrasound should therefore be limited to selected cases of IUGR that are most likely due to malnutrition, not diminished cell growth.

More recently there has been an attempt to directly analyze the fetus' internal circulation (the descending thoracic aorta or kidneys) and cranial circulation (the carotid or middle cerebral arteries). In fetuses with asymmetric IUGR there is evidence that blood flow to the head will remain stable at the expense of blood flow to the remainder of the body. The A/B ratios for cerebral waveforms in fetuses with distress have been noted to be lower because of the increased diastolic flow involved. Further work is needed to determine the true significance of a lower A/B ratio, and its predictive value in fetal compromise.

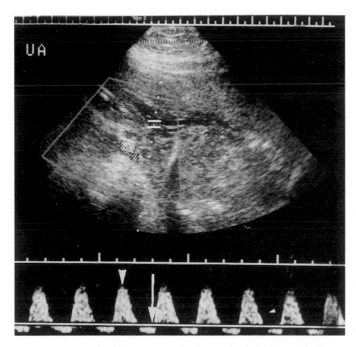

Fig. 8-4 Abnormal umbilical artery waveform obtained in a 34-week fetus. There is blunting of peak systole *(arrowhead)* and loss of end-diastolic flow, with actual reversal of flow *(arrow)*. A formal ratio cannot be obtained because the B, or end-diastolic, flow is below the baseline.

Biophysical Profile

Perinatal mortality is of clinical concern in the late third trimester. In premature deliveries 46% of the deaths are caused by the prematurity itself. In term deliveries, death is usually secondary to gross fetal anomalies (57%). In both settings, however, 17% of perinatal mortality (one out of every six fetuses) is caused by hypoxia.

The biophysical profile (BPP) is an extensively studied in utero test that can help in the prediction and management of fetuses with hypoxia. Five tests are used to determine the BPP: four of the fetus (acute hypoxia) and one of the amniotic fluid (chronic hypoxia). The four fetal tests evaluate the function of the heart, breathing, gross body movement, and overall tone. Of these, the heart rate study (the nonstress test [NST]) is typically performed in the obstetric department and makes use of an external monitor to analyze passive normal episodes of cardiac accelerations. The other four (breathing, gross body movements, tone, and amniotic fluid) are evaluated by an ultrasound examination.

The BPP uses a binomial grading system, with each variable assigned a 2 if present or a 0 if absent, for a maximum score of 10 and a minimum score of 0. The four fetal characteristics develop from different central nervous system centers. During embryogenesis the earliest developing center is fetal tone, followed by fetal movement, then fetal breathing movements, and last heart rate. Hypoxia appears to affect these centers in reverse order. Therefore, in addition to distinguishing chronic (amniotic fluid) from acute hypoxia, it is also possible to determine the degree of acute hypoxia by observing how many fetal characteristics are involved.

A normal fetus goes through sleep-wake cycles lasting 20 to 40 minutes. An important assumption of the BPP is that a fetus cannot be spontaneously awakened. When it is asleep, the normal fetus will resemble a compromised (hypoxic) fetus. However, the sleeping fetus will eventually awaken and start to move, and the compromised fetus will not. If during the 30 minutes the fetus responds appropriately, it is normal. In actuality most studies can be accomplished within 10 minutes. But, if the fetus is not moving, it is necessary to continuously observe the fetus for as much as 30 minutes to be certain that the fetus is not sleeping. If still unresponsive, the fetus is probably compromised. In actuality the absence of any response could still be questioned, as the normal cyclic changes last for as long as 40 minutes.

Specific definitions were given to each of the variables in the initial studies. Since that time, only the definition of gross body movements has remained unchanged; the definitions of the other four have changed. This is well described by Finberg and co-workers. For example, it has been suggested by one group that fetal tone too closely mirrors gross body movements and that fine body movements such as those of the hands should be used instead. Another group has suggested giving the fetus a "partial credit" of 1 (instead of 2) for any response that is somewhere between a full response and no response. Still another group has recommended using the contraction stimulation test, an active cardiac test requiring nipple stimulation or the administration of oxytocin.

These variations notwithstanding, there is a high degree of correlation between the BPP and the perinatal morbidity (fetal distress) and mortality (fetal demise). Fetal distress has a linear relationship to the BPP: there is almost no likelihood of fetal distress (<3%) associated with a BPP of 10, with this likelihood increasing steadily to 100% with a BPP of 0. Fetal death is tightly grouped at a score of 0 or 2, which means that only one characteristic can be normal. For a BPP score of 8 or 10, the negative predictive accuracy for a normal live outcome within 1 week of the test is 99.224%. Certain groups of high-risk mothers, particularly insulin-dependent diabetics, may need to be reexamined more than once a week. The intervening scores of 4 to 7, unfortunately, have not been analyzed fully.

It would be tempting to assume that all growth-retarded fetuses should have their BPP assessed. However, a number of fetuses with IUGR are not hypoxic and a number of hypoxic fetuses are not growth retarded. Therefore, although there is overlap in the characteristics of both, and many growth-retarded fetuses may be studied with BPPs, these two groups should not be considered the same.

A full BPP may not be needed in most cases, as the NST result is representative of the entire BPP. Although the positive predictive value for an abnormal BPP score is much greater than that for an abnormal NST result (56.6% versus 13.1%), the negative predictive value for a normal BPP score is virtually identical to a normal NST result (98.8% versus 98.0%). The NST should therefore be performed first, and only when the result is abnormal should the BPP be considered, thus saving time for ultrasound laboratories.

There is a distinct difference between the indications for a formal ultrasound obstetric examination and a BPP. The ultrasound examination is performed any time in pregnancy to establish fetal age and to evaluate for gross anomalies; the BPP is performed to evaluate fetal function in the late second trimester and third trimester.

Summary

When the gestational age is known, weight and abdominal circumference are helpful predictors of IUGR. When the gestational age is not known or uncertain, the only consistently useful characteristic for the analysis of symmetric growth retardation is slow interval growth.

Multiple additional characteristics are potentially available for determining asymmetric growth retardation: an abnormal head-to-body proportion, slow interval growth, decreased volume of amniotic fluid, abnormal Doppler signal. All must be evaluated because each case of asymmetric IUGR differs in its presentation and in its abnormal characteristics.

The BPP is a valuable test for predicting both normal (nonhypoxic) fetuses and impending fetal demise. The cardiac portion of the test should be performed first. The definition of the characteristics and the scoring systems need to be standardized, however.

MACROSOMIA

Large for gestational age and *macrosomia* are terms that are used interchangeably, but there is no consistent definition for them. Both are defined as a baby who is either above the 90th percentile by weight, or weighs more than either 4000 or 4500 g. Although a macrosomic or large for gestational age fetus will have an uncomplicated in utero life, problems can develop at the time of delivery.

These large fetuses are typically constitutionally symmetrically large, with fat distributed evenly over the entire body. In contradistinction, an asymmetrically large fetus has fat distributed more to the shoulders and body. This finding is commonly associated with gestational and mildly insulin-dependent diabetes in the mother, and such babies are at risk for shoulder dystocia during delivery. If a vaginal delivery is attempted, the head can be delivered without difficulty, but the shoulders may impact. If excessive traction on the neck is required to disengage the shoulders, this can cause injury to the newborn, most commonly an Erb's palsy (neurologic damage to the brachial plexus). At times, despite the use of all aggressive obstetric maneuvers, the results of delivery may be disastrous.

Estimated fetal weight alone cannot predict the disproportionality of the shoulders and body, and therefore tells the clinician little about the potential for dystocia. In addition, because there is a minimum of a 10% error in the calculation of the fetal weight, the fetus would have to weigh at least 4400 g to truly weigh more than 4000 g, and therefore potentially macrosomic or large for gestational age.

There have been attempts to measure the head, the head-to-body ratio, and shoulder size (from the neck to the edge of the shoulder) for the prediction of dystocia. This work is incomplete and has not been uniformly successful. At present, therefore, macrosomia can only be inferred from the estimated fetal weight and clinical suspicion.

Key Features

Neonates with small birth weights, usually defined as below the 10th percentile, are considered small for gestational age. These children can be either constitutionally small or growth retarded.

Intrauterine growth retardation (IUGR) varies in incidence, but on average affects 5% of the population and no greater than 10%.

There are two types of IUGR: diminished cellular growth, leading to a symmetrically small fetus (usually occurring in the first or early second trimester), and fetal malnutrition, leading to an asymmetrically small fetus (usually occurring in the third trimester). If the malnutrition is extreme, however, the asymmetric fetus may appear symmetric.

If the accurate fetal age is known, either from an early ultrasound examination or accurate menstrual dates, or both, then the measured abdominal circumference and calculated fetal weight can be used to determine if the fetal size and weight are appropriate.

When the accurate age is not known, additional less sensitive and specific characteristics for identifying IUGR are interval growth, the head-to-body ratio, the amniotic fluid volume, and the Doppler velocity waveform. Of these, only interval growth can be used for assessing both types of IUGR.

The volume of amniotic fluid can be evaluated either subjectively (by scanning the entire uterine content) or by a four-quadrant measurement called the *amniotic fluid index*. Subjective analysis is as accurate as the index and is of particular value in borderline cases.

Doppler evaluation makes use of a ratio of peak systole and end-diastole from the arterial waveform. As diastole decreases, the ratio increases, and the fetus is then at greater risk for circulatory problems. This has been evaluated for the uterine and particularly the umbilical arteries. More recently the fetal circulation has been studied, but no specific conclusions have been drawn.

The biophysical profile (BPP) can predict perinatal mortality by detecting in utero hypoxia (17% of all fetuses).

The BPP consists of five tests, four fetal ones for identifying acute hypoxia and the amniotic fluid for identifying chronic hypoxia. Each characteristic is rated as 2 if normal and 0 if absent, for a total score of from 0 to 10.

The fetus with a BPP score of 7 or more can be considered "safe" in most cases for a week, but is at risk for impending demise if the score is less than 4. Intervening numbers still indicate risk, but usually not the danger of sudden demise.

The two most sensitive BPP tests are the cardiac test for acute hypoxia (the nonstress test) and amniotic fluid analysis to assess for chronic hypoxia.

The terms *large for gestational age* and *macrosomia* can be used interchangeably. There are three definitions: a weight exceeding 4000 or 4500 g, or findings that place the fetus above the 90th percentile.

There are no problems with a macrosomic fetus in utero. At delivery, particularly if it is asymmetrically large (fat distributed more in the shoulders and body), the fetus is at risk for shoulder dystocia.

SUGGESTED READINGS

Benson C, Baltzman DH, Jones TB: FL/AC ratio: poor predictor of intrauterine growth retardation, *Invest Radiol* 20:727, 1985.

Benson CB et al: Intrauterine growth retardation: diagnosis based on multiple parameters—a prospective study, *Radiology* 177:499, 1990.

Brar HS et al: Cerebral, umbilical, and uterine resistance using Doppler velocimetry in postterm pregnancy, *J Ultrasound Med* 8:187, 1989.

Divon MY et al: Intrauterine growth retardation: a prospective study of the diagnostic value of real-time sonography combined with umbilical artery flow velocimetry, *Obstet Gynecol* 72:611, 1988.

Finberg HJ et al: The biophysical profile: a literature review and reassessment of its usefulness in the evaluation of fetal well-being, *J Ultrasound Med* 9:583, 1990.

Geirsson RT, Patel NB, Charisie AD: Intrauterine volume, fetal abdominal area and biparietal diameter measurements with ultrasound in prediction of small-for-dates babies in a high-risk obstetric population, *Br J Obstet Gynaecol* 92:936, 1985.

Geirsson RT, Patel NB, Christie AD: Efficacy of intrauterine volume, fetal abdominal area and biparietal diameter measurements with ultrasound in screening for small-for-dates babies, *Br J Obstet Gynaecol* 92:929, 1985.

Goldstein RB, Filly RA: Sonographic estimation of amniotic fluid volume: subjective assessment versus pocket measurements, *J Ultrasound Med* 7:363, 1988.

Hill LM et al: The transverse cerebellar diameter cannot be used to assess gestational age in the small for gestational age fetus, *Obstet Gynecol* 75:329, 1990.

Manning FA, Platt LD, Sipos L: Antepartum fetal evaluation: development of a fetal biophysical profile, *Am J Obstet Gynecol* 136:787, 1980.

Murao F et al: Detection of intrauterine growth retardation based on measurements of size of the liver, *Gynecol Obstet Invest* 29:26, 1990.

Pollack RN, Divon MY: Intrauterine growth retardation, and etiology, *Clin Obstet Gynecol* 35:99, 1992.

Rochelson B et al: The significance of absent end diastolic velocity in umbilical artery velocity waveforms, *Am J Obstet Gynecol* 156:1213, 1987.

Rochelson BL et al: The clinical significance of Doppler umbilical artery velocimetry in the small for gestational age fetus, *Am J Obstet Gynecol* 156:1223, 1987.

Sholl JS et al: Intrauterine growth retardation risk detection for fetuses of unknown gestational age, *Am J Obstet Gynecol* 144:709, 1982.

Trudinger BJ et al: Fetal umbilical artery velocity waveforms and subsequent neonatal outcome, *Br J Obstet Gynaecol* 98:378, 1991.

Trudinger BJ et al: A comparison of fetal heart rate monitoring and umbilical artery waveforms in the recognition of fetal compromise, *Br J Obstet Gynaecol* 93:171, 1986.

Trudinger BJ et al: Fetal umbilical artery flow velocity waveforms and placental resistance: clinical significance, *Br J Obstet Gynaecol* 92:23, 1985.

Vintzileos AM et al: The fetal biophysical profile and its predictive value, *Obstet Gynecol* 62:271, 1983.

First-Trimester Ultrasound

For a Key Features summary see p. 206.

The first trimester, defined as the interval between the last menstrual period and 12 weeks' gestation, is the most challenging diagnostic period in pregnancy. The key to any first-trimester test is to prove the existence of a normal intrauterine pregnancy (IUP). However, miscarriages (spontaneous incomplete or complete abortions), ectopic pregnancies, hydatidiform moles, and even unrelated pelvic pathologic conditions such as pelvic inflammatory disease and endometriosis may confuse this analysis.

The two most important diagnostic studies are the urine or blood pregnancy test and the ultrasound examination. The pregnancy test employs the β subunit of human chorionic gonadotropin (βhCG) and is highly specific for identifying a pregnancy. There are virtually no qualitative false-positive or false-negative diagnoses. If quantitated, the βhCG levels correlate well with embryonic age. Ultrasound is also invaluable in diagnosing IUPs. The combined use of transabdominal (TA) and transvaginal (TV) techniques has allowed the routine diagnosis of an early IUP.

In the first trimester the conceptus is called an *embryo;* later in pregnancy the term *fetus* is used instead. Throughout pregnancy, *gestational age, embryonic age,* and *menstrual age* are used interchangeably. All are sono-graphically defined as the age of the conceptus based on the first day of the normal last menstrual period (LMP). The LMP would seem to be an accurate method of defining the beginning of pregnancy. Its use, however, has many pitfalls. First, as much as 20% of women are uncertain about their menstrual dates, primarily because they have irregular periods or oligomenorrhea, or because they cannot recall their LMP. Second, the use of menstrual dates assumes a regular 28-day cycle. However, if, for example, a woman has a regular cycle, but it consists of 35 days, the LMP will create a 7-day error. Although the LMP could be accurate in any individual patient, its overall accuracy in the population as a whole is no better than ±2.5 weeks at the 95% confidence level (2 standard deviations). First- and second-trimester ultrasound, on the other hand, can determine gestational age to within ±1 week at 2 standard deviations.

THE GESTATIONAL SAC AND ITS MEASUREMENT

TA ultrasound scanning is performed suprapubically through a distended urinary bladder. The gestational sac can be identified by 5 weeks, with the embryo seen by 6.5 weeks; in some instances both can be identified earlier. Because there is usually a lag between identification of the gestational sac and the embryo, analysis of the gestational sac is important, especially before embryonic visualization.

The gestational sac is an anechoic space surrounded by a hyperechoic rim. Only the anechoic space is measured. In the early first trimester, before 7 weeks, the sac is often round and its diameter can be determined by a single measurement (Fig. 9-1). Later in the first trimester, the sac becomes more ovoid, and this is usually caused by pressure from the distended urinary bladder (Fig. 9-2). An average or mean gestational sac diameter (MGSD) is then obtained by determining the mean of three orthog-

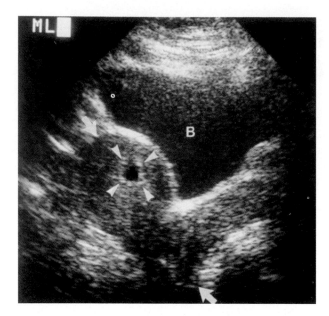

Fig. 9-1 Normal sagittal midline image of the uterus *(arrows)* at 5 weeks. Scanned transabdominally a well-defined round, anechoic gestational sac *(arrowheads)* with a hyperechoic rim is identified in the upper part of the uterine body. *B,* urinary bladder.

onal (perpendicular) measurements: the long axis and maximum anteroposterior diameter (perpendicular to it) obtained from the sagittal image and the width obtained from the transaxial view.

The gestational sac (using the MGSD) grows in a linear fashion. In the earliest ultrasound studies, some dating back to the late 1960s, a 10-mm sac was found at 5 weeks and it increased to 60 mm by 12.2 weeks (see Chapter 7, Table 7-1). More recently the early first-trimester measurements have been reevaluated (see Chapter 7, Table 7-2). Although differences have been found on both TA and TV studies, with all MGSDs smaller on TV studies, particularly those obtained between 5 and 6 weeks (Table 9-1), these differences are of uncertain origin. The TA and TV scanners are not the source of the differences, as both have been shown to be capable of similar measurement precision. The differences are also unlikely to be of clinical significance. They represent only a 1-week variance (compare the 11-mm size found by Daya and coworkers at 6 weeks with the 10-mm measurement noted by Hellman and coworkers at 5 weeks, as shown in Table 9-1). This is within the accuracy range of ±1 week.

In a simple formula preferred by some observers, the fetal age is computed in days using an MGSD rendered in millimeters. When the average sac is small (<15 mm), the fetal age is equal to 30+ MGSD. When the sac is large (>15

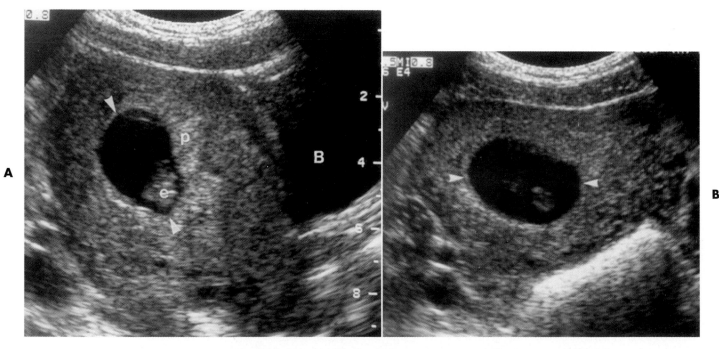

Fig. 9-2 Normal sagittal **(A)** and transaxial **(B)** images of a 7.1-week gestation. Scanned transabdominally the sac *(arrowheads)* is ovoid. A well-defined embryo *(e)* is identified within the sac. The hyperechoic placenta *(p),* a combination of chorionic villi and decidua basalis, is forming on the anterior surface of the sac. *B,* urinary bladder.

mm), the fetal age is equal to 31+ MGSD. This calculation yields numbers that approximate the data of Cadkin and McAlpin (Table 9-1).

THE EMBRYO AND ITS MEASUREMENT

The embryo can be identified routinely by TA imaging at 6.5 weeks. In almost all cases heart motion can be detected when the embryo is seen. It is not often necessary to use M-mode tracing to document heart motion; rather, observation with real-time ultrasound will usually suffice.

The embryo grows curvilinearly from 6 to 12 weeks, slowly at first with faster growth after 9 weeks. Its measurement, the crown-rump length (CRL), is performed along its longest observed axis. Both skilled and unskilled examiners are able to obtain accurate and consistent CRLs at any time in the first trimester. When the embryo is visualized at 6 to 7 weeks, it is difficult to identify the embryonic anatomy or even to differentiate the two ends of the embryo (the crown from the rump); by 8 to 9 weeks, the head and body can be identified (Fig. 9-3).

Findings from early studies on the accuracy of the CRL, performed in the 1970s, had suggested an accuracy of ±3 days in 95% of the pregnant population. Findings from recent studies have revealed a more realistic accuracy of ±5 to 7 days at 2 SD. The CRL can be less accurate after 12 weeks, in the second trimester, because the fetus can flex and extend and thus cause the measurement to vary. The biparietal diameter, on the other hand, is routinely imaged in the second trimester and has the same accuracy as the CRL up to 24 weeks. It is therefore recommended that the CRL be used until 12 weeks and the biparietal diameter thereafter.

In one of the earliest and best-regarded studies of TA ultrasound, the smallest routinely measured embryo was found to have a CRL of 6.7 mm at 6.3 weeks. This work has been reevaluated using both TA and TV ultrasound, most recently in 1991 (Chapter 7, Table 7-3). Unlike the MGSD, no significant measurement differences from previous studies have been found. The newer table, however, assigns a gestational age to embryos as small as 2 mm. This is equivalent to 5.7 weeks and permits earlier determination of the first-trimester age by approximately half a week.

COMPARISON OF GESTATIONAL SAC AND EMBRYO

There is potential value in comparing the MGSD to the CRL in the first trimester. This is comparable to evaluating the volume of amniotic fluid surrounding the fetus in the second and third trimesters. However, because the MGSD and CRL measurements come from different and unrelated tables, this analysis is limited. Nevertheless, ideally the gestational age indicated by these sac and embryo measurements should not be discrepant, and if the ages indicated by the two are found to be more than 1½ to 2 weeks apart, a follow-up study to evaluate normal growth is suggested.

In a recent study a direct comparison of the two was attempted, and a predictive value was found in subtracting the MGSD from the CRL (both rendered in millimeters). When the resultant value was 5 mm or more, all fetuses were found to be normal. When the value was less than 5 mm, almost all (94%) were aborted spontaneously, some of which were already abnormal at the time of the

Table 9-1   Comparison of gestational sac measurement between 5 and 6 gestational weeks

Gestational weeks	Mean gestational sac diameter (mm)		
	Hellman et al.* 1969, TA	Cadkin et al.† 1984, TA	Daya et al.‡ 1991, TV
5	10	5	2
5.5	13	8.5	6
6	17	12	11

TA, transabdominal; *TV*, transvaginal.

*Hellman LM et al: Growth and development of the human fetus prior to the 20th week of gestation, *Am J Obstet Gynecol* 103:789, 1969.

†Cadkin AV, McAlpin J: The decidua-chorionic sac: a reliable sonographic indicator of intrauterine pregnancy prior to detection of a fetal pole, *J Ultrasound Med* 3:539, 1984.

‡Daya S et al: Early pregnancy assessment with transvaginal ultrasound scanning, *Can Med Assoc J* 144:441, 1991.

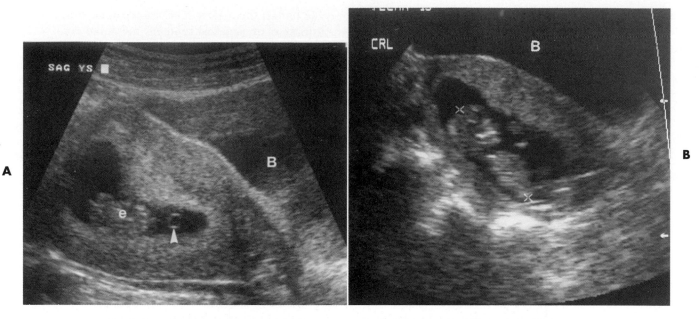

Fig. 9-3   Two transabdominal scans of embryos in the first trimester. **A,** An embryo *(e)* at 8.3 weeks. **B,** An embryo *(x)* at 11.6 weeks. With advancing size, definition of the embryo becomes more apparent, with **B** showing the head and some facial structures (in the upper left of the embryo) separated from the body. In the earlier gestation **B,** a yolk sac is also identified *(arrowhead).* *B,* urinary bladder.

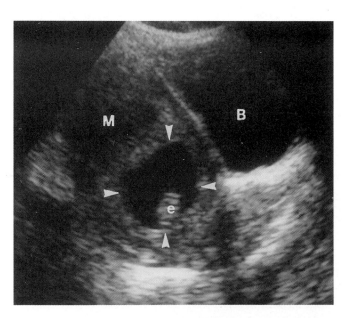

Fig. 9-4   Transabdominal sagittal image of a 6.6-week pregnancy shows a fundal fibroid *(M)* displacing the gestational sac *(arrowheads)* downward into the lower part of the uterine body. *e,* embryo; *B,* urinary bladder.

study. Although this direct comparison is valuable, all of the abnormal cases involved so little fluid that a measurement was not necessary. A larger study will be needed before the predictive value of this method can be determined.

THE NORMAL GESTATIONAL SAC

Until the embryo is identified, the gestational sac is the only available intrauterine structure that can be used to determine if a pregnancy exists and if it is developing normally. After implantation the gestational sac can first be identified as a hyperechoic, rounded area, and then as a small anechoic sac within the thickened decidua. This has been termed the *intradecidual sign.* It is seen before 5 weeks when the sac is still too small to indent the endometrial canal and to exhibit the other features of a larger gestational sac (see Fig. 9-14, *B*). The normal position of this early sac can also be confirmed.

After 5 weeks the appearance of the gestational sac can be evaluated more completely by a number of characteristics that are then evident: a double decidual sac (DDS), an anechoic space surrounded by a continuous hyperechoic rim that is 2 mm or more thick, a grossly spherical or ovoid shape without angulation, and growth of more than 1.2 mm/day. To evaluate growth, at least 5 days should separate the two studies so that a minimum of 6 mm of growth has occurred; adequate growth can only

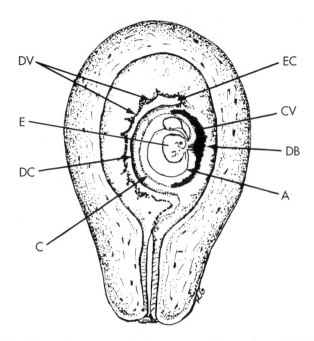

Fig. 9-5 The uterus in the first trimester. The embryo *(E)* is developing within the amniotic sac *(A)*. The chorionic sac *(C)*, containing the yolk sac, surrounds the amniotic sac. The chorionic villi *(CV)* and the decidua basalis *(DB)* will form the placenta. On the opposite side of the chorionic sac, the decidua capsularis *(DC)* is greatly thinned. Between it and the opposite decidua the decidua vera *(DV)* is the closed endometrial canal *(EC)*. The potential uterine normal spaces are the endometrial canal and the separation of the amnion from the chorion.

be analyzed effectively if the measurement error (1 mm on a single study and 2 mm on two studies) is minimized.

The position of the gestational sac is important (see Fig. 9-1). The sac should be situated in the upper uterine body, in a midposition between the uterine walls. A lower-lying gestational sac suggests a miscarriage (either an impending spontaneous pregnancy loss or one in progress), a cervical ectopic pregnancy, or the presence of a fundal fibroid displacing the sac downward (Fig. 9-4).

The DDS is also an important feature. As the embryo implants into the uterine wall, it causes a hyperechoic trophoblastic reaction; a secondary endometrial hyperechoic decidual reaction then occurs (Fig. 9-5). As the sac grows, it causes the endometrial canal to close, and the hyperechoic decidual reaction is interrupted by this apposed hypoechoic canal along part of its rim (Fig. 9-6). This DDS sign is seen in most normal early IUPs (>98%). Conversely, a hyperechoic rim without a DDS is more likely to occur in an abnormal pregnancy, and usually represents a pseudogestational sac of fluid within the endometrial canal secondary to an ectopic pregnancy (>70%). Less often it occurs in the setting of either a normal or abnormal IUP. Therefore, the finding of a DDS confirms a normal IUP; its absence does not rule out an IUP but strongly suggests the existence of an abnormality.

Further gestational sac analysis has revealed that an embryo and a secondary yolk sac (discussed later in this chapter) should be identified routinely when the sac reaches a certain size. In an evaluation of *abnormal* IUPs, a 100% positive predictive value is noted when the MGSD exceeds 25 mm without an embryo or exceeds 20 mm

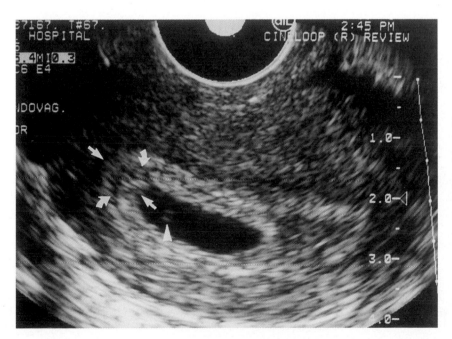

Fig. 9-6 The double decidual sac sign *(DDS)* of a normal intrauterine pregnancy. Transvaginal scan of an early gestational sac at less than 5 gestational weeks. The yolk sac *(arrowhead)* is seen but the embryo cannot yet be identified. The hyperechoic wall of the gestational sac *(small arrows)* is interrupted along part of its margin by a hypoechoic line *(curved arrows)* produced by the apposed endometrial canal.

without a yolk sac (Fig. 9-7). A considerably distorted sac is also 100% predictive of an abnormal IUP, with additional high positive predictive values (>90%) for a thin decidual reaction of less than 2 mm, a weak decidual amplitude and a low gestational sac position (Fig. 9-8).

POTENTIAL UTERINE SPACES OR COLLECTIONS

In addition to a normal gestational sac, other uterine findings can be seen: fluid within the endometrial canal, a normal chorioamniotic separation, a "vanishing twin," an implantation bleed, a necrotic fibroid, and a split-image artifact. These should be kept in mind during any first-trimester examination.

The endometrial canal is a potential space, apposed but patent throughout the first trimester (see Fig. 9-5). It is surrounded by a hyperechoic decidual reaction. Any fluid, usually blood, can cause the endometrial canal to distend and can outline the free margin of the gestational sac (the chorion and decidua capsularis), which has a well-defined thickness of 2 mm or more (Fig. 9-9).

The gestational sac is filled by the chorionic sac. Within it the embryo develops within the smaller amniotic sac (see Fig. 9-5). Ultimately the amnion will expand to the chorion and the two will fuse as late as 16 weeks. These two spaces can be likened to a balloon within a balloon, the smaller inner balloon the amniotic sac and the larger outer balloon the chorionic sac (Fig. 9-10). The normal amnion is a thin membrane (<1 mm). Some observers believe that the amnion is abnormal if it is unusually thick or "lumpy," or unusually large, or both. More

work in this area is needed to elucidate the nature and importance of these findings. The secondary yolk sac, when identified, develops within the chorionic space and is therefore completely separate from the embryo.

Additional intrauterine findings can sometimes be detected: a vanishing twin and an implantation bleed. The vanishing twin is an anechoic space that appears within the endometrial canal. It looks like (and is) a second gestational sac, but without an embryo. The contour of this second sac is often distorted, it is ovoid or curvilinear, and it is separated from the normal IUP by a membrane (Fig. 9-11, A). This diagnosis can only be suggested, not established, by an elevated βhCG level (above that for a normal singleton pregnancy) or by an earlier examination that had shown a twin pregnancy. An implantation bleed is bleeding that occurs within the uterine wall where the chorionic insertions attach into the endometrium (Fig. 9-11, B). It has been given many names, *implantation bleed* being the most common. An area of first-trimester bleeding can assume any degree of echogenicity, ranging from anechoic to hyperechoic, and is similar in concept to an abruptio placentae, seen later in pregnancy. Quite frequently an implantation bleed is only an incidental finding and is of no clinical concern, but, once detected, it should be followed to rule out propagation.

Rarely, fibroids, if necrotic, may resemble a gestational sac (Fig. 9-12). Fibroids are discussed more completely in the last section of this chapter.

One final potential pitfall that can arise in the evaluation of a first-trimester gestational sac is the split-image artifact. During TA scanning performed through a distended urinary bladder, a transaxial midline scan obtained immediately superior to the pubis may make a single ges-

Text continues on p. 201.

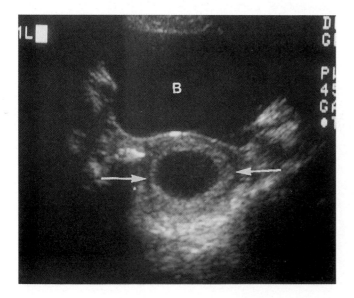

Fig. 9-7 Spontaneous incomplete abortion (miscarriage). In this transabdominal transaxial image of the uterus, the gestational sac *(arrows)* has a normal hyperechoic rim but without a double decidual sac sign. The sac averages 30 mm in diameter, but no embryo is identified. *B,* urinary bladder.

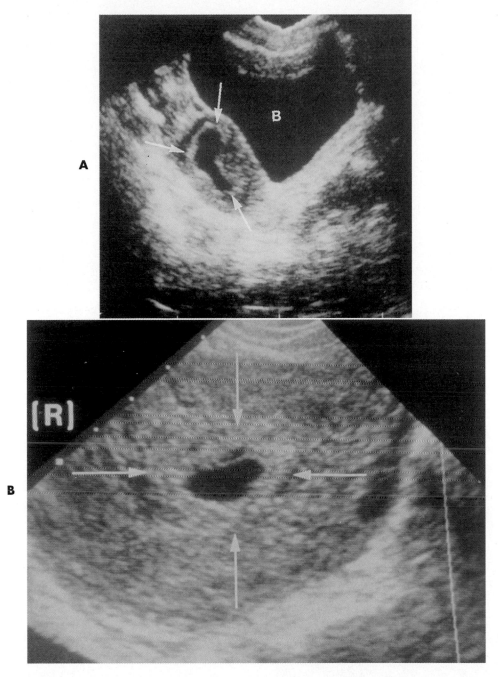

Fig. 9-8 Two cases of spontaneous incomplete abortions (miscarriages). In both arrows denote the gestational sac. An embryo is not identified in either. **A,** A transabdominal sagittal scan shows a markedly irregular and angulated gestational sac with a thinned and inconsistent hyperechoic rim. *B,* urinary bladder. **B,** A transvaginal image taken in a transaxial-coronal projection shows an irregularly thickened hyperechoic rim without well-defined margins and with hypoechoic to anechoic spaces.

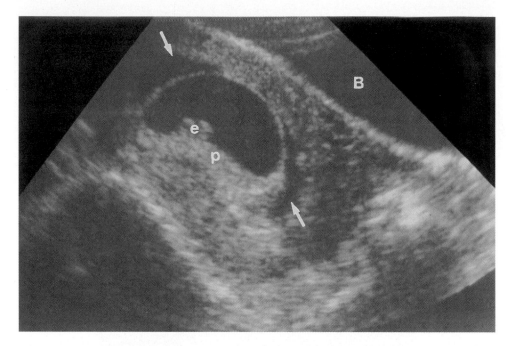

Fig. 9-9   Transabdominal sagittal scan of the uterus in an 8-week pregnancy. The woman had presented with active vaginal bleeding. A well-defined gestational sac is identified, containing a living embryo *(e)*. The forming placenta *(p)* is anchored to the posterior wall of the endometrium. Anechoic blood is seen superior and inferior to the sac *(arrows)*, spreading the endometrial canal and outlining the free surface of the chorionic sac and its decidua capsularis. *B*, urinary bladder.

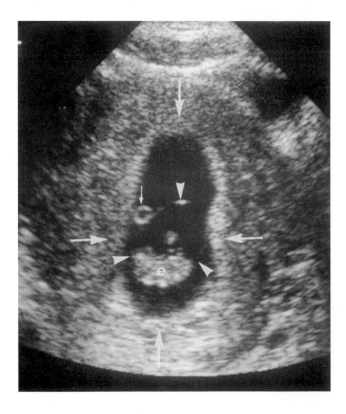

Fig. 9-10   Transvaginal transaxial-coronal image of a normal 7-week pregnancy. The chorionic sac fills the gestational sac *(arrows)*. Within it is the smaller amniotic sac *(arrowheads)* containing a living embryo *(e)*. Immediately above the embryo is hyperechoic tissue corresponding to a portion of the umbilical cord. The yolk sac *(small arrow)* is identified within the chorionic sac. Note the thinness of the amniotic membrane.

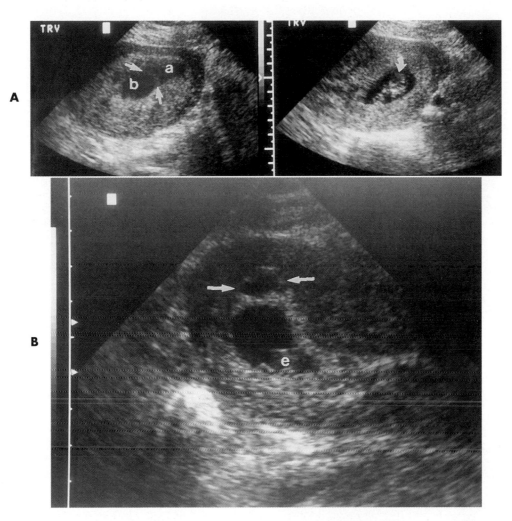

Fig. 9-11 Different first-trimester collections. **A,** A "vanishing twin." Two transaxial-coronal images are shown in this transvaginal study. In the left image two small anechoic spaces *(a* and *b)* are separated by a thick membrane *(arrows)* resulting from a previous dichorionic-diamniotic pregnancy. In the right image, more inferiorly, only sac *b* is seen, containing a well-defined embryo *(curved arrow).* Sac *a* is the resolving second sac of a former twin pregnancy, the thick membrane making this a dichorionic-diamniotic pregnancy. **B,** An implantation bleed. In this transabdominal midline sagittal scan a well-defined gestational sac is identified, containing a living embryo *(e).* Slightly superior and outside the sac a small hypoechoic to anechoic collection *(arrows),* noted within the uterine wall, disrupts part of the hyperechoic rim of the gestational sac. This finding is consistent with a bleed at the site of chorionic attachment.

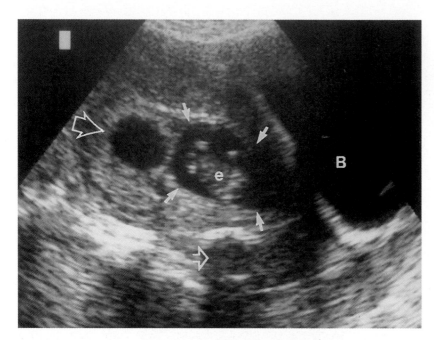

Fig. 9-12   First-trimester pregnancy with a necrotic fibroid. This transabdominal sagittal image of an 8-week pregnancy shows a well-defined gestational sac *(arrows)* in the lower part of the uterus with a normal embryo *(e)*. More superiorly a fibroid *(open large arrow)* is seen as a solid mass with a hypoechoic center that exhibits no distal acoustic enhancement. This mass is responsible for causing the unusually low gestational sac position. A second smaller fibroid with a hyperechoic rim of calcification *(small open arrow)* is seen posterior to the gestational sac. *B,* urinary bladder.

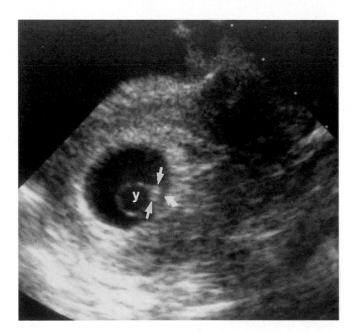

Fig. 9-13   Transvaginal scan of a normal 4.5-week pregnancy shows a well-defined gestational (chorionic) sac with a hyperechoic rim. Along one of its walls is a combination of three findings, termed the *double-bleb sign,* and these consist of two cystic spaces, the larger the secondary yolk sac *(y)* and the smaller *(curved arrow)* the amniotic sac, with a small 3-mm hyperechoic prochordal plate *(arrows)* of the developing embryo in between. Heart motion could already be identified.

tational sac appear as two. This illusion is caused by an optic lens effect: the ultrasound beam is focused between the two rectus abdominis muscles at the linea alba, and part of the beam is bent by the curvilinear fat pad located immediately below. This creates two partially separated, identical images. An artifact, rather than a twin gestation, is suggested by the unusually rectangular (instead of round or ovoid) shape of the uterus and the finding that the two sacs move together when the transducer is rocked from side to side. When the transducer is moved off the midline in a transaxial scan or into any sagittal plane, only a single gestational sac is identified, thus proving the artifact. If any doubt remains, TV scanning can also be performed.

TRANSVAGINAL SCANNING

TV scanning has had a significant impact on the evaluation of first-trimester pregnancies. After the probe is sterilized and placed into a latex sheath (usually a condom), it is inserted approximately halfway into the vagina. It does not routinely touch the cervix unless intentionally inserted farther, and its use is therefore not contraindicated in the first trimester, even in problem pregnancies. Although a careful TV examination can therefore be performed without undue concern, the obstetrician should be notified before the start of the examination if there is doubt about its appropriateness.

TV sonography is successful for three primary reasons. First, the study is performed with an empty or near-empty bladder. Any inconvenience having to do with the vaginal probe is far outweighed by the convenience of not needing a full bladder. Second, the study uses a high-frequency, short-focused transducer, which is capable of achieving better detail to a depth of approximately 8 to 10 cm. Third, landmarks can be evaluated in different planes, such as the coronal plane.

The TV technique has some pitfalls, however. First, because the probe is intracavitary (within the vagina), its positioning is limited. Second, a long-axis view of the uterus is sometimes the only consistently definable landmark. Third, any structure or mass that is more than 8 to 10 cm from the transducer face either cannot be identified or its full extent cannot be appreciated. Fourth, the ultrasound beam is usually angled anteriorly as it exits the TV probe. Although this angulation is useful for the long-axis examination of an anteverted uterus, a retroverted uterus may be imaged incompletely. It may be necessary to turn the transducer 180 degrees (then reverse the image on the ultrasound machine) so that posterior areas can be defined more clearly. Similarly, the probe may have to be turned 180 degrees when evaluating the adnexal regions so that both sides are identified fully.

THE VALUE OF TRANSVAGINAL VERSUS TRANSABDOMINAL STUDIES

In some very early IUPs, between 4 to 5 weeks, a double-bleb sign can be seen. By scanning the margins of the gestational sac (also the chorionic sac), two cystic structures may be identified: the smaller amniotic sac (closer to the wall) and the larger secondary yolk sac (farther away) (Fig. 9-13). Between the two, the prochordal plate of the developing embryo can be seen as a 2- to 4-mm linear hyperechoic disc, occasionally even with detectable heart motion. Although this double-bleb sign is not often seen, its position serves as a reminder that the initial development of the embryo takes place along the gestational sac margin.

Comparative studies have shown the value of the TV technique when TA scanning proves difficult. TV scanning is particularly helpful in unusually large women, when the distance from the anterior abdominal wall to the uterus is more than 10 cm, because it can add information, either by more clearly defining the gestational sac or by defining an embryo (Fig. 9-14). The TA and TV techniques have been directly compared in a prospective double-blind study that evaluated two normal first-trimester milestones (at the 100% cutoff limits): the size of the gestational sac needed to identify an embryo (not necessarily with heart motion) and the size of the embryo needed to see heart motion (Table 9-2). Transabdominally an embryo was always seen when the gestational sac was 27 mm or larger; transvaginally the sac only had to be 12 mm or larger to be seen. The value of TV ultrasound is clearly shown, as the embryo is identified by 5.3 weeks, more than 2 weeks earlier than detected by TA scanning! Some observers believe, however, that the definitive gestational sac size for identifying the embryo on TV images should be larger, either 16 or 18 mm. These are more cautious estimates representing gestational ages of 5.9 and 6.2 weeks, respectively, but are still considerably earlier predictors than those achieved by the TA approach.

In the same article, heart motion was detected 100% of the time transabdominally when the CRL was 9 mm or more (6.9 weeks), but on transvaginal images the embryo only had to be 5 mm or more (6.2 weeks) for heart motion to be detected. Heart motion could therefore be detected more than a half a week earlier on the TV images. Even earlier detection is possible, but not in every case.

The TA examination should not be abandoned, however. Instead it should be performed first. If it shows a normal IUP with normal heart motion, a TV study is rarely needed. If any of the findings are uncertain, however, TV imaging should be performed without hesitation to identify the embryo or its heart motion. If the abnormal findings persist, the pregnancy is most likely abnormal, and a follow-up study should be reserved for selected borderline cases.

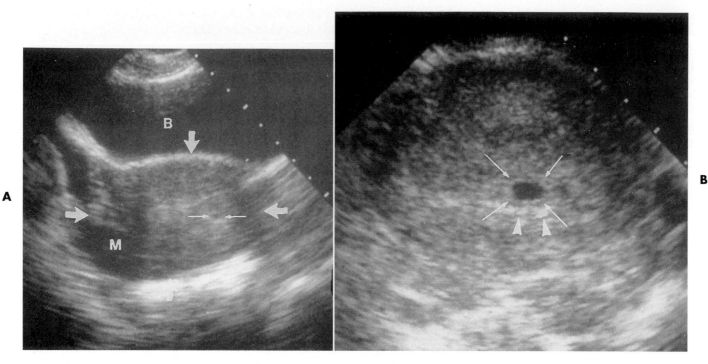

Fig. 9-14   Comparison of the transabdominal and transvaginal studies in a less than 5-week pregnancy. **A,** The transabdominal transaxial view shows a large bulky uterus *(arrows)*, with at least one hypoechoic solid mass, a fibroid *(M)*, identified on the right posterolaterally. A possible early intrauterine pregnancy is noted on the left *(small arrows)*. *B,* urinary bladder. **B,** The intradecidual sign. This transvaginal study in the transaxial-coronal projection shows a well-defined gestational sac with a normal hyperechoic rim *(small arrows)* embedded within the endometrium, adjacent to the apposed hyperechoic endometrial canal *(arrowheads)*. An embryo could not yet be identified.

Table 9-2   Analysis of first-trimester ultrasound findings in 100% of cases by transabdominal and transvaginal analysis

Ultrasound technique	Gestational sac size (mm) to identify embryo	Embryonic age (wk)	CRL size (mm) to identify heart motion	Embryonic age (wk)
Transabdominal	≥27	7.5	≥9	6.9
Transvaginal	≥12	5.3	≥5	6.2

From Pennell RG et al: Prospective comparison of vaginal and abdominal sonography in normal early pregnancy, *J Ultrasound Med* 10:63, 1991.
CRL, crown-rump length.

In the first trimester, at approximately 5 weeks, heart motion can be identified even before the heart is fully formed. Its rate is commonly 100 beats/min or more. By 8 weeks, and from then until term, the rate averages 140 beats/min, with a range of 120 to 180 beats/min. A bradycardiac heart rate of less than 90 beats/min at 5 weeks and less than 120 beats/min from 8 weeks on might imply impending fetal demise, and close observation of the pregnancy is then recommended. Faster heart rates have not been detected.

Because there is a known 20% to 25% spontaneous loss rate in the first trimester, does the early detection of car-

diac activity imply a "safe" ongoing pregnancy? A study by Levi and coworkers of embryos less than 5 mm (<6.2 weeks) revealed that, even when cardiac activity was detected, there was still a 24% miscarriage rate. When vaginal bleeding was present, spontaneous abortion occurred in 33%. Therefore, although it may be tempting to say that an embryo less than 5 mm with heart motion is normal (that it will progress normally to term) this diagnosis should be made cautiously. Even in asymptomatic women, this diagnosis should await the findings from a later examination, and it is probably safe to make this diagnosis only when the embryo exceeds 10 mm (>7.1

Table 9-3	First-trimester comparison of the serum βhCG levels (first international reference preparation) and ultrasound landmarks with gestational age

βhCG (IU/L)	Ultrasound landmarks	Gestational age
1,000	Gestational sac	32 days (<5 wk)
7,200	Yolk sac	36-40 days (5 to 6 wk)
10,000	Embryo with heart motion	40 days (<6 wk)

weeks). Conversely, some of the initial embryos smaller than 5 mm that showed no initial cardiac activity progressed normally to term. The initial absence of heart motion is therefore not always a poor prognostic sign.

The primary or primitive yolk sac develops and resolves early in the first trimester. By 2 weeks of implantation (4 menstrual weeks), it is no longer visible. The secondary yolk sac then develops, and it can be imaged as a 0.4-mm cystic structure by 4½ weeks (see Figs. 9-3, A, 9-6, 9-10, and 9-13). The secondary yolk sac exhibits slight curvilinear growth, increasing in average diameter to 4.0 mm by 10 weeks; after 11 weeks it begins to involute. Findings from normal studies have suggested that a normal yolk sac can be identified slightly less than 1 week before the normal embryo is seen. Transabdominally the normal embryo was detected by an MGSD of 25 mm, with the yolk sac routinely identified earlier by an MGSD of 20 mm. In another study, the embryo was seen transvaginally by an MGSD of 16 mm, but the yolk sac was identified by an MGSD of 8 mm. The authors of both articles stated that inability to identify the yolk sac (at its expected MGSD) was commonly associated with an abnormal pregnancy.

The characteristics of the yolk sac have been restudied, with most investigators corroborating these observations. However, the results from a continuation of the double-blind prospective study disagreed with these findings. In the study, there were cases in which both TA and TV studies (at the expected MGSD sizes) showed the yolk sac was not present but the pregnancies proved to be normal; there were other cases in which the yolk sac was present but the pregnancies were abnormal. It is therefore thought that the determination of a normal or abnormal pregnancy should await identification of the embryo and its cardiac motion.

A study conducted by Bree and coworkers analyzed the TV ultrasound and laboratory findings in first-trimester pregnancies (Table 9-3). Using the first international reference preparation for the βhCG values, TV ultrasound was found to identify the gestational sac when the βhCG exceeded 1000 IU/L (<5 weeks), the yolk sac when the βhCG was greater than 7200 IU/L (5 to 6 weeks), and the embryo when the βhCG exceeded 10,000 IU/L (slightly <6 weeks). Thus expected ultrasound landmarks could be identified at specific βhCG levels.

Fetal Anatomy

The ability of TA ultrasound to detect normal first-trimester fetal anatomic characteristics is limited. Only the embryo, its heart motion, and the differentiation of the head from the body have been consistently identified by 8 to 9 weeks. With TV imaging fetal anatomic characteristics are seen earlier and more completely. The embryo with its heart motion is routinely detected by 6 weeks, and the head can be distinguished from the body by 7 to 8 weeks. Additional analysis of intraembryonic structures is possible by 8 weeks. At 8 weeks two hypoechoic intracranial structures can be identified routinely: the forebrain (prosencephalon) and hindbrain (rhombencephalon) (Fig. 9-15, A). After 8 weeks the heart chambers and great vessels can (on occasion) be identified. Between 9 to 12 weeks a hyperechoic fullness can be identified routinely at the base of the umbilical cord, and this is due to normal midgut herniation (Fig. 9-15, B). Although an excess of soft tissue in this region has previously been diagnosed as an omphalocele, this diagnosis must be made cautiously; the soft tissue protrusion is normal when it is 7 mm or less in diameter, or less than one third the diameter of the adjacent abdomen. By 11 weeks the spine and extremities can be identified.

Because of the increased detection capabilities of TV imaging, one might consider performing a TV study during all first-trimester pregnancies. This is tempting, but, at present, no study has proved that the improved identification possible with TV ultrasound has clinical merits.

MULTIPLE GESTATIONS

The TA evaluation of multiple gestations often suffices to determine the number of gestations, cardiac activity, and the type of separating membranes. TV studies can be a valuable adjunctive first-trimester study, particularly when there are more than two gestations. The number and size of each embryo, and the type of interposed membrane can be evaluated more critically by TV scanning. Although each embryo is likely to be dizygotic or fraternal (dichorionic-diamniotic pregnancies) with a thick separating membrane, it is always possible to have a spontaneous monochorionic embryo with either a thin or no interposed membrane. This is discussed more completely in Chapter 16.

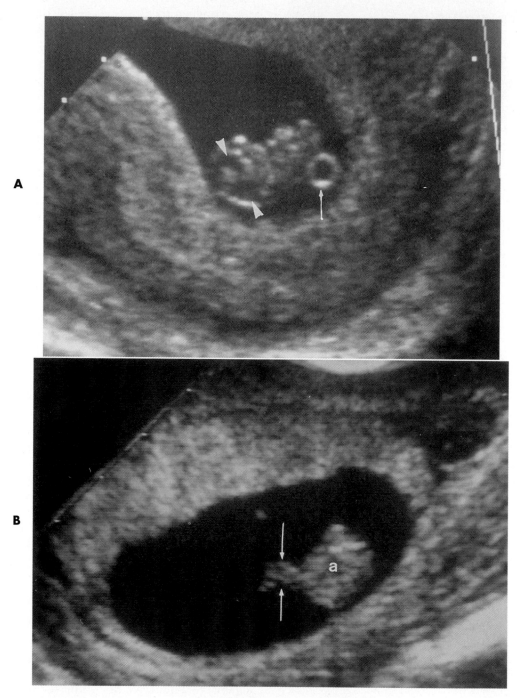

Fig. 9-15   Early normal embryonic anatomic features identified by transvaginal scanning. **A,** Long-axis image of an embryo shows two hypoechoic, well-defined structures within the head *(arrowheads)* corresponding to the normal forebrain and hindbrain. The yolk sac is also identified *(arrow)*. **B,** Transaxial view of the abdomen *(a)* at the umbilical cord insertion *(arrows)* showing the normal fullness of a midgut herniation at the base of the umbilical cord.

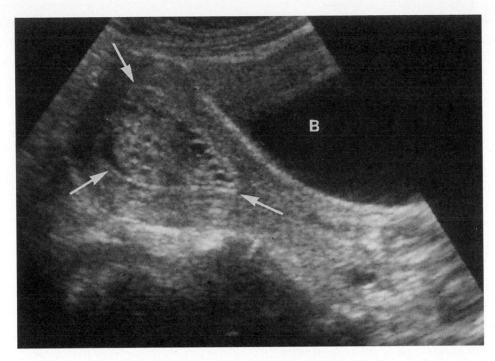

Fig. 9-16   Hydatidiform mole. This transabdominal sagittal midline image shows an enlarged first-trimester uterus. A markedly spread endometrial canal *(arrows)* is filled with hypoechoic and hyperechoic tissue. The extent of the tissue within the canal, combined with appropriate clinical and laboratory data, is consistent with the characteristics of a molar pregnancy. *B,* urinary bladder.

DOPPLER WAVEFORM ANALYSIS

Doppler waveform analysis has been used to examine the gestational sac wall. When an early first-trimester sac is identified (before the embryo is imaged) and found to be either normal or atypical, the arterial waveform can be studied to detect an elevation in peak systolic and in end-diastolic flow. Of the two, the end-diastolic flow appears to reflect the trophoblastic vascularity of an IUP, normal or recently aborted. A pseudogestational sac from an ectopic pregnancy or more long-term retained products of conception would not be expected to exhibit substantial flow within the uterus, although a similar trophoblastic Doppler pattern can, on occasion, be detected at an ectopic site. More work is needed to determine the positive predictive value of these observations.

OTHER ANOMALIES

Two additional first-trimester uterine anomalies should also be considered: hydatidiform moles and fibroids. If the uterus appears to be unduly large and has multiple hypoechoic and hyperechoic spaces filling and distending the endometrial canal (without a well-defined embryo), a hydatidiform mole is possible (Fig. 9-16). Although a spontaneous incomplete abortion would have to be considered, this distinction can usually be made on the basis of a markedly elevated βhCG level (often >100,000 IU/L) and the clinical symptoms. The possibility of invasion into the wall or of metastatic choriocarcinoma, or both, cannot, however, be determined by ultrasound. In approximately 50% of cases hydatidiform moles are accompanied by complex ovarian cystic masses (theca-lutein cysts), which are often bilateral. This is discussed more completely in Chapter 15.

Fibroids may markedly distort and enlarge the uterus (see Fig. 9-14). On occasion these fibroids may contain unusual necrotic cystic spaces. These can potentially be confused with an IUP or lead to the misdiagnosis of a second sac (see Fig. 9-12). Multiple fibroids can also greatly distort the position of the gestational sac (see Fig. 9-4), sometimes making it appear to be in an extrauterine (ectopic) position. If extensive, fibroids may precipitate miscarriage.

Key Features

In the first trimester the two most important diagnostic tests are the pregnancy test (the level of the β subunit of human chorionic gonadotropin) and the ultrasound examination.

Ultrasound identifies the gestational sac as an anechoic space surrounded by the hyperechoic rim. If it is round, only one measurement of the anechoic space is needed. If it is ovoid, three perpendicular measurements are obtained and averaged.

The discrepancy among different measurement tables in determining gestational age by the mean gestational sac diameter (MGSD) is approximately 1 week.

The first-trimester crown-rump length (CRL) and second-trimester biparietal diameter are equally accurate (±1 week) in predicting gestational age. These are superior to an optimal menstrual history.

It is suggested that the MGSD continue to be compared with the CRL throughout the first trimester.

The following characteristics are used in evaluating the gestational sac: correct uterine position, a double decidual sac sign, a continuous hyperechoic rim that is 2 mm or more thick, a grossly spherical or ovoid shape, and growth of more than 1.2 mm/day.

The finding of a DDS is highly predictive of a normal intrauterine pregnancy. Its absence is more suggestive of an ectopic pregnancy or a miscarriage.

Potential uterine findings that can cause confusion in the first trimester include fluid within the endometrial canal, chorioamniotic separations, a "vanishing twin," split-image artifact, implantation bleeds, and fibroids.

Transvaginal (TV) ultrasound has allowed earlier and occasionally more accurate assessment of the gestational sac and the embryo. It should be used whenever there is uncertainty after the transabdominal examination.

Care should be taken in rendering a definitive diagnosis of normal and abnormal pregnancies when the CRL is less than 5 mm.

Fetal anatomic characteristics are more completely identified by TV scanning. At present this has not translated into more precise first-trimester diagnoses, however.

TV scanning should be performed whenever there is a question about the number and type of multiple gestations.

Hydatidiform moles may present in the first trimester, occasionally mimicking a spontaneous incomplete abortion.

SUGGESTED READINGS

Benson CB, Doubilet PM: Slow embryonic heart rate in early first trimester: indicator of poor pregnancy outcome, *Radiology* 192:343, 1994.

Benson CB, Doubilet PM: Sonographic prediction of gestational age: accuracy of second- and third-trimester fetal measurements, *AJR* 157:1275, 1991.

Bowerman RA: Sonography of fetal midgut herniation: normal size criteria and correlation with crown-rump length, *J Ultrasound Med* 5:251, 1993.

Bree RL et al: Transvaginal sonography in the evaluation of normal early pregnancy: correlation with HCG level, *AJR* 153:75, 1989.

Bromley B et al: Small sac size in the first trimester: a predictor of poor fetal outcome, *Radiology* 178:375, 1991.

Cadkin AV, McAlpin J: The decidua-chorionic sac: a reliable sonographic indicator of intrauterine pregnancy prior to detection of a fetal pole, *J Ultrasound Med* 3:539, 1984.

Daya S et al: Early pregnancy assessment with transvaginal ultrasound scanning, *Can Med Assoc J* 144:441, 1991.

Dillon EH et al: Endovaginal US and Doppler findings after first-trimester abortion, *Radiology* 186:87, 1993.

Goldstein SR: Embryonic death in early pregnancy: a new look at the first trimester, *Obstet Gynecol* 84:294, 1994.

Hadlock FP et al: Fetal crown-rump length: reevaluation of relation to menstrual age (5-18 weeks) with high-resolution real-time US, *Radiology* 182:501, 1992.

Hellman LM et al: Growth and development of the human fetus prior to the 20th week of gestation, *Am J Obstet Gynecol* 103:789, 1969.

Hertzberg BS, Mahony BS, Bowie JD: First trimester fetal cardiac activity. Sonographic documentation of a progressive early rise in heart rate, *J Ultrasound Med* 7:573, 1988.

Kopta MM, May RR, Crane JP: A comparison of the reliability of the estimated date of confinement predicted by crown-rump length and biparietal diameter, *Am J Obstet Gynecol* 145:562, 1983.

Kurtz AB et al: Can detection of the yolk sac in the first trimester be used to predict the outcome of pregnancy? A prospective sonographic study, *AJR* 158:843, 1992.

Levi CS, Lyons EA, Lindsay DJ: Early diagnosis of nonviable pregnancy with endovaginal US, *Radiology* 167:383, 1988.

Levi CS et al: Endovaginal US: demonstration of cardiac activity in embryos of less than 5.0 mm in crown-rump length, *Radiology* 176:71, 1990.

Lindsay DJ et al: Yolk sac diameter and shape at endovaginal US: predictors of pregnancy outcome in the first trimester, *Radiology* 183:115, 1992.

Moore KL: *The Developing Human—Clinically Oriented Embryology,* Philadelphia, W.B. Saunders, 1982.

Nyberg DA, Laing FC, Filly RA: Threatened abortion: sonographic distinction of normal and abnormal gestation sacs, *Radiology* 158:397, 1986.

Nyberg DA et al: Ultrasonographic differentiation of the gestational sac of early intrauterine pregnancy from the pseudogestational sac of ectopic pregnancy, *Radiology* 146:755, 1983.

Nyberg DA et al: Distinguishing normal from abnormal gestational sac growth in early pregnancy, *J Ultrasound Med* 6:23, 1987.

Pennell RG et al: Complicated first-trimester pregnancies: evaluation with endovaginal US versus transabdominal technique, *Radiology* 165:79, 1987.

Pennell RG et al: Prospective comparison of vaginal and abdominal sonography in normal early pregnancy, *J Ultrasound Med* 10:63, 1991.

Robinson HP, Fleming JEE: A critical evaluation of sonar "crown-rump length" measurements, *Br J Obstet Gynaecol* 82:702, 1975.

Sauerbrei EE: The split image artifact in pelvic ultrasonography: the anatomy and physics, *J Ultrasound Med* 4:29, 1985.

Yeh H-C et al: Intradecidual sign: a US criterion of early intrauterine pregnancy, *Radiology* 161:463, 1986.

Yeh H-C, Rabinowitz JG: Amniotic sac development: ultrasound features of early pregnancy—the double bleb sign, *Radiology* 166:97, 1988.

CHAPTER 10

Fetal Central Nervous System: Head and Spine

For a Key Features summary see p. 234.

The overall frequency of congenital anomalies is 1:500 to 1:600 births. Central nervous system (CNS) abnormalities constitute the majority, and include anencephaly and spina bifida, both with an incidence of 1:1000 births, and encephalocele, with an incidence of 1:4000 births. If a woman has had a previous child with a CNS defect, the risk for another CNS anomaly (of any type) in a subsequent child increases to greater than one in 50. If she has had 2 previous children with CNS defects, the risk then exceeds one in 10.

In general CNS anomalies are large and obvious. However, small subtle defects may also occur. Because any abnormality can lead to a clinically significant deficit, a careful sequential evaluation of the head and spine is indicated in all pregnancies.

ANENCEPHALY

Anencephaly is a lethal anomaly caused by lack of development of the fetal brain. It is one of the easiest CNS anomalies to recognize. By the beginning of the second trimester, at 12 to 14 weeks, the normal fetal head with its bright calvarium and its intracranial structures, in particular the lateral ventricles, choroid plexus, and thalami, are routinely identified (Fig. 10-1). Using transvaginal (TV) scanning, it is likely that these structures can be routinely identified earlier, perhaps as early as 9 to 10 weeks. For now, however, it is still prudent to delay the definitive diagnosis of an abnormality until the early second trimester.

Inability to identify the normal calvarium and intracranial structures should prompt a consideration of anencephaly (Fig. 10-2). If it proves difficult to find the calvarium, scans from the cervical spine to the skull base can be obtained, and these should always identify a normal head. If not, anencephaly is diagnosed. On occasion hyperechoic ill-defined soft tissue can be identified (without the normal surrounding calvarium) above the normal facial structures. This is a variant of anencephaly. It is termed *angiomatous stroma* or *area cerebrovasculosa*, and represents the residuum of a dysmorphic brain (Fig. 10-2, *B*).

A pathologic entity called *acrania* has been confused with anencephaly. In it the calvarium is absent but the brain is normal. Acrania is a questionable entity, but need not be considered seriously because of its extreme rarity (1:100,000 cases). If it is present, it is an isolated anomaly and will not recur. In contradistinction, anencephaly is commonly associated with anomalies of the spine, including spinal dysraphism (a completely opened spine), and it is also associated with an increased incidence of CNS recurrence.

Infrequently an anencephalic fetus may not be studied until late in pregnancy, occasionally not until term. If the calvarium and intracranial structures are difficult to identify, particularly if the head is either in an unusually high breech position under the mother's ribs or in a deep vertex presentation below the pubic symphysis, the examiner may be tempted to deem the head normal but technically difficult to image. Instead, failure to identify the

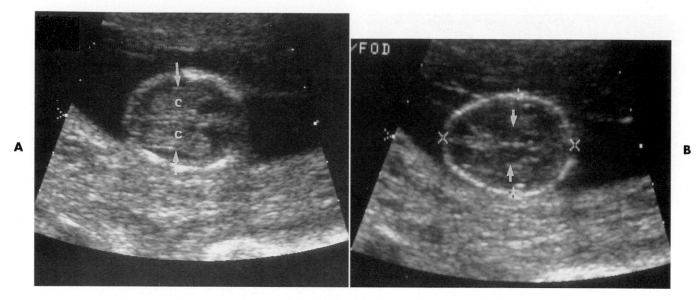

Fig. 10-1 Transaxial views of the normal fetal head in a 14-week fetus. Note the normally bright surrounding calvarium. **A,** At the level of the bodies of the lateral ventricles *(arrows),* the choroid plexus *(c)* completely fill the ventricles. **B,** Slightly lower at the level of the thalami *(arrows),* the place to measure the biparietal diameter from leading edge to leading edge (+) and frontooccipital diameter from outer edge to outer edge *(x)* are shown. A cephalic index can be obtained using these two measurements.

normal head, regardless of fetal position, should make the examiner suspect anencephaly. This diagnosis can be confirmed by a translabial or TV study, if the fetal head is in the vertex presentation.

POLYHYDRAMNIOS

Polyhydramnios is a frequent secondary finding in cases of anencephaly. It can be determined subjectively by observing increased amniotic fluid. Either measurement of a single anteroposterior fluid pocket (>8 cm) or a four-quadrant measurement (>24 to 25 cm) (see Table 8-2) can also be performed. If the amniotic fluid is so extensive as to also cause the placenta to "thin," this indicates the fluid is markedly increased in quantity (Fig. 10-3).

Polyhydramnios has many causes (Table 10-1). Approximately one third of the cases are idiopathic (not associated with anomalies), and the polyhydramnios is then usually mild. On occasion it can be moderate or even marked. In the remaining 67%, maternal or fetal problems, or both, are present. Women with diabetes mellitus, typically gestational but also mildly insulin dependent, may have polyhydramnios. This is usually mild, but may be pronounced. The amount of amniotic fluid in multiple gestations is increased because of the composite fluid from each gestation. Although this increase is often mild to moderate, polyhydramnios may be marked in the settings

of complicated monochorionic pregnancies (e.g., twin-twin transfusions) and uncomplicated monoamniotic pregnancies.

The remaining cases are caused by fetal abnormalities, either structural anomalies or fetal hydrops. These anomalies often result in failure of normal swallowing and consist of severe CNS abnormalities, obstruction of the gastrointestinal tract (usually from the hypopharynx through the upper jejunum), marked chest narrowing or chest masses, and even congenital severe hypotonia. In general the more severe the polyhydramnios, the more likely an anomaly. On the other hand, polyhydramnios is not always present, even when expected. In early cases of anencephaly, the amniotic fluid is often normal in quantity (see Fig. 10-2). Even at term polyhydramnios is not always present. Therefore the finding of polyhydramnios necessitates a careful search for an abnormality (although none may be present); the finding of normal amniotic fluid does not rule out an abnormality. Hydrops is discussed later in this chapter and in Chapter 11.

NORMAL ANATOMY OF THE HEAD

Normal structures can be identified outside of the calvarium. They are usually the following: subcutaneous tissue, skin, hair, and ears. All are inconstant findings and should not be confused with a pathologic condition.

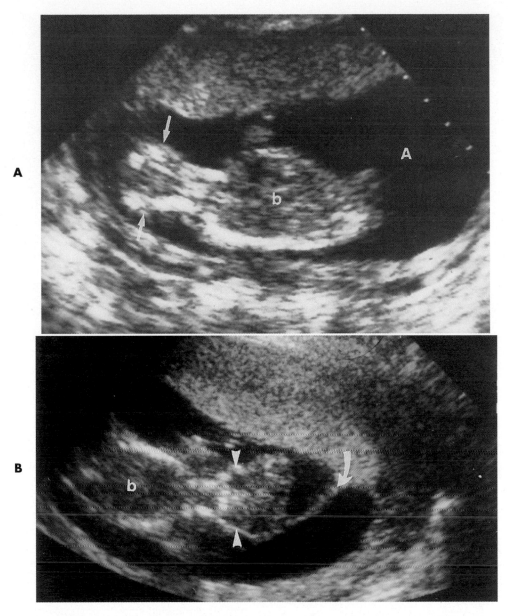

Fig. 10-2   Two different cases of anencephaly in the early second trimester. **A,** A long-axis view in a 15-week fetus. Arrows denote the incompletely formed skull. Note the normal amount of amniotic fluid *(A). b,* fetal body. **B,** A 14-week fetus, one of a set of twins. There is ill-defined hyperechoic tissue superior to the normal orbits *(arrowheads),* without a normal calvarium. This is angiomatous stroma of the dysmorphic brain. The curved arrow denotes the thick membrane of a dichorionic-diamniotic twin pregnancy.

Transaxial images of the thalami and occasionally of the midbrain are common starting points for analysis of the head (Fig. 10-4). Both structures are hypoechoic, and the thalami are round and the midbrain is heart shaped. At the level of the thalami, the normal cavum septa pellucidum is frequently seen. It is a cystic structure immediately anterior to the thalami. It should not be confused with the third ventricle, which is normally slitlike, situated between the two thalami (or midbrain), and less than

2 mm in diameter; the third ventricle is often not identified until the third trimester.

An accurate measurement of the head can be obtained at either of these levels, using the biparietal diameter (BPD) or head circumference (HC), or both. These midline structures must be imaged in the midline. Otherwise the scan plane is oblique and not truly transaxial. Standard measurement tables for the BPD and head circumference allow estimation of gestational age, and both a

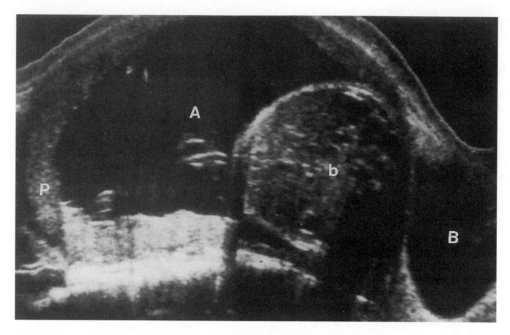

Fig. 10-3   Marked polyhydramnios in the third trimester. A static long-axis scan shows a significant increase in amniotic fluid *(A)*. Note the thinned placenta *(P)* stretched along the fundus and posterior aspects of the uterine wall. The fetal body *(b)* is large, consistent with a macrosomic fetus in a woman with known gestational diabetes. *B*, urinary bladder.

Table 10-1 Causes of polyhydramnios	
Cause	**Approximate Percentage**
Idiopathic	33
Maternal—diabetes mellitus	25
Multiple gestations	10
Fetal	
Anomalies*	20
Hydrops	12

*Central nervous system, gastrointestinal, thoracic, skeletal, chromosomal, cardiac.

mean and a range around that mean should be reported. In the second trimester, up to 24 weeks, the accuracy of the BPD and head circumference is ± 5 to 7 days, similar to that of the first-trimester crown-rump length. After 24 weeks, this accuracy decreases, and by the third trimester is only ± 3 to 4 weeks. To be certain that the BPD measurement is technically correct, the transaxial view should also take the head shape into account by calculating a cephalic index (see Fig. 10-1, *B*). If the head is too round (brachiocephalic) or oval (scaphocephalic) and the shape falls outside the normal range, the head shape should be corrected by an area-corrected BPD calculation. This is discussed more completely in Chapter 7.

The obstetric guidelines also recommend evaluation of the lateral ventricles. By 7 menstrual weeks, the lateral ventricles have formed from the prosencephalon, and once formed remain relatively constant until delivery. Subsequent head enlargement is caused by growth of the brain parenchyma around these ventricles. Because the lateral ventricular size is constant, the atria are measured for the following reasons: they are easy to identify (particularly the one farthest from the transducer), they can be routinely imaged in the transaxial plane (with the transducer angled slightly posteriorly), and they are most sensitive to the development of early hydrocephalus (Fig. 10-5, *A*).

Each atrium is measured perpendicular to its walls, as an inner-to-inner measurement (middle-to-middle can also suffice) (Fig. 10-5, *A*). From 14 to 38 weeks, its mean is constant at 7.6 mm. Care is needed not to measure off-axis and not to measure from outer edge to outer edge; if this happens, an error of up to 10% is possible. In one of the first studies, the normal atrium was found to not exceed 10 mm at a standard deviation (SD) of 4 (>99%). Recent studies have shown a variation in the upper limit of normal at different stages of gestation. Although these findings are not all in agreement, 10 mm is probably only 2 to 3 SD (95%) greater than the norm, with 12 mm closer to 4 SD. More work is needed to establish this upper limit. An additionally helpful sign in borderline cases (between 9 and 12 mm) is the amount of hyperechoic choroid

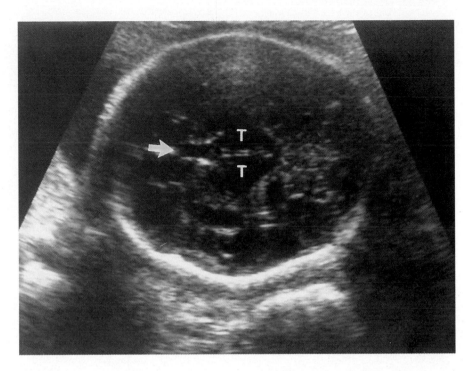

Fig. 10-4 Normal transaxial view of the brain at the thalami *(T)* in this late second-trimester image. This is the ideal position for obtaining the biparietal diameter and head circumference. The normal cavum septa pellucidum *(arrow)* is closer to the front of the head, toward the reader's left. Between the thalami are two parallel lines, representing the slitlike third ventricle.

plexus filling the lateral ventricles. In the second trimester, up to 16 weeks, choroid plexus are seen to completely fill the bodies of the lateral ventricles in a transaxial view (see Fig. 10-1); after 16 weeks, they are not as prominent. In the atria, however, the choroid plexus remain prominent, filling 60% or more. If true ventriculomegaly is present, the choroid plexus typically decrease in size (relative to the atria) and may also "dangle" downward in the enlarged atria (see Fig. 10-5, *B* and *C*). Further studies investigating the size of the atria and choroid plexus are needed.

HYDROCEPHALUS AND HYDRANENCEPHALY

Ventriculomegaly (enlarged lateral ventricles) is caused either by increased intraventricular pressure or by an ex vacuo phenomenon in which the formed ventricles expand to "fill in" the space previously occupied by brain parenchyma. The increased pressure is due to hydrocephalus; to "fill in" suggests the presence of brain underdevelopment or destruction. In both conditions, the atrio-occipital regions are usually affected first; more marked ventriculomegaly leads to dilatation of the entire lateral ventricular system (see Fig. 10-5).

Sonographically, hydrocephalus can be diagnosed definitively if at least one of the following additional findings is present: a disrupted falx echo, third ventricular dilatation, specific posterior fossa abnormalities, increasing ventriculomegaly, and head enlargement. In most cases of hydrocephalus, the size of the fetal head remains normal and is normally proportionate to the fetal body. The diagnosis on the initial study must then rely for confirmation on the further finding of a ruptured falx, third ventricular enlargement, or posterior fossa abnormalities, or a combination of these. A ruptured falx midline echo, imaged as a wavy line within the dilated ventricles, suggests the diagnosis of marked hydrocephalus (Fig. 10-6, *A*). An enlarged third ventricle becomes rounded and exceeds 2 mm in diameter (Fig. 10-6, *B*). Scans of the posterior fossa yield less information because the fourth ventricle is not always seen. Nevertheless, the appearance of the cerebellum and cisterna magna may be very helpful, and this is discussed later in the sections on the posterior fossa and on meningoceles and meningomyeloceles. A follow-up examination can show whether there has been further ventricular enlargement.

Although hydrocephalus can be diagnosed accurately, the precise level of obstruction cannot always be identified. As a rule of thumb, the level of obstruction is no higher than the lowest dilated structure, but may be even

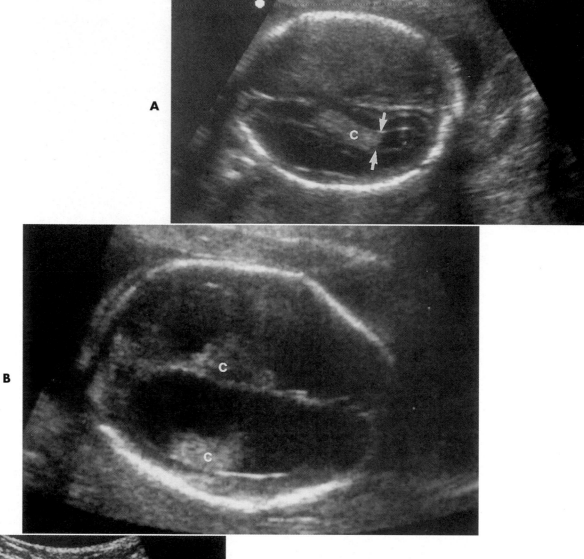

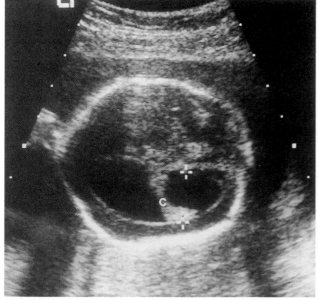

Fig. 10-5   Three different fetuses at 22 weeks. **A,** Normal transaxial view, tilted posteriorly toward the occiput to image the atria. The atrium farthest from the transducer is clearly identified. It is measured from the tips of the arrows, perpendicular to the atrium, and is completely filled with choroid plexus *(c)*. The near-side atrium is obscured by a reverberation artifact. **B,** Moderate to marked hydrocephalus. The choroid plexus *(c)* are at the most dependent portions of the dilated lateral ventricles. **C,** "Dangling" choroid plexus *(c)* within a dilated lateral ventricle (on the far side of the head). The measurement of this atrium is markedly enlarged to 20 mm (+). The near-side dilated ventricle is obscured by a reverberation artifact. In **B** and **C,** despite the hydrocephalus, the heads are normal in size and no polyhydramnios is present.

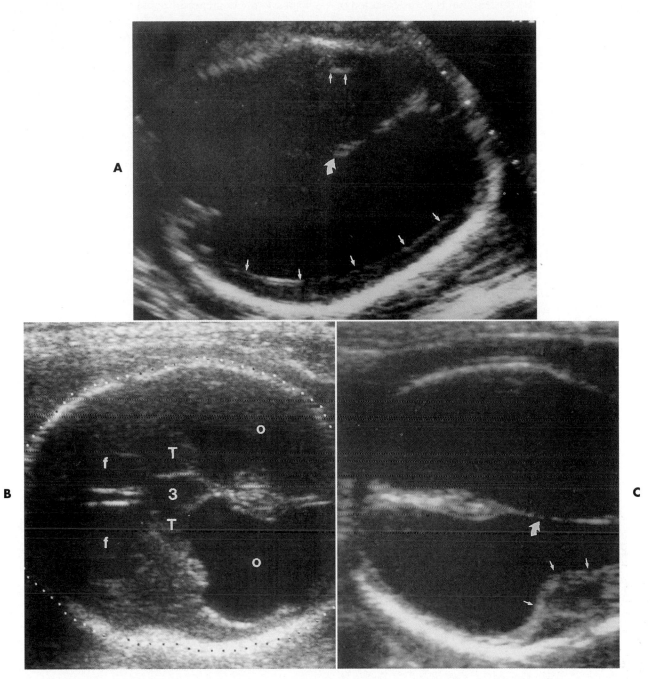

Fig. 10-6   Comparison of marked hydrocephalus to hydranencephaly in three third-trimester fetuses. **A,** Hydrocephalus. A disrupted falx midline echo is detected, with the edge denoted by a curved arrow. Despite the marked ventriculomegaly, a thin mantle of parenchyma can still be identified *(small arrows),* and this is better seen on the far side of the head. **B,** Hydrocephalus. Transaxial image of the head shows marked spreading of the thalami *(T)* caused by a markedly dilated third ventricle *(3).* The occipital horns *(o)* and the frontal horns *(f)* of the lateral ventricles are also markedly dilated. The enlarged head (compared with the body) is outlined by a dotted line. **C,** Hydranencephaly. There is an intact falx echo *(curved arrow).* Although a small amount of residual tissue *(small arrows)* still remains in the occipital region, the frontal and parietal regions on both the near and far side of the head do not have a mantle of cortical tissue. This is consistent with brain parenchymal destruction. The head is larger than the body.

lower. For example, the finding of lateral ventricular dilatation rarely means the obstruction is at the foramen of Monro; the obstruction in this instance is usually lower. If the lateral and third ventricles are dilated, in the absence of other intracranial abnormalities, the hydrocephalus may be at the aqueduct of Sylvius but is often at the level of the fourth ventricle or even part of a communicating hydrocephalus.

Head enlargement secondary to hydrocephalus is not a common finding but may occur in severe cases. Enlargement of any body part is somewhat arbitrarily defined, but is usually a measurement of 2 SD or more above the norm. In obstetrics, on average each 1 SD is equivalent to 3 mm. Therefore, for the head, a 2-SD enlargement represents a corrected BPD larger than the abdominal diameter (assuming a normal body size) by 6 mm or more. A circumference measurement takes π into account, and a 2-SD enlargement for a head circumference is a circumference of 6 mm or more times π, or 18 mm or greater than the abdominal circumference (again assuming a normal body size). Another approach is to use gestational age tables. If the true fetal age is known, the head needs to be larger than its expected size by 2 weeks or more.

In all cases of hydrocephalus, regardless of severity, there is always a residual rim or mantle of brain parenchyma (Fig. 10-6, *A* and *B*). This is in contradistinction to a condition called *hydranencephaly*, or "water head" (Fig. 10-6, *C*). Hydranencephaly results from destruction of the brain parenchyma, and is most commonly caused by a thrombosis of the middle cerebral arteries or an in utero infection. In this condition brain parenchyma is markedly decreased or absent in the frontal, temporal, and parietal regions, and the lateral ventricles expand to fill in the space left by the destroyed brain. The occipital lobes, posterior fossa, and brainstem regions are usually normal because the posterior cerebral circulation is not disrupted. Unlike the more common hydrocephalus, with its variable prognosis (even on occasion a normal one), hydranencephaly is a lethal condition.

The sonographic appearance of the brain in a fetus with hydranencephaly varies from the visualization of irregular areas (if the destruction is ongoing) to a complete absence of brain in the frontal and temporoparietal areas. No cortical mantle is visible. The head is typically enlarged and even continues to grow as the fetus matures. Although the reason for this enlargement is not known, the continued production of cerebrospinal fluid (with impaired resorption) must cause increased pressure, and this could be responsible for the enlargement. The falx midline echo is maintained.

MICROCEPHALY

Microcephaly has many causes. Among the most common are some of the TORCH infections (rubella, cytomegalovirus, and herpes simplex), developmental abnormalities (particularly holoprosencephaly), and genetic conditions (especially trisomies). Less commonly pollutants such as radiation, toxins, and heavy metals can be

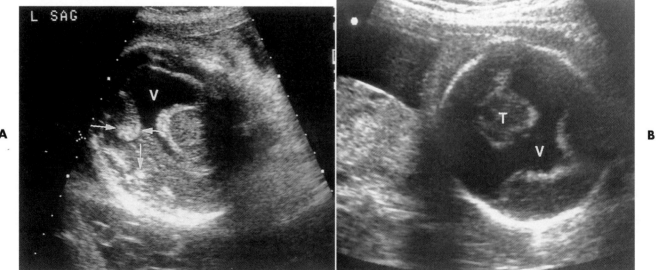

Fig. 10-7   Two cases of microcephaly. **A,** Cytomegalovirus infection at 22 weeks. The parasagittal image through the left lateral ventricle *(V)* shows a dilated ventricle and both periventricular and intraparenchymal hyperechoic calcifications *(arrows)* in a small head. Note that there is no distal acoustic shadowing. **B,** Alobar holoprosencephaly at 17 weeks. This coronal image shows fused thalami *(T)* and a single ventricle, or monoventricle *(V)*. Some ill-defined occipital tissue has formed superior to the ventricle. Hypotelorism (not shown) is also detected.

causative agents. The incidence of microcephaly is known from mental institution statistics to range from 1:6000 to 1:8500 births. However, not infrequently affected fetuses die in utero or in infancy and are not counted in these statistics. The true incidence is therefore undoubtedly higher.

For microcephaly to be diagnosed, the head must be smaller than expected. This is based on the same concept as that used to determine head enlargement (discussed in the previous section on hydrocephalus), except it is used inversely. Microcephaly must take into account a *clinically significant* small head, in that there must be both a small brain and mental retardation. In children in mental institutions, microcephaly was found to *always* be significant when the BPD or HC was more than 3 SD less than the norm. If the BPD or HC were decreased by 1 or 2 SD, the prognosis was variable and often normal.

At 3 SD below the norm the corrected BPD has to be 9 mm or more smaller than the abdominal diameter and the head circumference has to be 27 mm or more smaller than the abdominal circumference (assuming a normal body). Alternatively, the size of the head should lag behind that of the body by a gestational age of at least 3 weeks. Based on study findings, however, some believe that the sole use of BPD or HC measurements, or both, is not enough to permit accurate detection of microcephaly, and additional head measurements at different SD thresholds are also needed to make the diagnosis. More work is needed to shed further light on the merits of these measurements and perhaps to identify others.

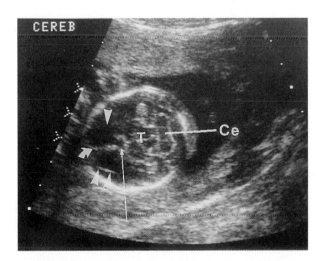

Fig. 10-8 Normal frontal horns and cavum septa pellucidum in a 16-week fetus. This transaxial image is tilted superiorly toward the frontal bone, still identifying the normal thalami *(T)*. Superiorly the cavum septa pellucidum *(arrow)* and the distinctly separated frontal horns *(arrowheads)* are seen. Note the intact intervening septum *(curved arrow)*. Posterior to the thalami, the posterior fossa including the cerebellum *(Ce)* can, as in this case, sometimes be identified.

If the lateral ventricles are seen to be prominent (ventriculomegaly) in conjunction with a small head, this is caused by loss of brain parenchyma, with the ventricles expanding to fill the void—the ex vacuo phenomenon. Concomitant intracranial calcifications, both periventricular and parenchymal, suggest the presence of cytomegalovirus infection (Fig. 10-7, *A*). If these are seen in a normal-sized head, however, toxoplasmosis may instead be the causative infection. These hyperechoic areas do not always shadow. In the correct clinical setting these areas may instead represent the tubers of tuberous sclerosis. If further differentiation is needed, an in utero or neonatal magnetic resonance imaging examination would be of value.

Holoprosencephaly is a midline developmental anomaly whose incidence cited in the literature varies widely, ranging from 1:2000 to 1:16,000 births. The brainstem and thalami are relatively well preserved. The telencephalon exhibits variable development, from the most severe alobar form, with a single underdeveloped amorphous ventricle (Fig. 10-7, *B*) to the least severe lobar form, in which only the frontal horns (of the lateral ventricles) are defective. In between, the semilobar form consists of only partial lateral ventricular development.

Holoprosencephaly is a first-trimester abnormality. The alobar form can be diagnosed by the early second trimester because of its obvious intracranial and frequently additional abnormalities: midline defects of the face (>80% of cases), heart, and abdomen. The semilobar form with its partially developed occipital horns and falx is also detected routinely in utero. Only the lobar form is difficult to diagnose. Aside from absent development of the frontal horns and cavum septi pellucidi, affected fetuses typically exhibit a normal-sized head and no other detectable anomalies. If suspected, a careful look for the frontal horns and cavum septa pellucidum is indicated. This is accomplished by a transaxial image of the head, which is tilted superiorly toward the frontal bone (Fig. 10-8).

FACIAL STRUCTURES

In the obstetric guidelines, routine analysis of the face is not recommended. However, a number of structures can be identified and their presence can be important because they form part of a constellation of findings in high-risk pregnancies.

Cleft lips and cleft palates are the most common congenital facial anomalies, and some observers have advocated a routine evaluation to search for them. A solitary cleft lip deformity occurs in 1:800 births; a combined cleft lip and palate occurs in 1:1300 births. These abnormalities may be either isolated or associated with significant abnormalities, including trisomies and holoprosencephaly. The clefts vary in severity from involvement of

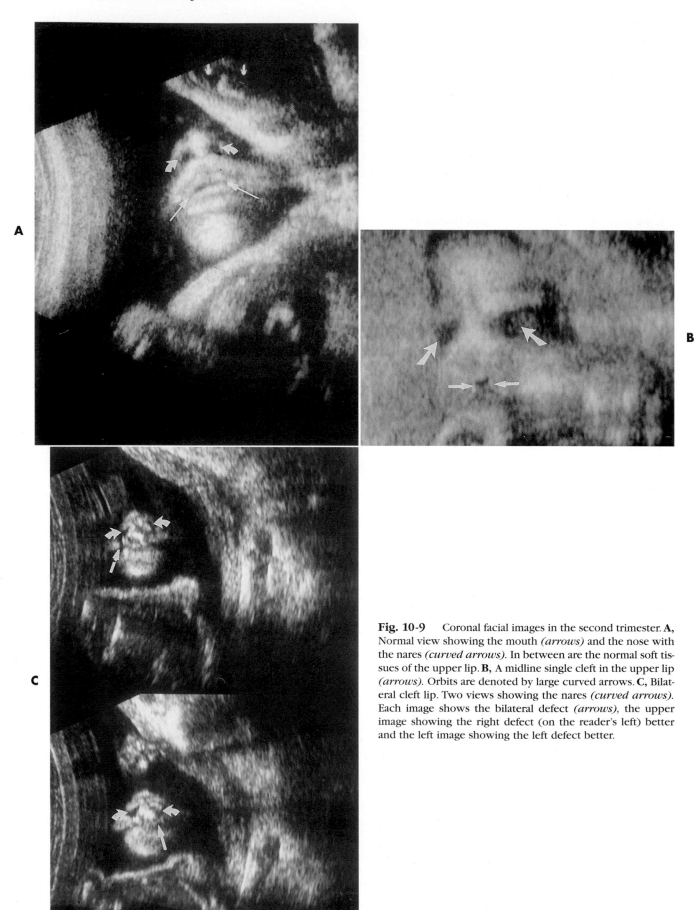

Fig. 10-9   Coronal facial images in the second trimester. **A,** Normal view showing the mouth *(arrows)* and the nose with the nares *(curved arrows).* In between are the normal soft tissues of the upper lip. **B,** A midline single cleft in the upper lip *(arrows).* Orbits are denoted by large curved arrows. **C,** Bilateral cleft lip. Two views showing the nares *(curved arrows).* Each image shows the bilateral defect *(arrows),* the upper image showing the right defect (on the reader's left) better and the left image showing the left defect better.

only the soft tissues of the upper lip to posterior extension into the hard and even into the soft palate. Occasionally the palate can be affected without involvement of the upper lip. If only an isolated soft palate abnormality is present, it is often not diagnosed in utero.

Cleft defects can be single (central or eccentric) or bilateral, with bilateral clefts more deforming and more likely to be associated with additional abnormalities. By scanning through the face in a coronal or transaxial plane, or both, depending on fetal position, the normal soft tissues of the lip and the hyperechoic hard bony palate can be identified (Figs. 10-9 and 10-10). Although both planes are good for visualizing lip anomalies, the transaxial projection is usually better for identifying abnormalities of the palate. As might be expected, the larger the defect, the easier the detection.

The orbital distance can be determined by scanning either transaxially or coronally. The hyperechoic bony rims of the orbits can be identified and an outer-to-outer diameter (OOD) obtained (Fig. 10-11). The OOD shows proportionate growth to the BPD and to the gestational age; measurement tables are available for these comparisons. Difficulties with this measurement occur because the edges of the rims can be difficult to define and errors of at least 2 to 3 mm are not uncommon. Nevertheless, a small OOD (hypotelorism) and a large OOD (hypertelorism) can be diagnosed.

There have been rare instances of the detection of a small chin (micrognathism), a finding sometimes associated with trisomy 13. Care must be taken in rendering this diagnosis, however. A true midline sagittal view of the face is necessary to establish it (Fig. 10-12). Because the

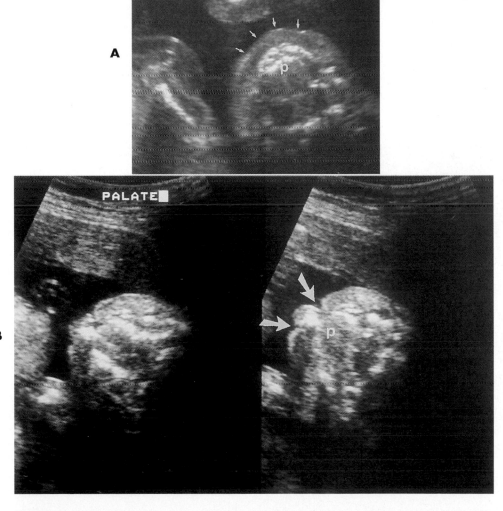

Fig. 10-10   Transaxial view of the upper lip and hard palate in the mid–second timester. **A,** Normal hard palate *(p)* with normal anterior soft tissues *(small arrows).* **B,** Bilateral cleft lip *(arrows)* with a normal hard palate *(p).*

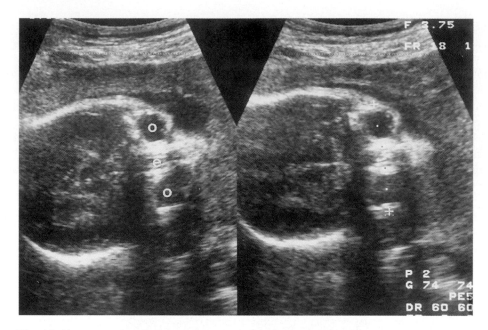

Fig. 10-11 Normal transaxial view of the orbits in the second trimester. In the left image, the orbits *(o)* and the intervening ethmoid sinus region *(e)* are noted. In the right image, the outer orbital diameter *(OOD)* from the outer edges of the bony orbits is shown (+ and *dotted line*).

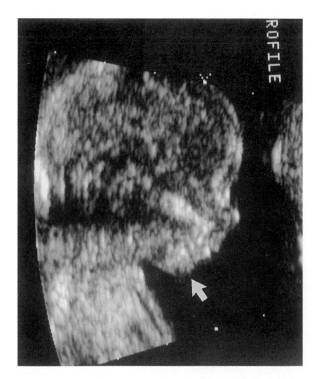

Fig. 10-12 Normal midline profile of the fetal face in a 26-week fetus. Arrow denotes the area of the normal chin. Note that it is mildly curved inward, even in a normal fetus.

mandible may normally appear somewhat small, only total flattening can be safely interpreted as abnormal.

Facial tumors have also been sonographically detected. They are primarily isolated anomalies, and yet can still be quite deforming and extensive. Hemangiomas are common; they are usually hyperechoic and somewhat compressible. Typically, no Doppler signal is detected because the blood flow in the tumor is too slow. Teratomas are solid tumors, either confined to the face or extending into the neck and even to the thoracic outlet. Concomitant polyhydramnios may be present, and is caused by an inability to swallow normally. If large, teratomas can obstruct the airway and lead to serious respiratory problems at birth.

ENCEPHALOCELE

Encephalocele is a midline abnormality that falls into two categories: those that contain only meninges (meningoceles) and those that also contain brain (encephaloceles). Its severity is primarily related to the amount of brain within the defect. Exposed brain is often dysmorphic, so there may be a significant CNS deficit, even if the area of exposed brain is surgically repaired. In addition, the incidence of additional associated abnormalities, both structural and chromosomal, is relatively high.

Encephaloceles range in size from a small bubble of meninges that extends through the calvarium to the en-

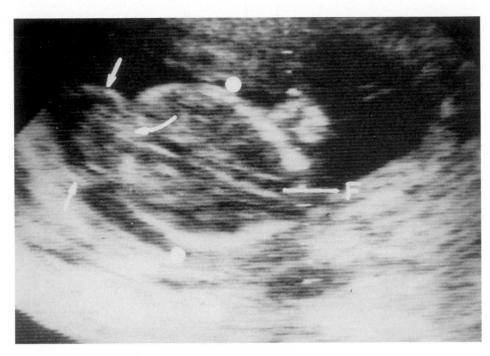

Fig. 10-13   Posterior encephalocele in an 18-week fetus. Transaxial view of the fetal head, scanned through the area of the lateral ventricles, shows a large posterior defect *(curved arrow)* in the occipital bone with an encephalocele *(arrows)* containing both meninges and brain. *F,* falx.

tire brain (and meninges) being located outside a collapsed calvarium. In the latter, identification of the collapsed head can be difficult; scans from the cervical spine to the skull base may be needed for this purpose.

In the United States population, particularly in the non-Asian population, at least 80% of the encephaloceles are posterior, extending through a defect in the occipital bone (Fig. 10-13). However, an encephalocele can occur anywhere along the midline, including at the top of the head and anteriorly into the ethmoid sinus region. The ethmoid abnormality, termed an *anterior encephalocele*, is much more common in an Asian population. It can be very subtle, and care must be taken when scanning the region of the nose, turbinates, and sinuses to make sure it is not overlooked (see Fig. 10-11).

THE POSTERIOR FOSSA AND NUCHAL SKIN

With the ability to evaluate the posterior fossa, important information has been added to the CNS examination. Although not now part of the routine obstetric study, it has been added to the next guideline update.

The posterior fossa is imaged starting with the standard transaxial view, with the transducer then being tilted backward toward the occiput, farther than the routine atrial image (Fig. 10-14). The bilobate cerebellum is identified by its two prominent hypoechoic lateral hemi-

spheres and its smaller midline hyperechoic vermis. Anterior to the vermis the normal fourth ventricle can be identified in up to 75% of normal fetuses. More posteriorly the cisterna magna is imaged between the cerebellum and the occiput. It is the largest cistern of the head and contains anechoic cerebrospinal fluid and sometimes normal hyperechoic strands, thought to represent arachnoid septa.

The cerebellum and cisterna magna have expected sizes. The cerebellum is measured transaxially from the outer edges of its hemispheres. It grows steadily as the head grows and its size correlates with the BPD and the gestational age. The cisterna magna, measured from the back of the cerebellar vermis to the inside of the occiput, is normally between 2 and 10 mm. The fourth ventricle is always normal when it is slitlike and less than 2 mm in width. In a recent article, Baumeister and co-workers recently reported that they found the normal fourth ventricle increases with gestational age in both its anteroposterior dimension and width. In width, the fourth ventricle can be 8 mm by term; its shape can be triangular, ovoid, or "boomerang" at any time during the second and third trimester. Confirmation of these findings are needed.

The cisterna magna can become abnormally too small or too large. When it is too small, less than 2 mm or obliterated, a neural tube defect is almost always present. This is caused by an Arnold-Chiari type II malformation with downward herniation of the cerebellar hemispheres into or through the foramen magnum. This is discussed more completely in the section on meningoceles and meningomyelocclcs.

When the cisterna magna is enlarged, a Dandy-Walker malformation (or its variant), an abnormal karyotype, or both, are present. In the setting of Dandy-Walker anomalies, the posterior fossa abnormality (previously inaccurately called a "cyst" or primarily "fourth ventricle en-

largement") is caused by dysgenesis (small) or agenesis (absence) of the vermis (Fig. 10-15). With agenesis, the cerebellar hemispheres become more widely separated and elevated. The cisterna magna and occasionally the fourth ventricle enlarge.

A single transaxial posterior fossa view of the bilobate cerebellum is not always sufficient to rule out a subtle vermis abnormality. A smaller defect may still be present,

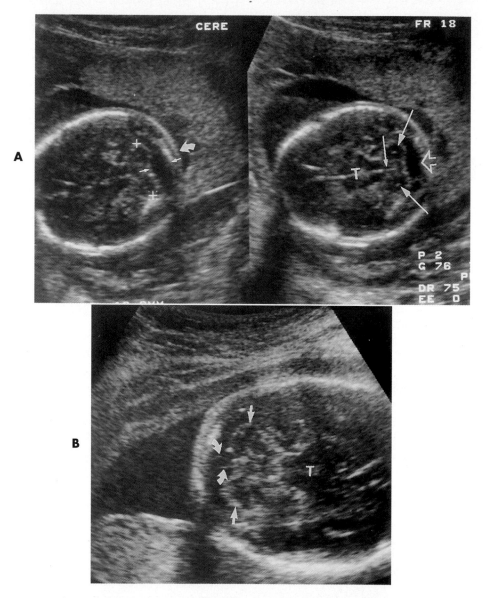

Fig. 10-14   Normal posterior fossa in two 20-week fetuses. The images are obtained in a true transaxial view, slanted posteriorly toward the occiput. **A,** The right image shows the cisterna magna *(open arrow)* and the normal bilobate cerebellum. The hypoechoic cerebellar hemispheres *(large arrows)* and the small, midline, more hyperechoic vermis can be seen. Anterior to the vermis is the slitlike fourth ventricle *(small arrow).* The left image shows a measurement of the bilobate cerebellum (+). Small arrows denote the measurement of the cisterna magna, from the posterior-most aspect of the vermis to the inside of the occipital bone. The curved arrow shows the normal nuchal skin outside the occipital bone. *T,* thalami. **B,** Normal arachnoid strands *(curved arrows)* are seen within the cisterna magna. The outer margins of the cerebellum are denoted by arrows. *T,* thalami.

usually toward the inferior (lower) margin of the vermis (Fig. 10-15, *B*). Unfortunately no landmarks are available to assure more complete posterior fossa imaging. In addition, developmental and technical factors need to be taken into account when imaging the posterior fossa. Because the cerebellum is not completely formed until the mid–second trimester, the diagnosis of subtle abnormalities, in particular an underdeveloped vermis, should be delayed at least until 18 weeks' gestation. Also, only true transaxial images should be used. Semicoronal views should be avoided because they can create a false impression of an enlarged cisterna magna; in these projections, the nuchal skin appears falsely thickened (discussed later in this section), the fourth ventricle is not identified, or the cervical spine is imaged, or a combination of these findings is encountered (Fig. 10-16).

Dandy-Walker abnormalities are commonly associated with additional CNS midline abnormalities, including hydrocephalus of the lateral and third ventricles, encephalocele, and agenesis of the corpus callosum. Abnormalities of the fetal body, including cardiac and renal anomalies, are also found.

Finally, a normal thin rim of nuchal soft tissue can be identified immediately posterior to the occipital bone (see Fig. 10-14, *A*). This skin should only measure up to 6 mm in the second trimester, between 16 and 22 weeks. If scanning of the posterior fossa is performed strictly, not angled farther posteriorly toward the cervical spine (see Fig. 10-16, *A*), an increased nuchal skin thickness of greater than 6 mm is diagnostic for trisomy 21 (Down syndrome), with a 50% sensitive and a less than 1% false-positive rate.

Nuchal skin thickening noted earlier or later in the pregnancy needs further evaluation. Some observers consider a prominent nuchal skin thickness of 3.0 mm or more to be abnormal if found in the first trimester (up to 13 weeks), and this is caused by multiple chromosomal abnormalities, particularly Down syndrome and a non-"cystic" hygroma (often associated with Turner's syndrome). The risk for an anomaly persists even if the skin thickening appears to resolve on a repeat study. Conversely, a "pseudomembrane" of prominent nuchal skin is actually the adjacent normal amnion (unfused from the chorion), not skin thickening. After 22 weeks, and particularly in the third trimester, the nuchal skin often becomes redundant; no accurate means of performing nuchal measurement during this time is available.

THE CHOROID PLEXUS

The choroid plexus are easily compressible. A decrease in choroid plexus size can be caused by raised intraventricular pressure (hydrocephalus). The choroid

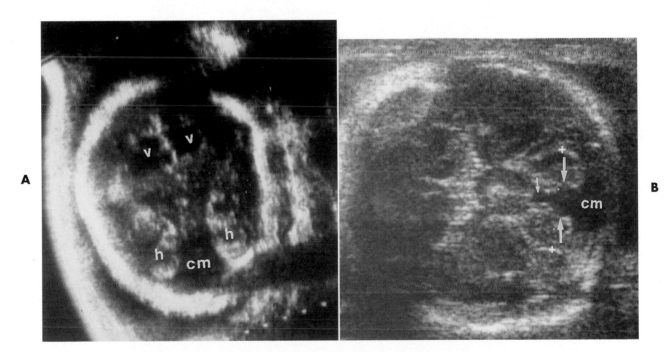

Fig. 10-15 Dandy-Walker malformations in two different patients. **A,** Coronally oriented view in a 34-week fetus. The cisterna magna *(cm)* is widely opened because of the complete absence of the vermis, and the cerebellar hemispheres *(h)* are widely displaced. Lateral ventriculomegaly *(v)* is also present. **B,** Transaxial view in a 24-week fetus showing an enlarged cisterna magna *(cm)*. Large arrows denote where the absent vermis should be. An enlarged fourth ventricle *(small arrow)* is also identified. The outer margins of the displaced cerebellar hemispheres (+) are shown.

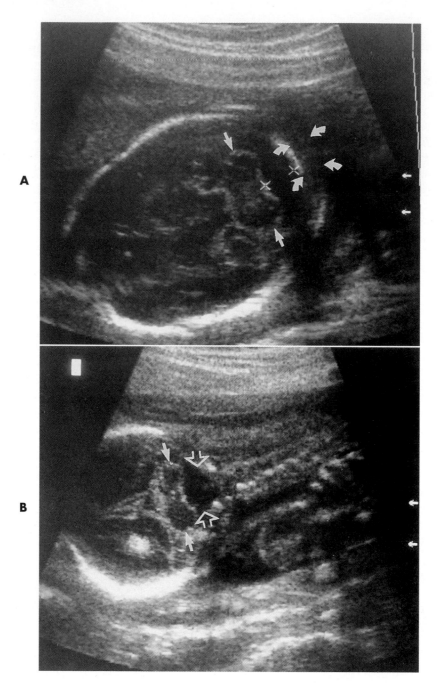

Fig. 10-16   Two scans of the normal posterior fossa, but incorrectly imaged in the semicoronal projection. This causes the cisterna magna to be falsely enlarged. **A,** The cerebellum *(arrows)* is normal. The cisterna magna *(x)* is larger than 10 mm. However, the fourth ventricle is not identified and the nuchal skin is falsely thickened *(curved arrows)*. **B,** The cisterna magna *(open arrows)* is falsely enlarged. With the fetal head toward the reader's left, identification of the spine reveals that this is a coronal rather than a transaxial projection. The normal cerebellum is denoted by arrows.

plexus are also a source of energy (in the form of glycogen) and appear to be important in the early developmental stages of the brain. Therefore, if hydrocephalus is not present, a decrease in size could suggest impaired brain development.

There has recently been intense interest in the study of choroid plexus cysts, particularly in the second trimester. Initial findings have suggested that these are variants, occurring in 1.8% to 3.6% of the normal population. However, other observers, most evaluating high-

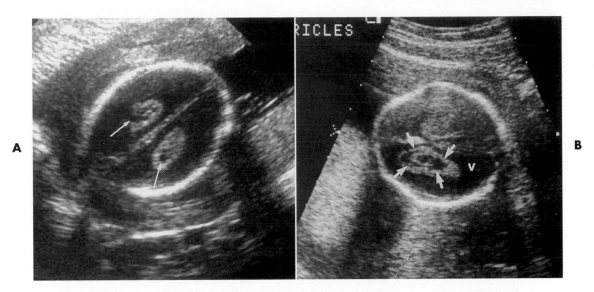

Fig. 10-17   Two different second-trimester fetuses with choroid plexus cysts. **A,** Normal fetus. Small simple cysts are seen bilaterally, two denoted by arrows. All are less than 1 cm in diameter and normally anechoic. No other abnormalities are noted. **B,** Fetus with trisomy 18. The far-side ventricle *(v)* is enlarged. The choroid plexus contains a large complex oval irregular cystic structure that exceeds 1 cm in diameter *(arrows)*. The near-side ventricle could not be imaged because of a reverberation artifact.

risk pregnancies, have found the cysts to be disproportionately associated with chromosomal abnormalities, particularly trisomy 18.

Certain ultrasound criteria for the assessment of these cysts have been evaluated: (1) cyst size and number, (2) cyst echogenicity—simple or complex (with internal echoes), (3) follow-up resolution, and (4) additional gross anomalies (Fig. 10-17). It is generally agreed that chromosomal analysis is needed when a fetus with a complex choroid plexus cyst (>1 cm), even without additional abnormalities, is encountered. Similarly, this is also so for a fetus with a simple cyst and structural anomalies. Whether the cysts are unilateral or bilateral and whether they resolve on follow-up study do not appear to change the risk.

An unanswered question persists: What is the risk of trisomy 18 in a fetus that has only simple small choroid plexus cysts? Although there is apparently still an increased risk, how great is it if the ultrasound examination findings are normal? Because fetuses with trisomy 18 often have structural anomalies (some very subtle), a complete ultrasound examination needs to include not only the routine study but also a thorough evaluation of the fetal face, all extremities (including the hands and feet), heart (complete examination not just a four-chamber view), the umbilical cord (for the presence of a single artery), and growth. Some observers consider that the configuration of the hands is particularly helpful. Although a normal fetus intermittently opens and closes its hands, and extends its fingers, a fetus with trisomy 18 al-

most always has a clenched fist that is maintained and overlapping fingers.

The risk associated with amniocentesis needs to be balanced against the benefit occurring from the detection of a chromosomally abnormal fetus. A second-trimester amniocentesis is associated with an average estimated pregnancy loss rate of 1:200, with some skilled obstetricians stating that it may be as high as 1:100! The approximate risk of having a child with trisomy 18 with only simple small cysts and without other abnormalities in the second trimester is uncertain. In addition, the ultrasound examination findings may be inaccurate for two reasons: subtle abnormalities may have been missed and others may not be detectable. The risk may also need to take into account a change in incidence with advancing maternal age. Although this issue has not been resolved, it is our opinion that the presence of a simple small cyst or cysts with otherwise totally normal findings from an extensive ultrasound examination needs only a follow-up study to rule out possible growth retardation.

Recently a serum triple screen of alpha fetoprotein (AFP), human chorionic gonadotropin, and unconjugated estriols, with maternal age adjustment, has been found helpful in detecting trisomy 18. In the second trimester, after fetal age has been established by ultrasound examination, up to 75% of the trisomy 18 cases have been correctly diagnosed, with few false-positive results. With further refinement, this test may help obviate or direct when amniocentesis is needed. Similar success with these same

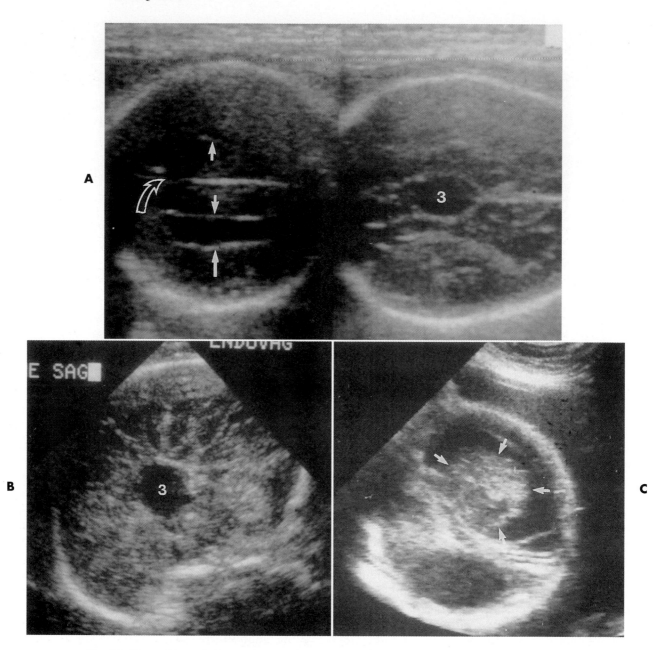

Fig. 10-18   Additional abnormalities of the head. **A** and **B,** Agenesis of the corpus callosum at term. **A,** Transabdominal transaxial views. On the right a high-riding enlarged third ventricle *(3)* is noted and on the left, more superiorly, there is spreading of the bodies of the lateral ventricles (medial walls denoted by small arrows and far-side lateral wall by large arrow). **B,** Sagittal midline transvaginal scan. The corpus callosum is absent and the enlarged high-riding third ventricle *(3)* is noted. **C,** Spontaneous third-trimester grade 3 intracranial hemorrhage. An oblique view through the occipital horns shows them to be dilated. A large heterogeneous hyperechoic mass *(arrows)* is seen in the near-side occipital horn.

serum markers has been experienced in the detection of trisomy 21.

Choroid plexus pseudocysts can occur. If the atrium of the lateral ventricle is imaged in an oblique/coronal rather than a true transaxial plane, ovoid hypoechoic structures may be seen to project into the choroid plexus from the adjacent corpus striatum. Although initially resembling cysts, they become oblong when the transducer is turned 90 degrees. Nelson and co-workers suggest that the overall incidence of choroid plexus cysts may therefore be overstated, thus changing the actual risk-benefit ratio and perhaps necessitating further studies to determine when amniocentesis is indicated in the evaluation of true choroid plexus cysts.

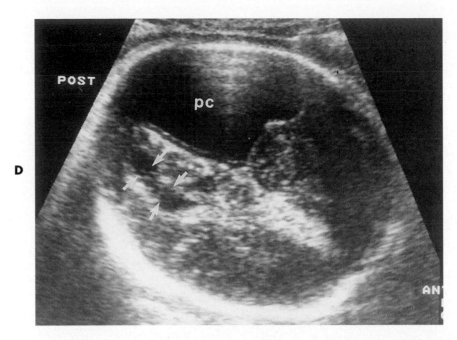

Fig. 10-18, cont'd.   **D,** Large porencephalic cyst *(pc)* in the left parietooccipital region in the distribution of the posterior cerebral artery. The occipital horn on the left is not identified because the "cyst" actually represents the enlarged ventricle filling the space of the destroyed brain. The normal right occipital horn is noted *(small arrows).* There is some evidence of a mass effect from the porencephalic area, with slight bulging of the midline toward the right.

OTHER HEAD ABNORMALITIES

Isolated midline CNS cystic structures can be detected by sonography. A dilated third ventricle without other obvious intracranial anomalies, especially if high in position, should suggest the diagnosis of agenesis of the corpus callosum (Fig. 10-18, *A* and *B*). If the cystic structure is posterior to the thalami or brainstem, an enlarged cistern, an arachnoid cyst, or a vascular malformation such as a vein of Galen aneurysm should be considered. A Doppler examination may be of value in settling the matter.

Intracranial hyperechoic areas may be seen infrequently. As previously discussed in the section on microcephaly, a calcified sequelae of in utero infection (see Fig. 10-7, *A*) or the tubers that form in tuberous sclerosis can occur. When hyperechoic areas without acoustic shadowing are seen either in the germinal matrix region or within the lateral ventricles, these are more likely areas of hemorrhage. Initially, intracranial hemorrhage was considered possible only in cases of direct trauma near term, when there was less amniotic fluid to protect the fetus. However, cases of spontaneous bleeding have now been reported that occurred in the middle to late third trimester, and the same neonatal intracranial hemorrhage grading system is used in this event: a grade 1 hemorrhage is within the germinal matrix, grade 2 is intraventricular bleeding, and grade 3 is associated with hydrocephalus.

When intraventricular, the hemorrhage can blend with and assume the appearance of an enlarged choroid plexus (Fig. 10-18, *C*).

Porencephalic cysts can also be detected in utero. Although the etiology is uncertain, brain parenchyma is lost typically in a vascular distribution (Fig. 10-18, *D*). The "cyst" communicates with and/or enlarges part of a ventricle (ex vacuo enlargement). The "cystic" area can vary in size, with some areas continuing to enlarge as the pregnancy progresses. The enlargement is presumably caused by the continued production (without resorption) of cerebrospinal fluid.

THE FETAL SPINE

AFP measurement has assumed considerable importance in screening pregnant women in the second trimester for the possible presence of open (not skin-covered) fetal anomalies. AFP is a normal fetal protein that is synthesized throughout fetal life, first in the yolk sac and then by the liver. Because it is excreted by the fetal kidneys, it can be identified in the amniotic fluid, with a normal fetal-to-amniotic fluid ratio of 1000:1. It is highest in concentration in the first trimester, and this decreases as the pregnancy progresses. AFP can also be detected in the maternal serum, caused by a transplacental diffusion

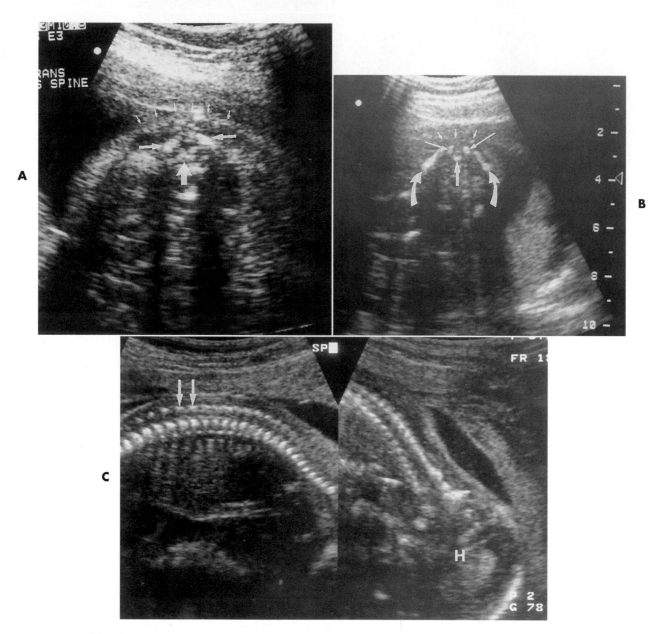

Fig. 10-19   Second-trimester views of a normal fetal spine. **A** and **B,** Transaxial views, **A** in the midabdomen and **B** at the area of the iliac crests *(curved arrows).* Large straight arrows denote the vertebral centrum; straight smaller arrows denote the posterior elements; and very small arrows denote the overlying soft tissue. There are two normal positions of the posterior elements: they either point inward toward each other, **A,** or remain parallel to each other, **B, C** and **D,** True sagittal views. **C** is a split image showing the fetal head *(H)* from the reader's right to the upper lumbar spine on the reader's left. Two of the partially imaged posterior elements are denoted by arrows in the left image. The normal overlying soft tissues are clearly identified. **D,** The lumbar and sacral region. The centra are ossified down to and including the S3 level *(large arrow).* The curved arrow denotes the lowest-most part of the spine, which has a normal lordotic curve. Note the normal overlying soft tissues and the lines within the spinal canal of the neural tube. **E,** Coronal view of the spine showing the parallel hyperechoic posterior elements, tapering to a point at the lower part of the sacrum *(curved arrow).* The straight arrow denotes one of the iliac wings, which on occasion may shadow and obscure the posterior elements.

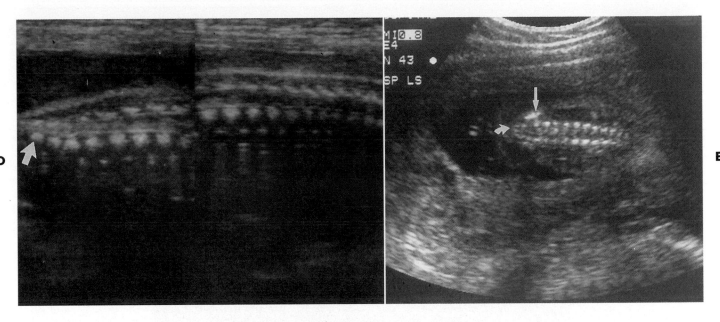

Fig. 10-19, cont'd.   For legend see opposite page.

gradient also of 1000:1. The level of maternal AFP in-creases as placental permeability increases and is normally highest in the second trimester.

There are normal bell-shaped distribution curves for the AFP levels in both the amniotic fluid and maternal serum, both related to fetal age. When there is an open fetal defect, the AFP level is elevated. The anomalies are usually neural (e.g., anencephaly, encephalocele, and spinal disorders). However, an open defect of any fetal part will cause an elevation in the AFP level; an abnor-mality affecting the anterior abdominal wall (omphalo-cele or gastroschisis) is an example of such a defect. Using an arbitrary cut-off level, which is different in different laboratories (between 2.0 to 2.5 multiples of the median or MOMs), the abnormal cases have higher levels. This cut-off needs to be adjusted for obese women and for those who have multiple gestations. Nevertheless, there is some overlap between the normal and the abnormal groups. In addition, a low serum AFP level can be used as a marker (after maternal age adjustment) for an increased risk of Down syndrome.

In the analysis of maternal AFP serum, false-negative (normal) results are very uncommon, and almost always occur in the setting of closed (skin-covered) fetal defects. False-positive results (elevated levels but not caused by fetal anomalies) are much more frequent and have been estimated to constitute upwards of 50% of the cases. The errors are mostly the result of inaccurate gestational dates, as older fetuses, particularly in the second trimester, have normally higher serum AFP levels. Pregnancies in which the levels are persistently elevated, without struc-tural anomalies, tend as a group to have a poorer progno-sis, particularly in the third trimester. This is discussed more completely in Chapter 15.

When elevated serum AFP levels are detected, two additional tests should be considered: (1) a thorough ul-trasound evaluation and/or (2) amniocentesis to obtain amniotic fluid for AFP and acetylcholinesterase measure-ments (the latter specific for neural tube defects). The ul-trasound examination must first be done to establish fetal age to determine whether the AFP level has been cor-rectly adjusted for fetal age. If it still proves elevated, there should be a thorough evaluation of the fetus, particularly the entire CNS and the anterior abdominal wall.

To perform a complete examination of the spine, every vertebral level from the cervical to the sacral region has to be studied (Fig. 10-19). At each level there are three hyperechoic bony structures (the anterior centrum and two posterior elements) and the overlying posterior soft tissues. However, for a neural tube defect to be detected, only the two posterior elements and the overlying soft tis-sues are important: the normal posterior elements should be parallel or point toward each other and the normal soft tissues should be uninterrupted and hypoechoic. If the fetus is in an ideal back-up and usually in a side posi-tion, transaxial images through the entire spine can be ob-tained that allow full visualization. Alternatively, if there are any technical or positional difficulties, the combina-tion of a midline sagittal view to evaluate the overlying soft tissues and the normal sacral lordosis and a coronal view to visualize the two parallel posterior elements, which taper to a point at the sacrum, can be used.

The spine can be identified clearly in most pregnan-cies by 16 weeks. By that time, the fifth lumbar vertebra is the most caudad level to be ossified. Thereafter the sacral spine ossifies sequentially every 2 to 3 weeks, so that S2 will not normally ossify until 22 weeks, with S3 through S5 ossifying even later. This observation would suggest that, at least in theory, abnormalities of the sacral bony structures may not be diagnosed before the late second trimester. In practice almost all except the must subtle defects can be identified accurately after 18 weeks' gestation.

NEURAL TUBE DEFECTS (MENINGOCELES/MENINGOMYELOCELES)

Neural tube defects are most common in the lumbosacral region. Termed *meningoceles* (if they contain only meninges) and *meningomyeloceles* (if they also have neural elements), there is always a splaying of the posterior elements and an abnormality of the overlying soft tis-

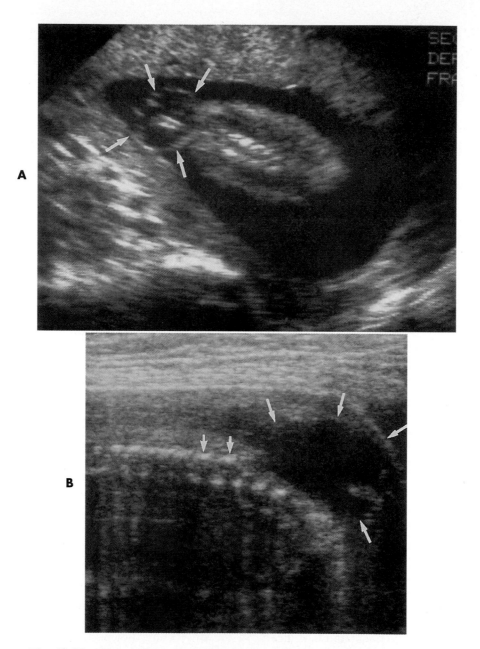

Fig. 10-20 Two neural tube defects. **A,** Meningomyelocele in a 20-week fetus. This coronal image of the lower part of the spine shows an anechoic (cystic) area *(arrows)* containing two hyperechoic lines. These lines are consistent with neural elements within the spinal defect. **B,** Meningocele in a 33-week fetus. In this sagittal image, the hyperechoic posterior elements on one side of the spine are seen down to the L5 level (L4 and L5 are shown by small arrows). A large cystic area *(large arrows)* distorts the soft tissues below this point and the posterior elements are no longer seen, as they have deviated outward.

sues. The soft tissue abnormality is either a "cystic" projection into the soft tissues (Fig. 10-20) or a flat defect (Fig. 10-21). The cystic projection is easy to identify, and the diagnosis can be made on the basis of the findings revealed by either a midline sagittal or a transaxial scan. If the cystic space is completely anechoic, most likely only a meningocele is present; if it is filled with thin hyperechoic strands, nerve roots (myeloid elements) are most likely present. It is not certain, however, if these strands always represent nerve roots, as arachnoid strands could give a similar appearance.

The extent of the defect is also important because the number of involved vertebral bodies can help predict its severity. If only several of the lower sacral verebrae are abnormal, the neurologic consequences will undoubtedly be less than those if the defect extends into the lumbar region. Because early in fetal life the neural tube occupies the entire length of the vertebral column and is still at S1 by the fifth month, a long sacral or lumbosacral defect affects many more neural levels than an abnormality in the same area acquires after birth (when the cord ends at L3). Ideally, particularly if the fetus is in a back-up presentation, the affected vertebrae can be accurately counted (Fig. 10-21).

Flat or subtle posterior soft tissue defects may be difficult to identify, particularly if the fetal back is against the uterine wall (obscuring soft tissue visualization) or if the fetus is in a face-up presentation (Figs. 10-21 to 10-23). In these situations, identification of the posterior (bony) elements assumes an even greater importance. These elements can be best evaluated in transaxial and coronal views. Their spreading is diagnostic for a neural defect.

Rarely an intraspinal hypoechoic to hyperechoic fatty tumor (lipoma) or a hyperechoic bony spur with shadowing (diastematomyelia) can be detected to further con-

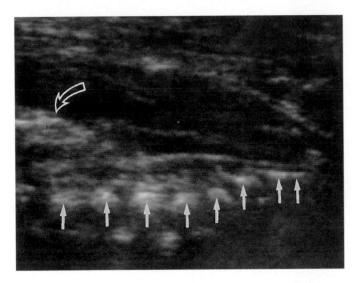

Fig. 10-21 Large, flat lumbosacral meningomyelocele in a 22-week fetus in back-up presentation. Arrows denote the vertebral centra from L1 (toward the reader's left) to S3 (toward the reader's right). The curved open arrow denotes the end of the normal soft tissues at the L1 level. Note that there are several hyperechoic strands, a finding consistent with neural elements.

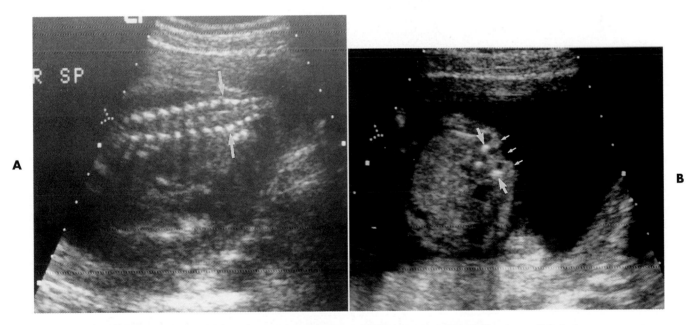

Fig. 10-22 Subtle flat meningocele in an 18-week fetus. **A,** Coronal view showing a slight bulge at the approximate L5-S1 level *(arrows).* **B,** Transaxial view at L5 showing the two posterior elements *(arrows),* which are deviated slightly outward, and the absence of the normal posterior soft tissues *(small arrows).*

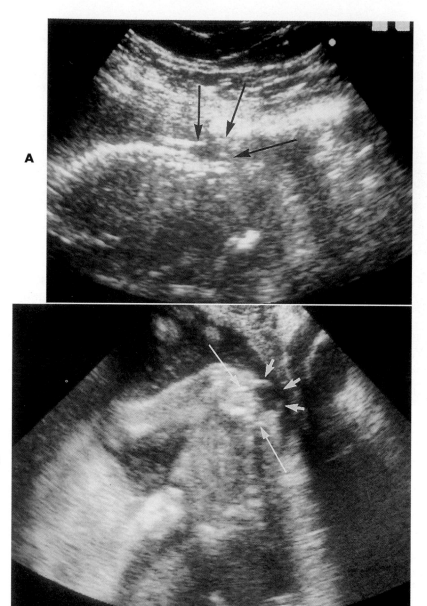

Fig. 10-23   Subtle small cystic meningocele in a 31-week fetus. **A,** This transabdominal sagittal view obtained in a very heavy woman suggests a small anechoic hypoechoic area *(large black arrows)* in the soft tissues of the lower part of the spine. The fetal head is toward the reader's left. The lack of amniotic fluid and closeness of the fetal back to the anterior uterine wall make visualization difficult. **B,** Transvaginal, transaxial view shows the posterior elements deviated outward *(long arrows)* and a definite "cystic" meningocele *(small arrows)* distorting the posterior soft tissues.

firm the spinal abnormality (Fig. 10-24, *A*). When the defect is severe, there may be an additional sharp angulation or deformity of the spine in the region of the abnormality (Fig. 10-24, *B*).

Whenever a neural tube abnormality is detected, the fetal head should be evaluated carefully. Three findings can be seen in this setting: hydrocephalus, the "lemon" sign, and the "banana" sign (Fig. 10-25). The banana sign is specific for spinal defects. It should theoretically be present in almost all, except the mildest, cases because it is the pathologic consequence of an Arnold-Chiari type II malformation. In it the cerebellum is pulled down, obliterating the cisterna magna, and the cerebellum is changed in shape from bilobate to a downward-curved C. With

today's technology, it should be seen in over 90% of the cases. In addition, there is at least a 50% incidence of associated hydrocephalus, presumably caused by obstruction at the outlet of the fourth ventricle. There is no direct correlation, however, between the extent of the spinal defect and the severity of the hydrocephalus.

The lemon sign is an unusual flattening of both frontoparietal bones, a fairly sharp indentation on both sides of the midline. Although its etiology is not known, the sign is present before 24 weeks in 98% of the open spinal defects; after 24 weeks, the sign is inexplicably present in only 13% of the affected fetuses. The sign is somewhat nonspecific. Some normal fetuses may have a milder, less indented, lemon configuration (1% to 2% of normal fe-

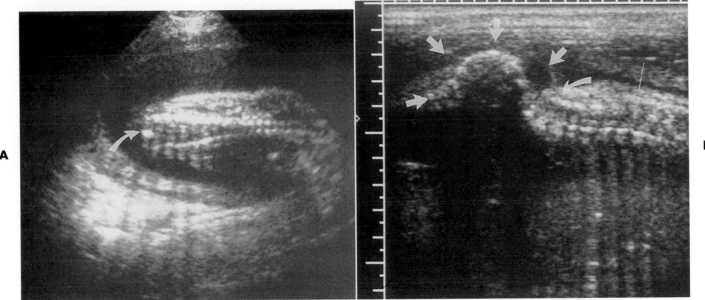

Fig. 10-24   Two cases of additional findings associated with meningomyeloceles. **A,** Diastemato-myelia. Coronal view with the fetal head toward the reader's right shows significant spreading of the posterior elements and a well-defined hyperechoic ossification *(curved arrow)* within the canal at the L5 level. **B,** Deformed spine at the point of the neural tube defect. This sagittal view shows the normal soft tissues and posterior elements down to the curved arrow at the L3 level. Below this, there is a marked spinal curvature with an overlying cystic area *(arrows).*

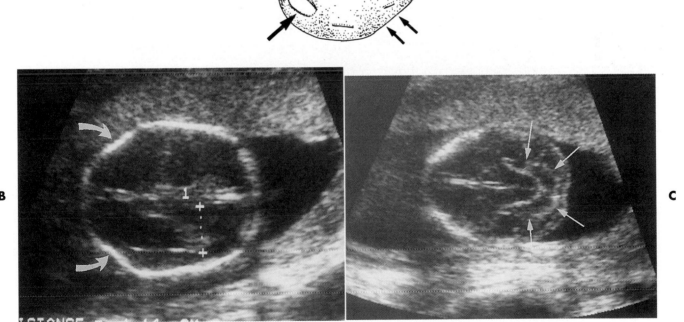

Fig. 10-25   Three head signs in cases of meningoceles and meningomyeloceles. **A,** The lemon sign with frontoparietal flattening *(small arrows)* and the banana sign of the curved cerebellum *(large arrows)* obliterating the cisterna magna. **B,** Transaxial scan showing frontoparietal flattening *(curved arrows)* and enlarged atria. (+), far-side atrium. **C,** Image of the posterior fossa showing the banana sign *(arrows).*

tuses before 24 weeks). It is also associated with other structural abnormalities, some not even related to the neural axis.

There are instances when the findings revealed by the initial examination of the spine are normal. However, if the banana and lemon signs are present (particularly the banana sign), and especially in association with hydrocephalus, a more careful evaluation of the spine is needed. It can be argued that a spinal defect must exist if the banana sign is detected.

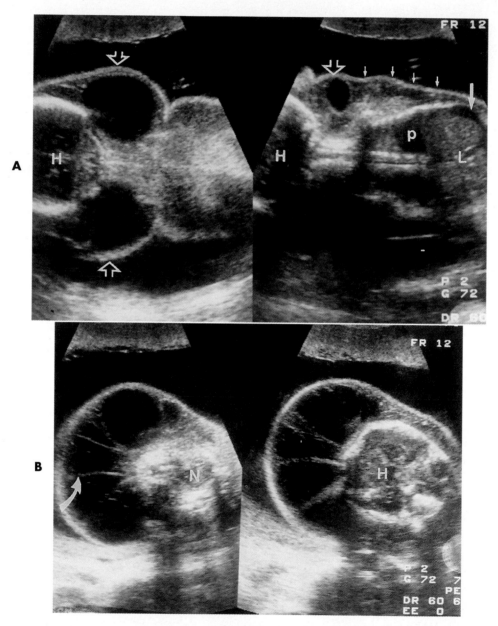

Fig. 10-26   Cystic hygroma with diffuse hydropic changes in a fetus with Turner's syndrome at 28 weeks. Two long-axis coronal views with the head *(H)* toward the reader's left and body toward the right. **A,** In the left image, a defect in the soft tissues of the neck represents a large cystic mass *(open arrows)* characteristic of cystic hygroma. In the right image, the liver *(L)* is surrounded by ascites *(arrow)*. Anechoic spaces in the thoracic cavity are consistent with pleural effusions *(p)*. One of the cystic areas of the hygroma is seen in the neck *(open arrow)*. Continued soft tissue thickness extends downward into the abdominal wall *(small arrows)*; these are findings consistent with diffuse edema. **B,** Two transaxial views of the head *(H)* and neck *(N)* region. The large cystic mass exhibiting a characteristic "spoked wheel" pattern extends posteriorly, one of the septations denoted by a curved arrow.

PARASPINAL ANOMALIES

Additional pathologic conditions may be detected in the paraspinal regions. A spoked-wheel–shaped cystic structure can be identified posterior and lateral in the soft tissues of the neck, with the underlying cervical spine normal. This pattern is characteristic for a lymphocele, and in this location (from the jugular lymph sac) is diagnostic of a cystic hygroma (Fig. 10-26). Although these hygromas can be isolated anomalies (unilateral or bilateral), they may also be part of a diffuse hydropic lymphatic obstruction, and occur in conjunction with additional signs of skin thickening and fluid in body cavities (e.g., ascites) (Fig. 10-26, *A*). Cystic hygromas are highly deforming; at least 50% are associated with chromosomal abnormalites, the best known of which is Turner's syndrome (XO karyotype). When hydropic changes are present, ultimate fetal or neonatal demise is a certainty.

Lymphoceles do not always originate from the jugular lymph sac, however. They can occur in any area of the body and, though deforming, are not associated with chromosomal abnormalities or diffuse obstruction.

In the low back a mass with a variable proportion of solid areas (from mostly cystic to completely solid) can be identified adjacent to the sacrum. The solid components and the location of the mass make the diagnosis of a teratoma likely. It most commonly originates from the sacrum and coccyx, and is therefore termed a *sacrococ-cygeal teratoma* (Fig. 10-27). These teratomas may be divided in four types, from completely external (type 1) to completely internal (type 4). Type 4 is the most difficult to diagnose. In utero these teratomas can be markedly deforming but are not predisposed to malignant degeneration. Only after birth, if they are not removed, is malignancy possible. The significance of these tumors is governed by the extent to which the surrounding area is either directly involved or compressed. They may also occur in other areas of the body unrelated to the spine.

There has been an attempt to evaluate the neurologic deficit caused by lumbosacral spinal defects and sacrococcygeal teratomas by observing the movement of the lower limbs and the filling and emptying of the urinary bladder. At present these observations have not proved to be accurate predictors of function or outcome.

TRANSVAGINAL CENTRAL NERVOUS SYSTEM IMAGING

There are times when transabdominal scans cannot adequately evaluate the fetal structures occupying the lower uterine segment. In this event TV scanning should be considered. Its higher resolution capability and different scanning planes, frequently coronal and sagittal, can permit identification or more complete analysis of the fetus (see Figs. 10-18, *A* and 10-23).

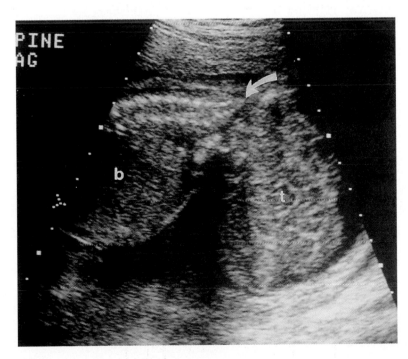

Fig. 10-27 Sacrococcygeal teratoma, type 1. This sagittal long-axis midline view of the sacrum of a 28-week fetus shows the large hyperechoic, completely exterior solid teratoma *(t)* at the lower-most part of the fetus. It extends below and does not involve the fetal spine. The lower-most tip of the normal spine is denoted by a curved arrow. *b*, fetal body.

Key Features

Anencephaly is easily diagnosed by the absence of normal calvarium and brain above the orbits. Occasionally, hyperechoic ill-defined soft tissue can be identified, a variant called *angiomatous stroma.*

Polyhydramnios has many causes. It is directly related to fetal anomalies in approximately 20% of cases, and is caused by the absence of fetal swallowing. In general the more severe the anomaly, the more severe the polyhydramnios.

Polyhydramnios may be present in otherwise normal pregnancies. Conversely, the amount of amniotic fluid may be normal even when it is expected to be increased.

The BPD up to 24 weeks' gestation has an accuracy of ±1 week. After 24 weeks, the accuracy decreases, and it is ±3 to 4 weeks by the third trimester.

When a BPD is being evaluated, the head shape must also be considered. If the head is too oval or round, a correction factor must be included in the calculation or a circumference obtained.

The lateral ventricles are evaluated at the atria. The transverse measurement should be ≤12 mm and the choroid plexus should occupy $\geq60\%$.

Increased intracranial pressure (hydrocephalus) can be diagnosed by the presence of progressive ventriculomegaly and/or an enlarged head. In most cases the head size is normal and proportionate to the body. Other additive signs include a ruptured falx echo, third- or fourth-ventricular enlargement, and certain posterior fossa abnormalities.

Regardless of the severity of the hydrocephalus, there is always a thin remaining mantle of cortex. In hydranencephaly, caused by destruction of parenchyma in the frontal and parietotemporal regions, there are either irregular hyperechoic areas of tissue (if the process is ongoing) or a complete absence of brain.

Microcephaly is clinically important when >3 SD below the norm, when BPD is discrepant from the body by 9 mm, and/or when the head circumference is discrepant from the body by 27 mm.

Holoprosencephaly is a midline development anomaly that occurs in one of three forms: alobar, the most severe (frequently associated with many additional anomalies), semilobar, and lobar. The lobar form frequently goes undiagnosed in utero.

Facial anomalies, although not discussed in the obstetric guidelines, can be diagnosed. These include the outer orbital diameter abnormalities, cleft lip and palate, small chin, and facial tumors.

Encephaloceles are frequently posterior defects that protrude through the occipital bone. They can occur anywhere in the midline, including the ethmoid region. They are commonly associated with additional structural and chromosomal abnormalities.

The posterior fossa has a normal bilobate cerebellum and a cisterna magna. A loss of cisterna magna and/or a change in shape of the cerebellum to a "banana" configuration is strong if not definitive proof of a spinal defect.

An enlarged posterior fossa is almost always associated with a chromosomal abnormality and/or a Dandy-Walker abnormality.

A thin rim of nuchal skin can be detected posterior to the occipital bone in the second trimester. Any enlargement >6 mm in the second trimester is diagnostic for trisomy 21.

The choroid plexus may contain cysts, and these may be normal variants. However, if any other abnormality is present or if the cysts are complex or large, the possibility of chromosomal abnormalities, in particular trisomy 18, is likely.

Intracranial hemorrhage can occur in utero in the middle to late third trimester.

The fetal spine can be evaluated by a combination of AFP measurements (in serum or amniotic fluid) and ultrasound examination.

Ultrasound studies can evaluate the spine in three projections. Spinal defects consist of a posterior element and overlying soft tissue (flat or cystic) defects.

Secondary abnormalities of the head, the "lemon" and "banana" sign and hydrocephalus, often occur with spinal defects.

Paraspinal abnormalties include teratomas and cystic hygromas.

SUGGESTED READINGS

Alagappan R et al: Distal lateral ventricular atrium: reevaluation of normal range, *Radiology* 193:405, 1994.

Ball RH et al: The lemon sign: not a specific indicator of meningomyelocele, *J Ultrasound Med* 3:131, 1993.

Baumeister LA et al: Fetal fourth ventricle: US appearance and frequency of depiction, *Radiology* 192:333, 1994.

Benacerraf BR, Frigoletto FD Jr, Greene MF: Abnormal facial features and extremities in human trisomy syndromes: prenatal US appearance, *Radiology* 159:243, 1986.

Benson CB, Doubilet PM: Sonographic prediction of gestational age: accuracy of second- and third-trimester fetal measurements, *AJR* 157:1275, 1991.

Bromley B, Benacerraf BR: Fetal micrognathis: associated anomalies and outcome, *J Ultrasound Med* 13:529, 1994.

Bromley B, Frigoletto FD Jr, Benacerraf BR: Mild fetal lateral cerebral ventriculomegaly: clinical course and outcome, *Am J Obstet Gynecol* 164:863, 1991.

Budorick NE, Pretorius DH, Nelson TR: Sonography of the fetal spine: technique, imaging, findings, and clinical implications, *AJR* 16:421, 1995.

Cardoza JD, Goldstein BB, Filly RA: Exclusion of fetal ventriculomegaly with a single measurement: the width of the lateral ventricular atrium, *Radiology* 169:711, 1988.

Chervenak FA et al: Fetal cystic hygroma. Cause and natural history, *N Engl J Med* 309:822, 1983.

Chervenak FA et al: A prospective study of the accuracy of ultrasound in predicting fetal microcephaly, *Obstet Gynecol* 69:908, 1987.

Chinn DH et al: Sonographically detected fetal choroid plexus cysts. Frequency and association with aneuploidy, *J Ultrasound Med* 10:255, 1991.

Crandall BF, Robinson L, Grau P: Risks associated with an elevated maternal serum alpha-fetoprotein level, *Am J Obstet Gynecol* 165:581, 1991.

Damato N et al: Frequency of fetal anomalies in sonographically detected polyhydramnios, *J Ultrasound Med* 12.11, 1993.

Estroff JA, Scott MR, Benacerraf BR: Dandy-Walker variant: prenatal sonographic features and clinical outcome, *Radiology* 185:755, 1992.

Farrell TA et al: Fetal lateral ventricles: reassessment of normal values for atrial diameter at US, *Radiology* 193:409, 1994.

Goldstein I et al: Sonographic evaluation of the normal developmental anatomy of fetal cerebral ventricles: I. The frontal horn, *Obstet Gynecol* 72:588, 1988.

Goldstein RB, Filly RA: Prenatal diagnosis of anencephaly: spectrum of sonographic appearances and distinction from the amniotic band syndrome, *AJR* 151:547, 1988.

Goldstein RB, LaPidus AS, Filly RA: Fetal cephaloceles: diagnosis with US, *Radiology* 180:803, 1991.

Heiserman J, Filly RA, Goldstein RB: Effect of measurement errors on sonographic evaluation of ventriculomegaly, *J Ultrasound Med* 10:121, 1991.

Hertzberg BS et al: The three lines: origin of sonographic landmarks in the fetal head, *AJR* 149:1009, 1987.

Hertzberg BS et al: Normal sonographic appearance of the fetal neck late in the first trimester: the pseudomembrane, *Radiology* 171:427, 1989.

Hertzberg BS, Kay HH, Bowie JD: Fetal choroid plexus lesions. Relationship of antenatal sonographic appearance to clinical outcome, *J Ultrasound Med* 8:77, 1989.

Hilpert PL, Hall BE, Kurtz AB: The atria of the fetal lateral ventricles: a prospective study of normal size and choroid plexus filling, *AJR* 164:731, 1995.

Jeanty P et al: The binocular distance: a new way to estimate fetal age, *J Ultrasound Med* 3:241, 1984.

Johnson ML et al: Evaluation of fetal intracranial anatomy by static and real-time ultrasound, *J Clin Ultrasound* 8:311, 1980.

Keogan MT, DeAtkine AB, Hertzberg BS: Cerebellar vermian defects: antenatal sonographic appearance and clinical significance, *J Ultrasound Med* 13:607, 1994.

Knutzon RK et al: Fetal cisterna magna septa: a normal anatomic finding, *Radiology* 180:799, 1991.

Kopta MM, May RR, Crane JP: A comparison of the reliability of the estimated date of confinement predicted by crown-rump length and biparietal diameter, *Am J Obstet Gynecol* 145:562, 1983.

Kurtz AB ct al: Ultrasound criteria for in utero diagnosis of microcephaly, *J Clin Ultrasound* 8:11, 1980.

Laing FC et al: Sonography of the fetal posterior fossa: false appearance of mega-cisterna magna and Dandy-Walker variant, *Radiology* 192:247, 1994.

Mahony BS et al: The fetal cisterna magna, *Radiology* 153:773, 1984.

Manelfe C, Sevely A: Neuroradiological study of holoprosencephalies, *J Neuroradiol* 9:15, 1982.

Mayden KL et al: Orbital diameters: a new parameter for prenatal diagnosis and dating, *Am J Obstet Gynecol* 144:289, 1982.

McLeary RD, Kuhns LR, Barr M Jr: Ultrasonography of the fetal cerebellum, *Radiology* 151:439, 1984.

Monteagudo A, Reuss ML, Timor-Tritsch IE: Imaging the fetal brain in the second and third trimesters using transvaginal sonography, *Obstet Gynecol* 77:27, 1991.

Nadel AS et al: Isolated choroid plexus cysts in the second-trimester fetus: is amniocentesis really indicated, *Radiology* 185:545, 1992.

Nelson NL, Callen PW, Filly RA: The choroid plexus pseudocyst: sonographic identification and characterization, *J Ultrasound Med* 11:597, 1992.

Nyberg DA et al: Holoprosencephaly: prenatal sonographic diagnosis, *AJNR* 8:871, 1987.

Pandya PP et al: First-trimester fetal nuchal translucency thickness and risk for trisomies, *Obstet Gynecol* 84:420, 1994.

Patel MD et al: Isolated mild fetal cerebral ventriculomegaly: clinical course and outcome, *Radiology* 192:759, 1994.

Pilu G et al: Sonographic evaluation of the normal developmental anatomy of the fetal cerebral ventricles: II. The atria, *Obstet Gynecol* 73:250, 1989.

Pretorius DH, Drose JA, Manco-Johnson ML: Fetal lateral ventricular ratio determination during the second trimester, *J Ultrasound Med* 5:121, 1986.

Sheth S et al: Prenatal diagnosis of sacrococcygeal teratoma: sonographic-pathologic correlation, *Radiology* 169:131, 1988.

van den Hoff MC et al: Evaluation of the lemon and banana signs in one hundred thirty fetuses with open spina bifida, *Am J Obstet Gynecol* 162:322, 1990.

For a Key Features summary see p. 251.

The obstetric guidelines recommend a routine four-chamber view of the heart. When the fetal position is appropriate, other views of the heart and images of the great vessels can also be obtained. These structures are easily identified because they are anechoic, pulsate, and have intraluminal movement of blood.

In the normal fetus the nonaerated lungs and the mediastinum blend together to assume a uniform hyperechoic echogenicity. To identify pulmonary and mediastinal abnormalities, there must be a change in the echogenicity or a shift in an anechoic structure, particularly cardiac displacement.

HEART

Rate and Rhythm

Heart motion defines a living conceptus, and its detection is of paramount importance in obstetric analysis. It is routinely identified by real-time observation during the early first trimester. At 5 to 6 weeks the heart rate av-erages 100 beats/min, rising to 140 to 160 beats/min by 8 weeks. This is discussed more completely in Chapter 9.

The same heart rate is then maintained throughout the remainder of intrauterine life, normally not decreasing below 120 beats/min or increasing above 180 beats/min. However, in the second, and especially in the third, trimester, a transient bradycardia can be normal, provided that it does not go below 60 beats/min or last longer than 15 to 20 seconds. Other rates and all arrhythmias should be considered abnormal.

Although the antenatal guidelines do not recommend routine hard-copy documentation of heart motion, an M-mode examination is suggested in any abnormal situation. M-mode is preferable to real-time sonography because, as a tracing, it can be analyzed more precisely. The ideal M-mode examination should be performed through an atrium and ventricle, and include its atrioventricular valve.

All heart motion abnormalities should be examined for five properties: (1) rate, (2) rhythm—constant or variable, (3) normal atrial-to-ventricular association, (4) structural abnormalities—cardiac and noncardiac, and (5) evidence of fetal hydrops. The most common arrhythmia is produced by premature atrial contractions. These are usually benign but, if very frequent, can predispose to the development of a supraventricular tachycardia (Fig. 11-1). All other conduction abnormalities must be closely observed and occasionally treated.

If a well-defined bradycardia or tachyarrhythmia is observed, a short M-mode tracing is sufficient for documentation. On occasion the heart rate may be normal and yet, because of unexplained hydrops, an intermittent conduction abnormality is suspected. A longer period of observation is then necessary.

Normal Structure

To identify cardiac position, it is often easiest to start with the standard transaxial view of the upper abdomen, which also identifies the stomach, and to move the transducer slightly toward the fetal head, still keeping a transaxial orientation. Normally both the heart and stomach arc on the fetus' left side. The right and left sides of the fetus can be determined from the fetal presentation (cephalic or breech) and by the position of the fetal spine; with practice this assessment can be done quickly and accurately.

The transaxial image of the lower chest of the fetus identifies the four-chamber view. After birth the apex of the heart points downward and the four-chamber view cannot be obtained in a transaxial projection. However, in utero the normal liver is proportionately much larger than it is after birth and elevates the cardiac apex.

The timing of the cardiac study is important. Transabdominally the heart chambers are usually not identified clearly before 16 weeks; however, by 18 to 22 weeks it is possible to satisfactorily identify the intracardiac anatomic characteristics 95% of the time. This can still be difficult if the fetus presents in a back-up position or is more than 8 to 10 cm from the transducer (usually in women of large girth or with polyhydramnios). In selected suboptimal cases, if the fetal thorax is close to the lower uterine segment, a transvaginal cardiac study can be attempted.

In the four-chamber view the cardiac apex points toward the fetus' left side at an angle of approximately 45 degrees (Fig. 11-2). The right ventricle is the most anterior chamber. Occasionally, particularly when the fetus is positioned obliquely, it may be difficult to identify the right ventricle. A simple and usually successful approach

to establishing chamber identity is as follows: In the transaxial view the descending thoracic aorta is immediately anterior and slightly to the left of the spine. Directly anterior to the aorta is the left atrium. From the left atrium, the right atrium and then their corresponding ventricles can be determined.

The four-chamber view (Fig. 11-2) permits identification of the ventricles and their interventricular septa, the atria with their ostium secundum and foramen ovale, and the atrioventricular valves (mitral and tricuspid). The overall sizes of the atria and ventricles, both during systole or diastole, should exhibit a 1:1 relationship throughout the second and third trimesters. If needed, measurement tables are available, with the chamber sizes measured at their inner margins just above and below the atrioventricular valves.

The transverse dimension or circumference of the heart, taken at the level of the atrioventricular valves, should not exceed 50% of a comparable measurement of the fetal thorax. This is similar to the expected heart size relative to the thorax seen after birth on a posteroanterior chest radiograph.

Structural Abnormalities

If the mother has a family history of congenital heart disease, the risk of a cardiac anomaly, but not necessarily of the same type, is increased in a subsequent child. Recurrence is increased by 10% if one parent, by 3% if one

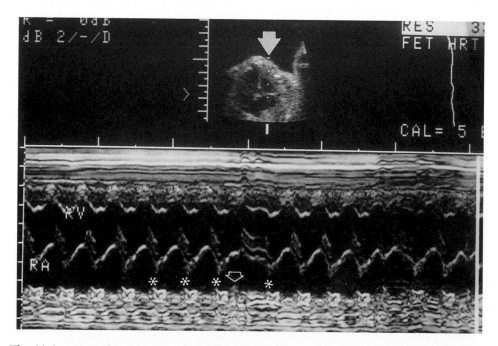

Fig. 11-1   M-mode tracing of the fetal heart in a 22-week fetus with premature atrial contractions. The ultrasound image shows the position of the M-mode tracing through the right side of the heart, starting at the arrow and extending along the dotted line. The M-mode tracing shows the right ventricle (RV) and the right atrium (RA) separated by the tricuspid valve. At the bottom of the tracing asterisks denote normal contractions. Note the normal association between the atria and ventricles. The open arrow denotes a premature atrial contraction followed by a prolonged pause.

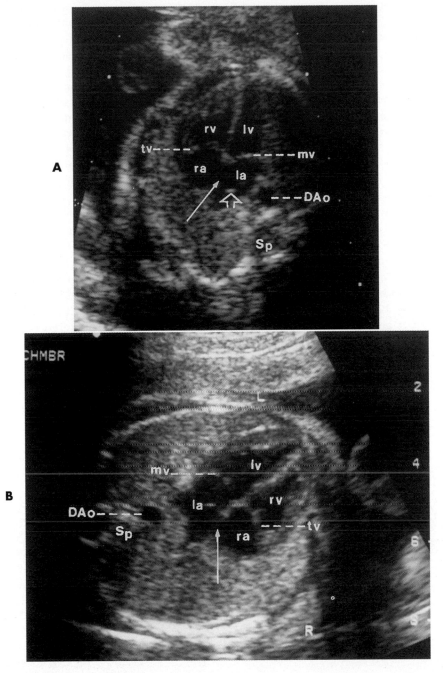

Fig. 11-2   Two normal four-chamber cardiac views in 20-week fetuses, both in diastole. Transaxial views of the lower chest show the "apical" **(A)** and the "parasternal" **(B)** four-chamber views. The normal interventricular septum is seen between the right ventricle *(rv)* and the left ventricle *(lv).* The normal ostium secundum with a patent foramen ovale *(arrow)* is seen between the right atrium *(ra)* and the left atrium *(la).* In addition, the flap of the foramen ovale *(open arrow)* is seen in **A.** Note that in **A** the membranous part of the interventricular septum, near the mitral valve *(mv)* and tricuspid valve *(tv),* appears very thin and almost absent. This is an artifact caused by the perpendicular orientation of that part of the septum to the ultrasound beam. With a change in orientation, such as that in **B,** the septum is shown to be normal. *DAo,* descending thoracic aorta; *Sp,* fetal spine; *R* and *L,* the right and left sides of the fetus, respectively, in **B.**

sibling, and by more than 15% if two siblings are affected. The highest incidence of recurrence, up to 25%, has been observed in the setting of fetuses with a hypoplastic left heart.

Using only the four-chamber view, the overall detection rate for significant cardiac anomalies approaches 70%. However, the rate reported by some observers has been less, as low as 50%. Therefore, although the four-chamber view is valuable, it has limitations. It is only able to detect certain anomalies, and typically only the larger ones. These are listed by frequency (likelihood) of detection (Box 11-1).

These anomalies can be classified into those affecting cardiac position (e.g., situs inversus and ectopia cordis), cardiac septae (e.g., ventricular septal defect), cardiac chambers (e.g., ventricular hypoplasia and Ebstein's anomaly), and masses (e.g., rhabdomyomas). Most are visualized directly; the presence of others is only inferred by the identification of a constellation of cardiac findings (e.g., that observed in the setting of pulmonary atresia). Because of its association with omphaloceles, ectopia cordis is discussed in Chapter 12.

The four-chamber view is good for identifying large septal defects, particularly if ventricular or atrioventricular (Fig. 11-3). Small ventricular and most atrial defects (because of the normally patent foramen ovale) go undiagnosed in utero. On an apical four-chamber view the region of the membranous septum, which is near the insertion of the mitral and tricuspid valves, may appear decreased in echogenicity or even absent (see Fig. 11-2, *A*). This is an artifact that is technically caused by the perpendicular orientation of this thin area to the ultrasound beam. Any change in transducer position proves the septum is normal (see Fig. 11-2, *B*).

Abnormal cardiac chambers are usually diagnosed on ultrasound studies. The "enlarged" right atrium that occurs in Ebstein's anomaly, a combination of the right atrium and the atrialized right ventricle, is readily detected (Fig. 11-4). Ventricular hypoplasia involving either the right or left ventricle is often diagnosed, provided a proper technique is used (Fig. 11-5). In a true transaxial four-chamber view, the apices of both normal ventricles are seen to extend to the cardiac apex. Although an off-axis (not transaxial) scan might incorrectly suggest ventricular asymmetry, the position of the ventricular apices would still be normal. In contradistinction, in the setting of a true ventricular hypoplasia the affected ventricular chamber is smaller and its apex shortened.

The four-chamber view can also identify cardiac masses. In particular, but rarely, rhabdomyomas have been diagnosed (Fig. 11-6). These masses, typically associated with tuberous sclerosis, are hyperechoic and arise from the muscle of the walls or septa. If large, they can compress and narrow the cardiac chambers.

Box 11-1	**Abnormal Four-Chamber Heart View: The Frequency (Likelihood) of Cardiovascular Abnormality Detection**

FREQUENTLY DETECTED

Hypoplastic right or left ventricle
Single ventricle
Atrioventricular (endocardial cushion) defect
Large ventricular septal defect
Double-outlet right ventricle
Ebstein's anomaly
Pulmonary atresia
Cardiac tumors
Ectopia cordis
Situs inversus

LESS FREQUENTLY DETECTED

Large atrial septal defect
Tetralogy of Fallot
Cardiomyopathy
Aortic stenosis (severe)
Coarctation of aorta (severe)

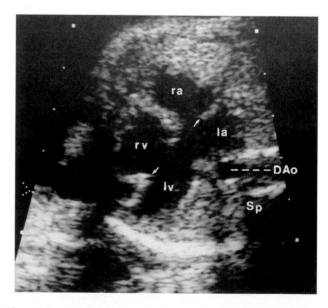

Fig. 11-3   Large atrioventricular septal defect (*A-V canal*) in an 18-week fetus. Transaxial view of the lower chest shows a four-chamber view of the heart. A large defect (*arrows*) is noted at the upper part of the ventricular septum between the right ventricle (*rv*) and left ventricle (*lv*). It extends into the atrial septum separating the right atrium (*ra*) from the left atrium (*la*). The tricuspid and mitral valves do not attach normally at the septum. *DAo,* descending thoracic aorta; *Sp,* fetal spine.

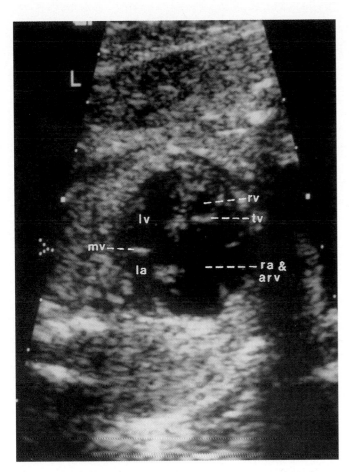

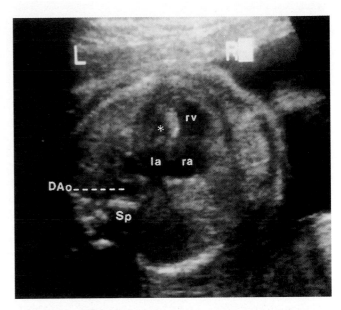

Fig. 11-5   Hypoplastic left ventricle in an 18-week fetus. Transaxial image of the lower chest shows a four-chamber view of the heart. All the chambers are normal, except the left ventricle. Compared with the right ventricle *(rv)*, the left ventricular chamber *(asterisk)* is much smaller and its apex foreshortened, not extending to the cardiac apex. *la,* left atrium; *ra,* right atrium; *DAo,* descending thoracic aorta; *Sp,* fetal spine; *L* and *R,* left and right sides of the fetus, respectively.

Fig. 11-4   Ebstein's anomaly in a 16-week fetus. Transaxial image of the lower chest shows a four-chamber view of the heart. The "right atrium" appears markedly enlarged, actually a combination of the right atrium and an atrialized right ventricle *(ra & arv)*. The right ventricle *(rv)* is markedly smaller than normal and the tricuspid valve *(tv)* inserts in a much lower position. The left-sided chambers are normal. *lv,* left ventricle; *la,* left atrium with a normal interposed mitral valve *(mv)*; *L,* left side of the fetus.

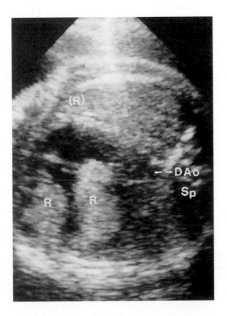

Fig. 11-6   Rhabdomyomas, indicated by an *R,* in a 20-week fetus. These were incidental findings in a fetus without tuberous sclerosis. Transaxial view of the lower chest shows a four-chamber view of the heart. Large hyperechoic masses are identified that distort the left-sided cardiac chambers and the septum. *DAo,* descending thoracic aorta; *Sp,* fetal spine; *(R),* right side of the fetus.

Infrequently, small hyperechoic foci can be seen in either ventricle, the left more than the right. These represent papillary muscle calcification, are of unknown cause, and are probably benign. Although an increased incidence of chromosomal abnormalities has been noted in association with histologically detected calcifications, this has not been associated with sonographically detected calcifications.

The four-chamber view often overlooks small or subtle intracardiac defects. In addition, the four-chamber view cannot identify the aorta and pulmonary arteries. To overcome these shortcomings, additional images have been proposed that are not described in the obstetric guidelines. The simplest two are a short-axis view of the great vessels at the base of the heart and a long-axis view of the left ventricular outflow tract. The base view, obtained by moving the transaxial four-chamber view cephalad, identifies the normal perpendicular origins of the pulmonary artery and aorta (Fig. 11-7). It is important to identify proper great vessel orientation, as this rules out the possibility of transposition of these vessels. The normal proportion of the overall sizes of the pulmonary artery and aorta is 1:1 throughout the second and third trimesters; size disproportionality can identify a number of abnormalities (Box 11-2). Occasionally the pulmonary bifurcation can also be identified, not uncommonly together with identification of the patent ductus arteriosus.

The long-axis view of the left ventricular outflow tract is obtained by scanning the left ventricle and turning the transducer toward the fetus' right shoulder (Fig. 11-8). This view analyzes the continuity of the left ventricle with the ascending thoracic aorta and permits more complete evaluation of the ventricular septum. More ventricular septal defects and overriding of the great vessels (commonly seen in the setting of tetralogy of Fallot) can be identified in this way. When these two views are added to the four-chamber view, the percentage of cardiac anomalies detected, as cited in most series, increases to greater than 80%. However, the aortic arch and descending thoracic aorta, ductus arteriosus (in the long axis), and the pulmonary veins are still not imaged.

If an examiner identifies a cardiac abnormality but does not feel convinced of the diagnosis, videotape recording of the heart is recommended. This permits better documentation than does freeze-frame imaging alone, and allows for later review and consultation, if needed.

Recently, color flow Doppler studies, often with pulsed-Doppler analysis, have been employed in the cardiac examination. Although a Doppler study allows determination of blood flow and its direction, as well as analysis of valvular regurgitation, it has had only limited diagnostic impact.

In women with a high incidence of recurrent cardiac anomalies in their offspring (>10%), an early transvaginal heart study can be performed at 12 to 14 weeks. This study is limited by the small size of the fetal heart at this time, and by the position of the fetus and the difficulty in obtaining optimal cardiac views (Fig. 11-9). Nevertheless, in selected cases, early detection of large anomalies is possible. "Normal" findings, however, have to be evaluated

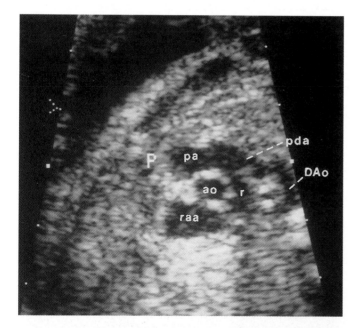

Fig. 11-7   Normal transaxial short-axis view of the great vessels at the base of the heart in a 20-week fetus. The pulmonary artery *(pa)* is seen curving around the ascending aorta *(ao)*, which is the normal configuration for these vessels. Note the 1:1 relationship in their diameters. The pulmonary artery then bifurcates into the right branch *(r)* and the patent ductus arteriosus *(pda)*, the latter extending back to the descending thoracic aorta *(DAo)*. The left branch is not identified; if seen, it would be found at a higher level. *raa,* right atrial appendage.

Box 11-2   Disproportionate Size of the Great Vessels

LARGE AORTA

Tetralogy of Fallot
Truncus arteriosus

SMALL AORTA

Coarctation
Hypoplastic left heart

SMALL PULMONARY ARTERY

Hypoplastic right heart
Ebstein's anomaly with pulmonary hypoplasia

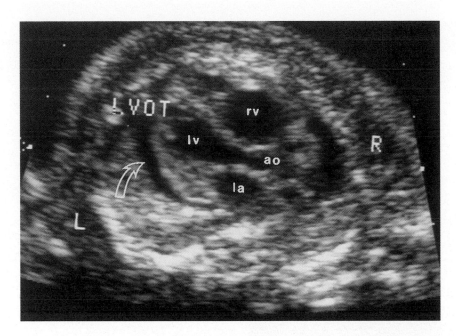

Fig. 11-8   Normal long-axis view of the left ventricular outflow tract *(LVOT)* in an 18-week fetus. There is normal continuity between the left ventricle *(lv)*, and the ascending aorta *(ao)*. Note a small pericardial effusion *(open curved arrow)* that is an incidental finding and of no clinical significance. *R* and *L,* right and left sides of the fetus, respectively; *rv,* right ventricle; *la,* left atrium.

cautiously, with a final diagnosis awaiting the results of a formal transabdominal study at 18 to 22 weeks. These studies should be videotaped for later review.

There are commonly extracardiac structural abnormalities associated with congenital heart disease, and meticulous attention to the rest of the fetus is therefore warranted. The karyotype of the fetus should also be determined when a cardiac abnormality is detected, because of the increased incidence of chromosomal abnormalities in this setting, particularly trisomies. If the cardiac structural abnormality is severe enough to be incompatible with life, an elective termination before 24 weeks should be considered. If not, these pregnancies should be observed serially for the assessment of fetal growth and for the detection of signs of heart failure—fetal hydrops. Medical treatment is available for certain cardiac arrhythmias (particularly digitalis and calcium channel blockers). This can be given to the mother, infrequently delivered into the amniotic fluid or rarely even directly into the fetus. Near term, decisions about the type of delivery and the type of hospital in which to deliver are important.

FETAL HYDROPS

Fetal hydrops (hydrops fetalis) is defined as excessive fetal body water. It is categorized as either immune or non–immune hydrops. Immune-mediated hydrops is caused by maternal exposure to certain fetal antigens, re-

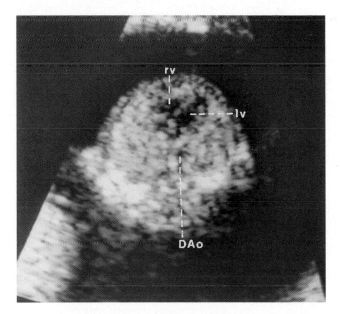

Fig. 11-9   Normal transvaginal, transaxial four-chamber view in a 13-week fetus. This image is captured from a real-time tape. The four-chamber view is incomplete. Although the right ventricle *(rv)* and left ventricle *(lv)* are identified, the interventricular septum is incompletely seen and the atria cannot be identified clearly. *DAo,* descending thoracic aorta.

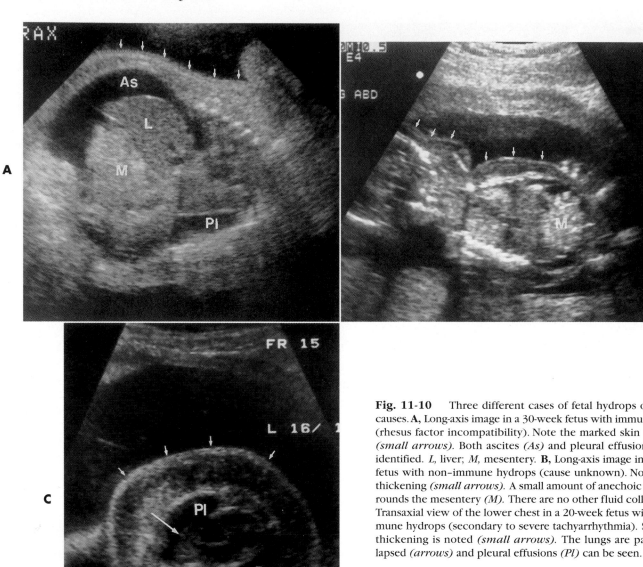

Fig. 11-10 Three different cases of fetal hydrops of different causes. **A,** Long-axis image in a 30-week fetus with immune hydrops (rhesus factor incompatibility). Note the marked skin thickening *(small arrows).* Both ascites *(As)* and pleural effusions *(Pl)* are identified. *L,* liver; *M,* mesentery. **B,** Long-axis image in a 15-week fetus with non–immune hydrops (cause unknown). Note the skin thickening *(small arrows).* A small amount of anechoic ascites surrounds the mesentery *(M).* There are no other fluid collections. **C,** Transaxial view of the lower chest in a 20-week fetus with non–immune hydrops (secondary to severe tachyarrhythmia). Severe skin thickening is noted *(small arrows).* The lungs are partially collapsed *(arrows)* and pleural effusions *(Pl)* can be seen.

sulting in a fetal hemolytic anemia. It is most commonly caused by rhesus (Rh) incompatibility.

Non–immune hydrops consists of a heterogeneous group of abnormalities. It can be divided into five categories: (1) cardiac (primary myocardial and high-output failure), (2) decreased plasma oncotic pressure, (3) increased capillary permeability, (4) obstruction of venous return, and (5) obstruction of lymphatic flow. The cardiac causes, constituting 22% to 40% of the non–immune cases, comprise severe arrhythmias (either intermittent or constant), structural anomalies, severe anemias, myo-

carditis, arteriovenous shunts (usually resulting from fetal or placental tumors), and the twin-twin transfusion syndromes (in multiple gestations). Decreased oncotic pressure resulting from decreased albumin formation or increased excretion (hepatitis or nephrotic syndrome, respectively), increased capillary permeability (anoxia), venous obstruction (congenital or space-occupying lesions), and generalized lymphatic obstruction (Turner's syndrome) may also lead to non–immune hydrops. In utero infections can present with fetal hydrops, usually caused by a combination of the causes just listed.

The classic sonographic findings of fetal hydrops are fluid in serous cavities (ascites, pleural and pericardial effusions), skin thickening (edema), placental enlargement, and polyhydramnios (Fig. 11-10). Hepatosplenomegaly may also be present, particularly in immune hydrops. In general the more severe the hydrops, the more numerous

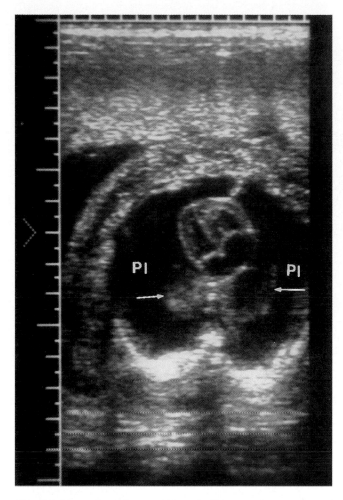

Fig. 11-11   Bilateral severe pleural effusions *(Pl)* in a 38-week fetus with fetal hydrops of unknown cause. Transaxial view of the lower chest shows a normal four-chamber heart. The lungs are completely collapsed *(arrows)* and there is marked skin thickening. A thoracentesis had to be performed before delivery.

The overall prognosis for fetal hydrops is variable. In immune conditions, particularly those caused by Rh incompatibility, fetal survival rates are high if appropriate aggressive treatment, including fetal transfusions, is instituted. In non–immune hydrops, the prognosis is poor unless the particular cause of the hydrops can be eliminated. This may only be possible in cases of severe arrhythmias controlled by medication or in anemias reversed by transfusions.

EXTRACARDIAC ABNORMALITIES

Major fetal thoracic extracardiac abnormalities can be detected by ultrasound. These abnormalities consist of congenital diaphragmatic hernias (CDH), cystic adenomatoid malformations (CAM), bronchogenic cysts, duplication cysts, pleural effusions, sequestrations, and rarely laryngeal atresia. Congenital lobar emphysema and congenital bronchiectasis are only detected after birth, not in utero.

To detect an extracardiac chest anomaly, either a shift in the cardiovascular structures (in particular the heart) or a change in echogenicity is needed. Commonly both are present. Any deviation of the heart without a mass is a suspicious sign for an unusual situs (situs inversus or indeterminus), and is often associated with cardiac anomalies. Although there are times when a right-sided heart is a normal variant, this is a diagnosis of exclusion.

Congenital Diaphragmatic Hernia

CDH is the most common intrathoracic, extracardiac fetal anomaly. It occurs sporadically, with an incidence of 1 in every 2000 to 3000 live births. It is strongly associated (16% to 56%) with abnormalities of all major organ systems and with an abnormal karyotype. If growth retardation is present, the incidence of associated anomalies increases to 90%.

CDHs are usually posterolateral in location (90%), and are then called *Bochdalek hernias.* They are typically unilateral, seven times more common on the left than on the right, and are rarely bilateral. The anteromedial, or Morgagni, hernia makes up the remaining 10%.

CDHs may be difficult to diagnose in utero. The typical presentation of a left-sided Bochdalek hernia is a cystic structure (the stomach) located on the left side of the chest, with no identifiable normal stomach bubble below the left hemidiaphragm. Often the heart is displaced upward or toward the right, or both (Fig. 11-12). Peristalsis or fluid-filled bowel loops within the chest are also diagnostic findings (Fig. 11-12, *B*); if the CDH contains only collapsed small bowel or mesentery, it is usually not detected. Left-sided hernias may also contain the spleen and left lobe of the liver.

and prominent the abnormalities. In any individual case, however, not all of these abnormalities are present and not all are of anticipated extent.

Ascites, pleural effusions, and rarely pericardial effusions may be the first findings in fetal hydrops (Fig. 11-11). On occasion, however, these findings may be isolated and caused by more local problems. For example, ascites may be secondary to a urinary tract rupture (urine ascites) or meconium peritonitis. A pericardial effusion is considered a normal finding if it is less than 2 mm in thickness (see Fig. 11-8). An isolated pericardial effusion, even when more prominent (between 2 and 7 mm) but without fetal structural anomalies, is not associated with an adverse fetal outcome. It is uncommon to have fetal hydrops occur with only skin thickening (without serous fluid collections). Skin thickening alone can be seen in gestational diabetes, sometimes in combination with placental enlargement and polyhydramnios.

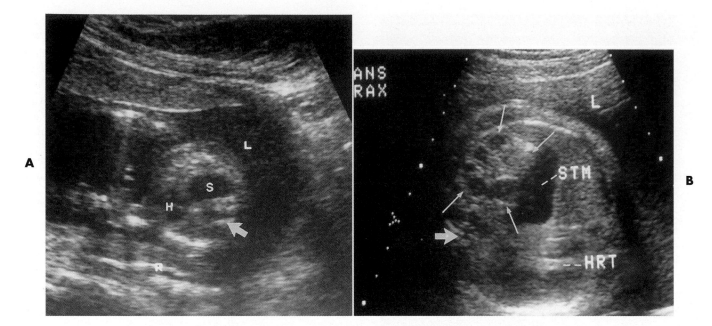

Fig. 11-12   Two cases of congenital diaphragmatic hernias, the left-sided Bochdalek type. **A,** Transaxial view of the lower chest in a 15-week fetus showing an anechoic structure, the stomach *(S)*, within the chest. It is displacing the heart *(H)* toward the right side of the fetus. *Arrow,* fetal spine; *L* and *R,* left and right sides of fetus, respectively. **B,** Transaxial view of the lower chest in a 30-week fetus shows the heart *(HRT)* displaced toward the right side of the fetus. In the left side of the chest *(L)* the stomach *(STM)* and multiple hypoechoic loops of small bowel and mesentery *(arrows)* are identified. *Large arrow,* fetal spine.

The right-sided Bochdalek hernias are usually more subtle. Typically only the liver herniates into the chest; its echogenicity is similar to that of the mediastinum and nonaerated lungs. If anechoic structures such as the hepatic vascular structures (the hepatic and portal veins), the gallbladder, and fluid-filled bowel also enter the chest, detection is easier. Unless the hernia is large, the position of the heart is frequently undisturbed.

Morgagni hernias typically herniate into the pericardial sac. They are often very difficult to diagnose because only the liver herniates and the cardiac position remains undisturbed. As with right-sided Bochdalek hernias, the diagnosis is made easier if the same anechoic structures also enter the pericardium or if a pericardial effusion is present.

Any CDH obstruction of bowel loops may lead to polyhydramnios. Additionally, shift of the heart may cause obstruction of venous return from the inferior vena cava, leading to ascites.

The prognosis for a CDH is often poor, even when it is only an isolated anomaly. CDHs are usually larger than they appear and often continue to enlarge as the pregnancy progresses. Pulmonary hypoplasia may therefore be an important secondary problem, and usually involves both lungs, especially when a significant cardiovascular shift is seen. Pulmonary hypoplasia is more completely discussed later in this chapter and in Chapter 13.

It would seem possible to diagnose a CDH by identifying a disruption in a hemidiaphragm. The hemidiaphragms, however, are curved, thin, hypoechoic bands that cannot be fully imaged and are often normally partially obscured by rib shadowing (Fig. 11-13). As might therefore be expected, the in utero defect has never been reported. It has been suggested, however, that paradoxical diaphragmatic motion (the hemidiaphragm on the affected side moving in the opposite direction with respiration) might serve to reveal a CDH.

Diaphragmatic eventration is a developmental abnormality caused by muscular hypoplasia or aplasia. It is not a true hernia, but represents an unusually elevated hemidiaphragm with the abdominal contents remaining intraperitoneally. The ipsilateral lung may be compressed secondarily. At least one lung will develop normally, however, unless the process is bilateral. An eventration is rarely associated with syndromes and triploidies.

Cystic Adenomatoid Malformation

CAM is a relatively uncommon dysplastic anomaly caused by hamartomatous involvement of the lung. In most cases the CAM involves only a sublobar area; less frequently an entire lung and rarely both lungs are affected. CAMs can be divided into three types (I to III) on the basis of histologic, gross, and clinical characteristics.

Type I is the most common, and consists of large cysts (2 to 10 cm in diameter) that are clearly identified by ultrasound (Fig. 11-14, *A*). In type II there are smaller macroscopic cysts, usually less <1.0 cm in diameter. Ultrasound detects some CAMs as cysts, with the remainder appearing as a hyperechoic mass (Fig. 11-14, *B*). Type III is the least common. It consists of multiple, small bronchiole-like structures (<0.5 cm in diameter) that are typically detected not as cysts, but as a hyperechoic mass (because of its multiple interfaces) (Fig. 11-14, *C*). The echogenicity of all three types of CAM permits intrathoracic detection. Theoretically, but not in practice, a type III CAM could be isoechoic with the surrounding tissues.

Prognosis is related to the size of the CAM and the presence of associated anomalies. Type I carries the best prognosis. Associated renal, gastrointestinal, and other pulmonary abnormalities occur in 25% of the cases, usually in the setting of type II CAMs. Type II therefore carries the worst prognosis. Type III CAMs are the largest and are therefore most likely to cause mediastinal shift and fetal ascites. These carry an intermediate prognosis. Chromosomal anomalies are not associated with any type of CAM.

Bronchopulmonary Sequestration

Bronchopulmonary sequestrations are less common than CDHs and CAMs, constituting 0.15% to 6.4% of all congenital pulmonary malformations. They form when a portion of the bronchopulmonary system develops separately. Sequestrations can be divided into two types on the basis of their pleural covering: the intralobar type without its own separate pleura, and the extralobar type with its own separate pleura. Sequestrations are often found in the lower lobes, in the posterior basal segments. They are more common on the left and are infrequently bilateral. Rarely they are found below the diaphragm. Significant anomalies are associated with both types: the less common extralobar type with 60% and the more common intralobar type with 14%.

Ultrasound often detects a bronchopulmonary sequestration as a hyperechoic mass at the lung base (Fig. 11-15). Very infrequently, cystic components may also be present. Classically the intralobar type is spherical and the extralobar type is conical or triangular; differentiation on the basis of shape, however, is unlikely. It is common for the extralobar type to present with fetal hydrops or as a mass associated with a pleural effusion.

Cysts

Primary bronchogenic (lung) cysts and duplication (gastrointestinal) cysts may also present as chest masses. They are commonly simple cysts and are usually solitary (Fig. 11-16). If large, they can cause cardiac displacement.

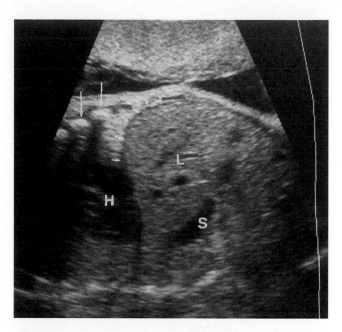

Fig. 11-13   Normal sagittal view of the left side of a 30-week fetus. The thin hypoechoic hemidiaphragm *(small arrows)* is only partially seen between the hyperechoic lung and heart *(H)*, above the diaphragm and the liver *(L)* below. Large arrows denote the lower ribs. *S,* fetal stomach.

Additional Comments

There is an overlap in the ultrasound features exhibited by extracardiac anomalies. When the mass has a primarily cystic appearance, it is more commonly a Bochdalek CDH (especially when left-sided), a type I or perhaps type II CAM, a bronchogenic or duplication cyst, or rarely a pulmonary sequestration. When the mass is primarily solid in appearance, either isoechoic or hyperechoic, it is more likely a Morgagni CDH, a type III CAM, or a bronchopulmonary sequestration.

There are cases in which an obvious extracardiac chest mass, detected early in the pregnancy, becomes less distinct toward term. There have even been reports of an extracardiac mass resolving by birth. If the mass does not grow, it becomes relatively smaller as the thorax grows. It is not certain if a mass detected by ultrasound can ever disappear. Instead the mass would more likely become so small by term that it would be concealed on a neonatal chest radiograph, and no further work-up performed. In either event, the continued normal growth of the chest is important, as it can prevent pulmonary hypoplasia. The heart (if initially displaced) can resume its normal position and signs of fetal hydrops may resolve.

Laryngeal Atresia

Laryngeal atresia is a rare lethal entity. It is an obstruction of the tracheobronchial tree occurring anywhere

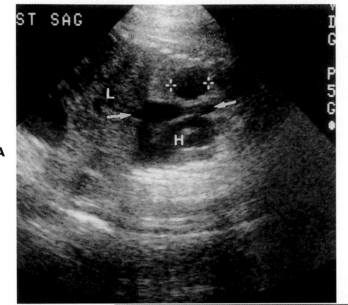

Fig. 11-14 Three cases of cystic adenomatoid malformations (CAMs). **A,** Type I CAM in an 18-week fetus. A sagittal-coronal view of the fetal body shows a well-defined cyst (+) surrounded by normal hyperechoic, nonaerated lung in the right hemithorax. There is slight displacement of the inferior and superior venae cavae *(arrows).* The heart *(H)* is in a grossly normal position. The echoes within the cyst are artifacts. *L,* liver. **B,** Type II CAM in a 32-week fetus. This is a sagittal view of the right side of the fetal body, with the fetal head toward the reader's right. A rounded mass containing both cystic and hyperechoic areas *(arrows)* can be seen in the right side of the hemithorax. This has caused considerable displacement of the heart (not visible on this scan). Surrounding the liver *(L)* is a significant amount of ascites *(As)* caused by impaired venous flow through the inferior vena cava. *P,* placenta. **C,** Type III CAM in a 22-week fetus. A transaxial view of the lower chest shows a hyperechoic mass *(arrows)* displacing the heart *(H)* toward the right side of the fetus. *Sp,* fetal spine.

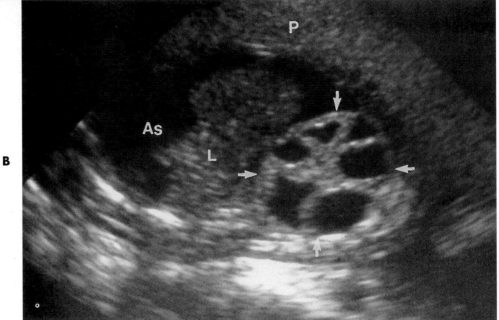

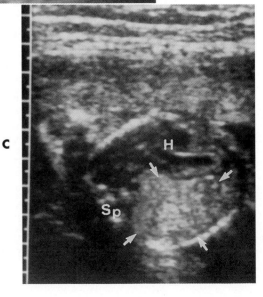

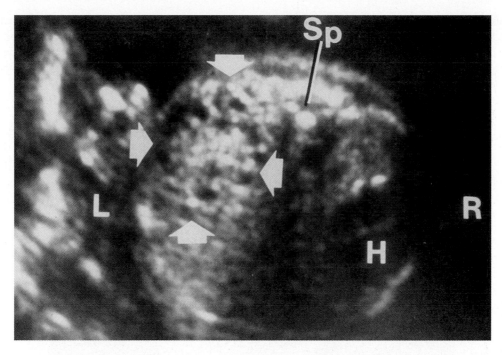

Fig. 11-15   Bronchopulmonary sequestration, the intralobar type. Transaxial view of the lower part of the chest in a 30-week fetus shows a mass *(arrows)*, which is primarily hyperechoic but with small cystic areas, in the left side of the chest. The heart *(H)* is displaced toward the right. *R* and *L*, right and left sides of the fetus, respectively. Note the similarity between this sequestration and a type III cystic adenomatoid malformation.

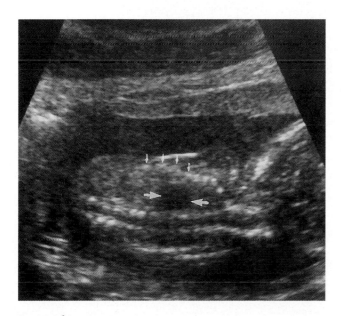

Fig. 11-16   Bronchogenic cyst in a 20-week fetus. Long-axis view of the fetus with its head toward the right shows a cyst *(large arrows)* within the fetal thorax, in the area of the right lung. The heart is not significantly displaced. Although this appeared to be a type I cystic adenomatoid malformation, a simple bronchogenic cyst was found at birth. *Small arrows,* ribs.

from the larynx to the bronchi. Rarely only one mainstem bronchus is involved. With obstruction, secretions from the lungs cannot be expelled. Both lungs (unless only one bronchus is involved) are found to increase in echogenicity and become enlarged, occasionally so large that they compress the heart and invert the hemidiaphragms (Fig. 11-17). The tracheobronchial tree can be identified as a tubular fluid-filled structure, which is filled with unexpelled secretions. Fetal hydrops and additional esophageal and tracheal abnormalities can also be present.

Pleural Effusions

Pleural fluid is readily detectable. It is typically anechoic, and occasionally hypoechoic, and is easily distinguished from the hyperechoic nonaerated lungs. When effusions are small, they are curvilinear collections (see Fig. 11-10). When larger, the effusions are more rounded and compress the lungs toward the hila (see Fig. 11-11). If they are large and left-sided, the heart can be displaced and compressed.

Pleural effusions are often bilateral and associated with fetal hydrops. Less commonly, pleural effusions may be unilateral and are then often an indication of a more localized pathologic condition such as an extracardiac mass (e.g., extralobar sequestration) or a chylothorax. A chylothorax is a lymphatic obstruction that is more common on the left. It cannot pathologically be diagnosed as chylous, however, because no fat is present within the in utero effusion.

Bilateral pleural effusions can be severe enough to compromise the fetal lungs in one of two ways: (1) if prolonged, they can cause pulmonary hypoplasia; and (2) if present at birth, the lungs (even if normal) cannot expand. In the latter case, a thoracentesis performed just before delivery may be necessary to allow aeration of at least one lung when the newborn attempts to breathe.

Pulmonary Hypoplasia

The bronchial tree is fully developed by 16 weeks of fetal life. The distal airways continue to develop, with 20 million terminal air sacs forming by birth. The alveoli de-

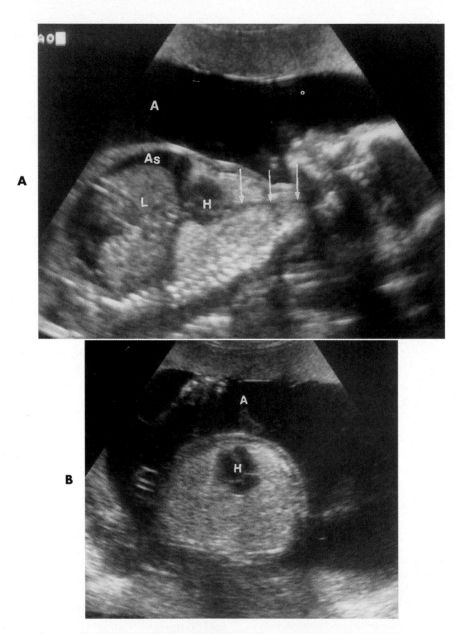

Fig. 11-17 Laryngeal atresia in a 28-week fetus associated with polyhydramnios. *A,* amniotic fluid. **A,** Long-axis sagittal view shows markedly hyperechoic enlarged lungs. A fluid-filled hypopharynx and trachea is identified *(arrows).* Ascites *(As)* surrounds the liver. *H,* heart; *L,* liver. **B,** Transaxial view through the fetal heart shows the heart *(H)* to be compressed by markedly hyperechoic enlarged lungs.

velop after birth and increase in number to 300 million by 8 years of age.

Anything that impedes the formation of the distal airways will cause the number of terminal air sacs, and ultimately the final number of alveoli, to be reduced. Any space-occupying process that compresses the lungs or any mass that involves part of the tracheobronchial tree will therefore inhibit lung development. Lung development also needs a large enough thoracic cage and a sufficient amount of amniotic fluid. A small chest or oligohydramnios, or both, will therefore also spawn underdevelopment of the lungs.

It may be difficult to predict when pulmonary hypoplasia is severe enough to be life-threatening. However, the more severe the visualized abnormality (by ultrasound) and the longer that it has been present, the greater the likelihood of serious pulmonary problems at birth.

This issue has not been resolved by the use of measurements. The thoracic-to-abdominal circumference ratio, consisting of the circumference taken at the level of the four-chamber view of the heart and of the standard upper abdominal circumference, respectively, is normal if it is more than 0.75. The lung-to-hemithorax diameter is normal if it is more than 0.75. The chest area minus the heart area divided by the chest area normally exceeds 0.62. None of these ratios, however, has shown a high degree of accuracy in predicting significant lung compromise.

Key Features

The normal nonaerated lungs and mediastinum are hyperechoic and blend together. An abnormality can be detected only by a change in echogenicity or by a mass effect on definable structures (usually the heart).

After 8 weeks the fetal heart rate normally ranges between 120 and 180 beats/min. Transient bradycardias are a normal variant. All other heart rates must be evaluated closely.

An M-mode examination of the heart is not a necessary part of a normal study. It is suggested, however, to document any abnormal condition.

All heart rate abnormalities should be examined in terms of rate, rhythm, the concordance of the atria to the ventricles, structural abnormalities, and fetal hydrops.

A routine four-chamber image of the heart, obtained on a transaxial view of the lower chest, evaluates the atria and ventricles, and their interposed septa. This view can detect up to 70% of significant cardiac anomalies.

Additional cardiac views improve the detection of abnormalities. These are an image of the base of the heart to evaluate the relationship and size of the aorta and pulmonary artery, and views of the ventricular outflow tracts.

Fetal hydrops (immune and non-immune) is caused by excessive fetal body water. Classically its presenting signs consist of serous cavity fluid, placental enlargement, and polyhydramnios. In any individual case, however, the number of abnormalities and their severity vary.

Cardiac causes of non-immune hydrops (22% to 40% of cases) are related to primary myocardial abnormalities and high-output failure. Severe arrhythmias and structural anomalies should be sought.

In utero infections may present as fetal hydrops.

Extracardiac in utero masses can be divided into those that are primarily cystic and those that are primarily solid. The primarily cystic masses are Bochdalek congenital diaphragmatic hernias (CDHs), type I and perhaps type II cystic adenomatoid malformations (CAMs), bronchogenic cysts, duplicated cysts, and pulmonary sequestration. The solid lesions are Morgagni and some Bochdalek CDHs, type III CAMs, and bronchopulmonary sequestration.

The heart is usually on the left side. Although there are occasions when the heart can be normal if on the right side, a right-sided or indeterminate situs is more often associated with cardiac and extracardiac anomalies.

The most common CDH is a left-sided posterolateral hernia (Bochdalek hernia). In its classic form the stomach is identified in the chest and the heart is displaced.

A CDH is generally more extensive than its sonographic appearance suggests. There is also an increased incidence of major organ abnormalities and an abnormal karyotype.

Pulmonary hypoplasia is caused by failure of normal bronchopulmonary development. Any space-occupying process that either compresses or involves part of the bronchopulmonary tree, a very small chest, and prolonged significant oligohydramnios can adversely affect lung development. It is not currently possible to predict the severity of the pulmonary hypoplasia, however.

SUGGESTED READINGS

Adzick NS et al. Fetal cystic adenomatoid malformation: prenatal diagnosis and natural history, *J Pediatr Surg* 20:483, 1985.

Adzick NS et al: Diaphragmatic hernia in the fetus: prenatal diagnosis and outcome in 94 cases, *J Pediatr Surg* 20:357, 1985.

Axel L: Real-time sonography of fetal cardiac anatomy, *AJR* 141:283, 1983.

Benacerraf BR, Pober BR, Sanders SP: Accuracy of fetal echocardiography, *Radiology* 165:847, 1987.

Bromley B et al: Fetal echocardiography: accuracy and limitations in a population at high and low risk for heart defects, *Am J Obstet Gynecol* 166:1473, 1992.

Bronshtein M et al: Early ultrasound diagnosis of fetal congenital heart defects in high-risk and low-risk pregnancies, *Obstet Gynecol* 82:225, 1993.

Bronshtein M et al: Fetal cardiac abnormalities detected by transvaginal sonography at 12-16 weeks' gestation, *Obstet Gynecol* 78:374, 1991.

Brown DL, Roberts DJ, Miller WA: Left ventricular echogenic focus in the fetal heart: pathologic correlation, *J Ultrasound Med* 13:613, 1994.

Brown DL et al: Sonography of the fetal heart: normal variants and pitfalls, *AJR* 160:1251, 1993.

Budorick NE et al: Spontaneous improvement of intrathoracic masses diagnosed in utero, *J Ultrasound Med* 11:653, 1992.

Copel JA, Pilu G, Kleinman CS: Congenital heart disease and extracardiac anomalies: associations and indications for fetal echocardiography, *Am J Obstet Gynecol* 154:1121, 1986.

Copel JA et al: Fetal echocardiographic screening for congenital heart disease: the importance of the four chamber view, *Am J Obstet Gynecol* 157:648, 1987.

DiSalvo DN et al: Clinical significance of isolated fetal pericardial effusion, *J Ultrasound Med* 13:291, 1994.

Dolkart LA et al: Prenatal diagnosis of laryngeal atresia, *J Ultrasound Med* 11:496, 1992.

Hagay A et al: Isolated fetal pleural effusion: a prenatal management dilemma, *Obstet Gynecol* 81:147, 1993.

Hernanz-Schulman M et al: Pulmonary sequestration: diagnosis with color Doppler sonography and a new theory of associated hydrothorax, *Radiology* 180:817, 1991.

Holzgreve W et al: Investigation of nonimmune hydrops fetalis, *Am J Obstet Gynecol* 150:805, 1984.

Johnson A et al: Ultrasonic ratio of fetal thoracic to abdominal circumference: an association with fetal pulmonary hypoplasia, *Am J Obstet Gynecol* 157:764, 1987.

Kirk JS et al: Prenatal screening for cardiac anomalies: the value of routine addition of the aortic root to the four-chamber view, *Obstet Gynecol* 84:427, 1994.

Marasini M et al: In utero ultrasound diagnosis of congenital heart disease, *J Clin Ultrasound* 16:103, 1988.

McGahan JP: Sonography of the fetal heart: findings on the four-chamber view, *AJR* 156:547, 1991.

Reid L: The lung: its growth and remodeling in health and disease, *Am J Roentgenol* 129:777, 1977.

Saltzman DH, Adzick S, Benacerraf BR: Fetal cystic adenomatoid malformation of the lung: apparent improvement in utero, *Obstet Gynecol* 71:1000, 1988.

Saltzman DH et al: Sonographic evaluation of hydrops fetalis, *Obstet Gynecol* 74:106, 1989.

Songster GS, Gray DL, Crane JP: Prenatal prediction of lethal pulmonary hypoplasia using ultrasonic fetal chest circumference, *Obstet Gynecol* 73:261, 1989.

Vintzileos AM et al: Comparison of six different ultrasonographic methods for predicting lethal fetal pulmonary hypoplasia, *Am J Obstet Gynecol* 161:606, 1989.

Weston MJ et al: Ultrasonographic prenatal diagnosis of upper respiratory tract atresia, *J Ultrasound Med* 11:673, 1992.

Wigton TR et al: Sonographic diagnosis of congenital heart disease: comparison between the four-chamber view and multiple cardiac views, *Obstet Gynecol* 82:219, 1993.

Fetal Gastrointestinal Tract

For a Key Features summary see p. 271.

The obstetric guidelines recommend measurement of the upper abdomen and identification of the stomach. The liver can be routinely imaged at this same level. The guidelines also recommend identification of the umbilical cord insertion. Although there are no other anterior abdominal wall landmarks, the entire wall should be evaluated.

Additional normal and abnormal gastrointestinal (GI) structures can be identified, but with varying success. It is common to diagnose abdominal masses, ascites, and upper GI tract obstructions, but anomalies of the small and large bowels are less frequently seen. It is unlikely for the spleen to be identified and rare for the pancreas (normal or abnormal) to be imaged.

THE UPPER ABDOMEN: LIVER AND STOMACH

The upper abdomen is either round or oval in a transaxial view (Fig. 12-1). With the spine identified posteriorly, the right-sided liver, which extends across the midline, and the left-sided stomach are constant landmarks. The umbilical portion of the left portal vein should always be positioned within the liver, equidistantly from the sides of the abdomen. The standard abdominal diameter and circumference measurements are obtained in this position, using the outer margin of the soft tissues of the abdominal wall. This is described in Chapter 7.

The fetal liver is normally prominent. Because of its glycogen store and hematopoietic activity, it is proportionately larger during gestation than in postnatal life, and is primarily responsible for the large size of the upper abdomen. The liver can enlarge further in the setting of a number of conditions, usually ones related to fetal hydrops, but also occurring in association with congenital infections and rarely hepatic infiltrating disorders. Conversely, the liver is smaller in the setting of asymmetric intrauterine growth retardation. To evaluate these changes, the liver length can be measured from its dome (immediately below the cardiac pulsation) to its caudal tip (Fig. 12-2). The right lobe of the liver is imaged by starting at the abdominal aorta and moving the transducer toward the right side of the fetus. The caudal tip of the liver is easy to identify; however, the dome may be more difficult to find if it is partially obscured by rib or upper extremity shadowing. Nevertheless, liver length may be a more sensitive way to assess liver size, and should be considered when conditions changing liver size are suspected, rather than relying solely on the upper abdominal measurement, (Table 12-1).

Liver echogenicity can also be assessed. As in postnatal life, the fetal liver has a normally uniform low-level echogenicity, interrupted only by blood vessels. In addition to the umbilical portion of the left portal vein, the main and right portal veins (see Fig. 12-1) and on occasion the gallbladder (Fig. 12-3) can be identified.

Liver masses and calcifications are rarely seen in utero. Cysts and hemangiomas are the most commonly identified tumors; cysts are typically anechoic and hemangiomas uniformly hyperechoic. Other benign (hemangioendothelioma and hamartoma) and malignant (hepatoblastoma and metastatic) masses have been reported. Discrete calcifications, with or without shadowing, have

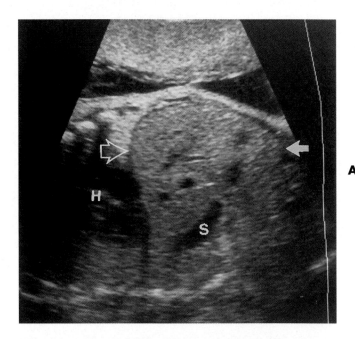

Fig. 12-1 Normal transaxial images of the upper abdomen. The outer margins of the soft tissues are measured *(x* and *+).* An arrow indicates the umbilical portion of the left portal vein, appropriately positioned within the liver. *S,* stomach; *Sp,* spine. **A,** Rounded abdomen in an 18-week fetus. Only one diameter measurement is needed. **B,** Ovoid abdomen in a 26-week fetus. Note the normal third-trimester increase in the amount of subcutaneous tissue. Because the abdomen is ovoid, two measurements perpendicular to each other are averaged to obtain the diameter. The curved open arrow denotes the right portal vein.

Table 12-1	Fetal liver measurement	

Gestational age (wk)	Long-axis measurement (mm)*	
	True mean	Range from 5th to 95th percentile
20	27.3	20.9 to 33.7
21	28.0	26.5 to 29.5
22	30.6	23.9 to 37.3
23	30.9	26.4 to 35.4
24	32.9	26.2 to 39.6
25	33.6	28.3 to 38.9
26	35.7	29.4 to 42.0
27	36.6	33.3 to 39.9
28	38.4	34.4 to 42.4
29	39.1	34.1 to 44.1
30	38.7	33.7 to 43.7
31	39.6	33.9 to 45.3
32	42.7	35.0 to 50.2
33	42.8	37.2 to 50.4
34	44.8	37.7 to 51.9
35	47.8	38.7 to 56.9
36	49.0	40.6 to 57.4
37	52.0	45.2 to 58.8
38	52.9	48.7 to 57.1
39	55.4	48.7 to 62.1
40	59.0	—
41	49.3	46.9 to 51.7

From Vintzileos AM et al: Fetal liver ultrasound measurements during normal pregnancy, *Obstet Gynecol* 66:477, 1985. From The American College of Obstetricians and Gynecologists.
*Measured in longitudinal plane from top of right hemidiaphragm to tip of right lobe of liver.

Fig. 12-2 Two normal long-axis images of the fetal liver. The caudad tip of the liver *(arrow)* is clearly noted. The dome (its superior margin) is sometimes indistinct. When not well seen, the lower-most part of the cardiac pulsation is used to define the superior liver margin. *H,* Heart. **A,** A 25-week fetus with a well-demarcated liver. The dome is clearly defined *(open arrow). S,* stomach.

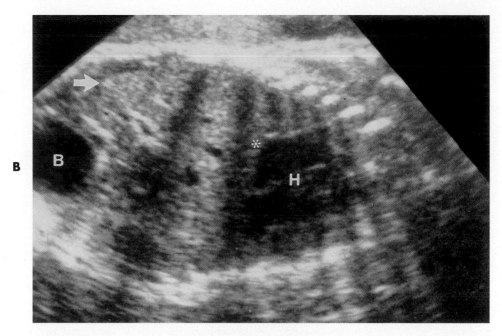

Fig. 12-2, cont'd. **B,** A 32-week fetus with an indistinct dome that is due to shadowing from the ribs. The superior margin is approximated by an asterisk. *B,* urinary bladder.

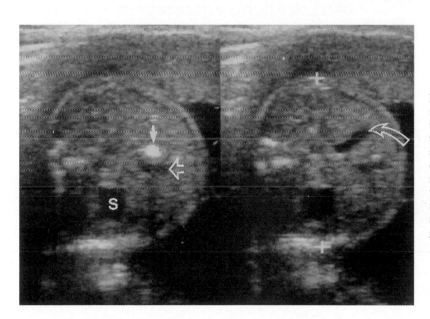

Fig. 12-3 Liver calcification of unknown cause (idiopathic) in a 22-week fetus. Two transaxial views of the liver are shown. The image on the left identifies a well-defined hyperechoic area *(arrow)* with distal acoustic shadowing, consistent with a parenchymal calcification. The remainder of the liver echogenicity is grossly normal. *Open arrow,* umbilical portion of the left portal vein; *S,* stomach. In the image on the right, the outer margin of the rounded abdomen is shown (+). A curved open arrow indicates a normal gallbladder.

also been identified (Fig. 12-3). Although some have no known cause, liver parenchymal calcifications have been detected from TORCH (specifically toxoplasmosis, cytomegalovirus, and herpes simplex) and varicella infections. Less commonly, benign and malignant liver tumors and peripheral liver emboli (caused by vascular accidents) calcify. Rarely, calcified thrombi can be identified within vascular structures, particularly within the portal veins. Any of these intraparenchymal calcifications should be easily differentiated from the occasionally seen peri-

hepatic calcifications of meconium peritonitis (described in a later section).

Between the liver and the anterior abdominal wall, a hypoechoic curved line can often be identified just inside the hyperechoic soft tissues. This is a normal variant (probably fat) and has been termed *pseudoascites* to distinguish it from true intraperitoneal fluid (ascites) (Fig. 12-4). Pseudoascites is seen only in the upper abdomen, but ascites is typically more widespread. Pseudoascites stops bilaterally at the ribs; ascites does not. Only the lu-

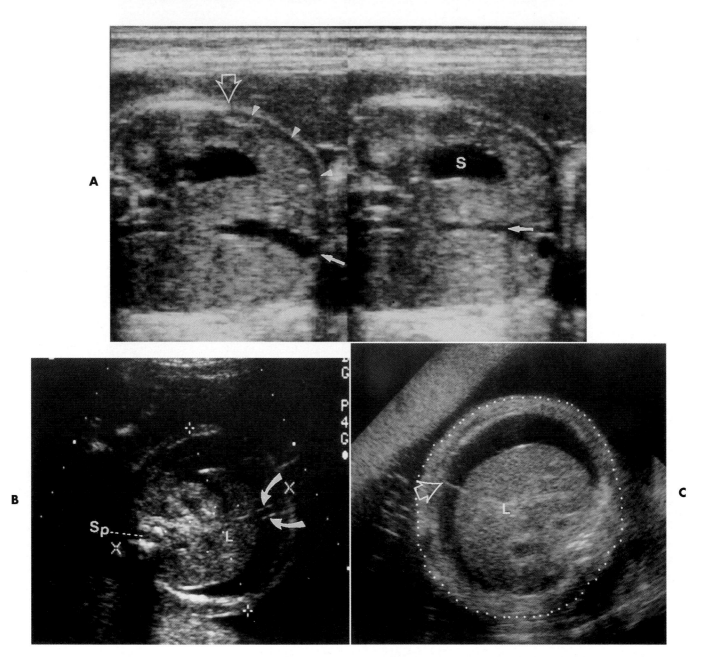

Fig. 12-4   Comparison of pseudoascites (a normal variant) with ascites. All of these are early third-trimester fetuses. **A,** Two images of the upper abdomen in a transaxial view showing pseudoascites. The image on the right shows the umbilical vein well positioned within the liver *(arrow).* The image on the left shows the bright anterior margin of a lower rib *(open arrow).* Extending anteriorly from the rib, inside the normal hyperechoic subcutaneous tissue, is a hypoechoic band *(arrowheads).* Note that at the umbilical cord insertion, at the anterior abdominal wall *(arrow),* only the anechoic internal margin of the vein can be seen. *S,* Stomach. **B** and **C,** Two different cases of fetal hydrops. Ascites is seen to extend anterior and lateral to the liver *(L)* and does not stop at the edge of the ribs. In addition, the outer margins of the umbilical vein *(curved arrows)* in **B** and the falciform ligament *(open arrow)* in **C** are surrounded by the ascites. There is increased subcutaneous skin thickening (edema). The outer margins of the abdomen are denoted in **B** (+ and *x*) and **C** *(dotted line). Sp,* spine.

men, not the outer walls of the extrahepatic intraabdominal portion of the umbilical vein (between the anterior abdominal wall and the liver), is normally identified. In the setting of ascites, the outer margins of this vein and of the falciform ligament are also seen.

The intraabdominal portion of the umbilical vein is normally small in caliber. It has parallel walls, and its diameter increases linearly from 3 mm at 15 weeks to 8 mm at term. A varix is an unusual enlargement of the extrahepatic portion of the vein (between the liver and anterior abdominal wall). It is typically observed to be large and round, even without the benefit of measurements (Fig. 12-5). A varix may not be benign. In a series reported on by Mahony and coworkers, there was associated fetal hydrops and early third-trimester intrauterine demise in 4 of 9 such cases.

The stomach is routinely identified as an anechoic (fluid-filled) structure. It ranges from a round 4-mm-diameter structure to an ovoid or kidney-shaped 4-cm-long structure (Fig. 12-6). Although not an absolute characteristic, its size is somewhat dependent on the stage of gestation, and it is typically larger in the third trimester. Occasionally, internal echoes are seen, and these are caused by swallowed "debris" from the amniotic fluid such as meconium or vernix caseosa.

The stomach fills in 10 to 45 minutes and empties in 5 to 30 minutes. The normal stomach is almost always identified, typically as soon as the abdomen is imaged. If not

seen or less than 1 cm in diameter (even though the latter finding could be normal), scanning should be repeated every 10 to 15 minutes for up to 1 hour (Fig. 12-7). If the stomach is still not identified or remains persistently small, there is a 50% or greater chance of there being an associated abnormality, with anomalies found in 100% of the nonvisualized cases after 19 weeks in one series. These anomalies are usually related to the inability of the fetus to swallow normally, and this is commonly associated with severe central nervous system and very high GI (esophageal atresia, facial clefts, and swallowing) abnormalities. The stomach may not be identified if significant oligohydramnios is already present (stemming from any cause); if the fetus has no amniotic fluid to swallow, a nonvisualized stomach may not be an abnormal finding. Polyhydramnios is usually present in the setting of a nonvisualized stomach. Its differential diagnosis is discussed in Chapter 10.

It is also important to assess the position of the stomach. It is typically on the left side, immediately below the heart (situs solitus) (see Fig. 12-2, *A*). If the stomach is on the right side or its position is indeterminate, this is commonly associated with complex structural abnormalities, particularly cardiac. If the stomach is identified within the chest, this indicates the presence of a diaphragmatic hernia (usually the left-sided Bochdalek type). This is discussed in Chapter 11.

HIGH GASTROINTESTINAL TRACT OBSTRUCTION

The high GI tract can be defined arbitrarily as consisting of the esophagus, stomach, and duodenum. The most proximal significant disorder is esophageal atresia, affecting 1 in 2500 to 4000 live births. There are five types of this disorder, the most common associated with a tracheoesophageal fistula. The incidence of additional anomalies in the setting of esophageal atresia is high (50% to 70% of cases), and these comprise cardiac abnormalities, especially atrial and ventricular septal defects (24%), other GI tract anomalies (28%), genitourinary tract disorders (13%), central nervous system disorders (7%), facial anomalies (6%), and chromosomal disorders, including trisomy 21.

The two classic findings in esophageal atresia are polyhydramnios and an absent stomach bubble (see Fig. 12-7). However, in any individual case one or both may be normal. The overall detection rate of esophageal atresia is therefore surprisingly low at 50%. Moderate to marked polyhydramnios, present in 60% to 90% of cases, may not be seen until after 24 weeks. The stomach (although usually small) appears grossly normal in 50% of cases, probably filling with swallowed amniotic fluid by means of the tracheoesophageal fistula.

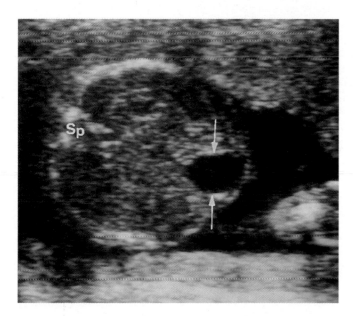

Fig. 12-5   Varix *(arrows)* in a 32-week fetus. The umbilical portion of the left portal vein, in its extrahepatic portion, is rounded and enlarged. *Sp,* spine. (From Mahony BS et al: Varix of the fetal intra-abdominal umbilical vein: comparison with normal, *J Ultrasound Med* 11:73, 1992.)

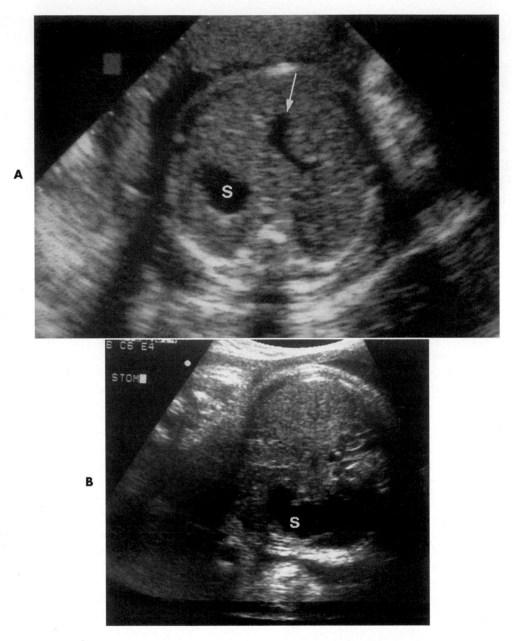

Fig. 12-6   Normally shaped stomachs (*S*) in second-trimester fetuses. **A,** An almost rounded stomach. The arrow denotes the umbilical portion of the left portal vein. **B,** A kidney-shaped stomach.

Although gastric obstruction is rare, duodenal obstruction occurs in 1 in 5000 pregnancies. It typically appears as two fluid-filled upper abdominal structures, the stomach and proximal duodenum, termed the *double-bubble sign* (Fig. 12-8). There is frequently also polyhydramnios. Duodenal obstructions are caused by intrinsic and extrinsic abnormalities: the intrinsic causes are atresia, diaphragmatic webs, and stenosis; the extrinsic causes are annular pancreas, malrotation, and bands. Duodenal atresia is the most common cause (42% of cases), and has a known link with trisomy 21 (33%). Other sonographic signs of Down's syndrome (although only rarely associated) should therefore be sought, in particular increased nuchal skin thickness and cardiac abnormalities.

LOW GASTROINTESTINAL TRACT OBSTRUCTION

The low GI tract can be defined arbitrarily as consisting of the jejunum, ileum, and colon. Jejunoileal obstructions are more common than those of the duodenum, oc-

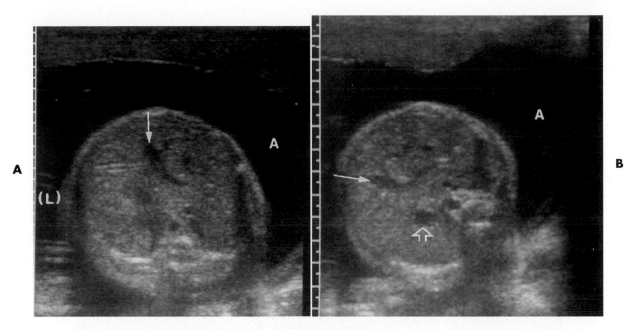

Fig. 12-7 Two different cases of esophageal atresia, detected in the early third trimester. **A,** A stomach could not be identified on the left side *(L)* of the fetus. The arrow denotes the umbilical portion of the left portal vein. *A,* amniotic fluid. **B,** A small stomach, approximately 5-mm in diameter *(open arrow),* can be seen on the fetus' left side, which failed to change size over the course of 1 hour. Note the increased amount of amniotic fluid in both cases.

curring in 1 in 3000 to 5000 live births. They are usually caused by atresia, stenosis, volvulus, and meconium ileus.

Sonographically, normal small bowel segments, occasionally exhibiting peristalsis, can be identified. These segments are more commonly seen in the third trimester and should not exceed 15 mm in length and 7 mm in diameter. Small bowel obstructions are not usually diagnosed in utero. If detected, they are typically not seen until after 24 weeks. Then, a proximal jejunal obstruction can present as an anechoic upper abdominal structure, either a single long tube or three adjacent "cysts" (the stomach, duodenum, and upper jejunum) (Fig. 12-9); a more distal small bowel obstruction can present as either a solitary dilated segment of bowel immediately preceding the point of obstruction or as multiple persistent loops of small bowel (Fig. 12-10). Amniotic fluid may be increased in volume. The reason for the usual paucity of bowel and amniotic fluid findings is not understood, but may be due to the intestinal resorption of amniotic fluid and subsequent renal excretion; resorption decreases the caliber of the small bowel, and both resorption and excretion maintain a normal amniotic fluid balance.

The large bowel is identified by its size, shape, position, and internal echogenicity (Fig. 12-11, *A*). Its normal diameter increases linearly from approximately 5 mm at 20 weeks to approximately 15 mm at term. Its maximum diameter should never exceed 20 mm. The normal colon typically appears tubular, and it is often identified by its

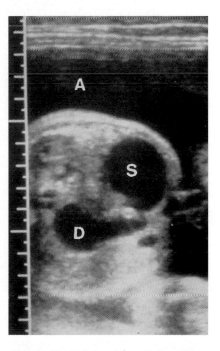

Fig. 12-8 Duodenal atresia in a 24-week fetus. Transaxial view of the upper abdomen shows a "double bubble" of the dilated stomach *(S)* and the dilated proximal duodenum *(D).* The amount of amniotic fluid *(A)* is increased.

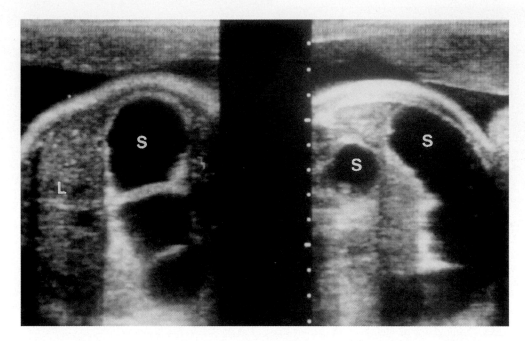

Fig. 12-9 Upper jejunal atresia in a 26-week fetus. Transaxial images show two different appearances of the jejunum in the same fetus. The image on the left shows three separate cystic structures—the stomach *(S)* in the upper part of the image, followed by the duodenum and upper jejunum. *L,* liver. The image on the right, obtained slightly lower, shows the long curvilinear structure of the three dilated segments down to the upper jejunum. Two portions of the curved stomach *(S)* are seen.

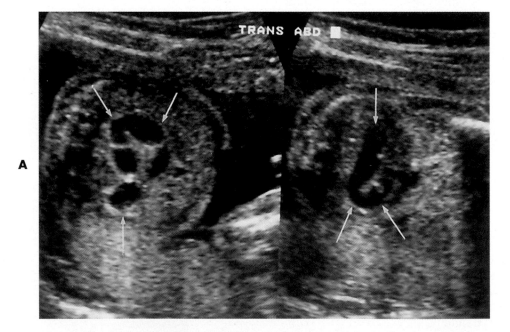

Fig. 12-10 Two cases of distal small bowel obstruction in the early third trimester. **A,** Two transaxial images of the lower abdomen showing a persistent focal dilated loop of distal jejunum *(arrows)*. The loop is longer and wider than is normal, and persists despite scanning for 30 minutes. Note the normal hyperechoic lines across the lumen of the bowel, the valvulae conniventes of the small bowel. *Continued.*

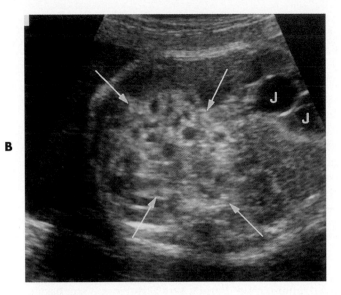

Fig. 12-10, cont'd. **B,** Ileal atresia. Note the mixed small bowel pattern on this transaxial view of the lower abdomen. Dilated cystic structures, toward the right, denote areas of jejunum *(J),* with multiple smaller anechoic spaces and hyperechoic mesentery consistent with additional matted loops of abnormal bowel *(arrows)* toward the left.

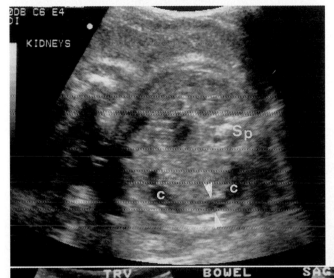

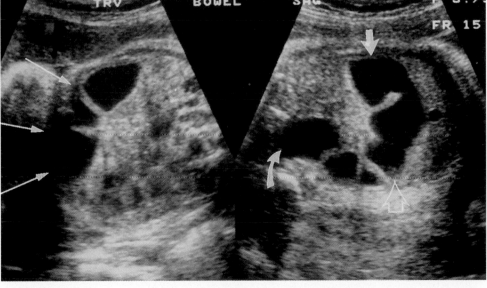

Fig. 12-11 The colon in two 37-week fetuses. **A,** Normal colon. The descending colon *(c)* is outlined along the left flank. The tips of the arrowheads denote the normal colonic width. The internal echogenicity in this case is both hyperechoic and hypoechoic. *Sp,* spine. **B,** Anorectal atresia. Two views of the fetal abdomen. On the left is a transaxial view of the midabdomen showing several dilated colonic loops extending along the edge of the flank *(arrows).* On the right is a sagittal-coronal view of the dilated colon extending from the rectum *(curved arrow)* up the left flank to the sigmoid flexure *(open arrow),* with the transverse colon dilated to the hepatic flexure *(short closed arrow).* Note that the hyperechoic septa do not extend completely across the bowel lumen, but exhibit the typical haustral markings of the colon. No other abnormalities were detected and the amniotic fluid was grossly normal in amount.

haustral markings. The ascending and descending colon are seen in the flanks, adjacent to and below the kidneys; occasionally the transverse colon can be detected in the midabdomen. The echogenicity of the colonic contents (meconium) can be divided into four stages: initially, in the second trimester (stage 1), it is hyperechoic, becoming progressively more anechoic by term (stage 4). Although the change in echogenicity may be a sign of maturity, any meconium echogenicity is likely to be normal, provided the colon size remains normal.

Large bowel abnormalities are rare, except in the anorectal region, where malformations occur in 1 in 5000 live births. Most are due to developmental stenosis and atresia (e.g., imperforate anus). Rarely the obstruction can be caused by a distal aganglionic segment (Hirschprung's disease) or by a sigmoid mechanical obstruction (usually a volvulus).

Anorectal atresia is associated with additional abnormalities more than 75% of the time. Because of their common embryogenesis, the genitourinary tract is often involved. Two groups of disorders have been described: the VACTERL syndrome of *v*ertebral, *a*nal, *c*ardiovascular, *t*racheoesophageal, *r*enal, and *l*imb anomalies, and the caudal regression syndrome of renal agenesis or dysplasia, sacral agenesis, and lower limb hypoplasia, and rarely including sirenomelia.

Sonographically, when a distal large bowel obstruction is present, the proximal colon usually dilates down to the anorectal region (Fig. 12-11, *B*). The position of these dilated loops and the presence of haustral markings typically confirm the diagnosis. The intraluminal echogenicity may not change, although the meconium may calcify. These calcifications may assume the appearance of punctate bright foci, and, because they are small, may not cause distal acoustic shadowing. Polyhydramnios is often present, although the reason for this is not understood. Associated multiorgan abnormalities should be sought.

MECONIUM ILEUS AND PERITONITIS, AND HYPERECHOIC BOWEL

Normal intraluminal bowel contents consist of swallowed amniotic fluid and a bowel mucopolysaccharide. This material is moved by peristalsis into the large bowel, where the fluid is resorbed, leaving meconium. Meconium is most prominent by the third trimester.

Meconium ileus is an impaction of unusually thick and sticky meconium. It typically occurs in the distal ileum, but on occasion may form within the colon. An impaction of abnormal meconium causes proximal bowel dilatation; more distally the bowel is typically collapsed. Almost all

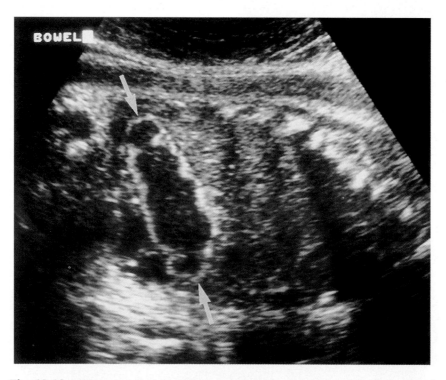

Fig. 12-12   Meconium ileus in a 37-week fetus with cystic fibrosis. A solitary dilated loop of ileum *(arrows)* is seen with a low-level internal echogenicity. Multiple punctate intraluminal hyperechoic areas are seen, consistent with meconium calcifications; because of their small size, distal acoustical shadowing is not seen. The remainder of the abdomen appears unremarkable.

infants with meconium ileus prove to have cystic fibrosis, an autosomal recessive disorder affecting Caucasians and occurring in 1 in 2000 births. Meconium ileus affects up to 15% of the infants with cystic fibrosis and, when present, is its earliest finding. Additional GI tract complications develop in 50% of cases, and consist of volvulus, atresia, bowel perforation, and meconium peritonitis.

Sonographically the dilatation of the proximal bowel in meconium ileus is not typically identified until the third trimester. The intraluminal echogenicity varies and is often heterogeneous (Fig. 12-12). The intraluminal meconium may sometimes calcify and present as punctate bright foci without distal acoustic shadowing. Polyhydramnios is frequently present.

Hyperechoic areas may on occasion be detected anywhere that small bowel is present, usually in the right lower quadrant. These areas, termed *hyperechoic bowel,* probably represent both small bowel and mesentery. No dilated loops of bowel are seen, only prominent echogenicity. Most observers consider these hyperechoic areas significant only if their echogenicity is comparable to or more so than that of adjacent bone, for example, if brighter than the iliac crests or spine. If this is found, there is then a statistically increased incidence of cystic fibrosis, a chromosomal abnormality, growth retardation, and perinatal death. Sonographically, hyperechoic bowel is often prominent if it takes up an area that exceeds 4 cm in diameter. It is often uniformly hyperechoic but

may be inhomogeneous (Fig. 12-13, *A*). Hyperechoic bowel may produce a mass effect on adjacent structures. Although there are instances in which this increased echogenicity may resolve spontaneously, this cannot be construed as a sign of normalcy. Therefore, when hyperechoic bowel is detected, a complete evaluation of all fetal structures to search for additional anomalies and at least one follow-up examination to look for growth retardation are indicated.

There are other instances, particularly in the mid–second trimester, when more subtle hyperechoic bowel can be seen. These areas are typically smaller (<2 cm in diameter), only vaguely identified (not as hyperechoic as the boney structures), without a mass effect, and most often transient (Fig. 12-13, *B*). These regions are better seen with some ultrasound equipment than with others, probably because of differences in the image processing. Although this finding has not been shown to be of clinical significance, the most prudent approach at present is still to obtain a careful fetal examination and an interval growth follow-up study.

Meconium peritonitis is an intense sterile chemical inflammation caused by leakage of the intraluminal bowel contents into the peritoneal cavity. Approximately 50% of cases are caused by an underlying bowel disorder, usually small bowel abnormalities such as atresia, volvulus, and meconium ileus. Some cases have no obvious cause (idiopathic) and are most likely the result of vascular com-

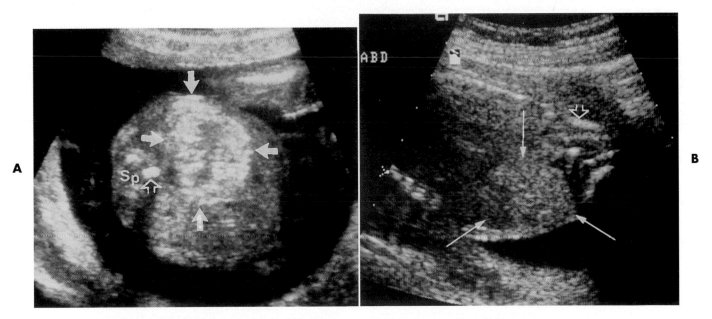

Fig. 12-13   Two cases of hyperechoic bowel in 20-week fetuses. **A,** Cystic fibrosis. Transaxial view of the lower abdomen shows a large, rounded heterogeneous mass *(arrows)* in the right lower quadrant. It is as echogenic as, or more so than, the vertebral centrum *(open arrow)* of the spine *(Sp).* **B,** Normal fetus. A vague hyperechoic area *(arrows)* is seen that is less echogenic than the iliac crest *(open arrow),* and without mass effect.

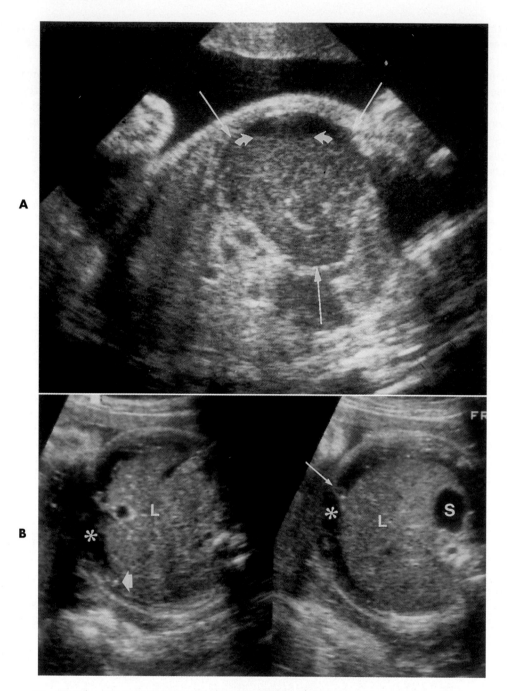

Fig. 12-14   Meconium peritonitis in two third-trimester fetuses. **A,** Pseudocyst with well-defined walls *(arrows)* in the midabdomen. Note the fluid-debris level *(curved arrows).* **B,** Two transaxial images of the upper abdomen showing ascites with internal echoes (*) curving around the anterior and lateral margins of the liver *(L).* In the right image the long arrow denotes the falciform ligament surrounded by ascites. In the left image the short arrow denotes two perihepatic calcifications, both hyperechoic and too small to cause an acoustic shadow (confirmed at birth). *S,* stomach.

promise of the bowel. The perforation can heal spontaneously. Intraperitoneal calcifications may develop within weeks.

Sonographically, the findings in meconium peritonitis are related to the extent of leakage and to the time interval before detection. Intraperitoneal calcifications do occur and have been reported in 85% of cases. They can be seen anywhere, particularly surrounding the liver and within the mesentery. In male fetuses, they can even extend through the process vaginalis into the scrotum.

<table>
<tr><td>

Box 12-1   Causes of Fetal Ascites

GENERALIZED
Fetal Hydrops*
Metabolic Storage Disease (e.g., Gaucher's, Wolman)

LOCALIZED
Genitourinary (Urine Ascites)*

Obstruction—most common at urethrovesicular junction*
Nephrotic syndrome
Ovarian cyst with torsion

Intestinal*

Meconium peritonitis*
Volvulus and atresia

Hepatic

Hepatitis and fibrosis
Biliary atresia

</td></tr>
</table>

*More common.

These calcifications are usually linear or clumpy, and typically exhibit acoustic shadowing. They are therefore different in appearance and position from parenchymal (organ) and meconium ileus (bowel) calcifications.

Meconium peritonitis may also present as a meconium pseudocyst (14% of cases) and as bowel dilatation (27% of cases) (Fig. 12-14, *A*). The extent of the dilatation may suggest the position (and sometimes even the cause) of the underlying bowel abnormality. Ascites is common, seen in 54% of cases, and usually contains internal echoes (Fig. 12-14, *B*). If ascites is the only or the predominant finding, other causes of ascites should be considered (Box 12-1). One type of meconium peritonitis, the fibroadhesive form, may be extensive yet difficult to diagnose because no mass is present. Polyhydramnios is likely in most cases (65%).

ANTERIOR ABDOMINAL WALL DEFECTS

There are four major anterior abdominal wall abnormalities: omphalocele, gastroschisis, pentalogy of Cantrell, and limb–body wall complex. All can be detected by careful evaluation of the anterior abdominal and lower thoracic wall. None involve intact skin, and therefore all cause the α-fetoprotein level in the serum and amniotic fluid to be elevated. After central nervous system anomalies, these defects are the most common fetal cause of an elevated α-fetoprotein level.

Omphalocele is the most common defect, occurring in 1 in 4000 live births. It is centrally positioned, caused by herniation of the intraabdominal contents into the base of the umbilical cord, and covered by a thin amnioperitoneal membrane. The frequently present ascites is confined within this membrane. Typically the umbilical cord inserts into the anterior part of the defect. If the omphalocele is large, however, the cord insertion may be turned to the side (Figs. 12-15 and 12-16). Occasionally a "cyst" of Wharton's jelly is also identified at the site of the cord insertion, and this is considered by some to be pathognomonic for this entity.

There are two categories of omphalocele. The larger defects contain liver (and usually also bowel), and their presence suggests failed primary abdominal wall closure. The abdomen in this setting is usually much smaller than normal because of the extracorporeal liver (Fig. 12-16), and there may be a marked scoliosis because the intraabdominal contents are not present to maintain fetal body shape. The smaller defects contain only bowel and probably represent a persistence of the primitive body stalk (failure of complete midgut rotation) (see Fig. 12-15). Unless obstructed, and causing secondary bowel dilatation, a small omphalocele might be missed. The volume of amniotic fluid may be normal, but is increased in one third of the cases. The first-trimester diagnosis of omphalocele is discussed in Chapter 9.

Theoretically a small omphalocele might be difficult to differentiate from an umbilical hernia. Both are defects that involve the base of the umbilical cord, but umbilical hernias rarely, if ever, occur in utero.

Omphaloceles are associated with a significantly increased incidence of chromosomal abnormalities, including trisomies. The mean incidence is 12% and is much greater in the setting of omphaloceles that contain only bowel. Other structural defects are also present in approximately 75% of cases. Concomitant complex cardiac (30% to 50%), other GI tract, and genitourinary tract anomalies are common. Associated central nervous system abnormalities and diaphragmatic hernia occur less frequently. The Beckwith-Wiedemann syndrome, an autosomal dominant disorder consisting of multiple anomalies including gigantism, renal tumors, hemihypertrophy, and macroglossia, accounts for 5% to 10% of all cases of omphalocele.

There is no normal "pot belly" appearance in a fetus. Any anterior abdominal wall "bulge," regardless of how subtle, must be considered abnormal. However, if during scanning the examiner inadvertently puts pressure on the fetal abdomen, an apparent bulge in the anterior abdominal wall (a pseudoomphalocele) may appear (see Fig. 12-16, *C*). The anterior wall appears intact, however, and releasing the pressure allows the abdomen to return to a more rounded appearance, without the anterior bulge. This is more likely to occur in the third trimester when the fetus is large. Very uncommonly a hemangioma at the base of the umbilical cord, of similar echogenicity to the bowel, could mimic a bowel-containing omphalocele.

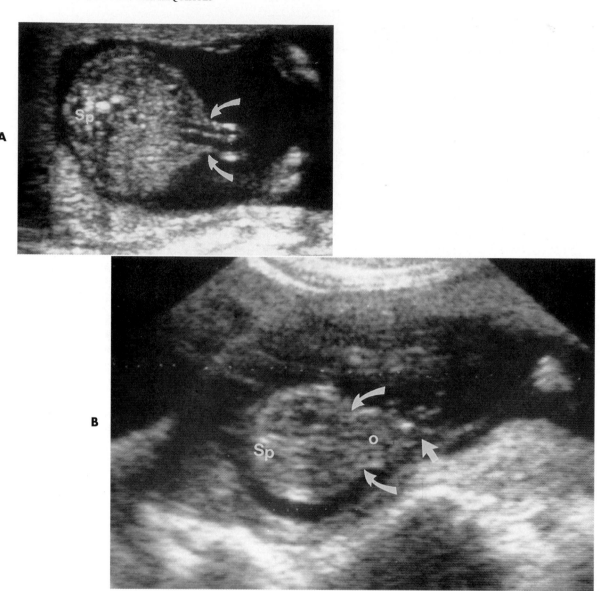

A

B

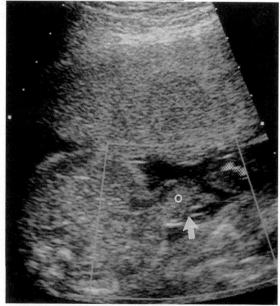

C

Fig. 12-15   The umbilical cord insertion in second-trimester fetuses, one normal and the others having small bowel-containing omphaloceles. **A,** Transaxial view showing the normal midline insertion of the umbilical cord *(curved arrows)* into the abdominal anterior wall. **B** and **C,** Small bowel-containing omphaloceles *(o).* In **B** the curved arrows denote the margins of the anterior abdominal wall defect with midline anterior extension of the abnormal contents. The arrow indicates the midline insertion of the umbilical cord into the omphalocele. In **C** the umbilical cord *(arrow)* inserts into the side of the omphalocele. *Sp,* spine.

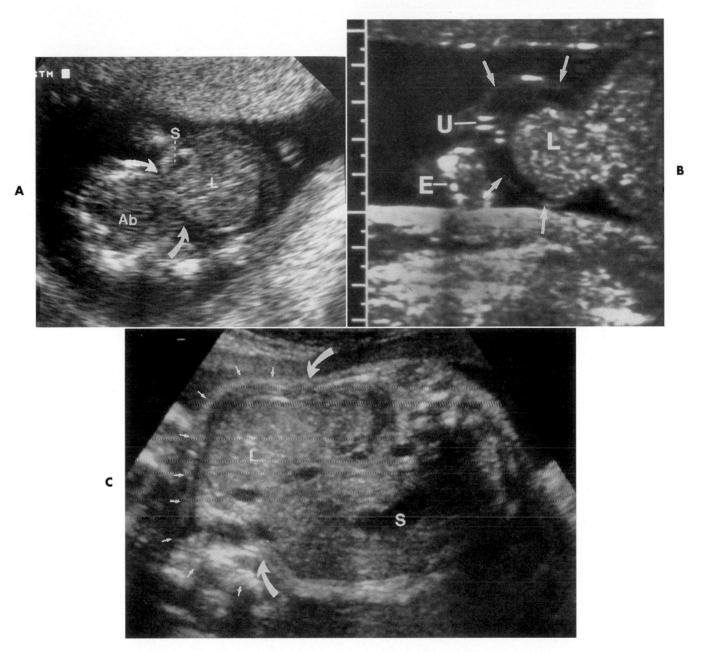

Fig. 12-16   Comparison of large omphaloceles with a pseudoomphalocele (a normal variant) in three third-trimester fetuses. **A** and **B,** Transaxial images showing large omphaloceles. In **A** the fetal abdomen *(Ab)* is markedly decreased in size, with both the liver *(L)* and stomach *(S)* protruding anteriorly into the defect. The margins of the defect *(curved arrows)* are noted. In **B,** not only liver but also anechoic ascites is contained within the amnioperitoneal membrane *(arrows)* of the omphalocele. The umbilical cord *(U)* inserts into the front of the omphalocele. *E,* an adjacent extremity. **C,** Pseudoomphalocele. Because of transducer pressure during scanning, the fetal abdomen has been inadvertently compressed between the anterior and posterior walls of the uterus, causing a false indentation *(curved arrows)* and a bulge. This bulge appears to contain liver *(L).* However, note the smooth normal margin of the anterior abdominal wall with its normal uninterrupted hyperechoic soft tissue *(small arrows).* When the pressure was released, the fetal abdomen resumed its normal configuration. *S,* stomach.

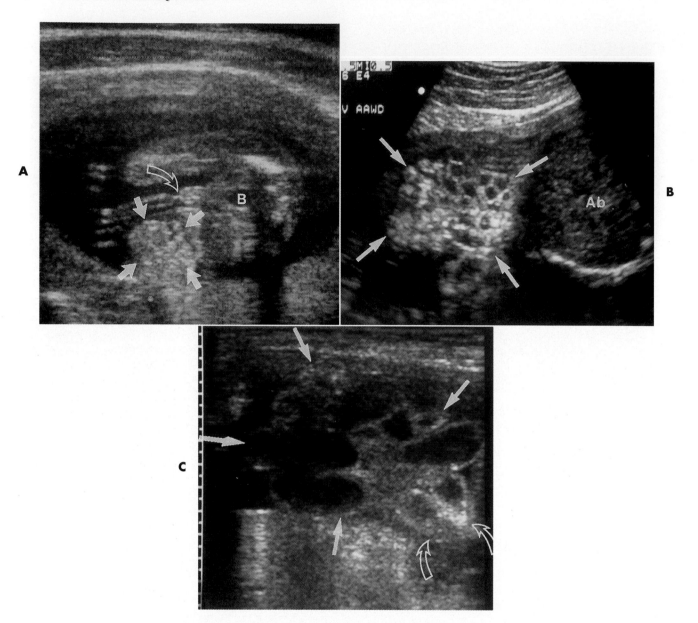

Fig. 12-17   Three cases of gastroschisis, all detected in the middle to late second trimester. **A,** Transaxial view through the lower part of the fetal abdomen shows the normal midline position of the umbilical cord insertion *(open curved arrow),* with the parallel lines of the umbilical cord extending into the amniotic fluid toward the left. In the right lower quadrant, separate from the cord insertion, a hyperechoic area is seen *(arrows)* extending outside the fetal body. *B,* urinary bladder. **B,** Transaxial view of the lower fetal abdomen *(Ab)* shows multiple mildly prominent small bowel loops *(arrows)* outside the right lower quadrant in the amniotic fluid. They have thickened hyperechoic walls. There was no evidence of bowel ischemia after delivery. **C,** Markedly dilated small bowel loops within a gastroschisis *(arrows).* The defect in the anterior abdominal wall in the right lower quadrant is denoted by curved open arrows. Although the bowel walls are not unusually thick, the loops of bowel are prominent, some more than 1 cm in diameter. This bowel was found to be necrotic at delivery.

Gastroschisis is a less common disorder, occurring in 1 in 10,000 live births. It is typically a small defect, less than 4 cm in diameter, extending through all layers of the abdominal wall. It should not be confused with an omphalocele because it is paraumbilical, typically in the right lower quadrant. Because it is not covered by a membrane,

the protruding loops of bowel float freely in the amniotic fluid and ascites cannot occur. Associated anomalies and aneuploidy are rare.

Although the defect is small, the amount of eviscerated bowel varies (Fig. 12-17). Small bowel always protrudes through the defect, and large bowel is often present. Protrusion of the stomach and parts of the genitourinary tract is uncommon. The extruded bowel may appear thicker and more dilated than usual. The remaining bowel may also dilate internally. At present there are no findings that can predict vascular bowel compromise, although small bowel dilatation may be the most suggestive if it exceeds 11 mm and compromise is likely if bowel dilatation exceeds 17 mm. If the bowel perforates within the abdomen, meconium peritonitis may occur. Polyhydramnios is infrequent, except when bowel obstruction is present. Care must be taken not to incorrectly mistake normal umbilical cord loops, adjacent to the abdomen, for a small gastroschisis.

The prognosis for both omphaloceles and gastroschisis is variable. If no additional structural or chromosomal abnormalities exist, the morbidity and mortality depend on the size of the defect and on the extent of the compromised bowel. The immediate problems in the neonatal period are related to heat loss and dehydration. A tertiary care center with facilities and experience to care for these newborns is therefore important for initial survival.

There is a uniformly poor prognosis for the other two anterior abdominal wall malformations: pentalogy of Cantrell and the limb–body wall complex. Ectopia cordis is a rare anomaly in which the heart is extrathoracic, causing it to pulsate against the amniotic fluid (Fig. 12-18, *A*). Although it can be divided into four or five types, the defect is usually thoracic (60% of the cases) or abdominal (30% of the cases). The less common thoracoabdominal form (7% of the cases) is associated with an omphalocele, a diaphragmatic defect, and a pericardiac defect, not infrequently in combination with additional cardiac anomalies; it is then termed *pentalogy of Cantrell*. The limb–body wall complex is a combination of abnormalities: a neural tube defect, an anterior abdominal wall defect, and limb anomalies. Although the spinal defect is not always present, severe scoliosis is common.

Amniotic bands can cause multiple and unusual fetal deformities. Although typically affecting the extremities, they can at times cause significant deformity of the abdomen and thorax (Fig. 12-18, *B*). Their diagnosis is usually only suspected on the basis of the asymmetry of the defects, as the bands are rarely, if ever, identified. The amniotic band syndrome is discussed in Chapter 14.

DISCRETE ABDOMINAL MASSES

Cystic masses are uncommon but can be identified within the fetal abdomen. In the midabdomen and lower abdomen, a cystic mass can be an ovarian cyst (in a female fetus), a mesenteric or duplication cyst, or a urachal cyst (originating from the dome of the bladder) (Fig. 12-19). If the mass is in the right upper quadrant, it may be associated with the liver or biliary system (choledochal cyst); if it is in the left upper quadrant, it may be associated with the spleen. Rare lymphangiomatous lesions have also been reported.

Complex and solid GI tract masses are rare, except when associated with meconium peritonitis (meconium pseudocyst). They are more often associated with the genitourinary tract, usually the kidney and adrenal, and are discussed in Chapter 13.

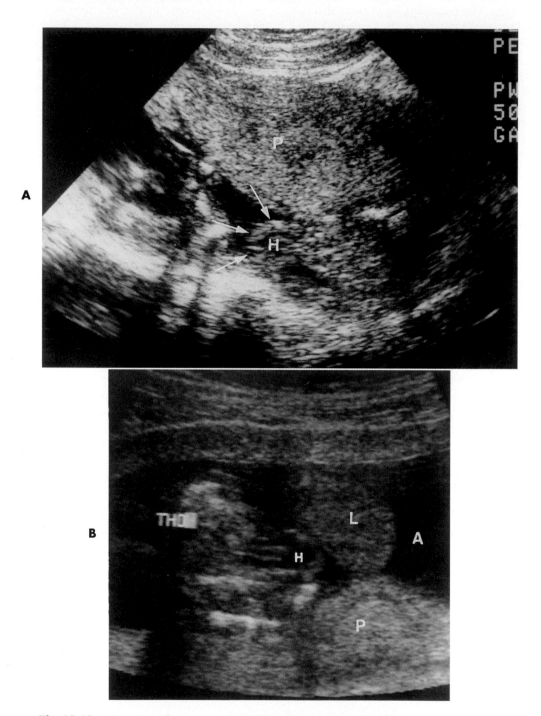

Fig. 12-18   Two cases of ectopia cordis. **A,** Thoracic ectopia cordis in a 24-week fetus. This oblique image of the lower part of the fetal chest fails to show a normal anterior chest wall. Instead the heart *(H)* is pulsating against amniotic fluid (arrows indicate the anterior margin of the heart). *P,* placenta. **B,** Ectopia cordis caused by the amniotic band syndrome. This image of a severe asymmetric deformity of the anterior thoracic *(THO)* and abdominal walls shows the heart *(H)* and liver *(L)* without an omphalocele floating in the amniotic fluid *(A)*. A severe scoliosis (not shown) was also present. *P,* placenta. (Courtesy Kathryn Gumbach, Baltimore, MD.)

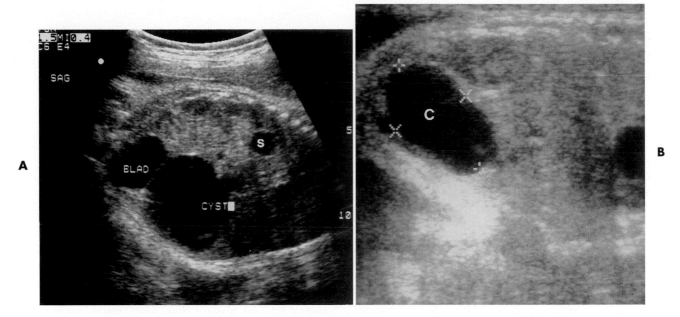

Fig. 12-19 Two cystic structures in the abdomen, both detected in the early trimester. **A,** Above the urinary bladder *(BLAD)* is a cystic structure *(CYST).* This is an ovarian cyst in a female fetus. *S,* stomach. **B,** Gastrointestinal duplication cyst *(C),* denoted in the right lower quadrant without other abnormalities *(x* and *+).*

Key Features

The standard upper abdominal image is obtained transaxially, just below the cardiac pulsation, where the umbilical portion of the left portal vein is within the liver. The liver and stomach can be identified routinely and appropriate abdominal measurements obtained.

The most common causes of an enlarged liver are fetal hydrops and infections. The most common cause of a small liver is asymmetric intrauterine growth retardation. Although both can be suggested by an abnormal abdominal measurement, a direct measurement of liver length may be a better way of evaluating liver size.

Pseudoascites, a hypoechoic band between the ribs in the upper abdomen, should not be mistaken for ascites.

An umbilical vein varix is probably not a benign entity, and has been associated with fetal hydrops and intrauterine demise.

The stomach is identified routinely. If not seen or persistently small, it is usually abnormal, caused by entities that reduce the ingestion of amniotic fluid.

High gastrointestinal (GI) tract obstructions of the esophagus and duodenum are associated with other anomalies and commonly with polyhydramnios.

Low GI tract obstructions of the jejunum and ileum may not exhibit in utero findings. On occasion a proximal dilated loop or polyhydramnios, or both, may be present.

Anorectal obstructions are commonly associated with multiple additional abnormalities, often presenting with proximal colon dilatation and polyhydramnios.

Meconium ileus, an impaction of abnormally thick inspissated meconium, usually occurs in the terminal ileum, but occasionally in the colon. It is commonly caused by cystic fibrosis.

Hyperechoic fetal bowel, with an echogenicity comparable to or greater than that of bone, has been associated with cystic fibrosis, chromosomal abnormalities, growth retardation, and perinatal death. At least one follow-up study is suggested. A subtle increase in small bowel echogenicity is probably a normal variant.

Meconium peritonitis, caused by leakage of meconium into the peritoneal cavity, leads to intraperitoneal calcifications. Meconium pseudocysts, bowel dilatation, ascites, and polyhydramnios are additional frequent findings.

The most common anterior abdominal wall defects are omphalocele and gastroschisis. Both are also associated with elevated α-fetoprotein levels.

Omphaloceles are defects that occur at the base of the umbilical cord and are covered by a thin amnioperitoneal membrane. They can be divided into two types: the larger containing at least liver and the smaller containing only bowel. An increased association with structural abnormalities and chromosomal abnormalities exists for both types.

Gastroschisis, usually paraumbilical in the right lower quadrant, does not have a covering membrane, so the protruding bowel floats freely in the amniotic fluid. There are no associated anomalies or an abnormal karyotype.

Discrete abdominal masses are usually cystic. In female fetuses they are usually associated with the ovary. In both male and female fetuses, they may be mesenteric, duplication, or urachal cysts. Complex or solid GI tract masses are usually associated with meconium peritonitis.

SUGGESTED READINGS

Babcock CJ et al: Gastroschisis: can sonography of the fetal bowel accurately predict postnatal outcome? *J Ultrasound Med* 13:701, 1994.

Bair JH et al: Fetal omphalocele and gastroschisis: a review of 24 cases, *AJR* 147:1047, 1986.

Bromley B et al: Is fetal hyperechoic bowel on second-trimester sonogram an indication for amniocenteses? *Obstet Gynecol* 83:647, 1994.

Dicke JM, Crane JP: Sonographically detected hyperechoic fetal bowel: significance and implications for pregnancy management, *Obstet Gynecol* 80:778, 1992.

Foster MA et al: Meconium peritonitis: prenatal sonographic findings and their clinical significance, *Radiology* 165:661, 1987.

Getachew MM et al: Correlation between omphalocele contents and karyotypic abnormalities: sonographic study in 37 cases, *AJR* 158:133, 1991.

Harris RD et al: Anorectal atresia: prenatal sonographic diagnosis, *AJR* 149:395, 1987.

Hashimoto BE, Filly RA, Callen PW: Fetal pseudoascites: further anatomic observations, *J Ultrasound Med* 5:151, 1986.

Haynor DR et al: Imaging of fetal ectopia cordis: roles of sonography and computed tomography, *J Ultrasound Med* 3:25, 1984.

Hertzberg BS: Sonography of the fetal gastrointestinal tract: anatomic variants, diagnostic pitfalls, and abnormalities, *AJR* 162:1175, 1994.

Lindfors KK, McGahan JP, Walter JP: Fetal omphalocele and gastroschisis: pitfalls in sonographic diagnosis, *AJR* 147:797, 1986.

Mahony BS et al: Varix of the fetal intraabdominal umbilical vein: comparison with normal, *J Ultrasound Med* 11:73, 1992.

Millener PB, Anderson NG, Chisholm RJ: Prognostic significance of nonvisualization of the fetal stomach by sonography, *AJR* 160:827, 1993.

Miro J, Bard H: Congenital atresia and stenosis of the duodenum: the impact of a prenatal diagnosis, *Am J Obstet Gynecol* 158:555, 1988.

Murao F et al: Detection of intrauterine growth retardation based on measurements of size of the liver, *Gynecol Obstet Invest* 29:26, 1990.

Nyberg DA et al: Echogenic fetal bowel during the second trimester: clinical importance, *Radiology* 188:527, 1993.

Nyberg DA et al: Fetal bowel. Normal sonographic findings, *J Ultrasound Med* 6:3, 1987.

Parulekar SG: Sonography of normal fetal bowel, *J Ultrasound Med* 10:211, 1991.

Patten RM et al: Limb–body wall complex: in utero sonographic diagnosis of a complicated fetal malformation, *AJR* 146:1019, 1986.

Paulson EK, Hertzberg BS: Hyperechoic meconium in the third trimester fetus: an uncommon normal variant, *J Ultrasound Med* 10:677, 1991.

Pretorius DH et al: Tracheoesophageal fistula in utero. Twenty-two cases, *J Ultrasound Med* 6:509, 1987.

Pretorius DH et al: Sonographic evaluation of the fetal stomach: significance of nonvisualization, *AJR* 151:987, 1988.

Scioscia AL et al: Second-trimester echogenic bowel and chromosomal abnormalities, *Am J Obstet Gynecol* 167:889, 1992.

Vintzileos AM et al: Fetal liver ultrasound measurements in isoimmunized pregnancies, *Obstet Gynecol* 68:162, 1986.

Vintzileos AM et al: Fetal liver ultrasound measurements during normal pregnancy, *Obstet Gynecol* 66:477, 1985.

Zilianti M, Fernández: Correlation of ultrasonic images of fetal intestine with gestational age and fetal maturity, *Obstet Gynecol* 62:569, 1983.

Fetal Genitourinary Tract

Normal Fetal Kidneys
The Urinary Bladder
Oligohydramnios and Pulmonary Hypoplasia
Bilateral Renal Anomalies
    Prognostic Indicators in Bilateral Obstruction
Unilateral Renal Anomalies
Megacalices, Megaureters, and Megacystis
The Adrenal Glands
Additional Pelvic Abnormalities
Fetal Sex

For a Key Features summary see p. 291.

Evaluation of the fetal urinary tract requires a study of the kidneys, urinary bladder, and amniotic fluid. The gross appearance of the kidneys helps in determining whether it is anatomically normal. Renal function, however, cannot be established except by observing the urinary bladder and amniotic fluid. The size of the bladder and its cyclic changes show that at least one kidney is producing an adequate volume of urine. The amount of amniotic fluid, which is primarily produced through urine excretion after 16 weeks, should also be appropriate. Any significant abnormality of *both* kidneys or the urinary bladder will cause oligohydramnios.

NORMAL FETAL KIDNEYS

The kidneys are situated paraspinally, caudad to the liver. Typically they have the same configuration as they do in postnatal life—round in transaxial views and ovoid in long-axis views. The identification of the kidneys (patterns 1 to 3) depends on when the study is performed (Fig. 13-1). Pattern 1 occurs in the early to middle second trimester. At this time the hypoechoic renal cortex is poorly delineated from both the weakly hypoechoic renal sinus and the surrounding perinephric tissues. Although the renal positions are therefore known, they are difficult to visualize. Pattern 2 occurs by the middle to late second trimester. At this time the kidneys and their cortices are better visualized because of the existence of increased hyperechoic interfaces (caused primarily by fat accumulation) in the perinephric and renal sinus regions. By the mid–third trimester further fat accumulation is responsible for causing pattern 3, which consists of even more distinct hyperechoic renal borders and sinuses. In addition, by the late third trimester, normal renal corticomedullary differentiation can often be identified.

Fetal position affects the degree of renal visualization. When the fetus is in a back-up position, both kidneys are easily detected. If the fetus is sideways to the transducer, only the closer kidney is easily identified. The farther kidney is usually at least partially obscured by shadowing from the spine. When the fetus is in a face-up position, it may be difficult to identify either kidney, particularly if the volume of amniotic fluid is decreased (degrading the ultrasound image) or if fetal limbs overlie and thus cause acoustic shadowing into the paraspinal regions.

It is typically unnecessary to measure the kidneys. A visual impression that they are less than one third the abdominal size often suffices. If a measurement is needed, the simplest is a transaxial ratio of the kidney to the abdomen. This ratio, which is constant throughout the second and third trimesters, is normally between 0.27 to 0.30. It is obtained by comparing circumferences, and anteroposterior or transverse diameters (Fig. 13-2). Although formal measurements of the renal length and anteroposterior dimensions are also possible, the examiner must be careful not to inadvertently let the kidney be foreshortened because of shadowing from the ribs, iliac crest, or extremities, and to obtain the anteroposterior measurement perpendicular to the renal length. This method is one which is a method similar to the technique described in Chapter 9 for measuring the mean gestational sac diameter.

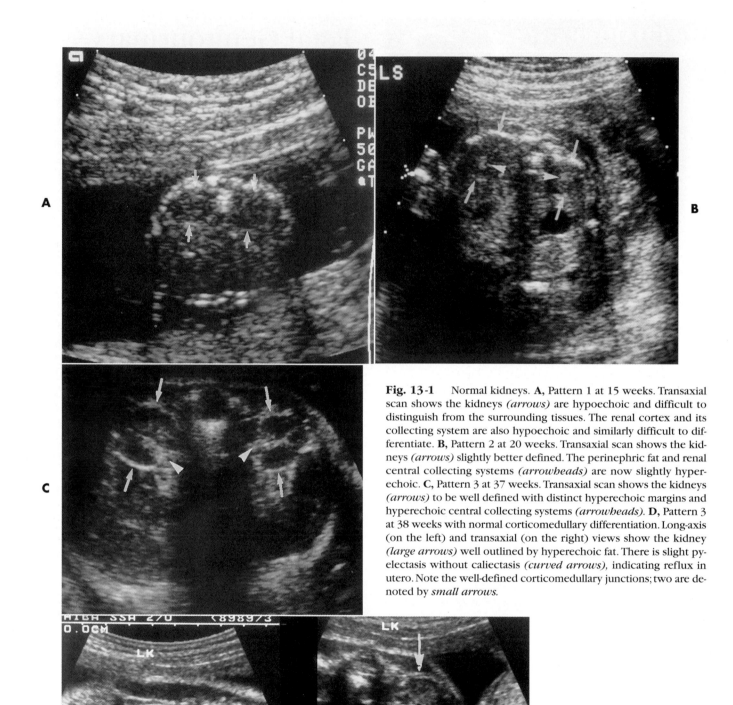

Fig. 13-1 Normal kidneys. **A,** Pattern 1 at 15 weeks. Transaxial scan shows the kidneys *(arrows)* are hypoechoic and difficult to distinguish from the surrounding tissues. The renal cortex and its collecting system are also hypoechoic and similarly difficult to differentiate. **B,** Pattern 2 at 20 weeks. Transaxial scan shows the kidneys *(arrows)* slightly better defined. The perinephric fat and renal central collecting systems *(arrowheads)* are now slightly hyperechoic. **C,** Pattern 3 at 37 weeks. Transaxial scan shows the kidneys *(arrows)* to be well defined with distinct hyperechoic margins and hyperechoic central collecting systems *(arrowheads)*. **D,** Pattern 3 at 38 weeks with normal corticomedullary differentiation. Long-axis (on the left) and transaxial (on the right) views show the kidney *(large arrows)* well outlined by hyperechoic fat. There is slight pyelectasis without caliectasis *(curved arrows)*, indicating reflux in utero. Note the well-defined corticomedullary junctions; two are denoted by *small arrows.*

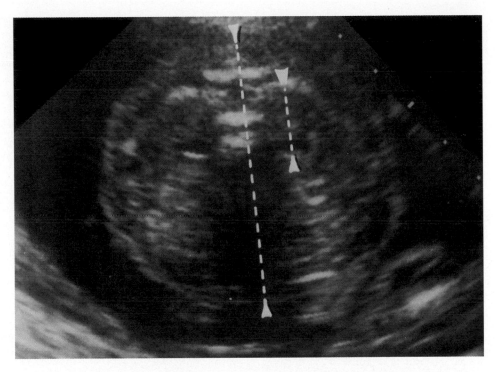

Fig. 13-2 Measurement of the kidneys. Transaxial scan of a normal 28-week fetus shows the anteroposterior dimension of the kidney compared with the anteroposterior dimension of the abdomen (at the same level), both denoted by arrowheads and dotted lines. The kidney-to-abdominal ratio is 0.30, which is within normal limits.

The renal sinus or central collecting system is indistinct (hypoechoic) in early gestation, becoming progressively more distinct (hyperechoic) by term (patterns 1 to 3) (see Fig. 13-1). In the third trimester an anechoic space may develop within this region. If only present medial to the margin of the kidney, it is an extra renal pelvis (a normal variant). If it spreads the renal sinus, it is termed *pyelectasis,* which may be either unilateral or bilateral (Figs. 13-1, *D,* and 13-3). Pyelectasis by itself is not indicative of hydronephrosis, which is a mechanical obstruction. Instead it represents reflux and is physiologically normal in the third trimester, provided it measures 7 mm or less in the anteroposterior dimension (occasionally up to 10 mm). The calices and ureters are not identified (if seen, this means they are dilated), the urinary bladder fills and empties normally, and the volume of amniotic fluid is grossly normal. Infrequently the urinary bladder decreases in size during the study, and, if the kidneys then show less pyelectasis, the diagnosis of normal physiologic reflux is confirmed. If any doubt of normalcy still remains, a follow-up study to look for progression is appropriate either later in the pregnancy or after delivery.

More recently, second-trimester pyelectasis has been studied (Fig. 13-3, *B*). Before 24 weeks, and perhaps up to 28 weeks, less prominent pyelectasis (≤4 mm) without caliectasis may be a sign of early obstruction. When detected, a follow-up study in 4 to 6 weeks is suggested. If the pyelectasis increases with developing caliectasis, hydronephrosis is present. If not, the pyelectasis is an earlier manifestation of normal physiologic reflux. A pyelectasis of 4 mm or more has been found to be associated with trisomy 21 when there are *other* ultrasound findings, such as nuchal thickening or skeletal abnormalities (femoral or humeral shortening).

THE URINARY BLADDER

The kidneys start to produce urine by 14 to 16 weeks. The urinary bladder should therefore be easy to identify from 16 weeks on, and often earlier than this. The bladder is an oval or circular anechoic pelvic structure. When normally distended, 2 cm or more in diameter, it can be identified in any view (Fig. 13-4). When smaller, a transaxial pelvic view allows more consistent visualization.

A nonvisualized or very small bladder in an otherwise sonographically normal fetus is most likely normal. However, the urinary bladder has a normal cycle of 60 to 90 minutes; if the bladder is not initially seen or is less than 1 cm in diameter, sequential pelvic scans obtained every 15 to 20 minutes for 1 hour are advised. If the bladder is still not identified (or small and unchanged), renal function is undoubtedly impaired, either stemming from a bilateral upper urinary tract abnormality or from a more general-

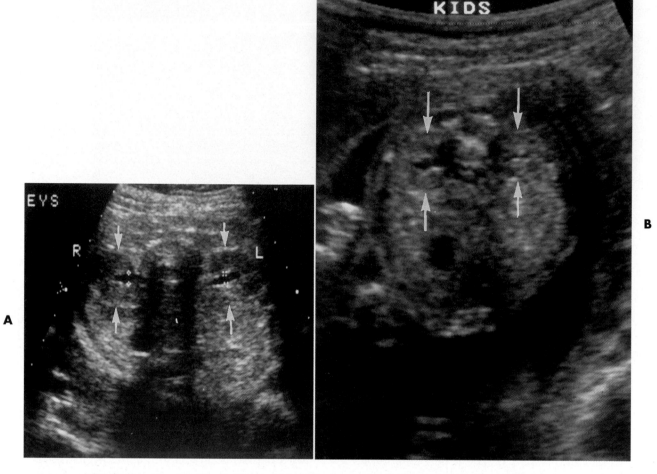

Fig. 13-3 Normal reflux in utero. **A,** A third-trimester transaxial scan through the kidneys *(arrows)* shows very mild anechoic spaces spreading the central collecting systems (+). This is consistent with pyelectasis, without extension into the calices, and measures only 5 mm in the anteroposterior dimension. **B,** Mid–second trimester scan shows the kidneys *(arrows)* to be poorly differentiated from the surrounding tissue. The central collecting systems are minimally spread (i.e., anechoic), the right kidney (on the left) measuring only 3 mm and the left kidney measuring only 1 mm in the anteroposterior dimension. There is no caliectasis.

ized process such as growth retardation. A small pelvic cystic structure need not always be the bladder. Rarely it might represent a fluid-filled loop of bowel (rectosigmoid colon or small bowel) or a subtle pelvic abnormality.

OLIGOHYDRAMNIOS AND PULMONARY HYPOPLASIA

Oligohydramnios has a number of causes involving different pathologic processes, each condition variable in severity and in its time of onset (Table 13-1; Fig. 13-5). Complete urinary tract obstruction, either bilaterally at the renal or ureteric level or unilaterally at the bladder or urethral level, will cause severe oligohydramnios, typically in the early to middle second trimester (Fig. 13-6). Bilateral renal absence (agenesis), or significant renal malfunction or malformation, will also cause early severe oligohydramnios (see Figs. 13-7 and 13-8).

The lungs need a number of factors to develop normally. One of them, amniotic fluid, is very important in that it has a direct positive effect on the development of the normal bronchial tree. Although amniotic fluid is primarily swallowed by the fetus, it must also be aspirated to aid lung formation.

Severe prolonged oligohydramnios has been unequivocally shown to lead to pulmonary hypoplasia. The severity and duration of the oligohydramnios are not at present uniformly predictive of pronounced pulmonary hypoplasia. However, marked prolonged oligohydramnios, particularly when beginning in the second trimester, always carries a very poor prognosis.

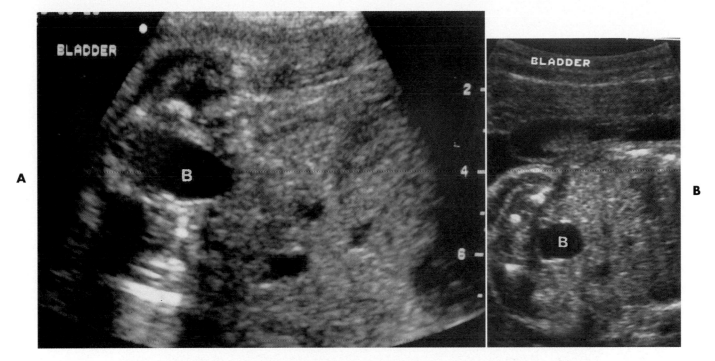

Fig. 13-4 Two normal shapes of the fetal urinary bladder *(B)*. **A,** An ovoid shape in a third-trimester fetus. **B,** A rounded shape in a second-trimester fetus.

Table 13-1 Causes of oligohydramnios

Causes	Trimester usually detected	Typical severity
1. Spontaneous rupture of membranes	Third	Mild to severe (sometimes normal)
2. Bilateral renal abnormality, dysfunction or obstruction	Second	Severe
3. Obstruction at the urinary bladder level or below	Second	Severe
4. Significant growth retardation, commonly asymmetric	Third	Moderate
5. Fetal demise, ≥5 days	Either	Variable
6. Abdominal pregnancy (rare)	Either	Variable (sometimes normal)

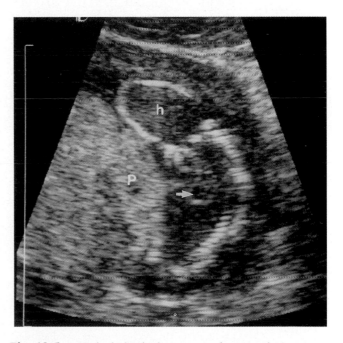

Fig. 13-5 Marked oligohydramnios in the second trimester in the setting of fetal demise. The fetus is in an unusual position, with the head *(h)* partially collapsed and the area where the heart is *(arrow)* showing no evidence of cardiac motion. *P,* placenta.

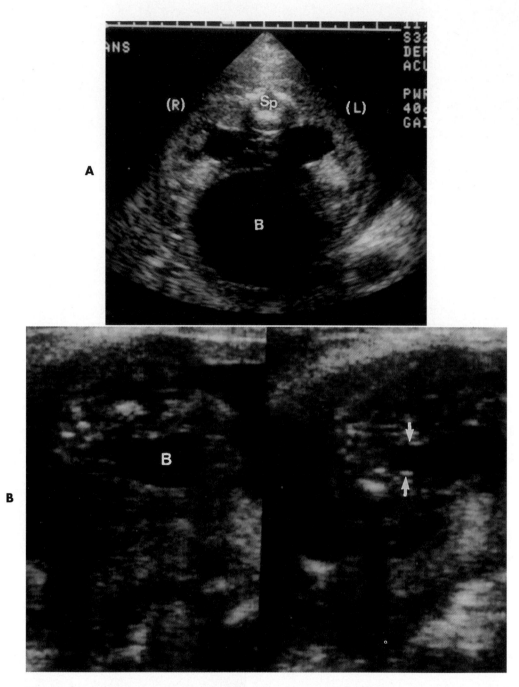

Fig. 13-6   Posterior urethral valves in a 23-week male fetus. **A,** Transaxial view through the area of the fetal kidneys shows both kidneys to have large anechoic spaces (in both paraspinal regions) and also shows a markedly dilated urinary bladder *(B)* extending out of the pelvis to the level of the kidneys. Note the marked absence of amniotic fluid. *Sp,* spine. **B,** Two transaxial images of the urinary bladder *(B).* On the right image, obtained slightly lower than the left image, a narrowing at the base of the bladder *(arrows)* is seen in the region of the proximal urethra. This "keyhole" appearance is consistent with a proximal urethral obstruction.

BILATERAL RENAL ANOMALIES

Urinary tract obstruction can occur at any level, from the kidneys to the urethra. Bilateral obstruction, however, is usually caused by a blockage at the bladder outlet, its cause either posterior urethral valves (in a male fetus) or urethral atresia (more common in a female fetus) (Fig. 13-6). This obstruction typically occurs early and is prolonged and severe, commonly leading to marked bilateral hydronephrosis. The renal parenchyma may be destroyed, leaving only large anechoic paraspinal sacs. Dilated ureters can often be seen as tubular structures in the lower abdomen. The urinary bladder is typically distended and may extend out of the pelvis to the level of the kidneys. A dilated proximal urethra is often seen as a keyhole-shaped structure caudad to the bladder (Fig. 13-6, B). The cause of the obstruction can be suggested by the fetus' sex. All cases are lethal because of the pulmonary hypoplasia that results.

Variants of bladder outlet obstruction exist. In some early cases, instead of severe hydronephrosis, there may be only renal pelvis dilatation or mild pelvocaliectasis. The urinary bladder may, on occasion, hypertrophy (rather than dilate) and be small and contracted. The keyhole appearance of the proximal urethra is not always present. If the obstruction is only partial, amniotic fluid may not be appreciably decreased in volume. Finally, urinomas, which are cystic structures situated next to the obstructed kidneys, may at times cause confusing appearances.

Bilateral renal agenesis, and much less commonly severe bilateral renal hypoplasia, always present with marked early second-trimester oligohydramnios. The urinary bladder is typically not seen, but it may be very small (<1 cm) and show no change on sequential scans, the contents either bladder mucosal secretions or residual urine (in cases of hypoplasia).

Renal agenesis is an autosomal recessive disorder with a one in four chance of future recurrence. It is always lethal because of the pulmonary hypoplasia that results. In the setting of agenesis, with limited analysis possible because of the degraded image caused by oligohydramnios, the kidneys would not be expected to be seen. However, paraspinal reniform structures with a size and echogenicity similar to those of the kidneys (particularly transaxially) are often identified (Fig. 13-7). These are the normally prominent adrenal glands that often descend into the empty renal beds.

Infantile polycystic kidney (IPCK) disease is a bilateral renal disorder, an autosomal recessive abnormality, that is typically manifested later in pregnancy (Fig. 13-8). "Polycystic" is actually a poor descriptive term, because the renal abnormalities in IPCK disease are not cystic, as in adult polycystic renal disease, but represent tubular ectasia. The kidneys in IPCK disease become progressively enlarged and uniformly hyperechoic, and their function decreases as the pregnancy progresses. However, the kidneys and volume of amniotic fluid are often relatively normal in the second trimester, with most of the findings occurring in the third trimester. The delay in onset of oligohydramnios may minimize (in some cases) the deleterious effect of the decreased volume of amniotic fluid on the developing lungs.

The adult form of polycystic kidney disease, which is rarely detected in utero, can present with hyperechoic kidneys (if the cysts are small) or with multiple cysts. In both infantile and adult polycystic disease, even if the kidneys are markedly enlarged, proof of their renal origin is their extension into the paraspinal regions. Abdominal masses that are not of renal (or adrenal) origin do not have a paraspinal component.

In IPCK disease, a careful analysis of the fetal head and hands is also suggested. In the Meckel-Gruber syndrome (Fig. 13-8, C) the infantile form of polycystic kidneys occurs in combination with an abnormality of the head, frequently an encephalocele or microcephaly, and polydactyly.

The prognosis in these fetuses is varied. Most die at or near birth of a combination of renal and pulmonary failure. Some survive into childhood and even adolescence, commonly then developing fibrosis of the liver. There are other cases, however, in which the fetuses exhibit IPCK disease in utero, and yet have relatively normal renal function at birth. It is uncertain whether these infants will ultimately go on to exhibit the full-blown IPCK pattern, or a milder form of the disorder, or whether they are a highly unusual normal variant. IPCK disease is therefore a difficult entity to diagnose early, its severity is difficult to determine, and the ultimate postnatal outcome is difficult to predict.

Prognostic Indicators in Bilateral Obstruction

Interest in obstructive uropathies centers around the possibility of surgical intervention. Theoretically the placement of a percutaneous catheter from a urinary obstruction into the amniotic cavity should partially or completely relieve the renal obstruction and increase the volume of amniotic fluid. Therefore it should prevent further renal and pulmonary damage.

At the time of initial detection an accurate determination of the extent of renal damage is important, that is, whether the kidneys are already dysplastic (irreversibly damaged). If not, an invasive procedure to lessen the obstruction could be considered. Two renal ultrasound characteristics have been found useful in predicting dysplasia in a fetus with an obstructive uropathy (and should also be of value in the evaluation of nonobstructed renal disorders). These are the renal cortical echogenicity and the

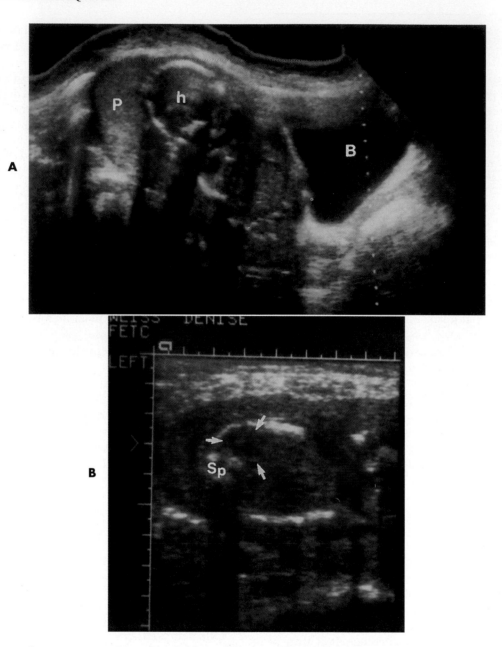

Fig. 13-7   Renal agenesis at 18 weeks. **A,** Static sagittal scan shows the fetus to be poorly visualized because of the marked oligohydramnios. *B,* maternal urinary bladder; *h,* fetal head; *P,* placenta. **B,** Transaxial real-time image in the region of the kidneys shows an ill-defined hypoechoic structure *(arrows)* in the left paraspinal region. The right paraspinal area is obscured by shadowing from the spine *(Sp).* Although the left side is reniform, the urinary bladder could not be identified over the course of an hour. The reniform shape was found at autopsy to be a normally prominent fetal adrenal gland. The immediate cause of death was pulmonary hypoplasia.

identification of cysts. When there is increased echogenicity (greater than that of the liver) or cysts (cortical or subcortical), or both, dysplasia is always present (Fig. 13-9). Conversely, normal echogenicity and the absence of cysts do not prove normalcy. Because of the importance of careful renal analysis and the difficulty in scanning when oligohydramnios is present, there may be selected cases in which the instillation of normal saline solution into the amniotic space may be necessary to better visualize the fetus.

Direct analysis of the fetal urine is often indicated. By percutaneous puncture, usually into the dilated urinary bladder but occasionally into an obstructed renal collecting system, urine can be obtained that can be analyzed for multiple biochemical characteristics, in particular the sodium content, the osmolality, and the total

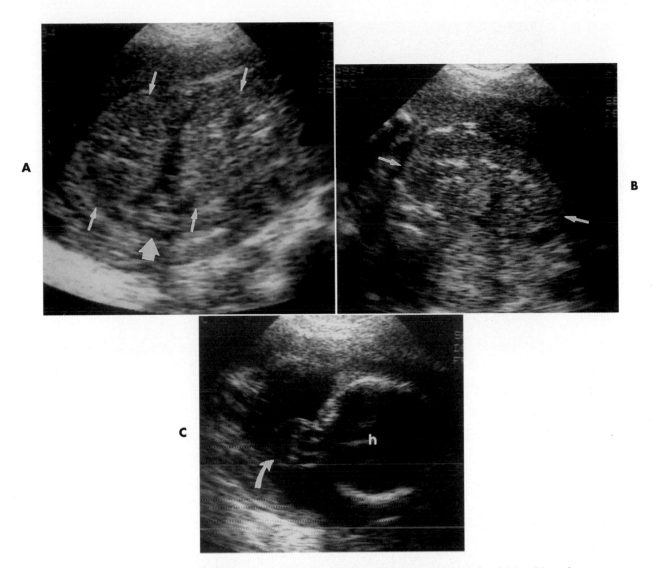

Fig. 13-8   Meckel-Gruber syndrome (infantile polycystic kidneys and encephalocele) in a 32-week fetus. Marked oligohydramnios is present and the urinary bladder cannot be identified. **A,** Transaxial view in the region of the kidneys shows two large paraspinal hyperechoic inhomogeneous structures *(arrows)* extending anteriorly. *Large arrow,* spine. **B,** Long-axis view of one of the hyperechoic structures shows a large reniform mass *(arrows)* with a slightly more hyperechoic center. **C,** Oblique view through the fetal head *(h)* shows a defect in the occiput with a posterior encephalocele *(curved arrow).* Polydactyly (not shown) was also present.

protein content. If these values are low, there is normal renal function. If they are elevated, serial punctures should be repeated to see if these values decrease, as they may have been initially falsely elevated because of water resorption in the setting of a long-standing obstruction. If they are still elevated, dysplasia exists. Additionally, the puncture can be used to obtain a sample for fetal karyotyping, either of the amniotic fluid or urine. There is a higher proportion of chromosomally abnormal fetuses in association with obstructive uropathies than in the general population.

The size of the abdomen does not appear to affect immediate neonatal outcome. If the obstruction is severe,

however, the abdomen may become much larger than normal, and after birth may result in a "prune belly" appearance (Eagle-Barrett syndrome). This consists of an abdomen with flaccid abdominal musculature, persistently dilated ureters, and, in some cases, abnormal bladder distention. When present, the likelihood of long-term morbidity is increased.

Intervention should be considered in selected cases only under the following circumstances: progressive oligohydramnios, relatively normal renal function, no other anomalies, and a fetus too immature to be immediately delivered (usually <34 weeks). The treatment consists of the placement of a pigtail catheter that extends

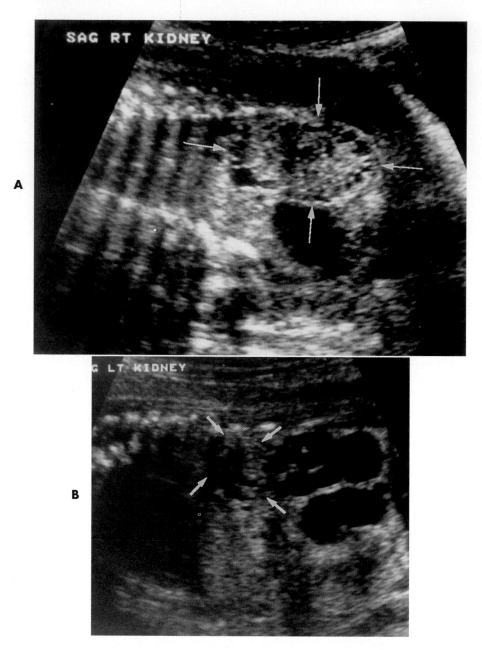

Fig. 13-9   Dysplastic (irreversibly damaged) kidneys in two different fetuses. **A,** Long-axis view through the right kidney *(arrows)* shows an ill-defined hyperechoic kidney that is more echogenic than the liver. Multiple cysts are identified in a cortical-subcortical distribution. **B,** Long-axis scan through the region of the left kidney *(arrows)* shows a hyperechoic shrunken kidney. Dilated cystic structures seen more caudally (toward the right) represent a large tortuous ureter in a male fetus with posterior urethral valves. This might be confused with a multicystic dysplastic kidney. The urinary bladder was not identified; it was markedly hypertrophied and was very small.

from the obstructed bladder (or less commonly from an obstructed kidney) into the amniotic space; it may first be necessary to instill saline solution into the amniotic cavity to provide a space for the catheter. These catheters do not always remain in place, and have been found in some cases either inside the fetus or in the amniotic space at birth. In other instances significant urine ascites has developed because of the puncture. Nevertheless, in some cases the procedure has been associated with no further deterioration in renal function. It is not possible to say if the procedure actually protected renal function.

The International Fetal Surgery Report has compiled a series of cases of treated obstructive uropathy. From 1980 to 1985, 73 cases were reported: 21 of posterior urethral valves, 3 of urethral atresias, and 3 of prune-belly syndromes (no other cause), with most of the remaining 46 of unknown cause. Chromosomal abnormalities occurred in six (8%). Only 30 (41%) of the fetuses survived, with the other 43 (59%) dying either as a stillborn or a neonate. Of the 29 neonatal deaths, 27 resulted from pulmonary hypoplasia. These poor results have made many examiners reluctant to perform invasive urinary procedures.

UNILATERAL RENAL ANOMALIES

Unilateral renal abnormalities are more common in fetal life than are bilateral anomalies. They are usually either a multicystic dysplastic kidney (MCDK) or a ureteropelvic junction (UPJ) obstruction. Both are relatively easy to diagnose in utero.

The MCDK is an enlarged paraspinal structure composed of multiple *noncommunicating* cysts. The cysts may vary in size, and usually look like a cluster of grapes (Fig. 13-10, *A*). No normal kidney is identified, but hyperechoic intervening tissue may be seen (Fig. 13-10, *B*, and 13-10, *C*). The MCDK is not expected to enlarge, so there is little need for a follow-up study, though some observers still prefer at least one additional examination. The ureter is atretic and is not identified. In contradistinction, the UPJ obstruction involves dilatation of the renal pelvis and calices (pelvocalciectasis). Both connect together to create the "glove" appearance of true hydronephrosis (Fig. 13-11). Because the obstruction is at the level of the renal pelvis, the ureter is normal in caliber and therefore not identified. Careful scanning, particularly in the transaxial and coronal planes, can always differentiate an MCDK from a UPJ obstruction by showing whether the cystic structures are separated (MCDK) or connected (UPJ). Rarely a dilated tortuous ureter may present as a cystic mass, thus mimicking an MCDK (see Fig. 13-9, *B*).

As long as the contralateral kidney is normal, the quantity of amniotic fluid will remain appropriate and the lungs will mature normally. However, for both entities there is a 20% incidence of a contralateral renal abnormality. This abnormality varies from subtle small (seemingly insignificant) cysts to another UPJ obstruction or a second MCDK. Very infrequently an MCDK can occur on one side and a UPJ obstruction on the other. Cysts are not normal in utero, and even solitary ones have been associated with renal dysplasia.

A very careful evaluation of both kidneys and the amniotic fluid is therefore indicated whenever a unilateral renal anomaly is discovered. As might be expected, bilateral severe renal anomalies with oligohydramnios are incompatible with life because of the renal and pulmonary failure that results. Occasionally this may be accompanied by additional abnormalities of the lower spine or lower extremities or by both (i.e., caudal regression syndrome). If the volume of amniotic fluid remains normal and the contralateral renal abnormality appears mild, however, the significance of the bilateral abnormalities may not be fully apparent in utero; problems will, however, usually be manifested by early childhood.

A unilateral obstruction may not always involve the entire kidney. A duplicated kidney may have an obstructed upper pole and a normal lower pole, the latter occasionally exhibiting normal reflux (Fig. 13-12). The upper pole obstruction is caused by an ectopic ureter, which typically inserts lower and more medially, toward the base of the bladder. On occasion a ureterocele (its distal end) can be identified as a cystic structure within the urinary bladder. However, even when the ureterocele is not seen, the disparity between the obstructed upper pole and the normal lower pole suggests this diagnosis. Amniotic fluid remains normal in volume unless the ureterocele obstructs urine outflow at the bladder base. This condition is rarely bilateral. Surgical removal of the upper pole moiety, either unilateral or bilateral, can be performed successfully after birth without further sequelae.

MEGACALICES, MEGAURETERS, AND MEGACYSTIS

Primary abnormalities of the calices (megacalices), ureters (megaureters), or the urinary bladder (megacystis) are rare. Normal calices and ureters are not identified, even in cases of reflux. When ureters are seen, they are dilated and appear as tubular structures in the lower abdomen and pelvis. If instead these prominent structures are thought to represent unusual loops of bowel or blood vessels, careful real-time observation to look for peristalsis and color flow Doppler to evaluate for blood flow should be performed. The urinary bladder is normally prominent without an upper limit of normal. The diagnosis of megacystis is therefore subjective.

Dilated calices, ureters, and urinary bladder are typically associated with obstructive uropathies. Dilatation of all three is most commonly a consequence of bladder outlet obstruction; dilatation of the calices and pelvis alone typically occurs in a UPJ obstruction. For megacalices to be diagnosed, usually a unilateral developmental anomaly, the renal pelvis and the ureter must be normal (not dilated).

When the ureters or bladder, or both, are considerably more dilated than the pelvocaliceal system, this may still represent the end stage of distal obstruction with dys-

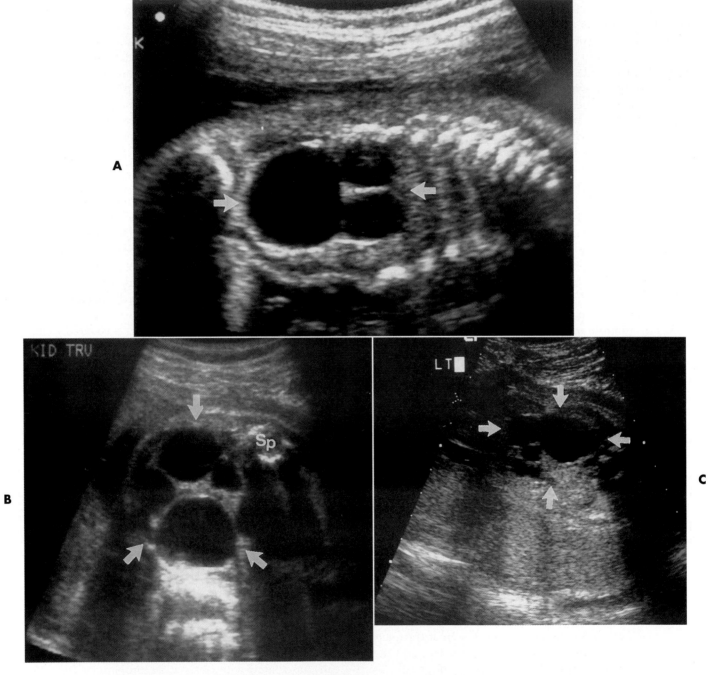

Fig. 13-10 Unilateral multicystic dysplastic kidneys in two different fetuses. **A** and **B** are from a 32-week fetus, **A** a long-axis view and **B** a transaxial view showing multiple discrete large cysts in the right renal bed *(arrows)*. *Sp,* fetal spine. **C,** Long-axis view in a 22-week fetus of the left renal bed showing no evidence of a normal kidney. Instead multiple discrete, separate cysts of varying diameter from 2 to 5 cm are identified *(arrows)*. Because all of the cysts have well-defined margins and do not interconnect, this should not be mistaken for hydronephrosis. Note the hyperechoic soft tissue between and around these cysts.

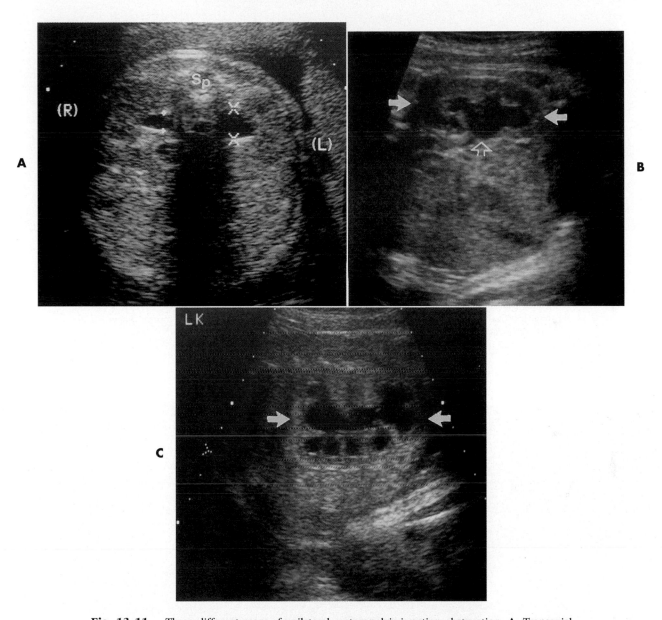

Fig. 13-11 Three different cases of unilateral ureteropelvic junction obstruction. **A,** Transaxial view of a 22-week fetus shows bilateral enlargement of the renal pelves. On the right *[(R)]*, the renal pelvis without caliceal dilatation (+) is 5 mm. This represents normal reflux. The left renal pelvis *[(L)]* is dilated to 9 mm *(x)*, however, although there was no caliectasis noted on this examination. Marked pelvocaliectasis was noted 5 weeks later on a follow-up study. *Sp,* fetal spine. **B,** Long-axis view of the left kidney *(arrows)* in a 25-week fetus shows pelvocaliectasis with the pelvis dilated to the area of the ureteropelvic junction *(open arrow).* The ureter was not identified, and therefore not dilated. **C,** Long-axis–coronal view of the left kidney *(arrows)* in a 34-week fetus shows multiple anechoic spaces, all connecting together. This pelvocaliectasis stops at the ureteropelvic junction.

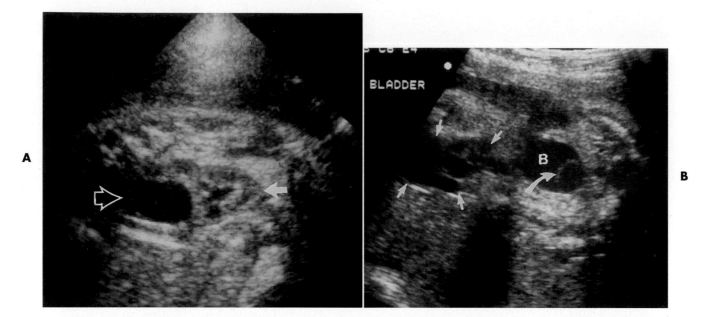

Fig. 13-12   An obstructed upper pole secondary to an ectopic ureter with ureterocele in a 32-week fetus. **A,** Long-axis view of the left kidney shows the lower pole *(arrow)* on the right, with very mild separation of the collecting system; this is secondary to normal reflux. The upper pole *(open arrow)* has a large cystic structure, a finding consistent with an upper pole obstruction. **B,** Long-axis midline image of the lower abdomen and pelvis shows the urinary bladder *(B)* with a cystic structure *(curved arrow)* at its base. This is the ureterocele. The dilated tortuous ureter is seen superiorly *(arrows).*

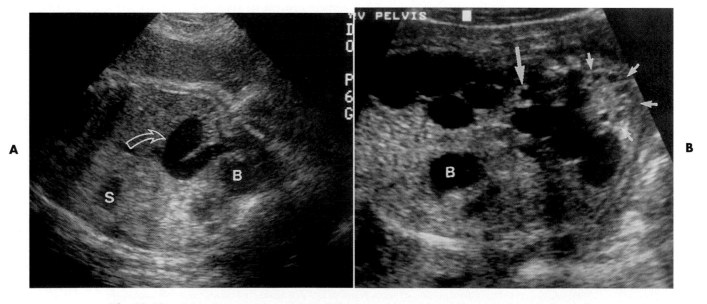

Fig. 13-13   Dilated ureters resulting from different causes. **A,** Megaureter in a 32-week fetus. Long-axis image of the left side of the fetus shows a large S-shaped, anechoic, tubular structure *(curved open arrow)* above the small (but normal) urinary bladder *(B).* This persisted without change, and with a normal-appearing kidney. *S,* stomach. **B,** Long-standing obstruction secondary to posterior urethral valves in a 38-week fetus. Transaxial-coronal view of the fetal abdomen shows a marked decrease in the volume of amniotic fluid. The upper part of the urinary bladder *(B)* and the fetal spine *(large arrow)* are seen. Multiple dilated cystic structures (the dilated ureters) are detected on both sides of the abdomen. The left kidney (on the right), denoted by small arrows, shows a small hyperechoic kidney with multiple cysts, a finding consistent with dysplasia.

plastic upper tracts (see Fig. 13-9, *B*). However, a diffuse mesenchymal disorder primarily affecting the ureters and bladder in the Eagle-Barrett (prune-belly) syndrome may instead be present (Figs. 13-13 and 13-14). This syndrome represents a group of disorders with different causes and presentations, which are often complex and frequently with poor prognoses.

On occasion the dilated urinary tract is associated with a normal or increased volume of amniotic fluid, rather than with oligohydramnios. A normal amniotic fluid volume suggests either a less severe functional problem of the ureters and bladder (perhaps still a mesenchymal abnormality) or only a partial (incomplete) obstruction. Polyhydramnios would not be expected in the presence of the urinary tract abnormality unless a postobstructive diuresis or an additional anomaly, usually of the gastrointestinal tract or central nervous system, was also present. A rare entity called *megacystis microcolon hypoperistalsis intestinalis,* for example, includes polyhydramnios, an enlarged bladder, and often enlarged ureters (see Fig. 13-14, *B*). Although not always identified, intestinal obstruction is the presumed cause of the increased volume of amniotic fluid.

THE ADRENAL GLANDS

The adrenal glands are normally quite prominent in utero, and are approximately one half the size of the kidneys. They are often not detected until the third trimester, when they are identified transaxially as thin disclike paraspinal structures located above the upper poles of the kidneys (Fig. 13-15). The adrenal glands can sometimes also be seen in long-axis views when they are ovoid or triangular. The length of the adrenal gland and its anteroposterior diameter have been evaluated. Measurements are usually not important and are frequently underestimated because rib shadowing often obscures at least part of the gland. The echogenicity of the adrenal glands is similar to that of the kidneys, with a hypoechoic cortex (periphery) and a hyperechoic medulla (center).

There are times when the adrenal glands can pose diagnostic problems. As previously discussed, when there is renal agenesis, the adrenals can assume an appearance in the renal bed mimicking that of the kidneys. The adrenal glands can also be abnormal. There have been documented cases of in utero adrenal hemorrhage (uni-

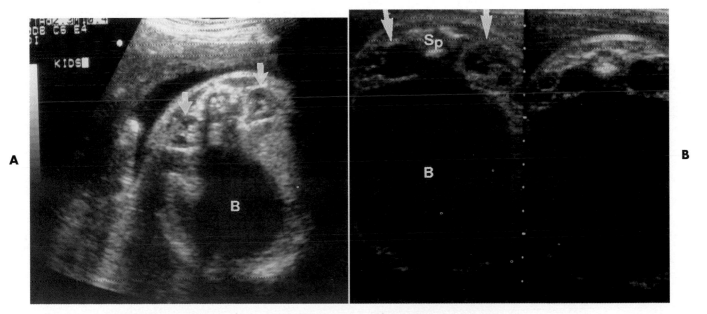

Fig. 13-14   Two cases of markedly dilated bladders (*B*), or megacystis. **A,** Primary megacystis of unknown cause in a 28-week fetus exhibits a "prune belly" at birth. The markedly prominent bladder does not appear to affect the ureters or the kidneys *(arrows).* Amniotic fluid is mildly decreased in volume. **B,** Megacystis microcolon hypoperistalsis intestinalis in a 38-week fetus. Two images in a transaxial view show cystic structures *(arrows)* on both sides of the fetal spine *(Sp),* a finding consistent with obstructed hydronephrotic kidneys. The dilated bladder, however, is much more distended than the kidneys. On different images the amniotic fluid was noted to be markedly increased in volume.

lateral or bilateral) and rarely a solid tumor, a neuroblastoma. Their differentiation is usually difficult, unless a considerable change in their size or echogenicity, or both, is noted on a follow-up study; this suggests an evolving hemorrhage. Even then tumors may undergo necrotic or hemorrhagic changes. If an adrenal mass is large, it can displace the kidneys such that the adrenal mass may be mistaken for a rare solid renal mass, the mesoblastic nephroma (a hamartoma), and the even rarer Wilms' tumor. A definitive diagnosis must often await neonatal evaluation.

ADDITIONAL PELVIC ABNORMALITIES

Structures posterior to the urinary bladder can occasionally be seen. The rectosigmoid colon, either normally filled with meconium or obstructed, can be identified as a tubular structure. This is discussed more completely in Chapter 12.

In a female fetus the normally prominent uterus (under maternal hormonal influence) can infrequently be identified. Although no measurements are available, the uterus would not be expected to be more than 3 cm in length. If the vagina is prominent and the uterus is teardrop shaped or ovoid, with an echogenicity that is cystic or complex, vaginal atresia with an obstructed vagina and uterus should be considered. This is termed either *hematocolpus* (if only the vagina is involved) and *hematometrocol-*

pus (if the uterus is also involved) (Fig. 13-16). Scans obtained more caudad may show a cystic structure (the distended vagina) bulging into the perineum. This can be corrected surgically at birth.

FETAL SEX

The external genitalia can often be identified by scanning the perineum. By 16 weeks, and sometimes earlier, the identification of a scrotum or penis clearly indicates the fetus is male (Fig. 13-17). Occasionally, anechoic fluid accumulates locally within the scrotal sac and outlines the testicles (hydroceles). This typically resolves spontaneously after birth.

In the female fetus, the labia are more difficult to image (Fig. 13-18). On occasion they can be prominent and sometimes mimic the scrotum. Care must be taken not to confuse the umbilical cord between the legs as part of the genitalia.

The overall accuracy of sex determination has not been fully established. There is obviously greater accuracy in the detection of males. This differentiation is not, however, of medical importance, unless a predisposition for a certain entity is of concern. For example, an obstructive uropathy caused by posterior urethral valves occurs only in a male fetus, and hemophilia (which cannot be detected in utero) occurs only in the male offspring of affected families.

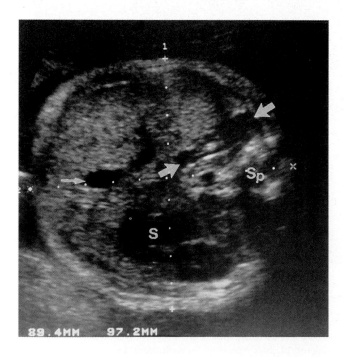

Fig. 13-15   Transaxial view, superior to the kidney, in a normal 32-week fetus. Large arrows denote a disclike structure adjacent to the fetal spine *(Sp);* this is a normal adrenal gland. Although different in shape, note the similar echogenicity of the adrenal gland to that of the kidney, with a hyperechoic center and a hypoechoic periphery. *S,* stomach; *small arrow,* umbilical portion of the left portal vein. Two measurements (+ and *x*) of the abdomen are shown.

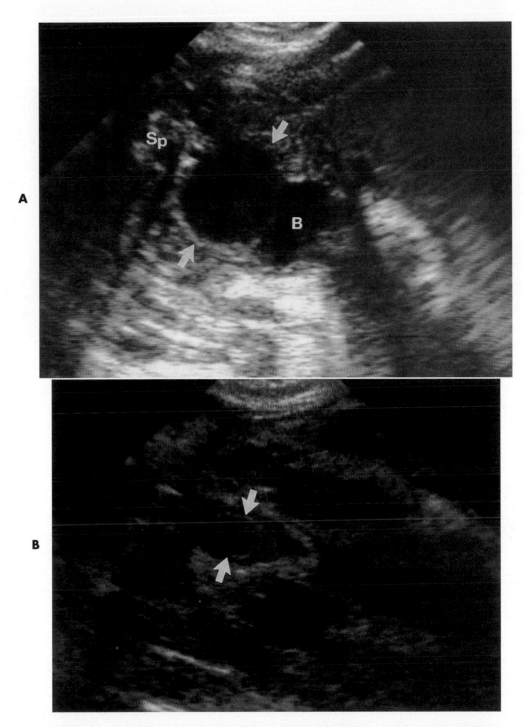

Fig. 13-16   Hematometrocolpus, secondary to vaginal atresia, in a term female fetus. **A,** Transaxial view of the pelvis shows a cystic structure *(arrows)* immediately posterior to the urinary bladder *(B)*. The bowel could be identified behind the cystic structure. The sagittal view (not shown) showed the cystic structure to be ovoid, a finding consistent with an obstructed uterus. *Sp,* fetal spine. **B,** Transaxial view through the perineum shows the cystic structure *(arrows)* extending down and spreading the labia, a finding consistent with an obstructed vagina.

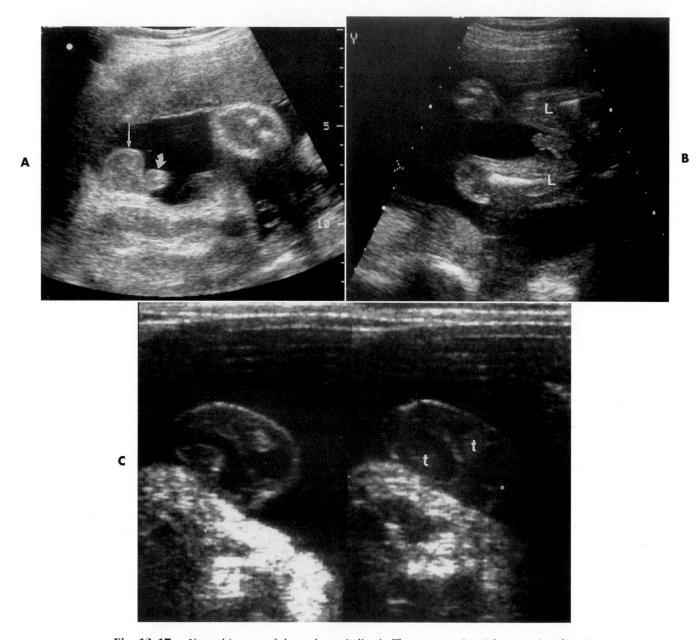

Fig. 13-17   Normal images of the male genitalia. **A,** The scrotum *(straight arrow)* and penis *(curved arrow)* are noted. **B,** Coronal view shows the penis between the fetus' legs *(L).* **C,** Benign hydroceles. These images of the scrotum shows the testes *(t)* surrounded by fluid.

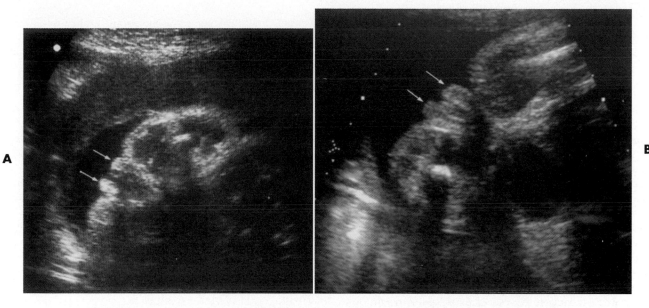

Fig. 13-18   Normal images of the female genitalia. **A,** Scan of the perineum shows the labia *(arrows).* **B,** Same view in a different fetus shows markedly hypertrophied labia *(arrows),* a normal variant. Their prominence can at times mimic the appearance of the scrotum.

Key Features

The kidneys, which are paraspinal in location, are progressively better seen throughout the second and third trimesters.

Measurements of the kidneys are not usually needed. The simplest is a transaxial ratio of the kidney to the abdomen (normally less than one third).

The renal sinus may have pyelectasis without caliectasis. This represents normal reflux in the third trimester if it measures less than 7 mm in diameter, with the remainder of the urinary tract and the volume of amniotic fluid normal.

Second-trimester pyelectasis (≤4 mm) is a normal finding. If greater than 4 mm, an evaluation for signs related to Down's syndrome and a follow-up examination to look for hydronephrosis are indicated.

The urinary bladder is identified routinely. If not, sequential scanning over the course of 1 hour is indicated. There are, however, infrequent cases in which a bladder is not seen, but this is a normal finding.

Oligohydramnios, particularly if severe and prolonged (starting in the second trimester), is often associated with a lethal condition, pulmonary hypoplasia.

The most common bilateral renal anomalies are urethral obstruction (usually posterior urethral valves), renal agenesis, and infantile polycystic disease.

An abdominal mass that extends to the paraspinal area is most likely of renal origin.

Two renal characteristics associated with dysplasia are increased echogenicity of the renal cortex (greater than that of the liver) and cortical cysts.

In a fetus with obstructed uropathy, even after shunting, (usually from the bladder to the amniotic fluid), the death rate still approaches 60%, with most of the infants dying of pulmonary hypoplasia in the neonatal period.

Unilateral renal problems are usually either a multicystic dysplastic kidney or ureteral pelvic junction obstruction. Twenty percent of the fetuses have an abnormality in the contralateral kidney.

If obstruction is identified in the upper but not the lower pole of the kidney, a duplicated kidney with an ectopic ureterocele should be considered.

Megaureter and megabladder may be related to functional abnormalities rather than obstruction. If they are associated with polyhydramnios, additional fetal abnormalities should be sought.

The normal adrenal glands can usually be identified in the third trimester. They become of diagnostic importance in the setting of renal agenesis, when they occupy the renal bed, and in the setting of adrenal masses, either neoplasms or hemorrhages.

A prominent vagina (and uterus) may present as a pelvic mass, termed *hematocolpus* (or *hematometrocolpus*).

SUGGESTED READINGS

Arger PH et al: Routine fetal genitourinary tract screening, *Radiology* 156:485, 1985.

Bowie JD et al: The changing sonographic appearance of fetal kidneys during pregnancy, *J Ultrasound Med* 2:505, 1983.

Clautice-Engle T, Pretorius DH, Budorick NE: Significance of nonvisualization of the fetal urinary bladder, *J Ultrasound Med* 10:615, 1991.

Cohen HL et al: Normal length of fetal kidneys: sonographic study in 397 obstetric patients, *AJR* 157:545, 1991.

Corteville JE, Gray DL, Crane JP: Congenital hydronephrosis: correlation of fetal ultrasonographic findings with infant outcome, *Am J Obstet Gynecol* 165:384, 1991.

Grannum P et al: Assessment of fetal kidney size in normal gestation by comparison of ratio of kidney circumference to abdominal circumference, *Am J Obstet Gynecol* 136:249, 1980.

Johnson MP et al: In utero surgical treatment of fetal obstructive uropathy: a new comprehensive approach to identify appropriate candidates for vesicoamniotic shunt therapy, *Am J Obstet Gynecol* 170:1770, 1994.

Kleiner B et al: Multicystic dysplastic kidney: observations of contralateral disease in the fetal population, *Radiology* 161:27, 1986.

Lewis E et al: Real-time ultrasonographic evaluation of normal fetal adrenal glands, *J Ultrasound Med* 1:265, 1982.

Mahony BS, Callen PW, Filly RA: Fetal urethral obstruction: US evaluation, *Radiology* 157:221, 1985.

Mahony BS et al: Fetal renal dysplasia: sonographic evaluation, *Radiology* 152:143, 1984.

Mandell J et al: Structural genitourinary defects detected in utero, *Radiology* 178:193, 1991.

Manning FA et al: Special report. Catheter shunts for fetal hydronephrosis and hydrocephalus, *N Engl J Med* 315:336, 1986.

Nimrod C et al: The effect of very prolonged membrane rupture on fetal development, *Am J Obstet Gynecol* 148:540, 1984.

Romero R et al: Antenatal diagnosis of renal anomalies with ultrasound. III. Bilateral renal agenesis, *Am J Obstet Gynecol* 151:38, 1985.

Romero R et al: The diagnosis of congenital renal anomalies with ultrasound. II. Infantile polycystic kidney disease, *Am J Obstet Gynecol* 150:259, 1984.

Willard DA, Gabriele OF: Megacystis-microcolon–intestinal hypoperistalsis syndrome in a male infant, *J Clin Ultrasound* 14:481, 1986.

CHAPTER 14

Fetal Musculoskeletal System

Femur Length Measurement and Its Uses
Skeletal Dysplasias
    The Four Major Types
        Heterozygous Achondroplastic Dysplasia
        Osteogenesis Imperfecta
        Achondrogenesis
        Thanatophoric Dysplasia
    Problems with the Diagnosis
    Other Associated Anomalies
Amniotic Bands and the Amniotic Band Syndrome

For a Key Features summary see p. 307.

The obstetric guidelines recommend imaging of a femur throughout the second and third trimesters, primarily to measure its length (Fig. 14-1, *A*). This measurement is then compared with measurements of the head and body to establish whether fetal proportionality is normal. The femur length (FL) can also be used to determine fetal age, particularly in the third trimester.

The other long bones can be analyzed as well; these comprise the other femur, the distal leg (tibia and fibula), the arm (humerus), and the forearm (radius and ulna) (Fig. 14-1, *B*, and 14-1, *C*). The obstetric guidelines do not recommend their routine imaging or measurement, but some observers consider it important to identify these four areas and to rule out gross absence or deformity of the long bones. Their relationship can be assessed quickly by estimating an approximate 1:1 length ratio between the bones of the forearm and the humerus, and between the bones of the distal leg and the femur. Measurement tables are also available, if needed. It is important to remember, however, that there is a slight difference in the length of the radius and the ulna and in the length of the tibia and the fibula (with the radius and tibia longer). If measured, each of these bones must therefore be evaluated individually (Fig. 14-1, *C*).

Other bones can also be assessed. The shape and digits of the hands and the configuration of the feet have been studied. The clavicles, ribs, and iliac crests can be identified, at least partially. The calvarium and spine are routinely evaluated as part of the obstetric guidelines, and this is discussed, along with the evaluation of facial structures, in Chapter 10.

The soft tissues, the subcutaneous fat and muscles, have not been well studied. Although the soft tissues are usually measured in the midarm or midthigh, the exact sites of measurement have not been firmly established. A diffuse thickening of more than 10 mm occurs in the setting of fetal hydrops and occasionally in the setting of maternal diabetes mellitus. Focal enlargement is usually secondary to a localized mass such as a hemangioma or lymphangioma (a lymphatic obstruction). If blood flow can be detected by Doppler waveform analysis, then a vascular tumor such as a teratoma is likely. The absence of detectable blood flow, however, is a nondiagnostic finding because avascular tumors and tumors with very slow flow (such as hemangiomas) typically have no detectable Doppler signal. Rarely, focal swelling may be a sign of constriction caused by an amniotic band.

Nuchal skin thickness that exceeds 6 mm in the mid–second trimester and 3 mm in the first trimester is a sign of trisomy 21. This is discussed in Chapter 10.

There is no established lower limit for soft tissue thickness. Decreased thickness is expected in the setting of asymmetric growth retardation, a state of fetal starvation. At present this in utero diagnosis cannot be made, even with magnetic resonance imaging.

FEMUR LENGTH MEASUREMENT AND ITS USES

Skeletal dysplasias can be a varied and confusing conglomerate of anomalies, with more than two hundred types identified. Nevertheless, they are relatively uncommon, occurring in less than 2.5 of every 10,000 births. Most dys-

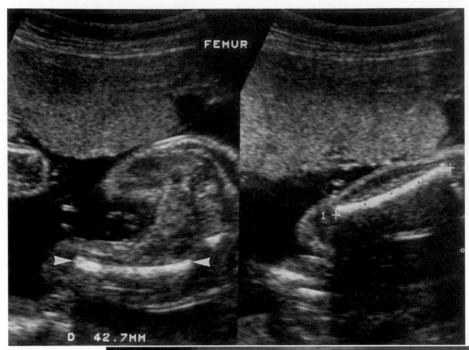

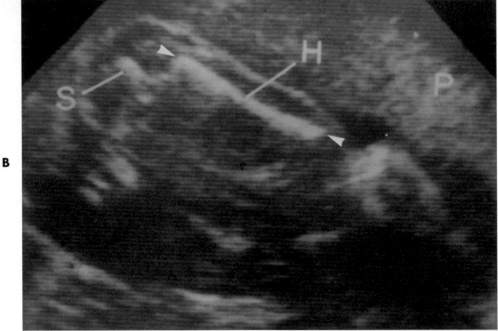

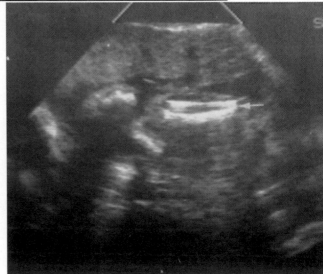

Fig. 14-1 Normal images of long bones in the mid–second trimester. **A,** Images of the femurs in one fetus. On the right the straight outer (lateral) margin of a femoral shaft is seen, measured from + to + along the dotted line. On the left the slightly curved inner (medial) margin of the other femur is seen. It is measured as a straight line (from the arrowheads), ignoring the curve. The femur farther away from the transducer may be incompletely visualized and inadvertently foreshortened. **B,** Image of the humerus *(H)* adjacent to the scapula *(S)* in another fetus. The measurement is taken along the shaft from the one edge to the other *(arrowheads). P,* placenta. **C,** The forearm in a third fetus shows the ossified radius and ulnar shafts, with the ulna farther from the transducer. The two bones are of different lengths; they align at the wrist *(arrow),* with the ulna longer at the elbow. Similarly, the tibia and fibula align at the ankle, with the tibia longer at the knee.

plasias present with short stature, the primary abnormality related to the length of the long bones. Because FL correlates directly with the length of the fetus, the routine FL measurement should detect most skeletal dysplasias.

The femur is measured linearly from one end of the ossified shaft to the other (along its diaphysis) (Figs. 14-1, *A,* and 14-2, *A*). Although there is also a thickness (depth) to the femoral shaft, this is usually not appreciated because the ultrasound beam is strongly attenuated after contacting the uppermost surface of the bone. Fibrous tissue surrounds the cartilaginous ends of the femoral shaft, at the nonossified head and at the condyles. If the ultrasound beam is perpendicular to the condylar fibrous tissue, an artifactual hyperechoic line is imaged extending from the end of the femoral shaft (Fig. 14-2, *B*). This line appears thinner than the rest of the shaft and should not be included in the measurement. Any change in the transducer orientation (off of the perpendicular one) will make it disappear. It has been termed the *distal femur point* and can be the source of an error in the calculation of fetal age of up to 2 to 3 weeks. Near term the normal distal femoral epiphysis begins to ossify. Although this will ultimately form the femoral condyles, it does not connect to the femoral shaft in utero, and therefore should not be included in its measurement (Fig. 14-2, *C*).

The primary use of the FL is in its proportionality to the biparietal diameter (BPD). For each BPD the FL has an expected mean and 2–standard deviation (SD) measurement. When there is a discrepancy between the measurement of one femur and the BPD, the other femur should be measured to determine if the process is unilateral or bilateral. When both femurs are too long (above +2 SD), this is a normal variant typically seen in the offspring of tall parents. If only one femur is elongated, this raises the possibility of unilateral hypertrophy, occasionally seen in the Beckwith-Wiedemann syndrome, which also includes visceromegaly and renal anomalies (including Wilms' tumors).

If only one femur is too short (below −2 SD), this is caused by femoral hypoplasia, often seen in the fetuses of diabetic mothers. If both femurs are short, either a constitutionally normally small fetus (frequently seen in the offspring of short parents) or a skeletal dysplasia should be considered. The differentiation between these two is usually possible and can be separated into two groups. The fetuses in the first group are normal and exhibit only very mild FL shortening, initially 4 mm or less below the −2 SD line (between −2 and −4 SD), with appropriate interval growth and no additional structural abnormalities. Only when the femur grows more slowly should heterozygous achondroplastic dwarfism be considered. The fetuses in the second group, all with skeletal dysplasias, have femurs more than 5 mm below the −2 SD line (often considerably below −4 SD). All have additional major abnormalities, including a narrow thorax, fractures, and decreased bone brightness.

Investigators have explored the possibility of using a shortened femur or humerus, or both, to predict chromosomally abnormal fetuses, in particular those with trisomy 21. The FL or its comparison (as a ratio) to the BPD has been used, with a cutoff of either −1.5 or −2 SD below the norm indicating an abnormality. Normally the FLs are distributed in a bell-shaped curve, with a certain percentage of normal cases falling outside any arbitrary cutoff. When 2 SD is taken as the limit, 5% of the normal cases lie outside it—2.5% above (2.5 per 100 cases) and 2.5% below (2.5 per 100 cases). For every measurement *below* −2 SD, there is therefore a possibility that, instead of a chromosomally abnormal fetus, it may be one of the 2.5 per 100 normal cases. When 1.5 SD is used instead, even more normal cases fall below the normal range, 6.5 per 100 cases. Therefore, unless there is significant separation of the normal from the abnormal cases, too much overlap occurs and differentiation is not consistent.

This in fact has been the problem. The majority of trisomy cases are "mixed in" with normal cases, even *above* the −2 SD cutoff, with only a small percentage falling below. When the femoral and humeral lengths are used to identify chromosomally abnormal fetuses, their positive predictive values (i.e., true-positive values divided by true-positive plus false-positive values) are very low at only 3.5. Although the detection of abnormal cases is relatively good (true positives), far too many normal cases are incorrectly shown to be abnormal (false positives). This is in contradistinction to a much higher positive predictive value of 44 for the finding of nuchal fold thickness of 6 mm or more in the detection of trisomy 21. The femoral and humeral lengths, separately or in combination with other characteristics, are therefore not accurate in predicting chromosomal abnormalities.

SKELETAL DYSPLASIAS

The in utero identification of skeletal dysplasias is important, as these are often associated with significant physical deformity or mental retardation, or both. Some are consistently lethal conditions, and all require genetic counseling before future pregnancies are undertaken. If they are severe, their in utero detection prompts two additional considerations: whether to electively terminate the pregnancy by the mid–second trimester or to avoid using any extraordinary maternal intervention (i.e., a cesarean section) at term. Most skeletal dysplasias are anticipated and studied because of a family history of an affected parent or sibling. On occasion, though, a dysplasia may be discovered fortuitously as an incidental finding during ultrasound examination.

Significant skeleton abnormalities can exhibit any of three osseous findings: shortened limbs, bony deformities (fractures or bowing, or both), and decreased bone brightness (demineralization). If the entire limb is shortened,

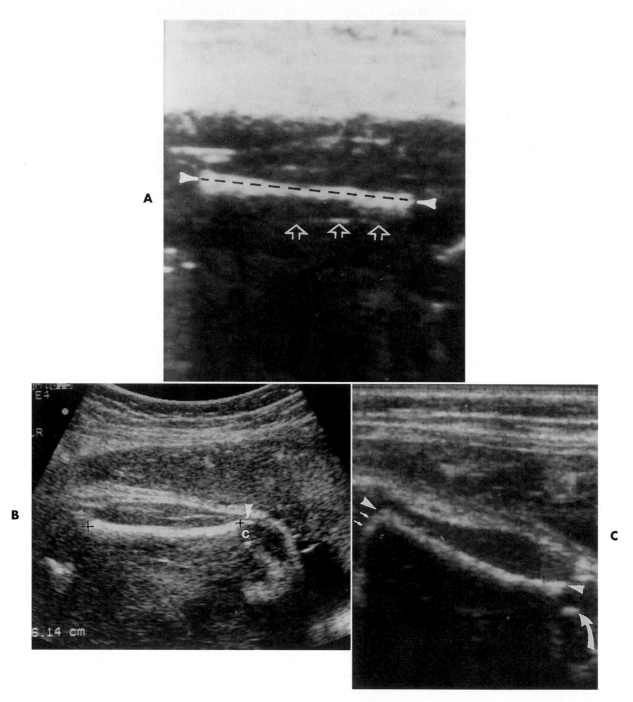

Fig. 14-2   Various properties of the normal femur shown in images obtained in three different fetuses. **A,** Femoral shaft in the second trimester. Its hyperechoic shaft (diaphysis) is denoted by arrowheads and a dotted line. Note that the thickness of the shaft can sometimes be seen *(open arrows)*. **B,** Femoral shaft in the mid–second trimester. Its hyperechoic shaft (diaphysis) is measured from one end to the other (+). Toward the right there is an apparent thin hyperechoic extension of the shaft *(arrowhead)*. This extension (an artifact) originates from the fibrous tissue surrounding the hypoechoic femoral condyle *(c)* when scanned perpendicularly. **C,** Distal femoral epiphysis in a 37-week fetus. In addition to the normal femur length (the diaphysis *[arrowheads]*),a small 5-mm-wide hyperechoic ossification center *(curved arrow)* is seen in the region of the femoral condyles. It is separate from the femoral shaft and should not be included in the femoral length measurement. The thickness of the shaft *(small arrows)* is seen at the femoral neck.

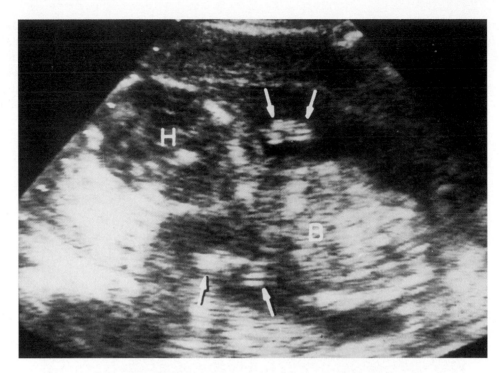

Fig. 14-3   The thrombocytopenia–absent radia syndrome, a rare micromelic skeletal dysplasia. Both the proximal and distal parts of the upper extremities are severely foreshortened, and only the area of the hands *(arrows)* is identified. *H,* fetal head; *B,* fetal body.

both proximally and distally, the skeletal dysplasia has a micromelic pattern (Fig. 14-3); if only the proximal segment is shortened, a rhizomelic type of dysplasia is present. Both will be detected by the FL measurement. Only the much less common isolated shortenings of the forearm and lower leg (mesomelia) and of the distal segment (acromelia) will be missed by sole analysis of the femur.

Fractures and bowing of the long bones are usually obvious. Only the medial (inner) aspect of the femoral shaft has a slight normal curve (see Fig. 14-1, *A*). If this curve is accentuated or occurs along any other margin of the femur, it is abnormal (Fig. 14-4, *A*). All other long bones are normally straight, and any bowing or fractures should be easily detectable and considered abnormal (Figs. 14-4 and 14-5). Fractures or the bowing of other bones such as the ribs, however, may be difficult to appreciate.

Bone brightness (mineralization) is an important feature, but often difficult to assess. Because quantification is not possible, the bones are considered abnormal if they are qualitatively decreased in brightness (Fig. 14-6). When in doubt, comparison with the scan of a normal fetus of the same gestational age, and ideally on the same machine (with appropriate technique), can be helpful to determine appropriate brightness.

Despite the large number of types of skeletal dysplasias, only four major types are encountered routinely.

They account for 66% of all dysplasias, and are thanatophoric dysplasia (28%), heterozygous achondroplasia (15%), osteogenesis imperfecta (OI; 14%), and achondrogenesis (9%). Heterozygous achondroplasia and approximately 50% of the cases of OI are nonlethal anomalies. Although all the other dysplasias are lethal, their impact on the number of perinatal deaths is not great. They are responsible for only 1 in every 110 deaths, with thanatophoric dysplasia accounting for 44%, achondrogenesis 18%, and osteogenesis imperfecta 13% of these deaths.

The Four Major Types of Dysplasia

Heterozygous achondroplastic dysplasia   Heterozygous achondroplastic dysplasia is the most common nonlethal skeletal dysplasia and is inherited as an autosomal dominant trait. One of the parents must be a heterozygous achondroplastic dwarf. When the other parent is normal, the chance of its occurrence in each offspring is 50%, with the other 50% normal. If both parents are heterozygous achondroplastic dwarfs, there is still a 50% chance of the child being a heterozygous dwarf, with the other 50% divided equally between a normal child and a child with the more severe form of the disorder, the lethal homozygous achondroplastic dysplasia.

The appearance of a heterozygous achondroplastic dwarf in children is obvious, with proximal limb shortening (rhizomelic dwarfism) and additional typical phenotypic and skeletal deformities. In utero, however, the diagnosis can be made only by detecting a shortened femur. It is recommended that the FL be plotted on a BPD-to-FL graph to enhance detection, as the initial shortening may be subtle and not fully appreciated by only comparing measurements or gestational ages. In addition, the FL, with its slower growth rate, may not decrease below -2 SD until the late second trimester. Therefore, if the fetus is at risk for achondroplasia, even when findings are initially

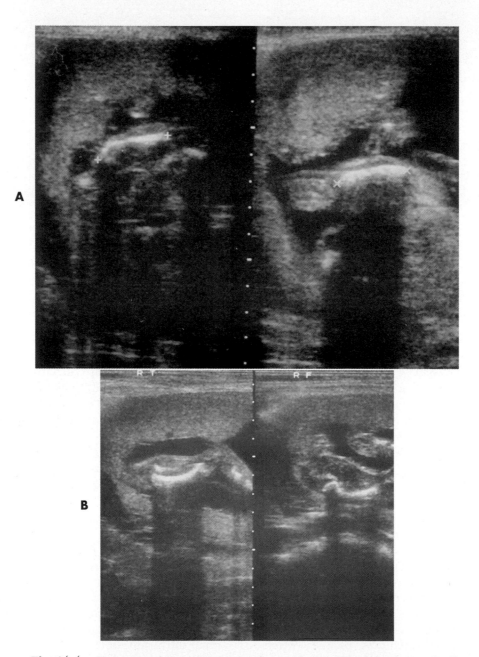

Fig. 14-4   Two cases of osteogenesis imperfecta with normal bone brightness. **A,** Abnormal bowing of the long bones of the left lower extremity in a 31-week fetus. The shaft of the femur, on the left (+), shows an abnormal curvature with angulation and thinning. The tibia, on the right *(x)*, is also bowed. Both extremities measure far shorter than would be expected for the gestational age of the fetus. **B,** Abnormal bowing of the right tibia and fibula in an 18-week fetus. There is a markedly abnormal curvature and foreshortening of the tibia (on the left) and of the fibula (on the right).

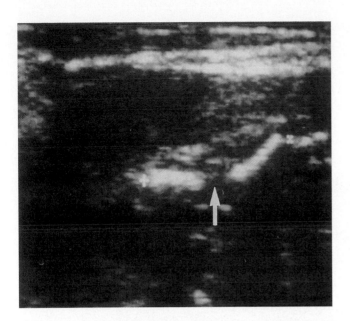

Fig. 14-5 Left femoral shaft fracture in an 18-week fetus with osteogenesis imperfecta. The approximate ends of the shaft are shown (+). A large hypoechoic space *(arrow)* is noted in its middle. The bone exhibits normal brightness.

normal in the early to middle second trimester, follow-up examinations should be continued up to 28 weeks before this type of dysplasia is ruled out.

Osteogenesis imperfecta There are four different types of OI, most inherited as an autosomal dominant trait. The in utero diagnosis can be made in one of two ways: the finding of deformities or of demineralization. With an appropriate family history, any fracture or abnormal bowing will establish the diagnosis of OI, assuming there has been no significant trauma to the fetus (see Figs. 14-4 and 14-5). Conversely, the diagnosis is not excluded if a normal fetus is identified, as a fetus with OI may be unaffected in utero or may only exhibit subtle, unappreciated deformities. Therefore an abnormal finding is always important; normal findings must be considered cautiously, particularly in a fetus at risk for a dysplasia.

Although osteoporosis is a hallmark of OI, the accurate ultrasound detection of bone brightness is variable. Obvious decreased brightness represents significant demineralization, and strongly suggests the existence of the most severe types of OI, usually lethal (see Fig. 14-6). Normal bone brightness, however, does not ensure that

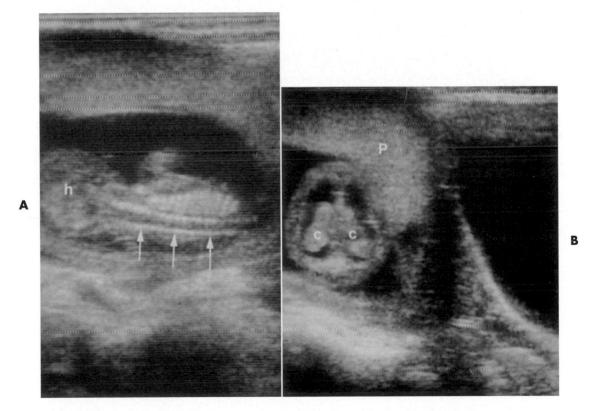

Fig. 14-6 Severe demineralization at 17 weeks in a fetus with osteogenesis imperfecta. **A,** Long-axis image of the fetal head *(h)* and body. Note the complete absence of normal mineralization of the calvarium. The spine *(arrows)* and ribs, though somewhat ossified, are also noticeably decreased in brightness. **B,** Transaxial view of the fetal head shows the normal choroid plexus *(c)* within the normal lateral ventricles, again with complete absence of calvarial ossification. *P,* placenta.

the bones will be found normal at birth. Without the appropriate history of OI, demineralization may instead suggest other rarer types of lethal dysplasias such as hypophosphatasia.

Achondrogenesis   Achondrogenesis is an autosomal recessive dysplasia, and is almost always lethal. The look of the newborn is that of a cherub, with very shortened extremities, short trunk, and a distended abdomen.

The long bones are all severely affected in a micromelic pattern, and are often deformed, with measurements needed only for the sake of thoroughness (Fig. 14-7, *A*). These long bones are of normal brightness.

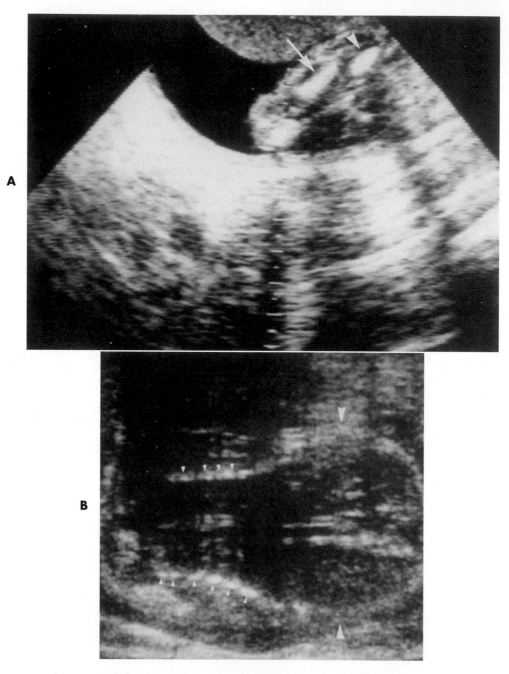

Fig. 14-7   Achondrogenesis at 16 weeks. **A,** Long-axis view of the arm shows a markedly shortened and deformed femur *(arrowhead)* and radius *(arrow)*. The normal brightness of the bones is maintained. **B,** Long-axis coronal view of the fetal body with the thorax toward the left. Note the marked demineralization of the ribs *(small arrowheads)*. The chest has a bell shape and is markedly narrowed compared with the abdomen *(large arrowheads)*.

The axial skeleton, however, can be either normal or markedly decreased in brightness. The chest can also be considerably narrowed, and may have a bell-shaped appearance (Fig. 14-7, *B*). When the chest is narrowed and the axial skeleton is of normal brightness, the differentiation of achondrogenesis from thanatophoric dysplasia may not be possible.

Thanatophoric dysplasia   Thanatophoric dysplasia is a lethal condition. The word *thanatophoric* derives from the Greek and means "death." It is a sporadic *noninherited* disorder, and the bones of the fetus exhibit a normal brightness. The limbs show severe shortening (and often deformity) in a micromelic pattern. Death is due to the markedly narrowed thorax, which gives the lungs little room to develop (Fig. 14-8); pulmonary hypoplasia results.

Ratios of the chest to abdominal measurements (usually circumferences) and intrathoracic ratios have been

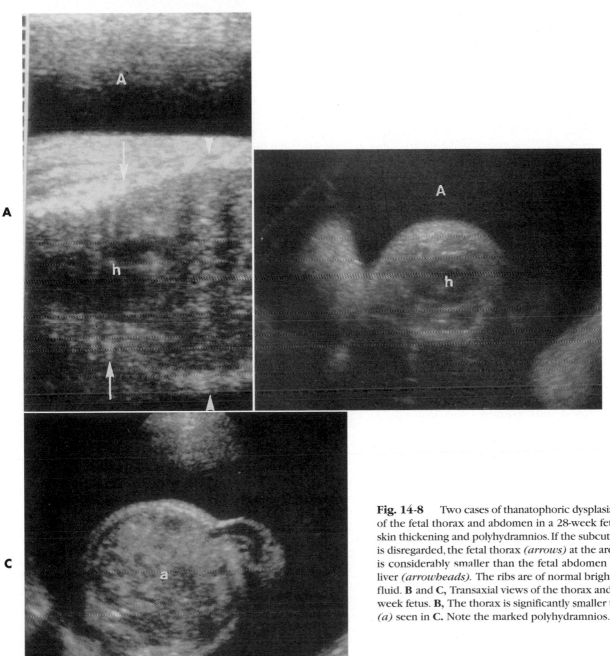

Fig. 14-8   Two cases of thanatophoric dysplasia. **A,** Coronal view of the fetal thorax and abdomen in a 28-week fetus shows marked skin thickening and polyhydramnios. If the subcutaneous thickening is disregarded, the fetal thorax *(arrows)* at the area of the heart *(h)* is considerably smaller than the fetal abdomen at the area of the liver *(arrowheads).* The ribs are of normal brightness. *A,* amniotic fluid. **B** and **C,** Transaxial views of the thorax and abdomen in a 20-week fetus. **B,** The thorax is significantly smaller than the abdomen *(a)* seen in **C.** Note the marked polyhydramnios.

evaluated in an attempt to predict when pulmonary hypoplasia will result. Although no definite predictive number has been found, the lower the ratio (i.e., the narrower the thorax), the greater the chance of serious pulmonary problems. This is discussed in Chapter 11. Moderate to marked polyhydramnios is also typically present, presumably caused by impaired swallowing secondary to the chest narrowing.

Problems with the Diagnosis

Because of the lack of information about dysplastic fetal growth, the in utero development of skeletal dysplasias is incompletely understood. Expected neonatal characteristics may not be present at the time of an ultrasound examination, and findings (even when present) may be too subtle to be appreciated. In addition, concomitant soft tissue abnormalities may not be detected. Despite these limitations, when an abnormal finding is discovered, particularly in the correct clinical setting, the diagnostic certainty is high.

The prediction of the lethality of any dysplasia is clinically important. Although there are no absolutes, other than knowledge of the type of dysplasia involved, certain ultrasound findings strongly suggest incompatibility with life. In addition to polyhydramnios, especially if moderate or marked, the following abnormalities (either occurring individually or in combination) should be sought:

1. Shortening of both the proximal and distal parts of the extremities (micromelia)
2. Marked skeletal demineralization (decreased brightness)
3. An unusually small thorax

Other Associated Anomalies

Because many skeletal dysplasias exhibit multiple characteristics, a thorough examination of the fetus should be performed, often going beyond the routine examination suggested in the obstetric guidelines (see Chapter 7).

The head should be analyzed for the presence of calvarial and facial abnormalities. The calvarium can be demineralized, and it can have a cloverleaf shape (the kleebattschädel deformity). This deformity is caused by the craniosynostosis of all the sutures, usually with associated mental retardation. It may be either an isolated anomaly or part of the thanatophoric dysplasia (Fig. 14-9). The face, too, can be affected. The outer orbital diameter may be abnormally increased or decreased. Cleft lips and palates can also be found.

The vertebrae can be demineralized in certain dysplasias. The spine may be deformed, particularly with a sharply angled scoliosis or kyphosis. If there is no evidence of a meningocele or meningomyelocele, the de-

formity may instead be caused by vertebral body developmental anomalies, that is, segmentation and fusion defects. Although often difficult to appreciate in utero, these problems can occur at any vertebral level, particularly in the thoracolumbar region (Fig. 14-10). Developmental anomalies are commonly isolated occurrences, but can be associated with additional structural anomalies, frequently multiple, such as the VACTERL syndrome (*v*ertebral, *a*nal, *c*ardiac, *t*racheal, *e*sophageal, *r*enal, *r*adial, and *l*imb anomalies).

Abnormalities of the hands can at times be diagnosed, but a meticulous scanning technique is needed for this. It is important to image not only the five metacarpals but also their phalanges (Fig. 14-11, *A,* and 14-11, *B*). This can be particularly difficult because, as is often the case, the hands move rapidly. Nevertheless, if more than five fingers are counted, polydactyly is present. The extra digits are usually on the ulnar side (adjacent to the little finger), and may be so rudimentary that they are difficult to appreciate (Fig. 14-11, *C*). Occasionally the distal edge of the fifth metacarpal may be mistaken for an extra digit. Syndactyly is skin or bony fusion of adjacent digits such that a trident type deformity of the hand may be seen, with the second and third fingers and the fourth and fifth fingers closely aligned. Clinodactyly is the sharp deviation of the fingers. Ectrodactyly, lobster-claw deformity, may also be identified (Fig. 14-11, *D*). A constantly clenched

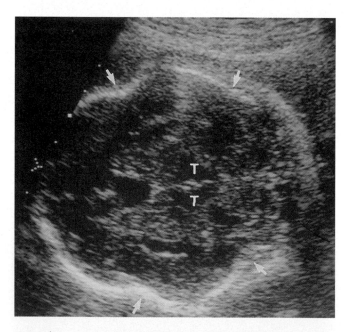

Fig. 14-9   Cloverleaf skull (kleebattschädel deformity) in a 20-week fetus, an isolated deformity not associated with thanatophoric dysplasia. Transaxial image of the fetal head through the area of the thalami *(T)* shows an unusual configuration of the calvarium. Arrows indicate unusual indentations in the frontal and parietal regions bilaterally, causing the head to be configured into three lobes.

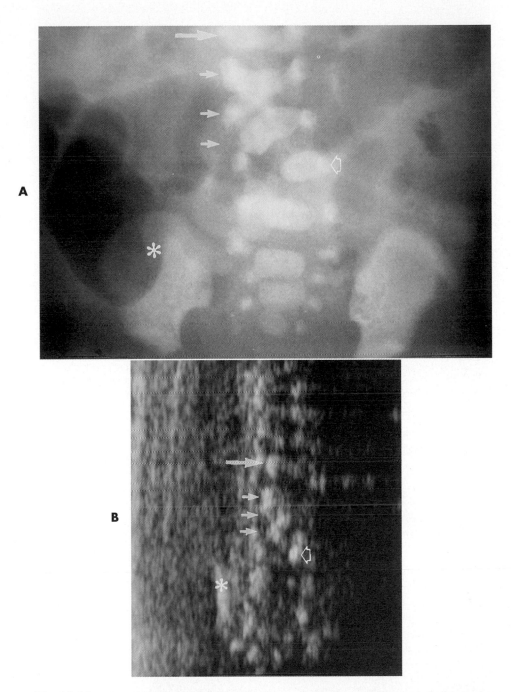

Fig. 14-10   Complex segmental-fusion anomaly in a 22-week fetus. This was an isolated anomaly and not associated with additional fetal abnormalities. **A,** Anteroposterior abdominopelvic radiograph obtained at birth. **B,** Coronal image of the lumbosacral spine. Both images are oriented in the same plane. The large arrow indicates the last normal lumbar vertebral body and the asterisk denotes the right iliac crest; arrows show a deformed vertebra and the open arrow shows a hemivertebra.

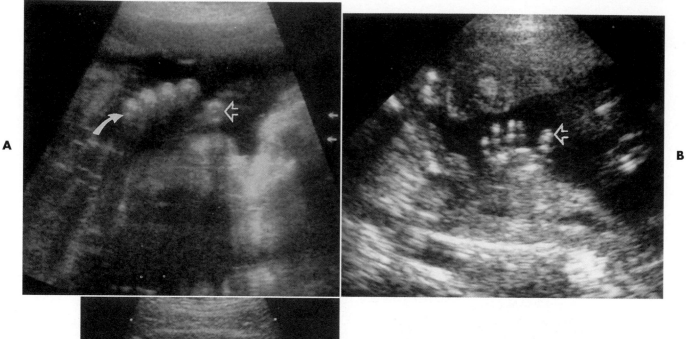

A

B

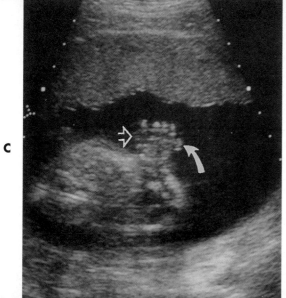

C

Fig. 14-11 Four different fetuses, all at approximately 20 weeks. **A,** A normal hand, with the images obtained at the heads of the metacarpals (open arrow denotes the first metacarpal). On the opposite (ulnar) side *(curved arrow),* a small sixth hyperechoic area was identified. Although initially thought to be a rudimentary sixth finger, further scanning found it to be part of the head of the fifth metacarpal. **B,** A normal hand, with the scan of the phalanges showing all five fingers and most of their phalanges (open arrow indicates the thumb). **C,** Polydactyly. A rudimentary sixth finger *(curved arrow)* is identified on the ulnar side of the hand. The open arrow identifies the region of thumb, which was normal but only partially imaged. **D,** "Lobster claw" deformity in the ectrodactyly–ectodermal dysplasia–clefting syndrome. As part of a complex series of anomalies, there are defects in the midportion of both the hands and feet. On this image only three partially formed fixed digits are detected in a claw configuration.

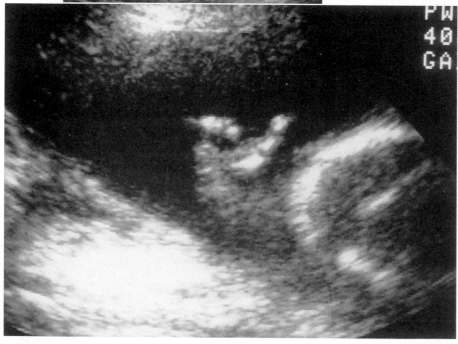

D

hand, especially with overlapping fingers, is seen in trisomy 18. Although some of these hand abnormalities can be isolated occurrences, they are not infrequently associated with generalized dysplasias.

Normally the hands and feet are positioned neutrally and move freely (Figs. 14-11, *B,* and 14-12, *A*). Clubhands and clubfeet are seen as sharply flexed distal extremities, remaining in fixed positions (Fig. 14-12, *B*). Although club-

bing can be found in the setting of skeletal dysplasias, it can also be associated with musculoskeletal or neurologic conditions, and is then called *arthrogryposis.* Prolonged severe oligohydramnios can also lead to secondary arthrogryposis, presumably caused by lack of fetal movement and the fixed position of the extremities. Arthrogryposis is not a true skeletal dysplasia, but nevertheless causes significant deformity.

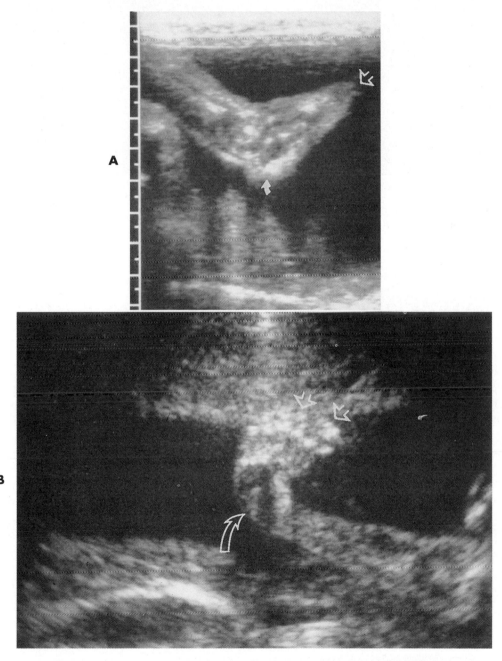

Fig. 14-12 A normal and abnormal foot, both in 24-week fetuses. **A,** Long-axis image of a normal left foot showing the heel *(curved arrow)* and toes *(open arrow).* The foot moved freely at the ankle. **B,** Clubfoot. There is an unusual angulation at the ankle *(open curved arrow)* and this foot remained in a fixed position. The toes are denoted by open arrows.

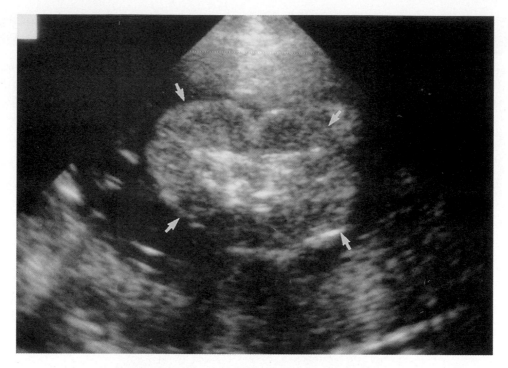

Fig. 14-13   Amniotic band syndrome at 35 weeks. This image of the right foot was markedly deformed showing only irregular hyperechoic structures (the normal bones cannot be identified) surrounded by marked soft tissue swelling *(arrows)*. The amniotic bands were not seen.

AMNIOTIC BANDS AND THE AMNIOTIC BAND SYNDROME

The fetus normally resides within the amniotic cavity, surrounded by a fused amnion and chorion. Rarely, because of conditions that are not well understood, there can be a rent or break in the amnion, with the fetus then entering the space between the two membranes. Although this may not cause problems, there is a potential for the thin amniotic membrane to encircle fetal parts as bands. As these fetal parts grow, their motion can be restricted and deformed by these bands.

Amniotic bands are rarely detected because they are less than 1 mm thick. However, the gross deformities, a late manifestation of the bands, can be seen, and the am-

niotic band syndrome can then be diagnosed. These bands can involve any part of the fetus. When involving the limbs, strangulation, deformity, and even amputation with pronounced soft tissue swelling are possible (Fig. 14-13). Unfortunately, when detected at such a late stage, the abnormalities cannot then be corrected.

The amniotic band syndrome is an isolated *noninherited* anomaly, and is therefore not likely to recur in subsequent pregnancies. These deformities are not part of the spectrum of either skeletal dysplasias or any standard anomaly, and can usually be distinguished by their unusual appearance and asymmetry.

In the case of amniotic sheets, synechiae extend into the amniotic fluid. Because of their thickness, the sheets should not be mistaken for amniotic bands. This is discussed more completely in Chapter 16.

Key Features

Measurement of the femur is a routine part of the obstetric examination.

The primary use of the femur length (FL) is to determine its proportionality with other fetal structures, especially the head.

In the third trimester the accuracy of the FL is approximately equal to that of the head measurement. Fetal age can be determined from the FL.

The following two aspects of the femur should not be included in the FL measurement: the distal femoral point and the distal femoral epiphysis.

If one femur measures abnormally short or long, the other femur should be measured to see if the process is unilateral or bilateral.

If both femurs are found to be short, usually a constitutionally normal fetus can be differentiated from one with dysplasia. Interval growth assessment and evaluation of the remainder of the fetal structures, or both, are usually necessary.

The femoral and humeral lengths do not have enough of a positive predictive value to be of use in predicting chromosomal abnormalities.

The value of ultrasound in the investigation of skeletal dysplasias is primarily in three areas. It can detect shortened limbs, fractures or bowing, and decreased bone brightness (demineralization).

Heterozygous achondroplasia can be evaluated in utero only by FL measurement and its interval growth. It is expected to be abnormal by 27 to 30 weeks.

Osteogenesis imperfecta can only be detected if fractures, abnormal bowing, or demineralization is present.

An abnormal finding almost always establishes the diagnosis of a dysplasia. Normal findings must be considered cautiously.

Achondrogenesis involves severe shortening of the limbs and exhibits a micromelic pattern. There are varying degrees of demineralization to the axial skeleton and chest narrowing.

Thanatophoric dysplasia is a noninherited condition in which the bone brightness is normal. There is severe limb shortening and significant chest narrowing, usually in combination with pronounced polyhydramnios.

If a fetus is being evaluated for a dysplasia, careful evaluation of the rest of the fetus is necessary, including the remainder of the skeleton.

Amniotic bands, a rent in the amnion, are virtually never detected. However, their late manifestation of structural abnormalities can often be seen.

The amniotic band syndrome can usually be distinguished from skeletal dysplasias and developmental abnormalities because the deformities that result are usually markedly asymmetric and unusual in appearance.

SUGGESTED READINGS

Benacerraf BR, Frigoletto FD Jr: Sonographic observation of amniotic rupture without amniotic band syndrome, *J Ultrasound Med* 11:109, 1992.

Benacerraf BR et al: Sonographic scoring index for prenatal detection of chromosomal abnormalities, *J Ultrasound Med* 11:449, 1992.

Benson CB, Doubilet PM: Sonographic prediction of gestational age: accuracy of second- and third-trimester fetal measurements, *AJR* 157:1275, 1991.

Bulas DI et al: Variable prenatal appearance of osteogenesis imperfecta, *J Ultrasound Med* 13:419, 1994.

Burton DJ, Filly RA: Sonographic diagnosis of the amniotic band syndrome, *AJR* 156:555, 1991.

Camera G, Mastroiacovo P: *Birth prevalence of skeletal dysplasias in the Italian multicentric monitoring system for birth defects.* In Papadatos CJ, Bartsocas CS, editors: *Skeletal dysplasias.* New York, 1982, Alan R. Liss.

Chinn DH et al: Ultrasonographic identification of fetal lower extremity epiphyseal ossification centers, *Radiology* 147:815, 1983.

Dicke JM et al: Fetal biometry as a screening tool for the detection of chromosomally abnormal pregnancies, *Obstet Gynecol* 74:726, 1989.

Goldstein RB, Filly RA, Simpson G: Pitfalls in femur length measurements, *J Ultrasound Med* 6:203, 1987.

Hashimoto BE, Filly RA, Callen PW: Sonographic diagnosis of clubfoot in utero, *J Ultrasound Med* 5:81, 1986.

Kurtz AB, Wapner RJ: Ultrasonographic diagnosis of second-trimester skeletal dysplasias: a prospective analysis in a high-risk population, *J Ultrasound Med* 2:99, 1983.

Kurtz AB et al: In utero analysis of heterozygous achondroplasia: variable time of onset as detected by femur length measurements, *J Ultrasound Med* 5:137, 1986.

Kurtz AB et al: Usefulness of a short femur in the in utero detection of skeletal dysplasias, *Radiology* 177:197, 1990.

Mahony BS, Filly RA: High-resolution sonographic assessment of the fetal extremities, *J Ultrasound Med* 3:489, 1984.

Mahony BS et al: The amniotic band syndrome: antenatal sonographic diagnosis and potential pitfalls, *Am J Obstet Gynecol* 152:63, 1985.

Merz E, Kim-Kern MS, Pehl S: Ultrasonic mensuration of fetal limb bones in the second and third trimesters, *J Clin Ultrasound* 15:175, 1987.

Pretorius DH et al: Specific skeletal dysplasias in utero: sonographic diagnosis, *Radiology* 159:237, 1986.

CHAPTER 15

Placenta, Umbilical Cord, and Cervix

For a Key Features summary see p. 339.

The placenta should be evaluated as part of the second- and third-trimester examination. Its position, size, and echogenicity can be assessed, and any evidence of hemorrhage, infarction, or mass noted. Although not specifically mentioned in the guidelines, the cervix should be analyzed for possible incompetence and the umbilical cord imaged. Doppler waveform analysis may be helpful in selected cases.

THE NORMAL PLACENTA

The early embryo (the blastocyst) embeds into the endometrium. It then sends out fingerlike projections called *chorionic villi*. In response, the entire endometrium undergoes a decidual reaction. Although most of the villi and decidua atrophy, the chorion frondosum and adjacent decidua basalis proliferate, forming the placenta by the middle to late first trimester.

Sonographically the placenta can be identified as early as 7 to 8 weeks, and is routinely imaged by the end of the first trimester. The placenta is best appreciated when fundal, anterior, or lateral in position; when it is in a poste-

rior position, the fetus often overlies and frequently obscures full visualization. The placenta has a uniformly moderate echogenicity (Fig. 15-1). On its surface, abutting the amniotic fluid, the chorionic plate (the chorioamniotic membrane) appears as a bright specular reflector. On its inner border with the uterine wall, the combined hypoechoic myometrium and interposed basilar layer is identified as a hypoechoic band, and is best seen in a placenta which is anterior in position. Although the basilar plate (also called the *decidua basalis* or *decidua basalis compactum*) cannot be distinguished from the myometrium, it contains numerous feeding maternal blood vessels, which can be identified by Doppler studies. Serosal veins can be seen outside and adjacent to the uterus, particularly laterally. These veins, which are often large, always conform without a mass effect to the outer contour of the uterus (Fig. 15-2).

Placental thickness is usually evaluated subjectively. If a measurement is needed, it is taken at its midposition, perpendicular to the placental surface from the chorionic plate to the beginning of the myometrial basilar layer. When the umbilical cord inserts into the middle of the placenta, the measurement can be taken at its insertion site (Fig. 15-3). Precise upper and lower values are not available, but the thickness is always normal if it is between 2 and 4 cm throughout the second and third trimesters. Care must be taken not to measure either obliquely or near a uterine contraction, as the placental size can be altered in both instances, usually creating a false impression of enlargement.

The placenta is a very vascular organ and consists of two blood supplies. From the fetus umbilical arteries (typically two) carry blood through the umbilical cord from the fetal hypogastric arteries to the placenta and one umbilical vein carries blood back to the fetal left portal vein. From the mother, branches of the uterine arteries (from the maternal hypogastric arteries) carry blood through the myometrium (the arcuate and radial arteries), through

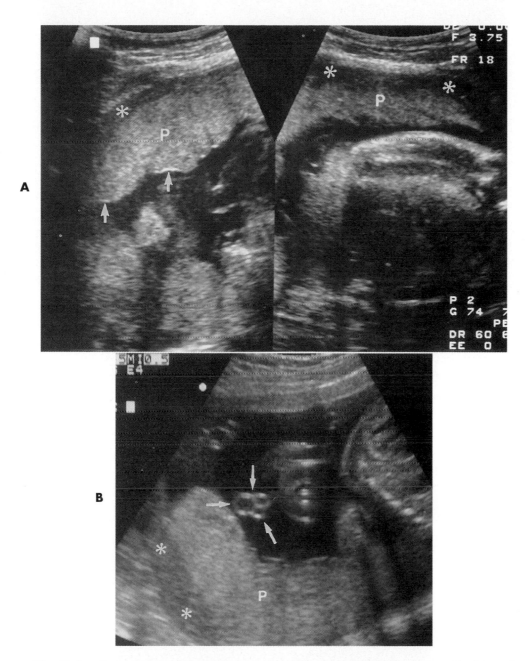

Fig. 15-1   Two normal mid–second trimester placentas. **A,** Fundal-anterior placenta. Dual sagittal images are combined to show a homogeneous moderately hyperechoic placenta *(P)*. The chorionic plate *(arrow)* is a bright reflector when perpendicular to the ultrasound beam. Asterisks denote the hypoechoic myometrial-basilar layer. **B,** Posterior placenta *(P)* in a transaxial view. Note the transaxial image of a normal three-vessel umbilical cord *(arrows)* with its two smaller arteries and the one larger vein. Asterisks show part of the hypoechoic myometrial-basilar layer.

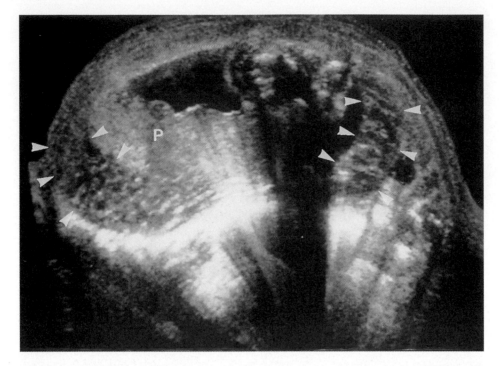

Fig. 15-2 Normal serosal veins. Static transaxial view of the gravid uterus shows large bilateral anechoic tubular structures outside the uterus *(arrowheads)*. Even when prominent these serosal veins do not distort the uterine shape. *P,* placenta.

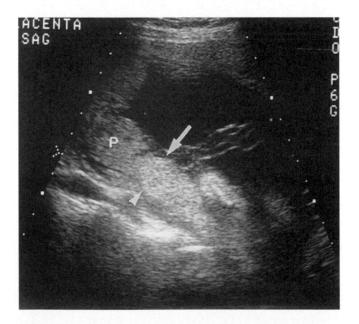

Fig. 15-3 Sagittal view of the normal uterus showing a posterior-fundal placenta. When the umbilical cord inserts into the middle of the placenta *(P)*, the placental thickness can be measured from its insertion site *(arrow)* to the beginning of the myometrial-basilar layer *(arrowhead)*. Note the normally "twisted" appearance of the umbilical cord.

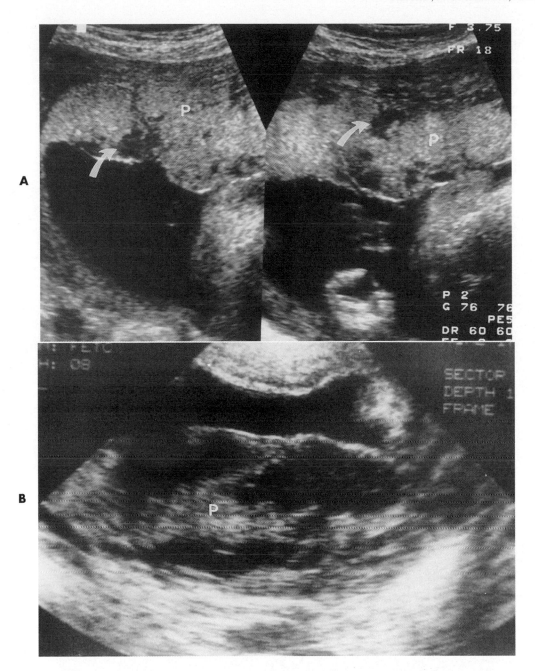

Fig. 15-4   Normal intervillous connections. Two different placentas *(P)* showing the extremes of normal maternal venous channels in the placenta. **A,** Dual sagittal images are combined to show subchorionic and deep placental hypoechoic focal areas *(curved arrows)* in an anterior placenta. **B,** There is a total distortion of the normally hyperechoic posterior placenta by large hypoechoic spaces, the spaces traversing the placenta from the basilar plate to the subchorionic region. In both cases slow movement of blood can be seen in these hypoechoic areas on a real-time evaluation.

the basilar plate (the spiral arteries), and into the placenta; maternal blood leaves by comparable veins. Within the placenta the two circulations intertwine (but do not admix). With their slow flows and large surface areas, maximum exchange of nutrients for wastes and oxygenated blood for deoxygenated blood can take place.

Normal maternal venous channels (without fetal inter-connections) are frequently seen as hypoechoic or anechoic spaces within the placenta. These are often focal and small, but may infrequently be numerous and large, rarely even traversing the placenta from the basilar plate to the subchorionic region (below the chorionic plate) (Fig. 15-4). Although given different monikers, including "venous lakes," they are best termed *intervillous connec-*

tions. Because they are filled with blood, rather than fluid, they do not exhibit distal acoustic enhancement. Blood flow can frequently be observed by real-time observation and confirmed (if needed) by its Doppler-detected venous flow.

The normal uniform placental echogenicity is defined as grade 0. In some women placental calcifications (hy-

perechoic foci) develop as the pregnancy matures (Fig. 15-5). Small diffuse, speckled calcifications constitute grade 1 changes. Grade 2 changes are similar to the grade 1 changes, but include larger calcifications lining the placenta adjacent to the basilar plate in a "dot-dash" configuration. Grade 3 changes are similar to the grade 2 changes, but are more extensive and thicker, separating the pla-

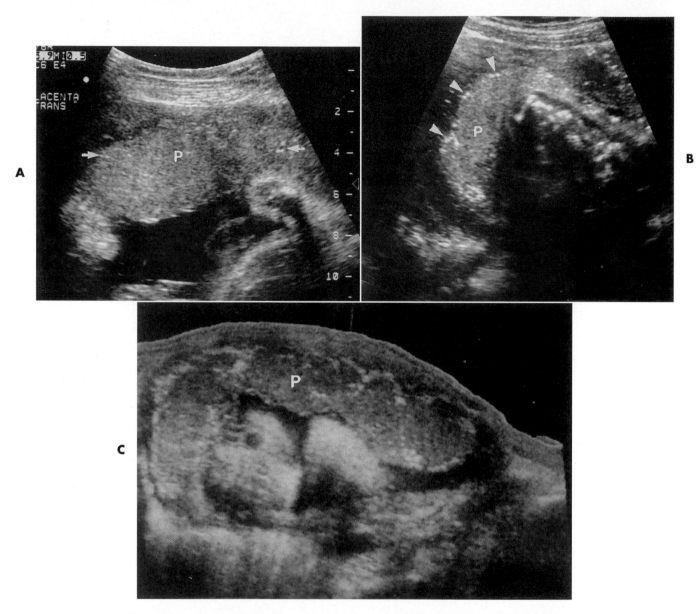

Fig. 15-5   Placental calcifications in normally maturing placentas. **A,** Grade 1 changes in a 31-week pregnancy. This transaxial image of an anterior placenta *(P)* shows small intraplacental hyperechoic foci (some shown by arrows) scattered throughout the homogeneous, moderately hyperechoic placenta. **B,** Grade 2 changes at 32 weeks. This sagittal image of a fundal placenta *(P)* shows larger hyperechoic foci in a "dot-dash" configuration (some denoted by arrowheads) along the basilar plate. Intraplacental foci are also present. **C,** Grade 3 changes in a 36-week pregnancy. This static sagittal image through the right side of the uterus shows an anterior-fundal placenta *(P)* exhibiting long hyperechoic areas along the basilar plate and extending into the substance of the placenta, dividing the placenta into areas called *cotyledons.*

centa into areas called *cotyledons*. Grade 3 calcifications can cause significant shadowing, making the placental echogenicity appear falsely hypoechoic to anechoic; increased gain will reveal its normal echogenicity. Although not officially stated, the placental grade is defined by its most advanced area. For example, if the placenta is grade 1 in one area and grade 2 in another, the placenta is classified as grade 2.

These grade changes are considered normal if they are identified at expected gestational ages: grade 1, 30 weeks or later; grade 2, 32 weeks or later; and grade 3, 34 weeks or later. Not all placentas undergo these changes, however. Up to 40% do not progress beyond grade 0 to 1 changes, with 45% maturing to grade 2 and only 15% maturing to grade 3. The lack of calcific changes is not significant, but, if calcifications occur too early, this may signify placental dysmaturity and possible growth retardation. More work is needed to elucidate the significance of these changes. This is also discussed in Chapter 8.

TROPHOTROPISM

Trophotropism is a unifying concept that explains the occurrence of unusual placental shapes, eccentric umbilical cord insertions, and changes in placental position (particularly in relation to the internal cervical os). Initially the placenta forms as a rounded disc, with the umbilical cord at its center, and each portion of the placenta attaches to its underlying endometrium. If there is equal and good vascularity furnished to all these attachments, the placenta remains unchanged in position throughout pregnancy. If, however, the blood supply is unequal, preferential trophoblastic villi will then proliferate into adjacent regions where the endometrial blood supply is better, with villous atrophy occurring in areas of poorer vascularity. The poorest vascularity is typically (but not always) in the lower uterine segment, in areas of uterine scarring, and near large fibroids.

In these conditions placental remodeling or trophotropism results, and the following changes can then take place:

1. The placenta can shift relative to the umbilical cord insertion, leaving an eccentrically situated cord insertion. The insertion site may then be anywhere from the placental center to its edge (a marginal insertion). In the most extreme cases the placenta may be remodeled so much that the cord insertion site may be outside the placental margin (termed a *velamentous cord insertion*).
2. Unusual placental shapes, including a bilobed placenta, can occur. Rarely a portion of the placenta (a succenturiate lobe) can separate from the main placental body.

3. A placenta previa can resolve in as little as a month. Sometimes fetal blood vessels remain over the internal cervical os, and this is termed a *vasa previa*. This is discussed later in the chapter.

THE UMBILICAL CORD

The umbilical cord is identified in the first trimester, and can therefore be readily evaluated throughout the second and third trimesters. Although its analysis is not part of the routine obstetric examination, basic knowledge of umbilical cord processes is important. They can be divided into six groups: placental insertion, cord length and twists, number of vessels, focal abnormalities, cord position, and fetal insertion.

The insertion of the umbilical cord into the placenta is considered normal if it is within the placental substance (Figs. 15-3 and 15-6). When the insertion site is marginal or velamentous, the umbilical cord's arteries and vein are connected by a pedicle to the placenta, covered by the chorioamniotic membrane. Typically asymptomatic during the pregnancy, a fetal catastrophe can develop at delivery, as these vessels are prone to rupture. In addition, a marginal or velamentous cord insertion near the internal os can fix the umbilical cord and, at delivery, cause it to present in front of the fetus. Called an *obligate cord presentation*, this can lead to cord prolapse, with potential loss of circulation to the fetus. Finally, a vasa previa may arise if these fetal vessels cross the internal os.

The umbilical cord length is also important. Cords that are too long or too short have been associated with problems of fetal circulation and fetal position. At present cord length cannot be measured accurately. Umbilical cord twists are normal, and the more uncommon untwisted cords have been found to be associated with a higher incidence of fetal circulatory problems (Figs. 15-3 and 15-7). Further work is needed, however, to determine the full extent of this risk.

The number of umbilical blood vessels has prognostic importance. This is easy to assess with a transaxial image of the cord, provided an adequate amount of amniotic fluid is present. More than 90% of singleton gestations have a normal three-vessel cord—two arteries and one vein (see Fig. 15-1, *B*). In the other 10% only two vessels (one artery and one vein) are identified (Fig. 15-8). Because it has been estimated that up to 50% of the pregnancies with two-vessel cords are associated with fetal structural abnormalities and growth retardation, a thorough fetal ultrasound evaluation is necessary, including evaluation of the posterior fossa, the face, and all the extremities, as well as a full cardiac examination.

The accurate diagnosis of a two-vessel cord, however, requires the identification of two vessels at three umbilical cord sites: near the placental insertion, in its middle,

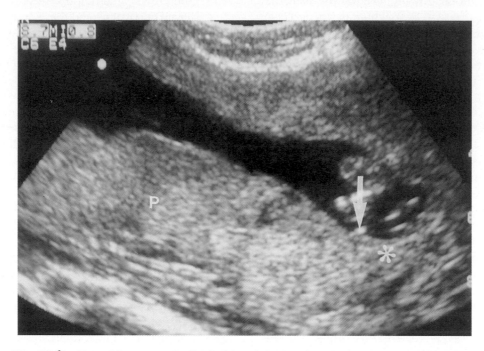

Fig. 15-6   Normal, but eccentrically placed, umbilical cord insertion *(arrow)*. On this sagittal oblique image, the posterior placenta *(P)* extends into the lower uterine segment (on the right). The umbilical cord insertion is still within the placental substance; an asterisk indicates the lower edge of the placenta.

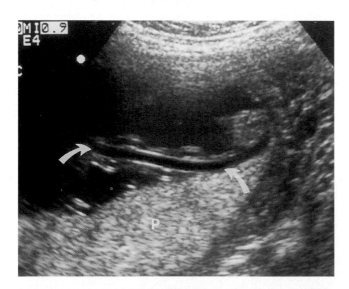

Fig. 15-7   "Untwisted" umbilical cord. Transaxial image of a posterior placenta *(P)*. Within the adjacent umbilical cord, a long segment of the umbilical vein *(curved arrows)* can be seen that does not exhibit its usual twisted appearance.

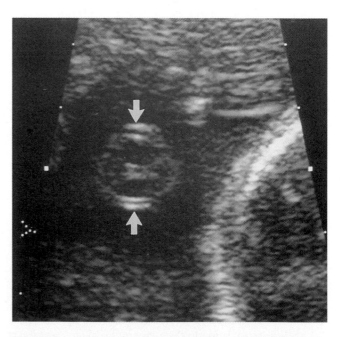

Fig. 15-8   Two-vessel umbilical cord. Transaxial image of the umbilical cord in its midposition *(arrows)* shows only one artery and one vein. Note the equal size of the artery and vein. In this case, there were no associated fetal anomalies.

and near the fetus. If the umbilical cord has two vessels in one part (most commonly near the placenta), with reconstitution to three vessels in the rest (most commonly near the fetus), then it is a normal three-vessel cord. An evaluation of the two fetal perivesicular (hypogastric) arteries can sometimes be helpful; the absence of one perivesicular artery confirms the absence of one umbilical artery. In multiple gestations a two-vessel cord is more common, and is actually a normal variant; nevertheless, some examiners still advocate a more careful fetal evaluation when this is discovered.

Diffuse cord abnormalities can occasionally be detected. The normal cord is usually less then 2 cm in overall diameter. An increase is most often caused by an excessive amount of the normal Wharton's jelly, and has been reported in the settings of maternal diabetes mellitus, fetal hydrops (secondary to edema), and rarely urachal (urine) extravasation. Umbilical blood vessel enlargement has not been reported.

Focal cord masses can be identified. These usually form close to the fetal insertion, are typically cystic (avascular), and usually represent either a focal thickening of Wharton's jelly (often associated with an omphalocele) or a developmental anomaly (e.g., allantoic duct or urachal remnants) (Fig. 15-9). Hematomas have also been reported. Rarely the cystic remnant of a blighted twin (from a di-

chorionic pregnancy) may arise adjacent to the placental insertion.

A hemangioma is the most common focal vascular cord anomaly. It typically has a uniform low-level echogenicity, similar to that of bowel-containing omphaloceles, and, if adjacent to the fetal body, could be a pitfall in the diagnosis of an anterior abdominal wall defect. Doppler waveform analysis is rarely of value, as the blood flow in the hemangioma is typically too slow to be detected (similar to the characteristics of hemangiomas elsewhere). If high flow is detected, particularly arterial, a rare vascular tumor could be present, and could put the fetus at risk for high-output failure.

The umbilical cord floats freely within the amniotic fluid and is often close to the fetus. It is common to identify the cord near the fetus' neck. It is also normal for the cord to fully encircle (or more) the neck at birth (20% of deliveries) without abnormal sequelae (Fig. 15-10). Therefore, although a nuchal cord is defined as at *least* encircling the neck once (confirmed by scanning the neck in the long axis and identifying two cross-sectional loops of cord), most observers *neither* look for *nor* report nuchal cords. Nevertheless, if the cord is fortuitously found to indent the soft tissues of the neck, this should be monitored as a sign of potential cord tightening.

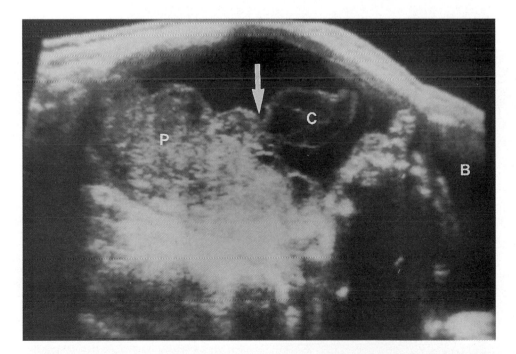

Fig. 15-9 Umbilical cord cystic *(C)* structure, diagnosed at birth as an allantoic duct remnant (a developmental anomaly). This static long-axis image of the gravid uterus shows a complex, predominantly cystic structure at the base of the umbilical cord, at its insertion *(arrow)* into a posterior-fundal placenta *(P)*. The remainder of the umbilical cord was normal. *B*, urinary bladder.

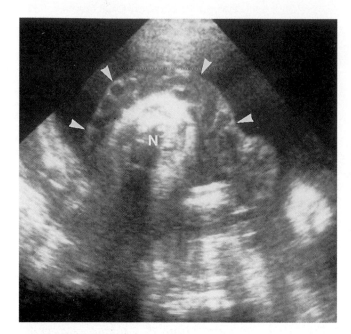

Fig. 15-10 Nuchal cord, identified as an incidental finding near term. Surrounding the fetal neck *(N)* in a transaxial view is a nuchal cord *(arrowheads)* encircling the neck more than 360 degrees. The fetus was delivered normally without incident.

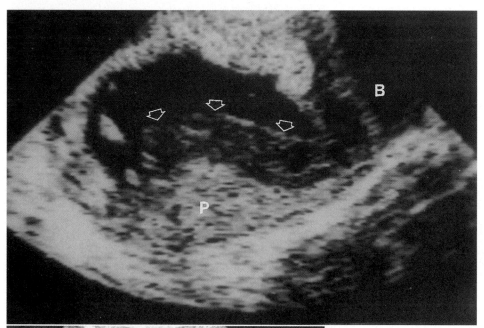

A

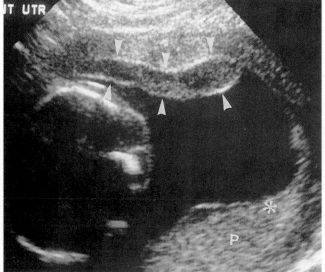

B

Fig. 15-11 Subacute subchorionic and submembranous bleeds in two different early third-trimester cases. Both images show the bleed to be hyperechoic and inhomogeneous. **A,** Subchorionic bleed. Long-axis image of the posterior placenta *(P)* shows a large collection (below the open arrows) that has stripped the chorionic plate from the underlying placenta. *B,* urinary bladder. **B,** Submembranous bleed. Transaxial image of the uterus shows a posterior placenta *(P)*. A collection *(arrowheads)* is noted on the anterior uterine surface, far away from the placental margin (*).

BLEEDING OCCURRING IN OR AROUND THE PLACENTA

Because the placenta is a very vascular organ, bleeding can occur spontaneously. Less commonly, iatrogenic bleeding can be caused by an intentional placental puncture for the purpose of biopsy or transfusion, or by an inadvertent or unavoidable placental puncture during amniocentesis. Regardless of the cause, the bleeding can occur at four sites. Three are directly related to the placenta, and these are subchorionic, intraplacental, and retroplacental. Retroplacental hemorrhages occur within the basilar plate and are also called *placental abruption* or *abruptio placentae*. The fourth type, a submembranous bleed, extends below the chorioamniotic membrane, similar to a subchorionic bleed, but in areas not directly related to the placenta; it is probably an extension of one of the other three types. Large bleeds commonly involve more than one area.

Blood classically evolves through three phases: in the acute phase it is hypoechoic to anechoic, in the subacute phase it is hyperechoic and inhomogeneous (as it organizes), and in the chronic phase it reverts to being hypoechoic to anechoic (as it lyses). Because bleeds can clot within minutes, the first observable phase may be a subacute hemorrhage. An occasionally helpful technique to prove a recent (acute) bleed is to bounce the transducer directly over the suspected area. If it quivers like jello or is compressible, then the blood has not yet organized. Rarely, blood entering an area of acutely active bleeding can swirl or spurt depending on the extent of its venous and arterial supply.

Subchorionic and submembranous bleeds are common (Figs. 15-11 and 15-12). They are usually of no clinical consequence, *unless* associated with the other two types. They are also asymptomatic *unless* vaginal bleeding is present. These bleeds range widely in size, from small localized collections to complete separation of the membranes from their attachment. There have been no reported cases of impaired fetal circulation resulting from even a subchorionic bleed that extends to the base of the umbilical cord. Their differential diagnoses include cysts (perhaps the sequelae of prior bleeds) and normal intervillous connections.

Women with abruptions (retroplacental bleeds) usually present with vaginal bleeding or significant pelvic pain, or both, and with tenderness over the uterus, sometimes localized to the region of the abruption. There can, however, be other causes for the same clinical symptoms: pain can result from a degenerating fibroid or adnexal torsion and bleeding can stem from a cervical abnormality such as polyps. Nevertheless, abruption must be considered seriously because of its potential to cause morbidity in the fetus and rarely in the mother. Concern should be

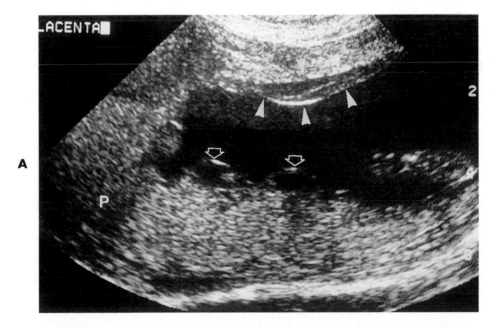

Fig. 15-12   Combined subchorionic and submembranous bleeds in two different cases. **A,** Acute bleed in a 25-week pregnancy. This long-axis image of a posterior-fundal placenta *(P)* shows small anechoic collections in the subchorionic region *(open arrows)* and a hypoechoic collection in the submembranous area *(arrowheads)*. When the transducer was bounced, both areas quivered, a finding consistent with an acute bleed.   *Continued.*

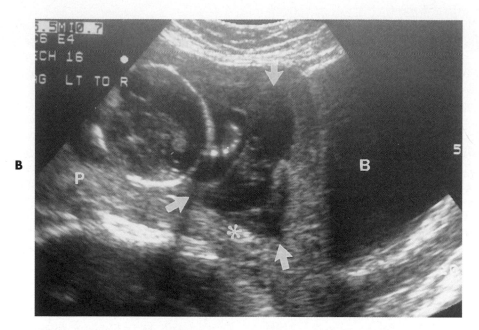

Fig. 15-12, cont'd.   **B,** Subacute to chronic collection *(arrows)* in the lower uterine segment of an 18-week pregnancy. On this long-axis view, the posterior placenta *(P)* extends into the lower uterine segment, its lower-most margin denoted by an asterisk. The bleed is in both the subchorionic and submembranous areas. *B,* urinary bladder.

heightened in the predisposing clinical settings of maternal hypertension, collagen vascular disease, and abdominal trauma. If the retroplacental hematoma remains in its initial basilar plate position, the bleed can range from a small focal to a large extensive collection (Fig. 15-13). If the blood dissects into other areas, its appearance varies. If the blood is predominantly expelled (by means of vaginal bleeding), the hematoma may shrink, occasionally so extensively that the placenta and surrounding area may appear normal. As already stated, the echogenicity of a hematoma is variable, from anechoic to hyperechoic. If it is isoechoic (a rare occurrence), it may make the placenta seem falsely enlarged (Fig. 15-14).

Bleeding may infrequently occur within the placental substance. Although these bleeds can exhibit variable echogenicity, they are typically less hyperechoic than the placenta. Unless a large portion of the placenta is involved, these bleeds should not limit fetal growth. If associated with retroplacental bleeds (a common occurrence), they can be more serious (see Fig. 15-13, *B*).

Hemorrhages near the chorionic plate can extend between and separate the amnion from the chorion. They can even enter the amniotic fluid (Fig. 15-15). In the first trimester bleeds can even cause the endometrial canal to distend (Figs. 15-16). The prognosis for any hemorrhage depends on its site and extent.

Bleeds can also recur and enlarge. Therefore, in the event of *any* clinically or sonographically suspected bleed, even with normal-appearing ultrasound findings, a follow-up study within 2 to 4 weeks is always indicated.

Doppler waveform analysis may prove to be of value in this setting. Because the maternal blood flow (through the spiral arteries) can be considerably disrupted, particularly in the setting of retroplacental or intraplacental bleeds, analysis of the maternal arterial waveforms in the basilar plate would seem important (see Fig. 15-13, *C*). Umbilical artery or intrafetal Doppler waveform analysis could also be of value in determining whether there is fetal compromise. More complete study of the use of Doppler analysis in the evaluation of placental bleeds is needed, however, before its true sensitivity and positive predictive value in this setting are known.

It is known that, when maternal serum α-fetoprotein *(MS-AFP)* levels are markedly elevated (≥5 multiples of the median), the risk of spontaneous fetal loss and growth retardation is increased. Some observers have found there is an association of all types of placental hemorrhage with elevated *MS-AFP* levels, and it has been postulated that any placental abnormality can increase fetal–maternal blood connections, and therefore *MS-AFP* levels.

PLACENTA ACCRETA, INCRETA, AND PERCRETA

The placenta normally attaches into the endometrium, with the intact endometrium serving as a barrier to deeper placental (trophoblastic) extension. If there is deficient endometrial decidua, there is an increased risk for further invasion. This can occur secondary to scarring

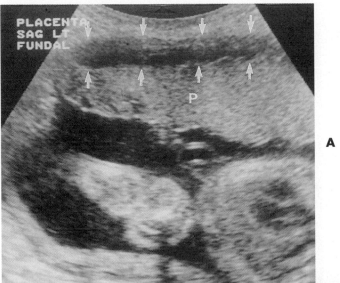

A

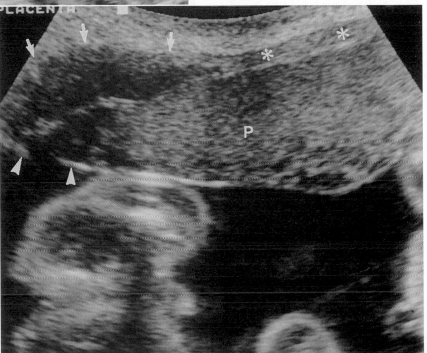

B

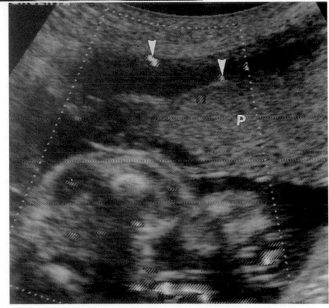

C

Fig. 15-13 Two cases of placental abruption in the mid–third trimester. **A,** A chronic anechoic retroplacental collection is noted on this long-axis image of the left uterine fundus. The anterior placenta *(P)* has been separated from the basilar plate and replaced by an anechoic collection *(arrows)*. This patient presented with mild pain over this area, without vaginal bleeding. **B** and **C,** Acute retroplacental bleed with extension into the intraplacental and subchorionic regions seen in two similar long-axis images of the anterior placenta *(P)*. In **B,** although the basilar plate in the uterine body is normal *(*)*, it is replaced by a large anechoic area at its fundal edge *(arrows)*. This bleed extends through the placental substance to the chorionic plate *(arrowheads)*. In **C** a gray-scale picture of a color flow Doppler evaluation shows only two areas of blood flow in the region of the abruption *(arrowheads)*, one at the outer edge of the basilar plate, now far removed from the placenta (on the left), and the other at the inner placental margin (on the right). This patient presented with vaginal bleeding; the fetus continued to grow and was delivered normally 8 weeks later.

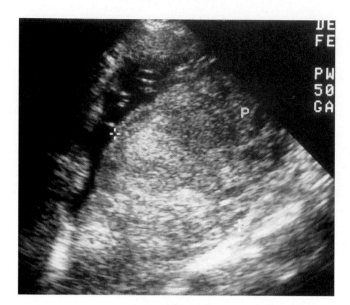

Fig. 15-14   Subacute placental abruption in a 38-week pregnancy. A sagittal image obtained to the right of midline shows a normal posterior placenta *(P)* in the uterine body. In the fundus the placenta is elevated and replaced by a heterogeneous (almost isoechoic) "mass" (+). This hemorrhage was initially misinterpreted to be an enlarged heterogeneous placenta.

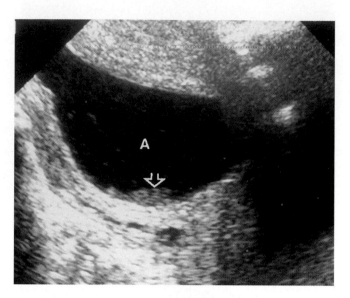

Fig. 15-15   Intraamniotic hemorrhage secondary to an attempted amniocentesis. Small hyperechoic foci (blood) are identified within the amniotic fluid *(A),* immediately after the margin of an anterior placenta (not shown) was inadvertently punctured. Some of the blood formed a clump in the most dependent portion of the amniotic cavity *(open arrow).*

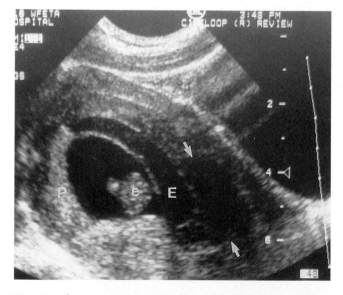

Fig. 15-16   First-trimester hemorrhage in a woman presenting with vaginal bleeding. This sagittal scan of the uterus shows an acute anechoic bleed in the submembranous region *(arrows)* anteriorly and within the endometrial canal *(E).* A living embryo *(e)* within the gestational sac and an uninvolved posterior fundal placenta *(P)* are also identified.

from previous cesarean sections or from endometrial canal instrumentation, and is defined as invasion *to* (accreta), *into* (increta), or *through* (percreta) the myometrium. Although not part of the definition, the intervening decidua basalis must also be invaded.

This penetration would prevent the placenta from separating normally during delivery, which would lead to extensive bleeding. Although the obstetrician may attempt a manual removal of the placenta, a hysterectomy is usually needed. With prior knowledge of the problem, delivery strategies can be planned to avoid an emergency operation.

The most common predisposing risk profile for this invasion is a history of a previous cesarean section, usually a low transverse incision, together with sonographic evidence of an anterior placenta and placenta previa. Considerable attention must be paid to the uterine hypoechoic myometrial-basilar layer in these women, particularly in the region of the anterior lower uterine segment (Fig. 15-17, *A*). If the hypoechoic layer cannot be identified adequately, or is present more superiorly but not inferiorly, this should raise suspicion of this abnormality. Transabdominal (TA) studies have shown that adequate urinary bladder distention is needed to orient the anterior lower uterine segment perpendicular to the transducer so that the serosal uterine surface can be studied.

The classic ultrasound finding indicating trophoblastic penetration is disruption or loss of the normal hypo-

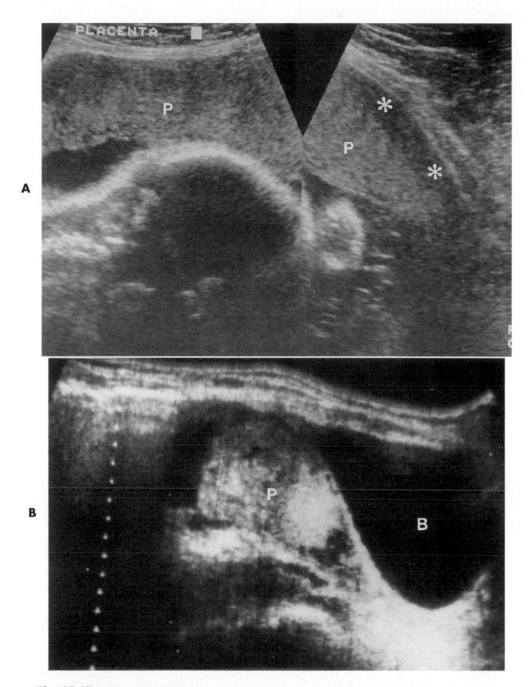

Fig. 15-17   Two transabdominal cases of anterior low-lying placentas, both in a sagittal view. **A,** Normal. An anterior placenta *(P)* is identified with its normal hypoechoic myometrial-basilar layer *(*)* in the lower uterine segment. **B,** Placenta accreta in a patient who had had a previous cesarean section. The anterior placenta *(P)* is inhomogeneous and bulky, and extends to the surface of the distended urinary bladder *(B).* The myometrial-basilar layer is obliterated.

echoic myometrial-basilar layer (Fig. 15-17, *B*). The additional detection of a thinned or interrupted serosa, focal masses, and prominent irregular venous spaces at or near the point of invasion further suggests the presence of this invasion. Although further differentiation of accreta from increta and percreta is not currently possible, interruption of the serosal surface makes either of these latter two, particularly percreta, more likely. Transvaginal (TV) ultrasound and Doppler imaging have not, at present, shown increased diagnostic accuracy.

PLACENTAL THICKNESS

Placental thickness normally decreases with increasing fetal age, with the midportion of a normal placenta remaining thicker than 2 cm. Abnormally thinned placentas are usually caused by maternal systemic vascular problems, that is, insulin-dependent diabetes, collagen vascular diseases (particularly the more severe cases due to microinfarctions), and severe hypertension, either essential or pregnancy induced. Because in theory, if not in practice, a thin placenta could lead to insufficient fetal nutrition and oxygenation, the fetus in such circumstances should be considered at risk for growth retardation and hypoxia. In the setting of marked polyhydramnios, the placenta can appear falsely thinned as it is stretched along the inner surface of an enlarged uterus.

Enlarged placentas (>4 cm thick) are most common in fetal hydrops. This can occur in the settings of blood group incompatibilities (immune hydrops), congenital anemias, particularly α-thalassemia, and congenital infections, particularly syphilitic and viral (nonimmune hydrops) (Fig. 15-18). Gestational maternal diabetes mellitus, for unknown reasons, can also cause an enlarged placenta, and this is commonly associated with a macrosomic fetus and polyhydramnios. In all cases follow-up studies are indicated to assess potential fetal problems. The placenta can appear falsely thickened in an isoechoic abruption or secondary to a contraction, the thickness in these instances more likely focal or transient, or both. Trophoblastic abnormalities (not to be confused with an enlarged placenta) are discussed later in the chapter.

UTERINE CONTRACTIONS

Myometrial contractions are common and can occur at any time during pregnancy. They are more likely to be focal in the first and second trimesters, becoming more generalized (Braxton Hicks) as term approaches.

Contractions can occur at any place within the uter-

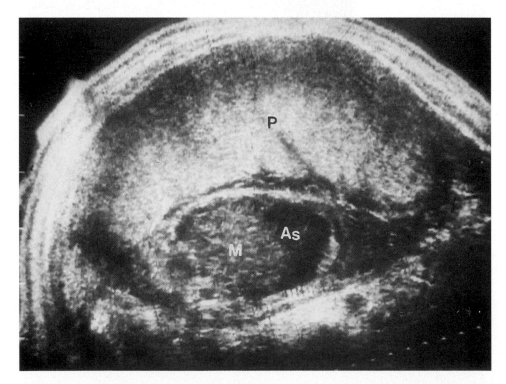

Fig. 15-18   Markedly enlarged placenta, secondary to α-thalassemia (a congenital anemia), in a 32-week pregnancy. A static transaxial image of the uterus shows a markedly enlarged placenta *(P)* that is 8 cm thick. A living fetus with hydropic changes is also noted, with ascites *(As)* displacing normal mesentery *(M)*; the fetus died at term.

ine wall. They are typically seen as rounded "masses" that are more hypoechoic than the placenta, and bulge into the amniotic space *without* changing the outer uterine contour (Fig. 15-19). Contractions are usually obvious and easy to differentiate from fibroids, which are typically more inhomogeneous and frequently distort the outer uterine contour. If located below the placenta, the contractions cause the placenta to bow into the amniotic space. If a contraction occurs in the lower uterine segment or cervix, when there is a low-positioned placenta, a placenta previa may be diagnosed incorrectly.

Contractions last variable amounts of time, from 5 minutes to rarely more than 1 hour, and usually do not need follow-up. However, if an "abnormality" is detected that could be a contraction (and uncertainty exists), a repeat study within 30 minutes can often show sufficient change to confirm the diagnosis. If the area persists, a longer interval of time, even an ultrasound study on another day, may infrequently be needed.

PLACENTA PREVIA

Placenta previa occurs in 1 in 200 to 400 deliveries and is more common in pregnancies after a cesarean section has been performed in an earlier pregnancy. It is a clinical term used at the time of delivery to define the position of the placenta in relation to the dilated and effaced cervix. By palpation and visualization, a low placental im-

plantation is found to encroach on the dilated *external* os in one of three ways: in a marginal previa the placenta extends to the edge of the os, in a partial previa the placenta partially covers the os, and in a complete previa the os is totally covered.

These terms have been modified in an attempt to make them applicable in the ultrasound diagnosis of placenta previa in utero (Fig. 15-20). With the closed *internal* cervical os (of the nondilated cervix) as the landmark, three ultrasound-based definitions are used: a low-lying placenta in which the placenta approaches but does not cover the os, a marginal previa in which the placenta extends to the edge but does not cross the os, and a complete previa in which the placenta extends over and for some distance beyond the internal os. The in utero distinction between a marginal and a partial previa is too subtle, and these terms are used interchangeably. A fourth type, a central previa, is a form of complete previa in which the placenta completely covers and is located centrally over the internal os. The definitions of all these terms are somewhat inexact and their meanings overlap. For example, it is not possible to consistently differentiate a marginal previa from a complete previa.

Two questions need to be asked. Because the cervix is closed (neither dilated nor effaced) during pregnancy, can ultrasound accurately detect a placenta previa? And, if placenta previa is detected in utero, can ultrasound predict whether it will be present at birth? The answer to both questions is "yes," provided a proper scanning technique

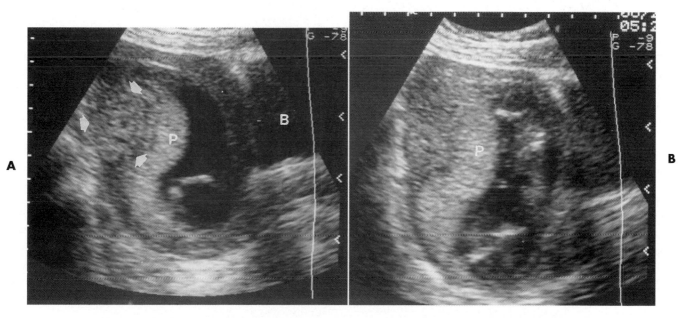

Fig. 15-19   Uterine contraction in the early second trimester. Two long-axis midline views of the uterus. **A,** On the initial study a hypoechoic contraction *(arrows)* has caused the posterior fundal placenta *(P)* to bulge into the amniotic space. Note that the outer uterine contour, toward the left, is unaffected. *B,* urinary bladder. **B,** Thirty minutes later there is a significant decrease in the size of the contraction. *P,* placenta.

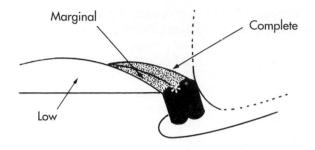

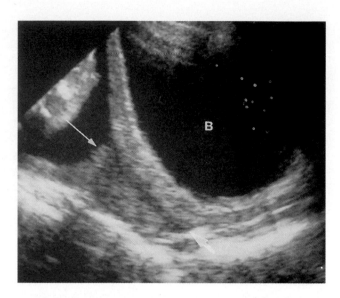

Fig. 15-21 Normal closed cervix in utero, identified by the transabdominal full-bladder technique in a 24-week pregnancy. A midline sagittal scan through a distended urinary bladder *(B)* shows the entire cervix. The closed internal os *(small arrow)*, the external os *(large arrow),* and the interposed thin hypoechoic endocervical canal are identified. In this case the cervix is not compressed by the distended urinary bladder.

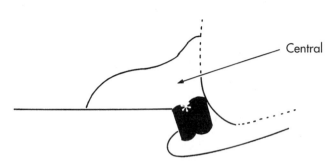

Fig. 15-20 In utero representation of a low-lying placenta and of three types of placenta previa. The upper diagram shows a low-lying placenta and both a marginal and complete placenta previa in relation to the closed cervix (shown in black) with an asterisk at the internal os. The lower diagram shows a central previa.

is used and trophotropism is taken into account. At any time in the pregnancy and using any technique, the finding of a placenta positioned *superior* to the lower uterine segment is an assurance that no previa will take place at any time during that pregnancy.

The lower uterine segment can be evaluated by the TA full-bladder technique, the TA empty-bladder technique, the TV empty-bladder technique, and the translabial (TL) empty-bladder technique. Although the TA approach should be attempted first, it is limited by its inability to always identify the internal cervical os (Fig. 15-21). In the second trimester, because the fetus is small relative to the amount of amniotic fluid, the os can usually be detected; as the pregnancy progresses, the fetus becomes relatively larger and frequently obscures this region. "Too much" placental tissue or "elevation" of the fetal parts in the lower uterine segment, or both, are diagnostic of a low-lying placenta and a probable placenta previa (Fig. 15-22). Placing the woman in the Trendelenburg position (head down) or pushing the fetus cephalad with gentle suprapubic transabdominal pressure, or the use of both maneuvers, may help in the identification of the internal os.

A full urinary bladder is valuable when performing TA

ultrasound because the bladder provides a sonic window for the visualization of all adjacent structures (including the lower uterine segment and cervix) and often displaces the fetus cephalad. However, the distended bladder can also compress and elongate both the cervix and the lower uterine segment, making them appear as one, as an elongated cervix (Fig. 15-23). A low-lying placenta can then falsely appear to abut on the cervix. This mistake can usually be prevented because the cervix then looks and measures too long. The length of the nondistorted cervix, measured along the endocervical canal from the internal to external os, varies with gestational age. Although the upper limit has not been fully worked out, it should typically not be longer than 5 cm (Table 15-1).

In the event of poor visualization or when a falsely elongated cervix is suspected, an empty-bladder technique should be used (Figs. 15-23 and 15-24). The TA examination can be repeated, with scans performed through the amniotic fluid, usually in a sagittal view angled downward from just below the umbilicus. However, the findings obtained by the TA empty-bladder technique can be difficult to interpret. Because the cervix then assumes a more vertical orientation and is more rounded, even a skilled examiner on occasion may have difficulty in its identification.

Therefore, if for either technical or anatomic reasons a previa can still not be ruled out, a TL or TV examination should then be performed. A midline sagittal scan with an empty urinary bladder can identify the internal cervi-

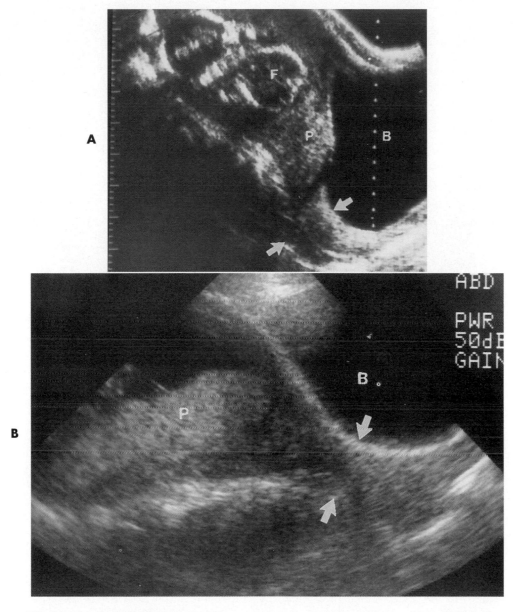

Fig. 15-22   Two transabdominal midline sagittal scans obtained in different patients. In both there is "too much" placenta overlying the lower uterine segment and cervix. The internal os is not identi-fied clearly. **A,** In this 20-week pregnancy the fetus *(F)* is displaced cephalad by a large amount of low-lying placenta *(P)*. The area of the cervix is denoted by arrows. *B,* urinary bladder. A central previa was present at birth. **B,** In this 28-week pregnancy a posterior low-lying placenta *(P)* overlies the area of the cervix *(arrows)*. A marginal previa was present at term. *B,* urinary bladder.

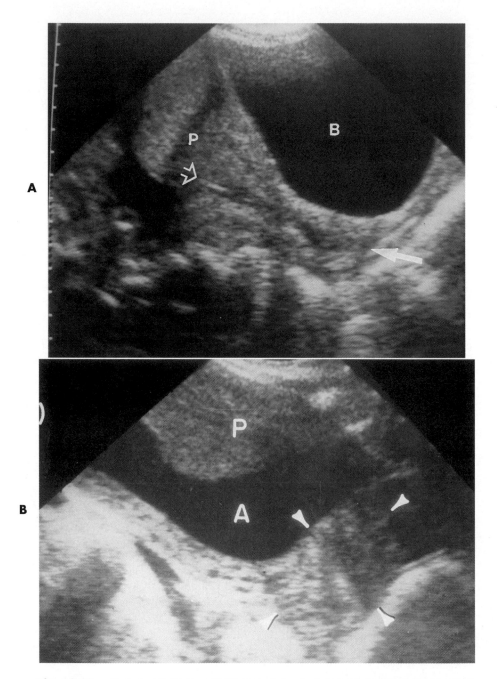

Fig. 15-23   Technical limitation of the transabdominal distended urinary bladder technique in a 32-week pregnancy. **A,** Sagittal midline scan through a distended urinary bladder *(B)*. The cervix and lower uterine segment are pressed together, making the anterior placenta *(P)* appear to be a placenta previa. With the large arrow denoting the external cervical os and the open arrow denoting the superior end of the compressed lower uterine segment, the entire length of 9 cm is too long for this to be a normal cervix. **B,** Sagittal midline scan after the urinary bladder is completely emptied. The nondistended cervix *(arrowheads)* can now be identified through the amniotic fluid *(A)*. The internal os is clearly separate from the anterior placenta *(P)*. Because the urinary bladder is empty, the cervix is now more squared and oriented more vertically.

cal os and lower uterine segment, and is almost always the only image needed to determine if a previa is present. Usually the bladder will still have some residual distention despite the sensation of an empty bladder, the small bladder providing a useful anatomic landmark. The TL approach should be attempted first because it is less invasive (Fig. 15-25). It involves placing the transducer on the perineum, on or outside the labia. If needed, the TV probe can then be used (Fig. 15-26). However, in cases of active bleeding and a suspected previa (or a cervical abnormality), care should be taken not to insert the TV probe too close to the external os. This is typically not a problem as the probe is usually inserted only halfway into the vagina.

Because trophotropism can cause significant changes in placental position, a previa is usually not formally diagnosed before 20 weeks (unless symptoms are present). When detected after 20 weeks, a follow-up study should be performed between 34 to 36 weeks (within 1 month of delivery) to determine if the previa is still present. If a woman is symptomatic, particularly presenting with vaginal bleeding, more frequent ultrasound studies are often necessary.

Blood vessels can be detected over the internal cervical os. Most occur at the margins of a low-positioned placenta and are caused by juxtaplacental or marginal

sinus blood vessels (Fig. 15-27). Some, however, stem from the fetal circulation as a marginal or velamentous umbilical cord insertion or a succenturiate lobe (if the vessels cross the internal os). While any may cause problems at birth, the ones from the fetal circulation may cause significant fetal blood loss at the time of delivery, even in an otherwise uncomplicated pregnancy. Blood vessels crossing the internal os can often be detected by ultrasound and, if needed, confirmed by Doppler examination.

Table 15-1   Cervical length*

Diagnosis	Cervical length (cm)
Upper limit of normal	5.0
Average	4.0
Lower limit of normal	3.0
Pathologically decreased	2.0

*Nondistorted cervix (measurements obtained with an empty maternal bladder). The cervical length is measured along the endocervical canal, from the external to internal cervical os.

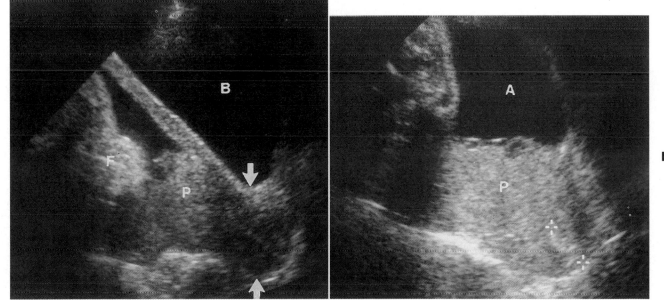

Fig. 15-24   Complete placenta previa, both before and after the urinary bladder is empty. These transabdominal midline scans were obtained in a 35-week pregnancy. **A,** The area of the cervix *(arrows)* is imaged incompletely through the distended urinary bladder *(B).* A posterior low-lying placenta *(P)* with an apparent complete previa is identified. The fetus *(F)* is displaced superiorly. **B,** After complete emptying of the urinary bladder, scans are obtained from just below the umbilicus through the amniotic fluid *(A).* The hyperechoic endocervical canal is more clearly identified (+) and a complete previa is confirmed. *P,* placenta.

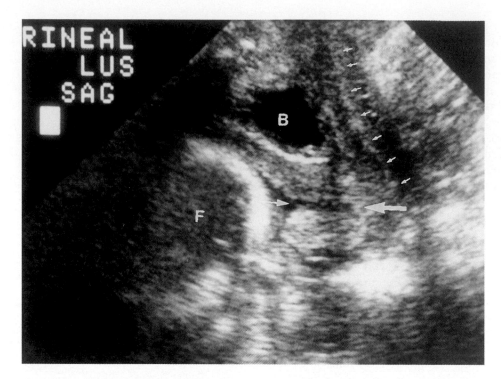

Fig. 15-25 Normal translabial scan findings in a 26-week pregnancy. This sagittal midline scan with only a minimally distended urinary bladder *(B)* shows the vaginal canal *(small arrows)*. In this case (as is most common) the normal cervix is at a right angle to the vaginal canal. The hypoechoic endocervical canal is identified from the external os *(large arrow)* to the internal os *(small arrow)*. The fetal head *(F)* is adjacent to the internal os and no previa is present.

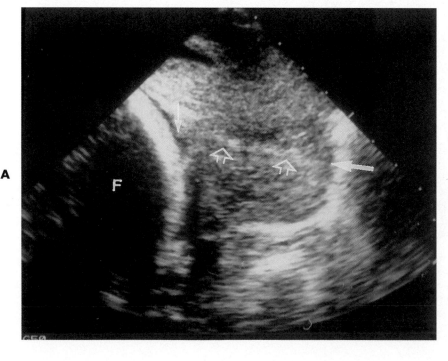

Fig. 15-26 Two transvaginal cases, both imaged with a midline sagittal scan. **A,** Normal findings in a 30-week pregnancy. The normal cervix is identified from the external os *(large arrow)* to the internal os *(small arrow)*. The open arrows denote a hyperechoic endocervical canal. The fetal head *(F)* is adjacent to the internal os and no previa is present.

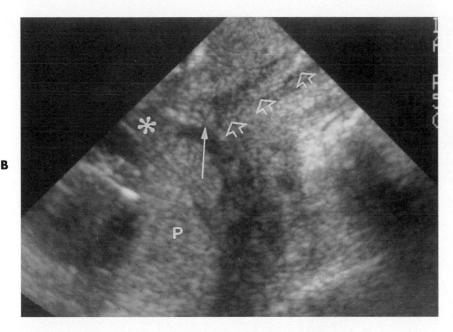

B

Fig. 15-26, cont'd.   B, Previa in a 32-week pregnancy. The hyperechoic endocervical canal *(open arrows)* and the internal os *(arrow)* are identified. A low-lying posterior placenta *(P)* extends over the internal os to the area of the asterisk. A marginal placenta previa is present. In this case (as is most common) the external os could not be identified.

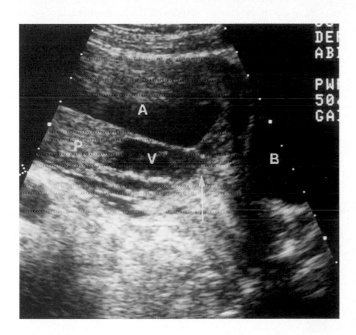

Fig. 15-27   Juxtaplacental or marginal sinus blood vessels at 34 gestational weeks. This transabdominal midline scan through a partially distended urinary bladder *(B)* and amniotic fluid *(A)* shows a low-lying posterior placenta *(P)*. Marginal sinus veins *(V)* cross from the lower edge of the placenta to the internal cervical os *(arrow)*. Blood could be seen moving within these veins on real-time evaluation.

THE CERVIX AND ITS EVALUATION FOR INCOMPETENCE

Ultrasound is able to identify the cervix and to evaluate it for possible incompetence. Although not mentioned in the guidelines, this analysis is important because incompetence increases the risk of preterm loss or delivery. Both the appearance and measurement of the cervix are important. A midline sagittal view is the optimal image for evaluating the cervix and for identifying its internal os, the thin hypoechoic (occasionally hyperechoic) endocervical canal, and, if possible, its external os (see Figs. 15-21, 15-25, and 15-26).

Normally the internal os is closed, with its "knuckles" apposed. In the event of incompetence, the cervical changes occur proximally to distally, with the internal os opening first. It is thought to be significantly dilated or spread when the os exceeds 1.0 cm in diameter (Fig. 15-28). The endocervical canal dilates next (from proximal to distal), thereby shortening the remaining cervical

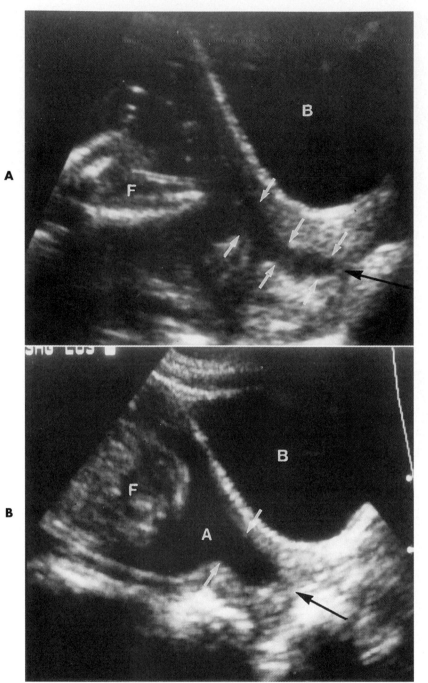

Fig. 15-28 Technical limitation in the evaluation of an incompetent cervix at 34 weeks. **A,** This sagittal midline transabdominal scan through a very distended urinary bladder *(B)* shows a falsely "closed" endocervical canal. It only appears slightly prominent *(arrows)*. Fetal parts *(F)* are identified in the lower uterine segment. *Large black arrow,* external os. **B,** After partial emptying of the urinary bladder *(B),* a markedly incompetent cervix is identified, extending from the widely spread internal os *(small arrows)* to within 1 cm of the external os *(black arrow)*. Amniotic fluid *(A)* enters the distended endocervical canal. Fetal parts *(F)* are again seen in the lower uterine segment.

length. Measured along its endocervical canal, the normal cervix averages 4.0 cm in length. The lowest acceptable length is 3.0 cm, and it is considered significantly (pathologically) shortened when it is only 2.0 cm long (see Table 15-1). Some observers have suggested also evaluating the lower uterine segment because its myometrium would be expected to "thin" before or in association with the cervical incompetence; this may be of value in subtle early cases, but more analysis is needed before its usefulness as a sign of incompetence is known.

In the event of more severe cervical incompetence, the endocervical canal opens fully and is replaced by anechoic amniotic fluid. Fetal parts and the umbilical cord can then descend into the dilated cervix (Fig. 15-29). If the cervix is maximally dilated, the entire endocervical canal opens to the external os and an "hourglass" deformity occurs in which the amniotic membranes are seen clinically to bulge into the vagina (Fig. 15-30). In these cases the appearance of the cervix, not its measurement, is most important.

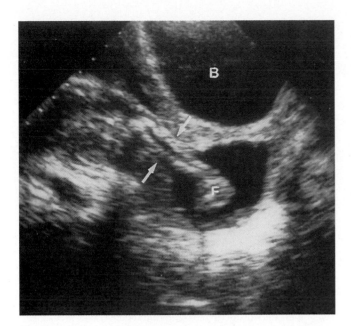

Fig. 15-29   An incompetent cervix. Transabdominal midline scan through a partially distended urinary bladder *(B)* shows a minimally compressed internal os *(arrows)*. The widely patent cervix, however, has allowed amniotic fluid and fetal parts *(F)* to enter the endocervical canal.

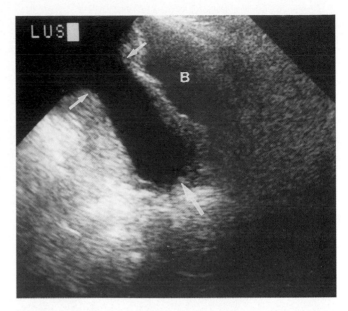

Fig. 15-30   The "hourglass" deformity of a severely incompetent cervix. Transabdominal midline scan through a minimally distended urinary bladder *(B)* in a 30-week pregnancy. The cervix is completely open from the internal os *(small arrows)* to the external os *(large arrow)*.

When incompetence is detected, the patient should *not* be moved. She should be ideally placed in a reverse Trendelenburg position, and the obstetrician notified immediately. In the event of an hourglass deformity, however, spontaneous pregnancy loss is usually imminent.

There is not always a correlation between the clinical and the ultrasound findings. This is understandable when one considers the different approaches of the examinations. Clinically the external os is identified and palpated, sonographically the internal os is imaged. When a "soft" cervix is diagnosed on physical examination by the introduction of a finger through the external os, the ultrasound findings may appear normal. On the other hand, the physical examination findings may be normal when ultrasound detects dilatation of the internal os and the proximal endocervical canal. In the latter case the clinician may not be overly concerned by the ultrasound findings, and may therefore be unwilling to act on them.

The TA full-bladder technique is often sufficient to make the diagnosis of incompetence. However, on occasion an incompetent cervix may appear normal (compressed, falsely closed, and even normal in length) because of the distended bladder (see Fig. 15-28). Therefore, if the patient has physical examination findings suggestive of incompetence or a history of incompetence in a past pregnancy, the findings yielded by the TA full-bladder examination may be misleading. The urinary bladder should then be emptied to allow a more complete evaluation of the cervix. Although a somewhat experimen-

tal maneuver, placing gentle pressure on the uterine fundus during cervical scanning may cause a compromised but closed cervix to open, thus confirming the diagnosis of incompetence.

Of the other two techniques, the TL empty-bladder study is usually preferred. It often images the entire cervix, including the external os, and the probe does not enter the vaginal canal (Fig. 15-31). When needed, however, an empty-bladder TV study, performed with the probe inserted into the midposition of the vagina, may yield additional information. Aggressive maneuvering of the probe, particularly deeper penetration, should be avoided.

When incompetence is suggested, particularly when subtle, follow-up studies at close intervals are needed. These patients may require bed rest, tocolytic medication to decrease uterine contractions, and a cerclage (surgical sutures placed around the cervix). These sutures are placed through the vagina, as high as possible around the proximal third of the cervix, to the level of the pars vaginalis. A cerclage is not possible, however, if fetal parts or umbilical cord are already present within the dilated cervical canal. Postoperatively the clinical examination findings become less precise. Ultrasound can then be used to evaluate the extent and possible progression of endocervical canal dilatation; the hyperechoic cerclage sutures can often be identified in these images (Fig. 15-32).

It is also important to evaluate the lower uterine segment and cervix for masses (i.e., fibroids). They may cause

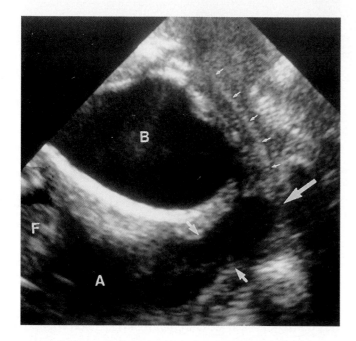

Fig. 15-31   Incompetent cervix detected by translabial scanning. In a 24-week pregnancy a sagittal midline scan obtained with a partially distended urinary bladder *(B)* shows the normal hyperechoic vaginal canal *(small arrows)*. The internal os *(medium-sized arrows)* is distended and there is amniotic fluid *(A)* entering a dilated endocervical canal. *Large arrow,* external os; *F,* fetal parts in the lower uterine segment.

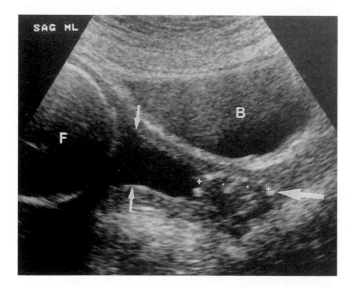

Fig. 15-32   Cerclage at 32 weeks. This transabdominal midline sagittal scan through a partially distended urinary bladder *(B)* shows hyperechoic sutures (+ and *dotted lines)* surrounding the lower part of the cervix. The cervix is closed from the cerclage to the external os *(large arrow)*. The proximal half of the cervix from the internal os *(arrows)* to the cerclage, however, is dilated and filled with amniotic fluid. *F,* fetal head in the lower uterine segment.

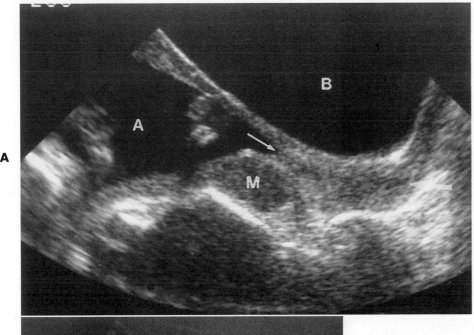

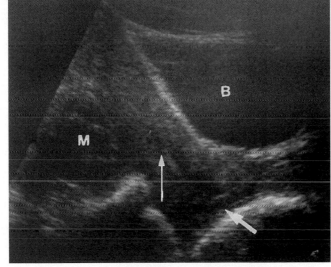

Fig. 15-33   Fibroids. Transabdominal midline sagittal scans, imaged through a distended urinary bladder *(B)*. **A,** Myoma *(M)* at 28 weeks. A small solid posterior mass is distorting the area of the lower uterine segment–cervix. The endocervical canal is identified from the internal os *(small arrow)* to the external os *(large arrow)*. *A,* amniotic fluid. **B,** Myoma *(M)* near term. A large hypoechoic solid mass is seen in the posterior body of the uterus, apparently narrowing the lower uterine segment. The cervix appears grossly normal, with the internal os *(small arrow)* and the external os *(large arrow)* identified.

obstruction (dystocia) to a normal delivery at term (Fig. 15-33). Cul-de-sac masses are usually ovarian in origin and, if large, can cause similar problems at birth.

HYDATIDIFORM MOLES AND HYDROPIC CHANGES

The clinical manifestations of a classic or complete hydatidiform mole are abnormal vaginal bleeding, hyperemesis gravidarum, preeclampsia, and occasionally thyrotoxicosis. Physical examination reveals a large-for-date uterus and rarely passage of vesicular tissue. The β subunit of human chorionic gonadotropin (βhCG) levels are markedly elevated.

Molar pregnancies are usually detected in the second and third trimesters (Fig. 15-34). They can, however, be discovered earlier. The ultrasound examination classically shows an enlarged uterus with uniformly hyperechoic tissue filling the endometrial canal. There is good through-transmission because of the multiple small cystic villi (hydropic changes), which are often too small to be identified. If these cystic spaces are large (>2 cm), they give the mole a more inhomogeneous appearance (Fig. 15-34, *A*). No fetus is seen. Pathologically a mole has three properties: hydropic swelling of the chorionic villi, absent or inadequate development of villous vascularization, and variable degrees of hyperplasia and anaplasia of the chorionic epithelium.

Hydatidiform moles are noninvasive in 85% of the cases and remain confined to the endometrial canal. Of the other 15%, 13% are locally invasive (termed *chorio-*

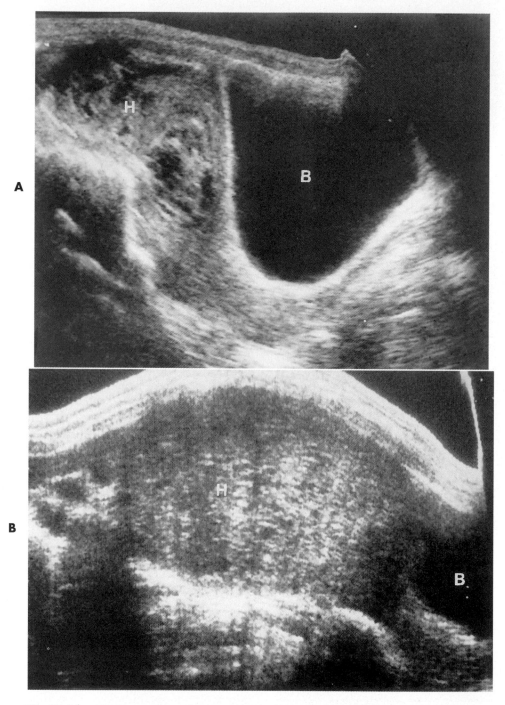

Fig. 15-34   Two cases of complete or classic hydatidiform moles *(H).* **A,** Static midline scan in an 18-week pregnancy shows a large inhomogeneous hyperechoic and hypoechoic mass filling and completely distending the endometrial canal. *B,* urinary bladder. **B,** Static sagittal midline scan in a 24-week pregnancy shows a large, uniformly hyperechoic mass with good through-transmission completely filling and distending the endometrial canal. *B,* urinary bladder. In neither case was a fetus identified.

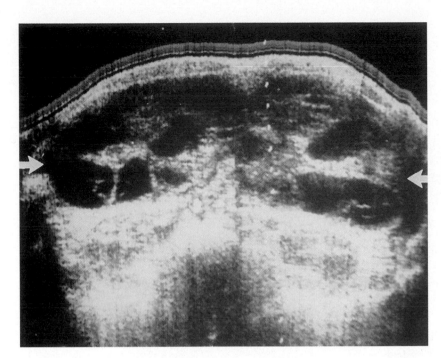

Fig. 15-35 Large theca-lutein cyst. This transaxial static image of the lower abdomen shows two large complex areas, with both cystic and solid components (their outer margins denoted by arrows), that is displaced out of the pelvis. The coexistent 18-week complete hydatidiform mole is not shown.

adenoma destruens) and extend into the myometrium. Only 2% metastasize as choriocarcinoma. Because of the clinical symptoms involved and their malignant potential, molar pregnancies are evacuated and observed closely for signs of recurrence by monitoring the βhCG levels.

In 50% of the molar pregnancies, coexistent multilocular ovarian cystic masses are identified. These are theca-lutein cysts and they can be unilateral or bilateral (Fig. 15-35). Theca-lutein cysts may occur de novo, but, when associated with a molar pregnancy, are commonly large. They can be so large as to be displaced out of the pelvis, above the uterus, and only identified by abdominal (not pelvic) scanning. There may be hemorrhage into any of the cystic components leading to changes in echogenicity. Ascites may also be present.

There are other types of trophoblastic pregnancies, and these consist of (1) two separate sacs, one representing a normal pregnancy and the other containing a complete mole; (2) a partial (incomplete) mole affecting part of the placenta with a coexisting living fetus (Fig. 15-36, *A*); and (3) hydropic degeneration of the placenta, either partial or complete, with a coexisting living fetus (Fig. 15-36, *B*, and 15-36, *C*). Although all can manifest similar symptoms and laboratory results, except without the passage of vesicular tissue, only the first possesses the significant malignant potential of a complete hydatidiform mole. Differentiation of the other two, the partial mole and the hydropic changes, may not be possible in utero. They both pose significant maternal problems during the pregnancy (preeclampsia or eclampsia) and at the time

of delivery (bleeding). Both are associated with significant potential fetal structural and chromosomal (particularly triploidy) abnormalities.

Molar and hydropic changes can be differentiated by careful pathologic evaluation. Placental hydrops does not exhibit the chorionic epithelial hyperplasia and anaplasia of a hydatidiform form.

Other abnormalities may infrequently mimic a partial hydatidiform mole or partial hydropic changes; these are an unresolved loculated abruptio placentae and an unusual-looking fibroid. Usually the clinical symptoms, physical examination findings, and βhCG levels will establish the difference. When uncertainty persists, chromosomal analysis and careful fetal evaluation may be indicated.

PLACENTAL INFARCTS

Placental infarcts can be solitary or multiple. Most are too small to be detected by ultrasound. When seen, they are classically hypoechoic and 1 to 2 cm in diameter. Some may be isoechoic or hyperechoic. All have a thick hyperechoic rim (Fig. 15-37).

The source of placental infarcts is not usually known, although they are more common in certain maternal vascular conditions such as collagen vascular diseases. If there are few infarcts, they should not impair fetal blood flow. If more than 50% of the placenta is affected, the pregnancy should be closely monitored for possible impaired fetal growth.

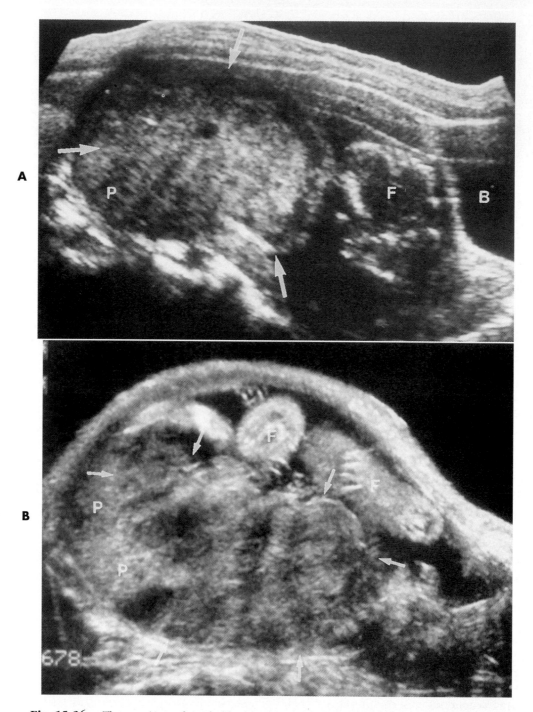

Fig. 15-36   Three variants of trophoblastic pregnancies. **A,** Partial (incomplete) mole with a co-existing living normal fetus. This static midline image in a 17-week pregnancy shows a normal posterior and fundal placenta *(P)*. A large bulky, predominantly hypoechoic and hyperechoic mass *(arrows)* is contiguous with the placenta. A normal fetus *(F)* is identified in the lower uterine segment. *B,* urinary bladder. **B,** Partial hydropic degeneration of the placenta with a coexisting living triploid fetus. This static sagittal image to the right of midline in a 28-week pregnancy shows part of a normal fundal placenta *(P)* with a large inhomogeneous mass *(arrows)* contiguous with the placenta. An abnormal living fetus (some of the limbs are shown by an F) is seen anteriorly.

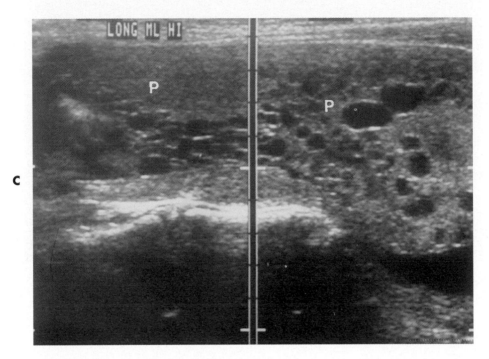

Fig. 15-36, cont'd.   C, Partial hydropic degeneration of the placenta in an 18-week pregnancy. A triploid fetus (not shown) was also present. The anterior placenta *(P)* has multiple cystic spaces. This is the infrequent but classic "swiss cheese" appearance of a hydropic placenta (courtesy Kathryn Grumbach, Baltimore, Md).

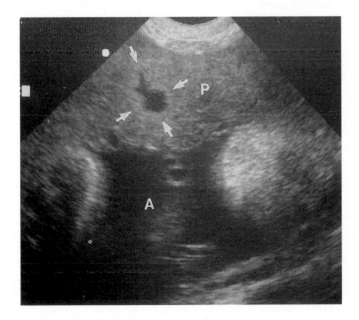

Fig. 15-37   Placental infarction in a 30-week pregnancy. This transaxial view shows an anterior placenta *(P)*. A well-defined mass *(arrows)* is identified that exhibits an irregular hypoechoic center and a thick well-defined hyperechoic rim, findings typical of an infarct. *A,* amniotic fluid.

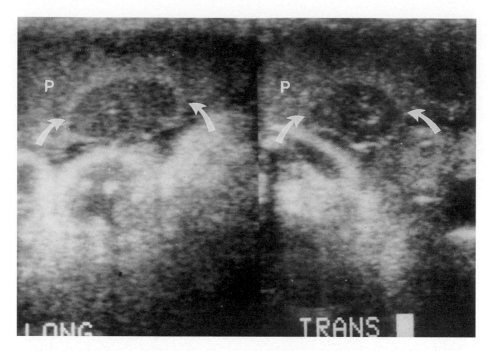

Fig. 15-38 Chorioangioma identified at 32 weeks. Longitudinal *(LONG)* and transaxial *(TRANS)* images of an anterior placenta *(P)* show a well-defined placental mass *(curved arrows).* The mass is oval and primarily hypoechoic, with some internal hyperechoic components. The mass causes the chorionic plate to bulge slightly. Doppler waveform analysis showed primarily venous flow with only a minimal arterial component.

PLACENTAL TUMORS

Chorioangiomas are placental vascular neoplasms that are well circumscribed and usually solitary. When small, they are typically slightly hypoechoic relative to the normal placental tissue (Fig. 15-38). When large, they are more commonly inhomogeneous. Chorioangiomas are either round or ovoid. Although they can be seen anywhere within the placental substance, they are more often at or near the chorionic plate, and usually bulge into the amniotic fluid.

Chorioangiomas have a variable but complete arterial-to-venous blood connection to the fetus (both have the same heart rate). The fetus is at risk for hydrops, with the risk dependent on the size of the chorioangioma and the amount of extra tissue the fetal heart needs to perfuse. If the heart cannot keep up, high-output congestive failure develops in the fetus. This blood flow can be evaluated by a combination of color flow and pulsed Doppler analysis; the more the arterial flow, the closer the pregnancy should be observed for signs of fetal hydrops.

It is usually easy to differentiate chorioangiomas from fibroids. Although both may indent the placenta, they are situated in different areas (placenta versus myometrium). However, the Doppler findings may be similar. Although most fibroids have little appreciable vascularity, some exhibit considerable arterial flow.

Key Features

The placenta normally has a low-level, uniform echogenicity with a thickness between 2 to 4 cm. On its surface is the thin hyperechoic chorionic membrane and on its inner border is the hypoechoic myometrial-basilar layer.

Trophotropism is a concept of placental remodeling, used to explain unusual placental shapes, eccentric umbilical cord insertions, and changes in placental position. Each part of the placenta normally attaches to the underlying endometrium. If the blood supply is uneven, villi proliferate into areas of better vascularity and atrophy in areas of worse vascularity.

The umbilical cord is considered normally positioned if it is within the placental substance. A marginal or velamentous cord insertion can cause serious fetal problems at delivery.

The umbilical cord normally contains three vessels, two arteries and one vein. A two-vessel cord is associated with a high incidence of fetal structural and karyotype abnormalities.

The placenta is a very vascular organ made up of maternal and fetal blood supplies.

Placental bleeding can occur in any of four sites, with large bleeds typically extending into more than one area and even into the amniotic fluid. Uncomplicated subchorionic and submembranous bleeds are benign; retroplacental and intraplacental bleeds can cause considerable fetal and infrequently maternal problems.

Placental accreta, increta, and percreta define the extent of trophoblastic proliferation beyond the normal endometrium and into or through the basilar layer. They most commonly occur in areas of scarring, and the classic ultrasound finding is disruption or loss of the hypoechoic myometrial-basilar layer. Women at highest risk are those who have had previous cesarean sections, and have an anterior placenta and a placenta previa.

A thin placenta is most commonly seen in the setting of maternal systemic vascular problems: hypertension, insulin-dependent diabetes, and collagen vascular disease. A thick placenta often occurs in the settings of fetal hydrops and gestational diabetes.

Contractions can occur anywhere within the myometrial wall. Although often obvious, they can cause uterine distortion and may make a low-lying placenta appear as a previa. Contractions usually change significantly in appearance within 30 to 60 minutes.

Placenta previa is diagnosed at birth and constitutes the position of the placenta relative to the *dilated* and effaced cervix. In utero the placenta is evaluated in relation to a *closed* internal os, and is classified as low-lying, marginal (partial), or complete. A form of complete placenta previa is a central previa, which is centrally located over the os.

The diagnosis of placenta previa should not be made prior to 20 weeks' gestation. If diagnosed, a repeat study within 1 month of delivery is suggested. There can be considerable placental movement (except in cases of central previas) even within a month of delivery. Only women with symptoms need to be evaluated more frequently.

A full urinary bladder may compress and elongate the cervix and lower uterine segment during transabdominal scanning, making a low-lying placenta appear to be a previa. Having the patient empty the urinary bladder, with scanning performed in any of three ways (transvaginally, transabdominally, and translabially) can confirm the existence of a previa.

Vasa previa is the presence of fetal blood vessels (not placenta) that cross the internal cervical os. This can occur in the settings of marginal or velamentous cord insertions, and succenturiate lobes.

The cervix can be evaluated for incompetence, a finding suggested when the cervix is less than 3 cm and definitely less than 2 cm. The ultrasound findings are an opened internal os and a dilated endocervical canal. In the most severe cases the amniotic membrane may bulge into the vagina.

When cervical incompetence is suspected, the patient should not be moved and the obstetrician should be notified immediately. The identification of fetal parts or umbilical cord within the dilated cervix is important, because this rules out the possibility of surgical intervention (cerclage), even if it is needed.

In diagnosing cervical incompetence there are not infrequent discrepancies between the physical examination findings, which rely on the detection of an abnormal external os, and the ultrasound findings, which rely on the detection of an abnormal internal os.

An incompetent cervix may look relatively normal during a distended urinary bladder study. When there is a clinical suspicion or a history of cervical incompetence, a nondistended bladder study (to eliminate cervical compression) should also be performed.

The classic or complete hydatidiform mole is noninvasive in 85% of the cases, locally invasive in 13%, and metastatic (as choriocarcinoma) in 2%. It presents as an enlarged uterus that is typically filled with hyperechoic tissue and that exhibits good through-transmission; larger cysts give the mole a more inhomogeneous appearance. No fetus is present.

Other types of trophoblastic disease can occur. One type consists of two separate sacs, with a normal pregnancy in one and a complete molar pregnancy (with malignant potential) in the other. A partial (incomplete) mole and hydropic placental changes, both coexisting with a living fetus, are associated with a very low malignant potential but a high risk of structural and chromosomal abnormalities.

Placental infarcts most commonly occur in certain maternal vascular conditions. They are usually small and not identified by ultrasound. They can be seen when 1 to 2 cm in diameter and display a hypoechoic center with a hyperechoic rim.

Chorioangiomas are vascular placental tumors with a complete arterial-to-venous connection to the fetus. Commonly there is little, if any, effect on the fetus. At its worst, high flow may lead to high-output failure and fetal hydrops.

SUGGESTED READINGS

Anderson HF et al: Prediction of cervical cerclage outcome by endovaginal ultrasonography, *Am J Obstet Gynecol* 171:1102, 1994.

Bowie JD, Andreotti RF, Rosenberg ER: Sonographic appearance of the uterine cervix in pregnancy: the vertical cervix, *AJR* 140:737, 1983.

Crandall BF, Robinson L, Grau P: Risks associated with an elevated maternal serum α-fetoprotein level, *Am J Obstet Gynecol* 165:581, 1991.

Farine D et al: Vaginal ultrasound for diagnosis of placenta previa, *Am J Obstet Gynecol* 159:566, 1988.

Finberg HJ, Williams JW: Placenta accreta: prospective sonographic diagnosis in patients with placenta previa and prior cesarean section, *J Ultrasound Med* 11:333, 1992.

Fleischer AC et al: Elevated alpha-fetoprotein and a normal fetal sonogram: association with placental abnormalities, *AJR* 150:881, 1988.

Grannum PAT, Berkowitz RL, Hobbins JC: The ultrasonic changes in the maturing placenta and their relation to fetal pulmonic maturity, *Am J Obstet Gynecol* 133:915, 1979.

Guzman ER et al: A new method using vaginal ultrasound and transfundal pressure to evaluate the asymptomatic incompetent cervix, *Obstet Gynecol* 83:248, 1994.

Harding JA et al: Color flow Doppler—a useful instrument in the diagnosis of vasa previa, *Am J Obstet Gynecol* 163:1566, 1990.

Harris RD, Barth RA: Sonography of the gravid uterus and placenta: current concepts, *AJR* 160:455, 1993.

Heifetz SA: Single umbilical artery. A statistical analysis of 237 autopsy cases and review of the literature, Perspect Pediatr Pathol 8:345, 1984.

Hertzberg BS et al: Diagnosis of placenta previa during the third trimester: role of transperineal sonography, *AJR* 159:83, 1992.

Hoddick WK et al: Placental thickness, *J Ultrasound Med* 4:479, 1985.

Hoffman-Tretin JC et al: Placenta accreta. Additional sonographic observations, *J Ultrasound Med* 11:29, 1992.

Jauniaux E, Campbell S, Vyas S: The use of color Doppler imaging for prenatal diagnosis of umbilical cord anomalies: report of three cases, *Am J Obstet Gynecol* 161:1195, 1989.

Kåregård, M Gennser G: Incidence and recurrence rate of abruptio placentae in Sweden, *Obstet Gynecol* 67:523, 1986.

Katz VL et al: The clinical implications of subchorionic placental lucencies, *Am J Obstet Gynecol* 164:99, 1991.

Kerr de Mendonça L: Sonographic diagnosis of placenta accreta. Presentation of six cases, *J Ultrasound Med* 7:211, 1988.

McGahan JP et al: Sonographic spectrum of retroplacental hemorrhage, *Radiology* 142:481, 1982.

Murakawa H et al: Evaluation of threatened preterm delivery by transvaginal ultrasonographic measurement of cervical length, *Obstet Gynecol* 82:829, 1993.

Smith DF, Foley WD: Real-time ultrasound and pulsed Doppler evaluation of the retroplacental clear area, *J Clin Ultrasound* 10:215, 1982.

Spirt BA, Kagan EH, Rozanski RM: Sonolucent areas in the placenta: sonographic and pathologic correlation, *AJR* 131:961, 1978.

Spirt BA et al: Antenatal diagnosis of chorioangioma of the placenta, *AJR* 135:1273, 1980.

Strong TH Jr, Finberg HJ, Mattox JH: Antepartum diagnosis of noncoiled umbilical cords, *Am J Obstet Gynecol* 170:1729, 1994.

Verdel MJC, Exalto N: Tight nuchal coiling of the umbilical cord causing fetal death, *J Clin Ultrasound* 22:64, 1994.

Zorzoli A et al: Cervical changes throughout pregnancy as addressed by transvaginal sonography, *Obstet Gynecol* 84:960, 1994.

CHAPTER 16

Twin (Multiple) Gestations

For a Key Features summary see p. 354.

Multiple births have a worldwide incidence, with twins occurring (on average) in 1 of every 85 births, and with triplets, quadruplets, and quintuplets occurring in 1 of every 7,629, 670,734, and 41,600,000 births, respectively. The incidence of multiple births varies by nation and by race. The highest and lowest birth rates for twin gestations are in South America: the maximum is in Chile at 1:51 and the minimum is in Venezuela at 1:294. Twin gestations in the United States vary by race, with incidences in blacks, whites, and orientals of 1:76, 1:86, 1:92 births, respectively.

The common lay terminology regarding fraternal and identical twins is well known. Fraternal twinning is caused by the production of two ova (dizygotic) and their separate fertilization. These twins can be of the same or different sex and are, in most instances, phenotypically dissimilar after birth. Identical twins are caused by the fertilization of one ovum (monozygotic) and then its separation. These twins are usually similar in appearance and are always of the same sex. The incidence of monozygotic twins noted in all twin studies is the same, one for every five twin gestations (20%). The variation in twins is therefore related to the incidence of dizygotic twinning. Fertility drug–induced pregnancies have been responsible for increasing the incidence of dizygotic gestations, by increasing the number of ova available to be fertilized.

Twin pregnancies are the focus of the remainder of this chapter, because twins have been studied the most completely and serve as a model for all multiple gestations. Larger numbers of gestations (e.g., triplets) exhibit similar growth and in utero complications as twin gestations. The major differences relate to the greater tendency for earlier delivery, and therefore for smaller babies.

CHORIONICITY AND AMNIONICITY

From a medical standpoint, the terms *dizygotic* and *monozygotic* do not fully describe twin pregnancies. Instead, it is more appropriate to determine their chorionicity and amnionicity, as this allows a more accurate anticipation of potential risk factors.

When two ova are fertilized separately (dizygotic twinning), each grows within its own sac, surrounded by its own amnion and chorion. As the two layers of the one sac abut on the two layers of the other, four layers appose and usually fuse. These four interposed layers define this type of twinning as *dichorionic-diamniotic* (Di-Di).

The separation of a single fertilized ovum (monozygotic twinning) can occur at any of four stages. In 20% to 30% of conceptions, the fertilized blastomere separates within the first day; these embryos also develop within their own chorionic-amniotic sacs and are therefore also Di-Di pregnancies. These two Di-Di groups are indistinguishable, except that half the dizygotic twins are of a different sex. Di-Di twins are affected by the least risk factors of any type of twinning because each embryo develops within its own environment and has its own placental circulation.

The remaining 70% to 80% of the monozygotic twins separate later, causing either a partially or completely shared environment and placental circulation. Almost all (70% to 75%) separate within 1 to 7 days after fertilization. The two embryos then share a common chorion but

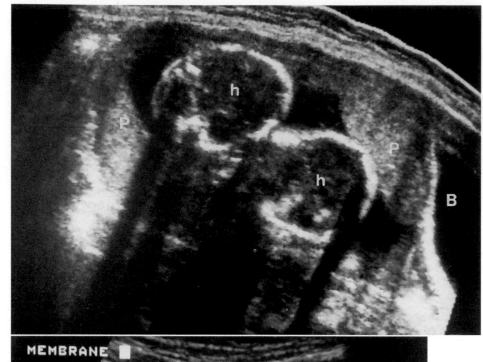

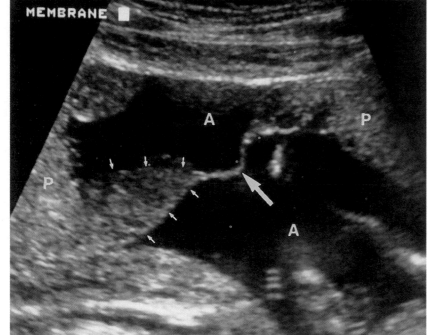

Fig. 16-1   Two late second-trimester dichorionic-diamniotic twin pregnancies. **A,** Static long-axis image shows separate placentas *(P),* one anterior and the other posterior-fundal. *h,* fetal heads; *B,* urinary bladder. **B,** Real-time transaxial image shows separate placentas *(P),* one toward the left and the other toward the right. Between the two is a thick well-defined membrane *(large arrow).* Note the triangular hyperechoic extension of the placenta *(small arrows)* along a margin of one of the placentas and into the amniotic space, an appearance consistent with the lambda sign. *A,* amniotic fluid.

have their own amniotic sacs. The two interposed amniotic layers define this type of twinning as *monochorionic-diamniotic* (Mono-Di), and the twins partially share the same environment.

When the monozygotic separation occurs still later, between 7 to 13 days (1% to 3% of the cases), the two embryos are then surrounded by a common amnion and chorion. They then completely share the same environment, with no interposed membrane, and this type of twinning is termed *monochorionic-monoamniotic* (Mono-Mono). This rarest group, less than 1% of twins,

separates after 13 days. Not only is this a Mono-Mono twinning but the embryos only partially separate. The twins are therefore conjoined (i.e., siamese).

TWIN GESTATIONS

There are two initial questions about twin gestations that need to be considered. The first one is why is it important to diagnose a twin gestation in utero? In the United States the overall perinatal death rate for singleton gestations is 33 in 1000; in twins the risk is increased fourfold to 138 in 1000. The anticipation of twin births is therefore important, with the following the most likely neonatal complications: prematurity, each twin being smaller than a singleton infant, and a prolapsed cord and ensuing anoxia in the second born twin. The second question is why classify the twins into different categories, by their amnionicity and chorionicity? The perinatal death rate in Di-Di twins versus that in Mono-Mono twins is 75 in 1000 versus 191 in 1000, respectively, a two and a half–fold increase for monozygotic twins. In addition to the complications for all twin pairs just mentioned, all monochorionic twins (whether monoamniotic or diamniotic) are at risk for twin-twin transfusions and acardiac twinning. The Mono-Mono twins, because they do not have an intervening membrane, are at risk for two further potential complications: entanglement of the umbilical cords and conjoining.

Therefore, not only should twins be detected, but also (if possible) they should be described in terms of their chorionic and amniotic membranes. When more than two gestations are detected, all are likely to be Di-Di gestations. However, careful analysis of each sac is needed because of the possibility of a spontaneous monochorionic gestation.

SECOND- AND THIRD-TRIMESTER EVALUATION

Many twin pregnancies are not detected before the second trimester. In the second and third trimesters, five characteristics can be used to determine the type of twinning: the number of placentas, the fetal sexes, the type of interposed membranes, the presence or absence of the lambda sign, and the volume of amniotic fluid. The amniotic fluid is discussed later under the complications of monochorionic pregnancies.

If two completely separate placentas can be identified, this assures the existence of a Di-Di pregnancy (Fig. 16-1). However, because of the physical constraints of the uterine cavity, it is common to identify only one placental site. This single-appearing placenta can be either the two separate but apposed placentas of a dichorionic pregnancy or the fused placenta of a monochorionic pregnancy (Fig. 16-2). At present these two cannot be differentiated; perhaps in the future, color flow Doppler may help show the separate or shared placental circulations.

Evaluation of the external genitalia is often not possible until the mid–second trimester. The detection of different sexes confirms Di-Di twinning. However, this determination is limited, as identification is not possible in all cases and only 50% of dizygotic twins are of different sexes. The evaluation of the external genitalia is discussed in Chapter 13.

The identification and type of the interposed mem-

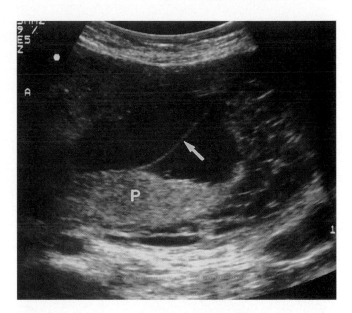

Fig. 16-2   A single-appearing placenta *(P)* in a mid–second trimester dichorionic-diamniotic twin pregnancy. The placenta represents two separate but apposed placentas. It cannot be differentiated from the fused placenta of a monochorionic pregnancy. The arrow shows an intermediately thick, interposed membrane.

brane have been well studied. A Di-Di membrane, composed of two layers of chorion and two layers of amnion, is characteristically well defined and thick, at least 2 mm in thickness (see Fig. 16-1, *B*). Although not often seen, when the two layers of one twin (its amnion and chorion) do not completely fuse to the two layers of the other, this finding is also characteristic of a Di-Di twinning (Fig. 16-3). A Mono-Di membrane, composed of only two thin layers of amnion, appears thin and wispy (like a spider web), and is approximately 1 mm thick (Fig. 16-4). In a Mono-Mono pregnancy, no interposed membrane can be detected (Fig. 16-5).

In all trimesters, a well-defined thick membrane is always a diagnostic sign of a Di-Di pregnancy. However, false-positive and false-negative diagnoses do occur. If a thin membrane is perpendicular to the ultrasound beam and the gain is set unusually high, it may appear falsely thick and mimic a Di-Di membrane (Fig. 16-6). Conversely, a thick Di-Di membrane can sometimes appear thinner, particularly in the third trimester, perhaps "thinned" or stretched by the increased volume of amniotic fluid (see Fig. 16-2). These membranes still appear intermediate in thickness and are almost always still Di-Di membranes. Last, although the absence of a membrane strongly suggests a Mono-Mono pregnancy, it is not always possible to appreciate a very thin diamniotic membrane, particularly late in pregnancy.

The lambda sign is so named because of the triangular-shaped area of hyperechoic placental tissue that extends between the two dichorionic sacs and that resem-

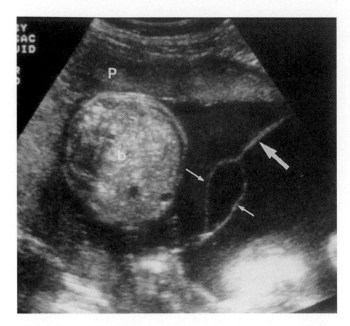

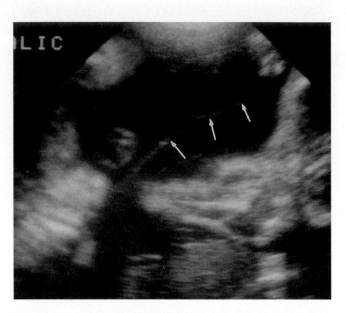

Fig. 16-3 Late second-trimester twin pregnancy with a nonfused dichorionic-diamniotic membrane. Although a thick well-defined membrane is identified *(large arrow)*, in one area *(small arrows)* the amnion and chorion of one sac are not fused with those of the other. The sac toward the left shows a fetal body *(b)* and its separate placenta *(P)*.

Fig. 16-4 Monochorionic-diamniotic twinning in the mid–second trimester. Sometimes difficult to identify, the thin wispy membrane *(arrows)* of only two layers of amnion can be seen separating the two sacs.

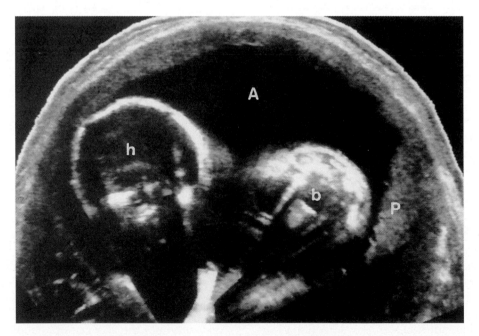

Fig. 16-5 Marked polyhydramnios in a late third-trimester monochorionic-monoamniotic twin pregnancy. This static transaxial image shows a significantly increased volume of amniotic fluid *(A)*. A single posterior placenta is mostly obscured by fetal shadowing from the head of one fetus *(h)* and the edge of the body of the other *(b)*. Part of the placenta *(P)* is seen toward the right, stretched along the margin of the distended uterine cavity. No interposed membrane is identified.

bles the shape of the Greek letter. This finding is seen only in Di-Di twinning. The lambda sign is particularly useful when a single placental site is detected (Figs. 16-1, *B*, and 16-7). It should not be present in a monochorionic pregnancy because a single chorionic membrane surrounds both sacs and prevents the placenta from extending between the sacs. In the second and third trimesters the lambda sign (also termed the *twin-peak sign*) accurately predicts a Di-Di pregnancy. However, its sensitivity and specificity have not yet been analyzed.

FIRST-TRIMESTER EVALUATION

Separate gestational sacs can sometimes be seen early in the pregnancy. These are a diagnostic sign of a dichorionic (Di-Di) pregnancy (Fig. 16-8, *A*). In addition, the membrane thickness, the number of placental sites, and the lambda sign can be used to analyze chorionicity and amnionicity in the first trimester. In a recent study of transabdominal ultrasound, two placental sites or a 2-mm-thick membrane, or both, were found to correctly diagnose Di-Di pregnancies in 82 of 85 cases (96%) (Fig. 16-8, *B*). This high accuracy suggests that the first trimester is the best time in pregnancy to establish chorionicity. Nev-

ertheless, an intermediate or thin membrane was found in seven Di-Di cases, indicating an overlap with monochorionic pregnancies. An appropriately thin membrane (and one placental site) was seen in 14 of 16 Mono-Di pregnancies (87%). However, of the other two cases, there was no membrane in one (overlapping a Mono-Mono pregnancy) and an intermediate membrane in the other (overlapping a Di-Di pregnancy). All four Mono-Mono pregnancies were appropriately diagnosed as not having an intervening membrane (Fig. 16-9).

The lambda sign was present in six of the 85 (7%) Di-Di pregnancies. It was also identified (without an apparent reason) in two of the 16 Mono-Di pregnancies (13%). Because anatomically the lambda sign should only be seen in Di-Di pregnancies, further study of this sign in the first trimester is needed.

A higher-frequency transducer is used in the transvaginal examination and different imaging planes of section are possible. This method should be used to reevaluate any apparently thin or absent membrane before the final diagnosis of a monochorionic twinning (with its increased risk) is made (Fig. 16-10). On the other hand, detection of two placental sites or a thick membrane, or both, confirms the presence of a dichorionic pregnancy, and there is no need for further evaluation.

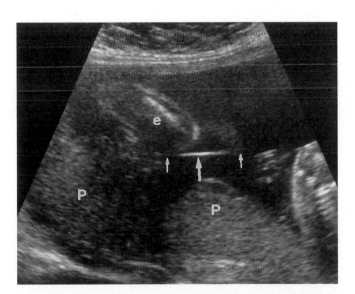

Fig. 16-6   Monochorionic-diamniotic twin pregnancy in the late second trimester. A single placenta *(P)* is identified posteriorly, partially obscured by shadowing from an overlying extremity *(e)*. Although the interposed membrane is thin and wispy *(small arrows)*, it is falsely thickened *(large arrow)* at a point where it is exactly perpendicular to the ultrasound beam. This is caused by increased gain, which can be suggested by the marked increase in "noise" or echoes within the amniotic fluid adjacent to the extremity. When the gain was lowered, the entire membrane looked thin and wispy.

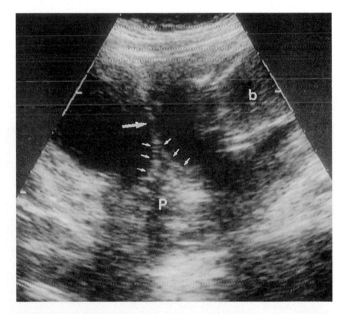

Fig. 16-7   Dichorionic-diamniotic membrane in a mid–second trimester twin pregnancy. The thick membrane is denoted by a large arrow. The lambda sign is seen *(small arrows)*, with placenta extending from a single posterior placenta *(P)* between the two chorionic sacs. One of the twin sacs, toward the right, shows a normal fetal body *(b)*.

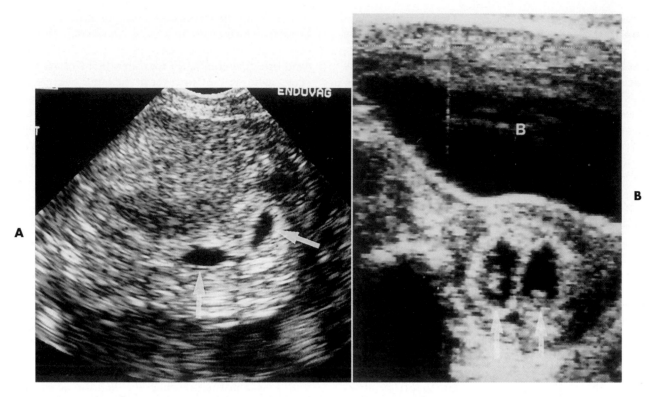

Fig. 16-8   First-trimester dichorionic-diamniotic twins. **A,** Transvaginal transaxial-coronal view of the uterus at 5 gestational weeks. Two well-defined separate gestational sacs *(arrows)* are identified. Although the sacs are normal, it is too early to identify the embryos. **B,** Transabdominal transaxial image of the uterus at 8 weeks shows two well-defined intrauterine gestational sacs *(arrows)* with a well-defined thick intervening membrane. *B,* urinary bladder.

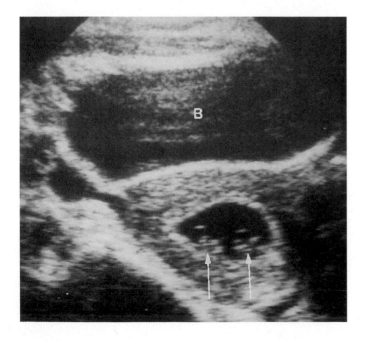

Fig. 16-9   Monochorionic-monoamniotic twin pregnancy at 8 gestational weeks. Transabdominal transaxial view of the uterus shows two well-defined embryos *(arrows)* within a single gestational sac. Separate yolk sacs are also seen, slightly superior to the embryos. No intervening membrane could be identified, and this was confirmed on a transvaginal study. *B,* urinary bladder.

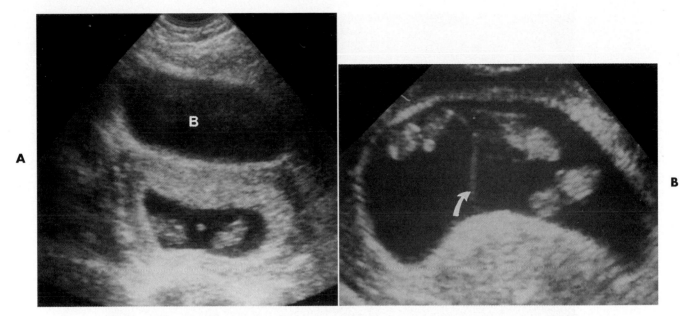

Fig. 16-10   First-trimester triplets identified at 9 gestational weeks. **A,** Transabdominal transaxial view shows apparent twins within a single gestational sac without an intervening membrane. This part of the study was technically limited because of the patient's large body habitus. *B,* urinary bladder. **B,** Transvaginal transaxial-coronal view shows three well-defined embryos, all with heart motion. Between two of the embryos, the one on the left and the one in the middle, is a well-defined thick di-chorionic-diamniotic membrane *(curved arrow).* No membrane could be identified between the middle embryo and the one on the right. This is consistent with monochorionic-monoamniotic (Mono-Mono) twinning. The discrepancy between the transabdominal and transvaginal images was probably caused by only imaging the Mono-Mono twins.

PITFALLS IN DIAGNOSIS

There are potential intrauterine spaces in the first trimester. These can mimic an abnormal second sac or falsely create the impression of a second sac, and are due to fluid within the endometrial canal, the normal chorioamniotic separation, an implantation bleed, a necrotic fibroid, and a split-image artifact. These are discussed in Chapter 9.

Additionally, the "vanishing twin" sign is the first-trimester demise of one of two twins, usually in a Di-Di and much less commonly in a Mono-Di pregnancy. One sac contains the surviving embryo, and the sac that is empty, without an embryo, is typically distorted. This, too, is discussed in Chapter 9.

In the second and third trimesters an unusually thick membrane called an *amniotic sheet* or *shelf* can sometimes be identified within the amniotic cavity, usually in a singleton gestation (Fig. 16-11). This is a synechia, a fibrous band caused prior to the pregnancy by endometrial instrumentation or infection, or by both. It extends into the amniotic space and is covered by a single layer of normal amnion and chorion. This shelf is too thick to be con-

fused with any other membrane, even a Di-Di membrane, and frequently exhibits two additional characteristics: a Y-shaped split at its endometrial margin and often a bulbus-free end within the amniotic fluid. The fetus typically moves freely and is unaffected by the shelf. Very infrequently, however, the shelf can extend across the amniotic cavity, appearing to divide it into two sacs, with the fetus then either unusually positioned or remaining only on one side of the shelf, or both. The fetus should still be normal at birth.

COMPLICATIONS OF DICHORIONIC PREGNANCIES

In dichorionic pregnancies the fetuses are in separate sacs. Each twin is unaffected by the other, except for the heightened risk of premature delivery with the lower birth weights that this entails and for possible complications at delivery. The incidence of structural anomalies and growth retardation in either twin is not greater than that in singleton gestations. However, each fetus must be studied carefully, as either or both could be abnormal.

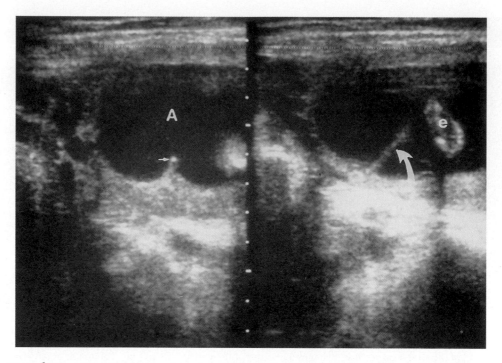

Fig. 16-11   Amniotic shelf or sheet detected in a late second-trimester pregnancy. Two images of the amniotic shelf, a fibrous synechia, are seen extending into the right side of the amniotic cavity *(A)*. In the righthand image this shelf is thicker than the typical dichorionic membrane and extends only partially into the amniotic cavity *(curved arrow)*. In the left image a small arrow denotes its bulbous end. A fetal extremity *(e)* is seen, which moved freely around this sheet.

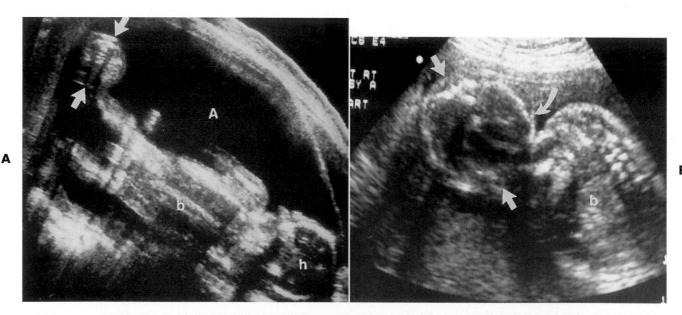

Fig. 16-12   Two examples of the twin-twin transfusion syndrome in monochorionic-diamniotic pregnancies. **A,** Static long-axis image of the uterus in the late second trimester shows two living fetuses. The larger fetus in the lower uterine segment *(h,* head; *b,* body) is in a markedly enlarged sac with polyhydramnios *(A,* amniotic fluid). The smaller fetus is "stuck" in the uterine fundus, its body denoted by arrows. Although a membrane could not be detected, this constellation of findings is consistent with a diamniotic membrane and severe oligohydramnios affecting the smaller fetus. **B,** Real-time oblique view of twin gestations in the early third trimester shows a normal fetus on the right, its fetal body *(b).* A grossly normal volume of amniotic fluid (not shown) surrounds this fetus. A smaller fetus on the left (the body denoted by arrows) is "stuck" in a sac with a decreased amount of amniotic fluid. A thin membrane *(curved arrow)* separates the twins.

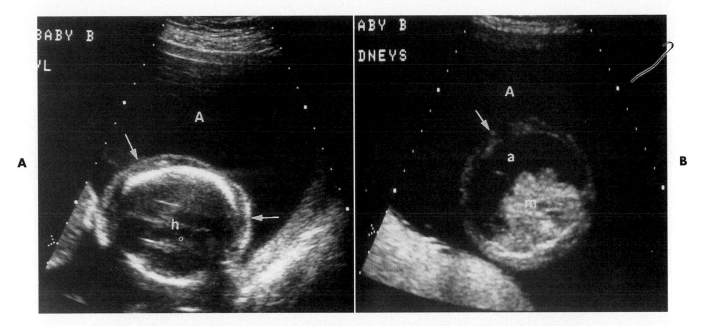

Fig. 16-13   A twin-twin transfusion syndrome in a monochorionic-diamniotic pregnancy in the early third trimester. Only fetus "B" is involved, showing signs of significant hydrops. **A,** A transaxial image of its head *(h)* shows markedly thickened skin *(arrows).* **B,** A transaxial view of its body, below the liver, shows mesentery *(m)* surrounded by ascites *(a)* and skin thickening *(arrow).* Polyhydramnios is present. *A,* amniotic fluid.

COMPLICATIONS OF MONOCHORIONIC PREGNANCIES

In all monochorionic pregnancies there is a single fused placenta with arterial and venous interconnections. Some of these interconnections are inconsequential to the twins; others are highly important. Although their extent should be able to predict the major vascular monochorionic twin risk factors, at present these interconnections cannot be fully assessed. Their significance must instead primarily be inferred from the detection of abnormal intrauterine findings, typically the late manifestations of the twin-twin transfusion syndrome.

The twin-twin transfusion syndrome occurs in 15% to 30% of the monochorionic twin gestations. In its full-blown (most severe) form, one fetus receives or "steals" blood, becoming larger and plethoric, frequently with hydropic changes; the other fetus gets less blood and becomes smaller and anemic (Fig. 16-12). Although a twin-twin transfusion can occur at any time after the first trimester, it is commonly not appreciated until the late second or early third trimester. The direction of Doppler flow in the umbilical arteries and veins is in the correct directions. Arterial flow is away from and venous flow is toward the fetus.

If the twins have their own amniotic sacs (i.e., a Mono-Di pregnancy), then differences in the volume of amniotic fluid can also be appreciated. In its most typical and severe form, polyhydramnios is associated with the larger fetus and oligohydramnios with the smaller fetus. The smaller twin appearing "stuck" or fixed to a margin of the uterine cavity by the thin diamniotic membrane. A number of variations can also occur. One fetus may look completely normal and the other smaller, both with a normal volume of amniotic fluid, or one fetus may look normal while the other smaller fetus is affected by significant oligohydramnios. It may be difficult to differentiate either of these patterns of findings from growth retardation of the smaller fetus. In another permutation one fetus may be normal and the other fetus larger or exhibit signs of hydrops, or both (Fig. 16-13). Preliminary studies of the fetal heart and blood vessels, in particular the right ventricular ejection fraction and the inferior vena cava Doppler waveform, have shown promise in determining potential fetal cardiovascular compromise. More work is needed, however, before these can be used as prognostic indicators.

Once the ultrasound findings of a twin-twin transfusion syndrome are detected, the prognosis is not good for either fetus, with the reported mortality rates frequently exceeding 50%; usually the prognosis is worse for the smaller fetus. Frequent follow-up examinations should be performed, as these fetuses are in a hostile environment and should be delivered as soon as clinically possible.

A rarer complication of a monochorionic pregnancy is a very unfortunate condition called *acardiac twinning.* In it one fetus is normal and the other, the acardiac twin, exhibits an unusual lack of development of a heart, usu-

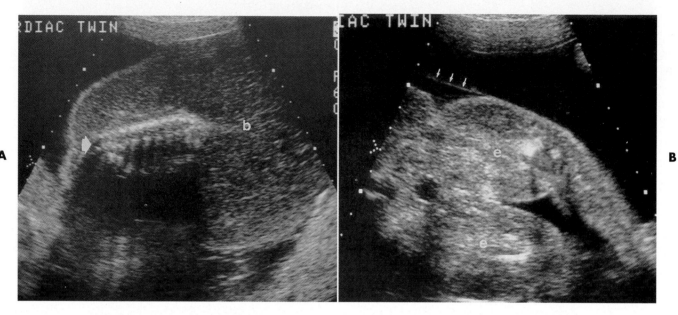

Fig. 16-14 Acardiac twinning in a monochorionic-diamniotic pregnancy. Two real-time images show the abnormal acardiac twin. **A,** The acardiac body *(b)* is seen as an edematous amorphous mass. Only the partially developed lower spine (arrow denotes its distal end) can be identified. **B,** The lower extremities *(e)* are identified with normal boney structures and edematous soft tissues. Small arrows denote thin diamniotic membrane.

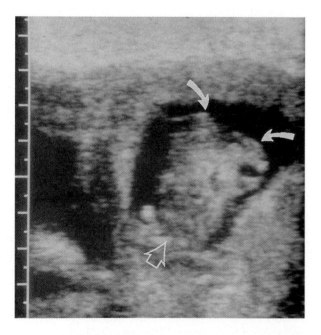

Fig. 16-15 First-trimester conjoined twins detected by transvaginal scanning. A thoracoomphaloischiopagus, with conjoined chests, abdomens, and pelves, is noted. The separated heads are denoted by curved arrows and the conjoined rest of the twins extends down to the rump *(open arrow).*

ally also without a head, upper extremities, and part of the thorax (Fig. 16-14). Marked skin thickening is usually present. The midtrunk through the lower extremities is typically less unaffected but can still be markedly abnormal. The shared blood supply is artery-to-artery and vein-to-vein with arterial blood flow *toward* and venous blood flow *away* from the acardiac twin. In addition to the detection of the gross physical abnormalities involved, Doppler waveform analysis can be used to demonstrate this reversed circulation to the acardiac twin.

The overall volume of amniotic fluid in a twin pregnancy is more than that for a singleton gestation. However, in most twin pregnancies, the volume of amniotic fluid for each fetus is normal. In the setting of a twin-twin transfusion syndrome, however, polyhydramnios may be present and significantly increased in the sac of the larger twin (see Fig. 16-12, *A*). In addition, severe polyhydramnios can occur in uncomplicated Mono-Mono pregnancies, but its cause is unknown (see Fig. 16-5).

Of the two additional monoamniotic complications, entangled umbilical cords cannot be diagnosed with any degree of certainty. The other complication, conjoined twins, can, however, be detected at any time in pregnancy (Figs. 16-15 through 16-17). Although the most common type is thoracopagus, in which the fetuses are joined at the chest, conjoining can occur anywhere from the head to the hips. The type of conjoining should not affect the survival of the twins in utero, but it is important in terms of the type of delivery used, and the twin's chances for separation and their quality of life after birth. At one extreme, if the connection is only at the pelvis, it is likely that the twins can be separated successfully. At the other extreme, connection of the heads with a shared brain parenchyma makes the chance of separation, with survival, highly unlikely for either twin. If the abdomens are conjoined, a combined umbilical cord containing two sets of blood vessels can sometimes be identified. There will always be two umbilical veins, but the number of umbilical cord arteries varies, from two to four.

INTRAUTERINE DEMISE IN TWIN PREGNANCIES

Embryonic loss is most common in the first trimester, affecting either one or rarely both pregnancies. As with singleton gestations, the loss of either of the twins occurs (on average) in 20% to 25% of the cases. Many of these demises go undetected, are typically not evident at birth, and have been described as the "vanishing twin" phenomenon.

When, more uncommonly, an intrauterine demise (of one of the twins) occurs in the second or third trimester, the fetal material is less likely to disappear. In the second trimester a small thin remnant of the dead twin can often be identified as residual bone and soft tissue, frequently along a margin of the uterine cavity. This is called a *fetus papyraceus*, with *papyracia* meaning "like paper." If the demise occurs in the late second or third trimester, the fetus undergoes autolysis and maceration and is clearly identified at the time of delivery (Fig. 16-18).

The risk to the surviving twin depends on the extent of the shared circulation. In a Di-Di pregnancy the risk to the surviving fetus is minimal, provided there are no other uterine problems such as subchorionic collections, or fibroids. However, when a later demise occurs, there is a risk of premature labor and of the macerated fetus obstructing delivery. In monochorionic gestations, because of their vascular interconnections, the surviving fetus is at considerably greater immediate potential risk of suffering twin embolization syndrome and disseminated intravascular coagulation. If, however, the demise has occurred more than 3 to 4 weeks earlier, this risk should be greatly decreased.

GESTATIONAL MEASUREMENTS OF TWINS

It is important to determine the fetal age of the twins. As with singleton pregnancies, this should be established at the first ultrasound examination, preferably before 24 weeks. Assignment of a single fetal age for both twins can at times be difficult, however. If the twins have the same measurements, the same crown-rump lengths or less commonly the same gestational sac sizes in the first trimester or the same biparietal diameters in the second trimester, establishing a single mean and range for both twins is straightforward. If there are discrepancies in the measurements, however, a single fetal age can be established by one of two methods: by averaging the means and taking the outer limits of the ranges, or by picking the mean and range closer to the menstrual dates, if the dates can be determined to be accurate. On all subsequent examinations the age of the twins is determined by adding the first established age to the number of intervening weeks since that study.

It is also important to establish the position of each twin and to keep this constant throughout pregnancy, perhaps by labeling the fetus "A" and "B." If problems develop for either fetus, such as discrepancies in measurements, structural abnormalities, or abnormalities in position, these can then be monitored without confusion as to which twin is affected.

Measurements and growth in twin pregnancies have not been as well studied as they have been for singleton pregnancies. The number of articles and the numbers of cases per study are much smaller. As might be expected, evaluation of the more uncommon triplet and quadruplet pregnancies is further limited by even smaller numbers of cases per series.

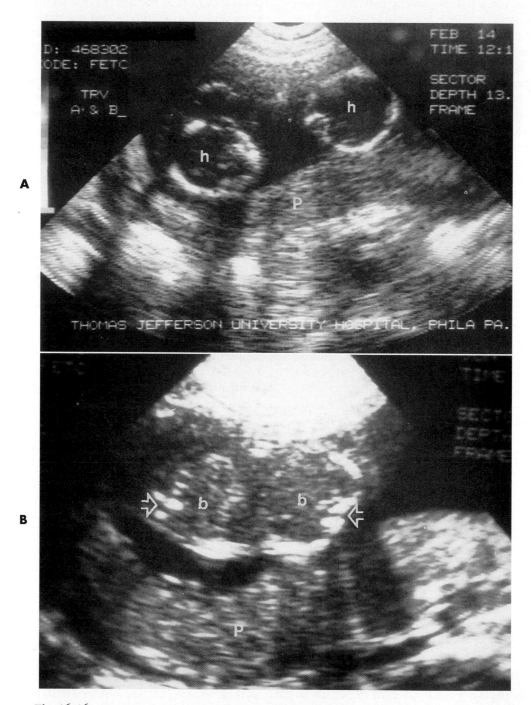

Fig. 16-16　Conjoined twins in the mid–second trimester. This transabdominal image shows twins affected by omphalopagus, connected anteriorly at the abdomen. **A,** The normally separated heads *(h)*. **B,** The bodies joined anteriorly *(b)*. Open arrows denote their spines. *P,* common posterior placenta.

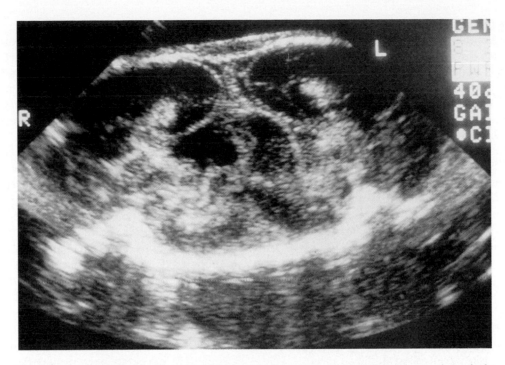

Fig. 16-17   Craniopagus detected in the mid–third trimester. Transabdominal scan through the joined fetal heads imaged coronally shows significant interconnection of the ventricles and brain parenchyma. Although not shown, the chests, abdomens, and pelves are all separate.

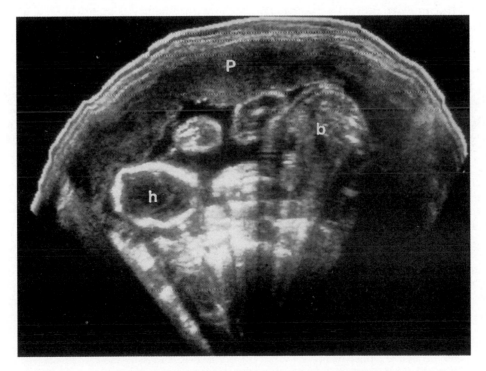

Fig. 16-18   Fetal demise in the early third trimester. Transabdominal transaxial scan shows a normal fetus with its normal body (b) on the right. On the left is the partially collapsed, ill-defined fetal head (h) of a deformed macerated dead fetus. Although no well-defined membrane could be detected, this was found at birth to have been a dichorionic-diamniotic (Di-Di) pregnancy. P, anterior placenta.

However, the literature on twin gestations is still quite extensive, and a number of issues about twins have been resolved. First, the growth of dichorionic and monochorionic twins is similar, provided there are no complications (such as a twin-twin transfusion syndrome). Second, twins closely parallel each other in their size and growth. Third, the growth of the twins closely parallels that of singleton gestations until at least 30 weeks. Fourth, if slowing of growth does occur after 30 weeks, it normally will not decrease below the lower 10th percentile for singleton growth. The findings from much larger studies on singleton gestations are therefore applicable to the analysis of twins, and the singleton measurement tables are also recommended for twin assessments (see Chapter 7).

Because twins parallel each other in their growth, can we define a range beyond which the twins can be considered discrepant in size? The biparietal diameters should normally be within 5 mm of each other, or 5%, and the interval growths within 3 mm per week of each other. These criteria are somewhat limited and have not been substantiated in strictly controlled studies.

Abdominal circumferences and weights have been evaluated in an attempt to predict twin growth discordance. Both are limited in their ability to identify discrepancy, even when wide discordances are found. At present, when the abdominal circumferences differ by more than 20 mm, the positive predictive value (true-positive value divided by the true-positive plus false-positive values) is only 80%. The positive predictive values for weight discrepancies of more than 20% are even more disappointing, only approaching 75%. Therefore, even when large measurement differences are used, 20% to 25% of the cases are still not correctly diagnosed!

If discrepancies in the twin biparietal diameters are detected (or in the abdominal circumferences), femur lengths should be analyzed more carefully. The femur length correlates directly with fetal length, and the lengthwise growth of twins does not slow, even in the late third trimester. Additionally, as twins crowd each other, particularly in the third trimester, the head and body measurements may become less accurate. Although discrepancies in the biparietal diameter can be partially corrected by either an area-corrected biparietal diameter or a head circumference, and an unusually shaped body partially corrected by an average abdominal diameter or circumference, these corrections only rectify inaccuracies in two dimensions. The third dimension of the head, from the vertex to the base, and of the body, from the diaphragm to the pelvis, cannot be corrected without the use of volume measurements; at present volume calculations have only been provided in small series and their validity is unsubstantiated. The femur length, on the other hand, is unaffected by crowding. Finally, in the third trimester, the femur length is as accurate as the head measurements in establishing fetal ages. Therefore, when the other measurements show discrepancies, if the femurs remain within 5 mm of each other and continue to grow normally, it is highly likely that the twins are developing normally.

Key Features

It is best to define twin gestations in terms of their chorionicity and amnionicity. This helps to predict the potential complications in utero and at the time of birth.

Twins in totally separate environments are surrounded by their own chorionic and amniotic membranes and are called *dichorionic-diamnionic* (Di-Di) *twins.*

When twins partially or completely share the same environment, they are monochorionic. If they still have their own amniotic membrane, they are *monochorionic-diamnionic* (Mono-Di) twins. If they completely share the same environment and membranes, they are *monochorionic-monoamnionic* (Mono-Mono) twins.

Five characteristics can be used to diagnose the type of twinning in the second and third trimesters: the number of placentas, the fetal sex, the type of interposed membranes, the presence or absence of the lambda sign, and occasionally the amount of amniotic fluid.

Separate placentas, different fetal sexes, or a thick Di-Di membrane, or a combination of these findings, confirms a Di-Di pregnancy.

In the first trimester a Di-Di pregnancy is diagnosed by membrane thickness or by the finding of separate placentas. Transvaginal scanning may be of value in determining membrane thickness.

The most common complication of monochorionic pregnancies is twin-twin transfusion. This has a variable presentation, but, in its most severe form, in a Mono-Di pregnancy, consists of a small twin in an oligohydramnic sac (a "stuck" twin) and an enlarged hydropic twin affected by polyhydramnios.

The identification of an in utero twin death and its complications are related to the trimester in which the death occurs and the type of twinning.

The following is known about twin gestational growth: it is similar regardless of the chorionicity and amnionicity, twins closely parallel each other in their growth, and twins closely parallel singleton gestations in growth until at least 30 weeks, when their growth usually slows down toward the lower 10th percentile.

When in doubt about the concordancy of twin growth, one should evaluate the femur lengths. If they are close (within 5 mm) and maintain parallel growth, growth in both twins is most likely normal.

SUGGESTED READINGS

Barss VA, Benacerraf BR, Frigoletto FD Jr: Ultrasonographic determination of chorion type in twin gestation, *Obstet Gynecol* 66:779, 1985.

Barth RA et al: Conjoined twins: prenatal diagnosis and assessment of associated malformations, *Radiology* 177:201, 1990.

Benson CB, Doubilet PM, Vivek D: Prognosis of first-trimester pregnancies: polychotomous logistic regression analysis, *Radiology* 192:765, 1994.

Blickstein I: The twin-twin transfusion syndrome, *Obstet Gynecol* 76:714, 1990.

Brown DL et al: Twin-twin transfusion syndrome: sonographic findings, *Radiology* 170:61, 1989.

Finberg HJ: The "twin-peak" sign: reliable evidence of dichorionic twinning, *J Ultrasound Med* 11:571, 1992.

Finberg HJ: Uterine synechiae in pregnancy: expanded criteria for recognition and clinical significance in 28 cases, *J Ultrasound Med* 10:547, 1991.

Grumbach K et al: Twin and singleton growth patterns compared using US, *Radiology* 158:237, 1986.

Hertzberg BS et al: Significance of membrane thickness in the sonographic evaluation of twin gestations, *AJR* 148:151, 1987.

Hill LM et al: The sonographic assessment of twin growth discordance, *Obstet Gynecol* 84:501, 1994.

Kurtz AB et al: Twin pregnancies: accuracy of first-trimester abdominal US in predicting chorionicity and amnionicity, *Radiology* 185:759, 1992.

Langlotz H, Sauerbrei E, Murray S: Transvaginal Doppler sonographic diagnosis of an acardiac twin at 12 weeks gestation, *J Ultrasound Med* 10:175, 1991.

Mahony BS, Filly RA, Callen PW: Amnionicity and chorionicity in twin pregnancies: prediction using ultrasound, *Radiology* 155:205, 1985.

Mahony BS et al: The "stuck twin" phenomenon: ultrasonographic findings, pregnancy outcome, and management with serial amniocenteses, *Am J Obstet Gynecol* 163:1513, 1990.

Naeye RL et al: Twins: causes of perinatal death in 12 United States cities and one African city, *Am J Obstet Gynecol* 131:267, 1978.

Randel SB et al: Amniotic sheets, *Radiology* 166:633, 1988.

Sauerbrei EE: The split image artifact in pelvic ultrasonography: the anatomy and physics, *J Ultrasound Med* 4:29, 1985.

Weissman A et al: Sonographic growth measurements in triplet pregnancies, *Obstet Gynecol* 75:324, 1990.

GYNECOLOGY

Pelvis and Uterus

For a Key Features summary see p. 386.

The female pelvis can be evaluated by two ultrasound techniques: transabdominal (TA) and transvaginal (TV). In the TA study, which is performed through a distended urinary bladder, transducers with frequencies of up to 5 MHz are used. These transducers can focus deep into the pelvis and can obtain an overview of the pelvic structures. In the TV examination, which is performed with the patient's bladder empty, transducers with higher frequencies of up to 7.5 MHz and capable of better near-field focusing are used. This allows for greater detail of the uterus and adnexa. However, the intracavitary position limits movement of the transducer and the ultrasound beam penetrates only 8 to 10 cm from the transducer face.

The TA study should be the first pelvic ultrasound examination, with the TV examination reserved for a more critical evaluation. For subsequent studies, because of prior knowledge of a patient's particular pelvic anatomy or pathologic condition, often only the more diagnostic of the two techniques is needed.

The pelvic examination is best initiated by first identifying the urinary bladder. With TA scanning the bladder is typically distended and is used as a "sonic" window to examine the adjacent gynecologic structures. Even when a patient has completely voided, often identifiable residual urine can be seen within the bladder. It is important to find the urinary bladder to rule out the presence of a large cystic or complex mass, usually of ovarian origin, that can occupy the lower pelvis. Although not common, such a mass may otherwise be inadvertently mistaken for the bladder (Fig. 17-1).

The uterus should then be identified in its long axis. This may not be in a true anatomic sagittal plane because the uterus can be deviated (normally) toward the right or left. Once the uterine long axis is established, parallel sagittal scans are then obtained to its right and left to evaluate the uterine margins and the adnexa. The transducer is then turned 90 degrees so that transaxial or transaxial-coronal images can be obtained. If the orientation is lost, which is a particular problem in TV scanning, the study should be restarted with a long-axis uterine image.

The direction of the ultrasound beam is important. A TA probe has end-firing transucers. The beam is emitted directly from its end like a flashlight beam, and the body part imaged is directly below the probe. Most TV probes, however, have transducers that emit the ultrasound beam at an angle of 30 to 60 degrees. This angle is not appreciated during scanning but is important. In the sagittal plane the beam is angled anteriorly and images an anteverted uterus. If the uterus is tilted posteriorly, full uterine visualization is not possible unless the probe is turned a full 180 degrees. The image can then be inverted back to its original position by pushing the appropriate button on the ultrasound machine. Similarly, in transaxial and transaxial-coronal views, when the transducer is turned to the right, the left side may not be imaged adequately unless the same 180-degree maneuver is used.

There are no gynecologic contraindications to the use of the TV probe. After the probe is appropriately soaked in an antibacterial and often antiviral solution and after a sheath (usually a condom) is placed over the transducer, the probe is typically inserted about halfway into the vagina. If carefully inserted, the probe will not touch the cervix. The TV study is therefore considered relatively noninvasive and, when clinically or sonographically needed, can be performed to evaluate pelvic abnormalities (i.e., cervical, uterine, and adnexal problems).

Doppler waveform analysis (color or pulsed) may be of value because it can help differentiate vascular from nonvascular tubular structures and can help define normal anatomic characteristics. Its use in the evaluation of adnexal masses is discussed in Chapter 18.

NORMAL FERTILE YEARS FINDINGS

Most women are examined during their fertile years, which are typically between 14 and 50 years of age. Menstrual cycles usually occur during these years. These cause the appearance of the endometrium and the ovaries to constantly change (discussed in Chapter 18) and result in some inconsistency in the vaginal findings.

During midline sagittal scanning, the vagina is usually identified as a thin hyperechoic line (Fig. 17-2, A). If blood or a tampon causes the canal to spread, it becomes thicker and is often more hypoechoic.

The endometrial stripe (or complex) is composed of the endometrial canal surrounded by two layers of endometrium. The brightness and thickness of this stripe varies and primarily depends on the time in the patient's menstrual cycle. During TA scanning a very distended urinary bladder may sometimes compress and distort both the myometrium and endometrium. Either TA scanning after the bladder has been partially emptied or TV scanning may be needed to more completely evaluate the pelvis.

At the end of menses the endometrial stripe is a discrete, very thin hyperechoic line, only 2 to 3 mm thick (Fig. 17-2, A). Between then and the onset of ovaluation, termed the *proliferative (estrogen) phase*, the stripe becomes thicker, as much as 8 mm, and remains uniformly hyperechoic and distinct (Figs. 17-2, B, and 17-3). Occasionally a striated appearance (also called the *triple layer*) may be detected; this consists of three hyperechoic lines surrounding two hypoechoic layers (Fig. 17-3, B). Although the overall thickness of both patterns is similar, the striated appearance seems to signify a time when the endometrium is more receptive to implantation. Fertility medications control the number of days of the proliferative phase and the timing of ovulation. If the proliferative phase is lengthened, the endometrial complex may be thicker (Fig. 17-3, B).

From ovulation until the start of the menses, termed the *secretory (progesterone) phase*, the endometrium thickens further, typically as much as 15 mm, but sometimes more than this (Fig. 17-4, A). Although uniformly hyperechoic, its boundaries are less well defined. As menses begins, the endometrium sloughs, the stripe thins, and the cycle starts again.

A thin hypoechoic layer, commonly called the *junctional zone*, is identified deep to the endometrium (see Figs. 17-2 through 17-4). It is anatomically either the boundary between the endometrium and myometrium or the innermost margin of the myometrium. Although not always detected by ultrasound, it is an important landmark. The junctional zone is distorted in the settings

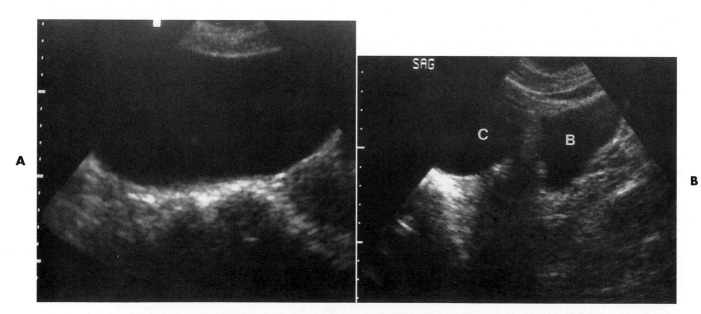

Fig. 17-1 Large ovarian cyst, initially mistaken for the urinary bladder. **A,** Transabdominal midline sagittal image with the urinary bladder empty. The large ovarian cyst looks like the bladder. **B,** Transabdominal midline sagittal image after urinary bladder *(B)* distention. The ovarian cyst (its lower part denoted by a *C*) has now been displaced more cephalad and is distinct from the bladder.

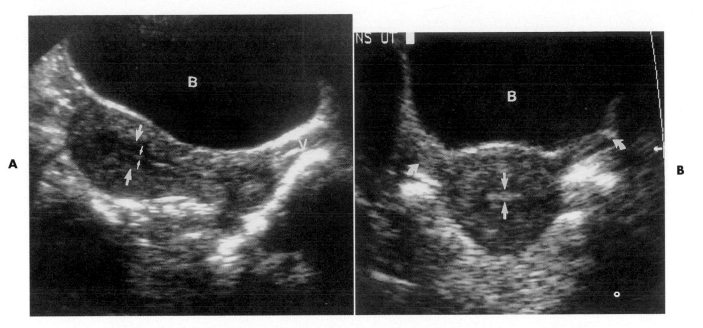

Fig. 17-2   Proliferative phase. Transabdominal images of the uterus in fertile women. **A,** This sagittal midline scan of the uterus obtained at the end of menstruation shows a thin (2-mm), hyperechoic endometrial stripe *(small arrows)*. The stripe is surrounded by the hypoechoic junctional zone *(large arrows)*. The myometrium is of intermediate echogenicity. Note that the fundus and body of the uterus (toward the left) are more prominent than the cervix. The vaginal canal *(V)* is normally thin and hyperechoic. **B,** Transaxial image obtained on day 10 in another patient shows a midline uterus with a slightly thicker (5-mm), discrete hyperechoic endometrial stripe *(arrows)*. The junctional zone is not as well seen. Parts of both adnexa are identified *(curved arrows)*. *B,* urinary bladder.

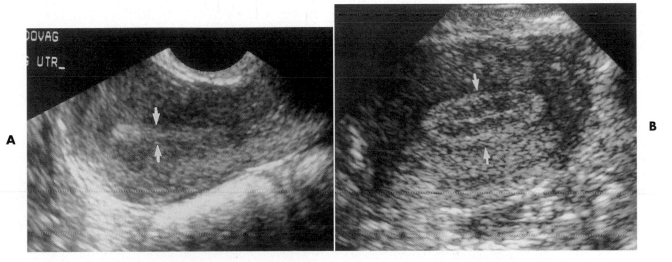

Fig. 17-3   Proliferative phase. Transvaginal images of the uterus in a fertile woman close to the time of ovulation (midcycle). **A,** Long-axis sagittal midline image shows the uterus with a discrete, 8-mm-thick, hyperechoic endometrial stripe *(arrows)*. Note the normal prominence of the uterine body and fundus. **B,** Transaxial-coronal view shows an endometrial complex with a striated appearance *(arrows)*. It is 14 mm thick, and this is caused by extended fertility medication. The surrounding hypoechoic junctional zone is partially identified.

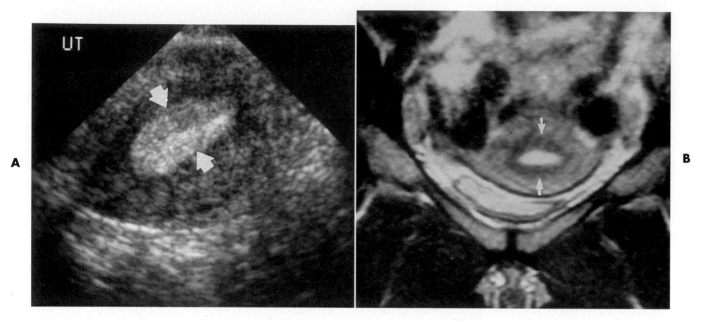

Fig. 17-4   Secretory phase. Transvaginal ultrasound study and magnetic resonance (MR) image in different fertile women with an endometrial stripe thickness of 15 mm. **A,** Transvaginal sagittal midline ultrasound image shows a uterus with a prominent hyperechoic endometrial stripe *(arrows)*. The margins are somewhat indistinct. Note the surrounding hypoechoic junctional zone. **B,** Transaxial, fast spin echo, T_2-weighted MR image shows the high-intensity endometrial complex surrounded by the low-intensity signal of the junctional zone *(arrows)*.

of adenomyosis (the uterine form of endometriosis), diffuse fibroids, and invasive endometrial carcinoma. The junctional zone is more consistently identified by magnetic resonance imaging (MRI), which can perhaps better differentiate among these processes (see Fig. 17-4, *B*).

The myometrium (the uterine muscle) is identified beyond the junctional zone. It is the largest component of the uterus and gives the uterus its shape. During the fertile years the uterine body and fundus are more prominent than the cervix (see Figs. 17-2 and 17-3). The normal myometrium has a uniform low-level echogenicity, which is less than that of the endometrium.

The serosal surface is usually not appreciated. Occasionally subserosal veins may appear as prominent anechoic spaces (Fig. 17-5). This is a normal variant, usually identified in parous women.

There is a wide range of normal uterine sizes, and these are due to a variety of factors, particularly previous pregnancies. The nulliparous uterus is classically 7 × 5 × 3 cm in its length, width, and anteroposterior dimensions, respectively, with the anteroposterior measurement obtained perpendicular to the uterine length (Table 17-1). In parous women the uterus is typically larger in all three dimensions, increasing with each pregnancy up to six. It may then be more than 10 cm long. Uterine size is not (in and of itself) an indicator of uterine abnormality;

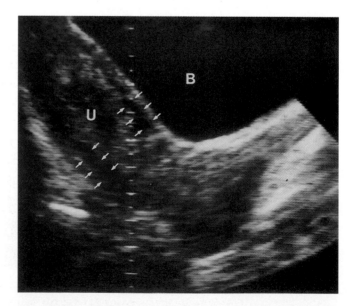

Fig. 17-5   Subserosal veins, a normal variant. Transabdominal midline sagittal image of the uterus *(U)* shows hypoechoic serpiginous structures between the myometrium and the serosal surface *(small arrows)*. *B,* urinary bladder.

if the echogenicity is normal and all uterine layers are maintained, the uterus is most likely normal. Age does not appear to affect uterine size.

The normal uterus has different normal positions. It is most commonly anteverted, with the entire uterus (from the cervix to the fundus) tilted forward toward the anterior abdominal wall. When the urinary bladder is distended during TA scanning, the anteverted uterus is often pushed backward into a more horizontal position. It is then perpendicular to the ultrasound beam and ideally positioned to be imaged through the bladder (Fig. 17-6). However, because the distended bladder can also compress and distort all (or part) of the uterus, empty-bladder scans may be needed to evaluate its true size and shape.

In some women the uterus is retroverted, that is, tilted posteriorly from the vaginal vault. For unexplained reasons, a retroverted uterus assumes a more globular shape, with the myometrium absorbing more of the ultrasound beam and giving the impression of a large hypoechoic fibroid (Fig. 17-7). The endometrium is often difficult to identify. By increasing the transducer gain the normal myometrial echogenicity and occasionally the endometrial complex can be appreciated better.

A less common normal variant position of the uterus is termed *flexion*. Rather than tilted entirely forward or backward, the uterine body is folded in on itself: anteflexed if folded anteriorly and retroflexed if folded posteriorly (Fig. 17-8). The overall ultrasound appearance is approximately the same as that of an anteverted and

Table 17-1	Normal anatomic uterine dimensions in adult women during their fertile years according to parity		

		Mean (± SD)	
Parity	Length (cm)	Anteroposterior dimension (cm)	Transverse dimension (cm)
0	7.7 (1.1)	2.9 (1.1)	4.7 (0.6)
1	8.6 (1.5)	3.5 (1.0)	5.0 (1.0)
2-3	9.2 (1.3)	3.9 (1.3)	5.6 (1.3)
4-5	9.4 (1.1)	4.2 (1.1)	5.8 (1.1)
6+	9.7 (1.1)	4.2 (1.1)	5.9 (1.1)

Adapted from Langlois PL: The size of the normal uterus, *J Reprod Med* 4:221, 1970.

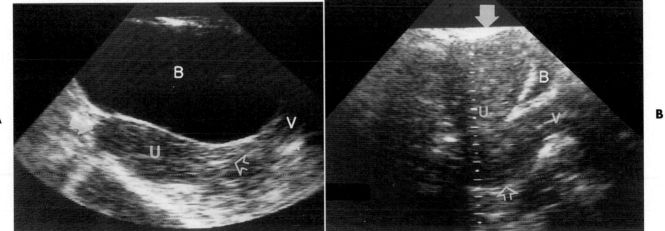

Fig. 17-6   The effect of urinary bladder *(B)* distention on the uterus *(U)*. Transabdominal sagittal images of the uterus. **A,** With a distended urinary bladder, the uterus is pushed into a more horizontal position, with its fundus *(solid arrow)* and cervix *(open arrow)* almost perpendicular to the transducer. The uterus is also compressed and flattened. **B,** After almost complete emptying of the urinary bladder, the uterus now assumes its "neutral" anteverted position and undistorted shape, with the fundus *(solid arrow)* more round and prominent than the cervix *(open arrow)*. *V*, vagina.

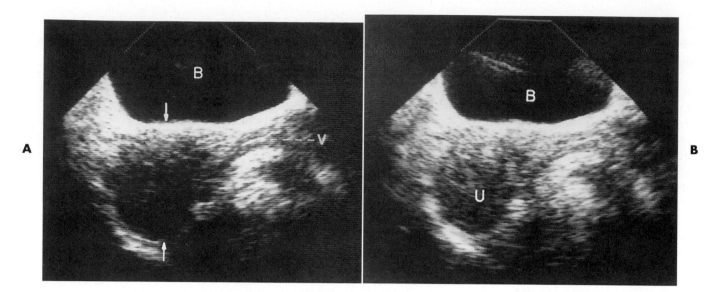

Fig. 17-7 Transabdominal sagittal midline images of a retroverted uterus. **A,** The retroverted uterus has a globular shape *(arrows)*. At normal gain settings the thickened myometrium absorbs the ultrasound beam and appears hypoechoic, almost as if it were a large fibroid. **B,** With increased gain, the normal myometrial echogenicity fills in and the uterus *(U)* appears normal. Note that the endometrial stripe cannot be identified. *V,* vagina; *B,* urinary bladder.

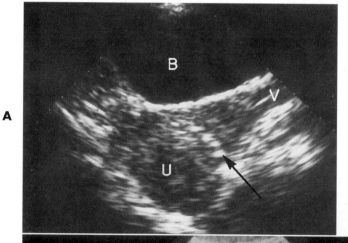

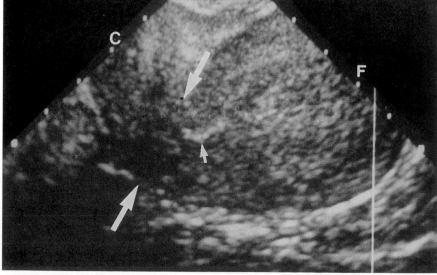

Fig. 17-8 Retroflexed uterus. **A,** Transabdominal sagittal midline image of the uterus *(U)* shows a hyperechoic band *(arrow)* in the middle of the uterine body at the point of flexion. *V,* vaginia; *B,* urinary bladder. **B,** Transvaginal sagittal midline image again shows the uterus flexed at the body *(large arrows)*. The cervix *(C)* is toward the left with the uterine fundus *(F)* toward the right. Part of the normal thin endometrial stripe is identified *(small arrow)*, which is not seen on the transabdominal image.

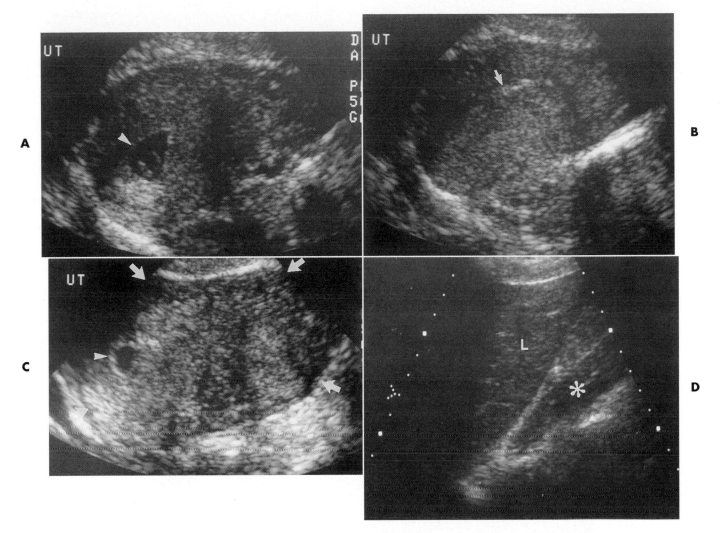

Fig. 17-9   Bicornuate uterus with agenesis of the right kidney, diagnosed during an early first trimester pregnancy evaluation. **A, B,** and **C** are transvaginal images of the uterus. **A,** Sagittal image of the right horn shows an early gestational sac *(arrowhead)* with a living 5.0-week embryo. **B,** Sagittal image of the left horn shows a normal thin, hyperechoic endometrial stripe *(arrow)*. **C,** Transaxial-coronal view shows an unusually "squared-off" uterus *(arrows)* with the intrauterine gestation noted in the right horn *(arrowhead)*. **D,** Transabdominal sagittal image of the right upper quadrant shows the normal liver *(L)*. The right kidney is absent, and only the right iliopsoas muscle (*) is identified.

retroverted uterus except that there is a sharp angle to both the uterine body and the endometrial complex (if seen) at the point of flexion. The gynecologist is often not able to differentiate version from flexion on the basis of clinical findings. If evacuation of the endometrial cavity is planned, knowledge of flexion is important because the angle may interfere with effective treatment of the upper part of the canal. With correct proble angulation, perhaps done under ultrasound guidance, more complete insertion is usually possible.

There are a number of congenital uterine anomalies, ranging from a simple uterine septation to a bicornuate and didelphic uterus. Occasionally only one horn of the uterus (a unicornuate uterus) develops. These are all re-lated to müllerian duct anomalies and are not uncommonly associated with ipsilateral renal anomalies. Although most uterine and cervical anomalies are detected on the basis of a combination of physical examination and hysterogram findings, an ultrasound examination may reveal (sometimes initially) the anomalies by showing two endometrial canals, two uterine horns, an unusually broad and "squared-off" uterus in a transaxial view, and ptosis or absence of a kidney (Fig. 17-9). TV ultrasound and MRI may help confirm the presence of a malformation.

TV imaging is not always needed when scanning the uterus. It should be used when expected TA findings are not detected or are equivocal, or when abnormal findings

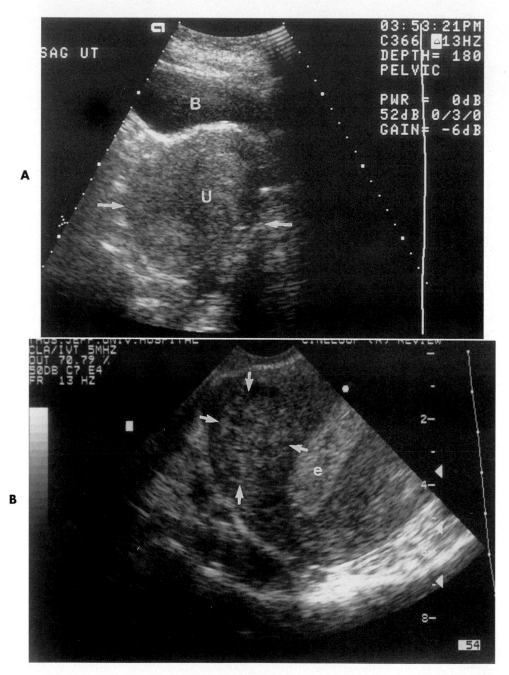

Fig. 17-10   Comparison of transabdominal and transvaginal techniques in the imaging of a fibroid uterus. **A,** Transabdominal sagittal image of the uterus *(U)* shows the fundus to be bulky but without a definite mass *(arrows)*. The endometrial stripe cannot be identified. *B,* urinary bladder. **B,** Transvaginal sagittal image of the uterine body and fundus shows a thickened hyperechoic endometrial stripe *(e)* and a heterogeneous, solid fibroid *(arrows)* in the fundus.

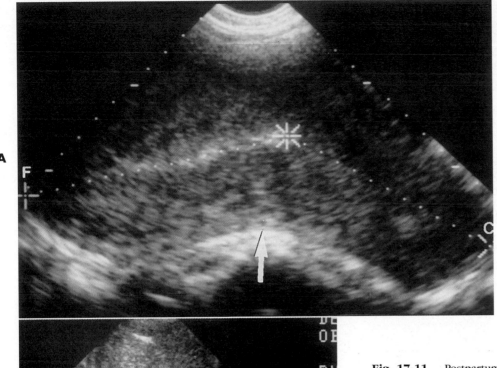

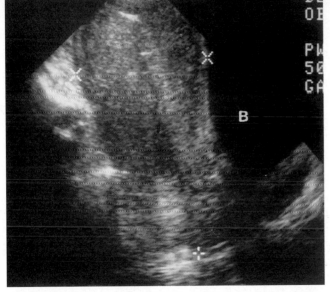

Fig. 17-11   Postpartum uterus. Transabdominal sagittal images showing measurements of the postpartum uterus. **A,** Early postpartum period. At 2 days the markedly enlarged uterus is scanned with a small-headed transducer, without compression. Two measurements are taken along the endometrial stripe, one from the fundus *(F)* to the angle at the sacral promontory *(star)* and the second from the sacral promontory *(star)* to the cervix *(C)*. When added together, the composite measurement is 20 cm. The sacral promontory is denoted by an arrow. (From Wachsberg RH et al: Real-time ultrasonographic analysis of the normal postpartum uterus: technique, variability, and measurements, *J Ultrasound Med* 13:215, 1994.) **B,** Midpostpartum period. At 3 weeks an image through a partially distended urinary bladder *(B)* shows an 11-cm uterus from the fundus (at the top of the image) to the cervix (+). *x,* anteroposterior dimension.

require further evaluation (Fig. 17-10). TV scanning permits different orientations, its resolution is better, and a more "neutral"-appearing uterus is possible because the bladder is not distended. The endometrial stripe is often more completely identified, especially when the uterus is retroverted or retroflexed (see Fig. 17-8). The stripe may occasionally appear thicker, perhaps because the bladder is not compressed.

POSTPARTUM FINDINGS

The postpartum uterus normally begins to involute immediately after delivery, and this continues for 6 to 7 weeks. Changes in uterine size can be evaluated transab-

dominally by measuring its length. In the most definitive postpartum study to date, at mean times of 1.4 days, 2.7 weeks, and 6.7 weeks, the uterus decreases in length from a mean ± 1 standard deviation of 19.9 ± 2.1 cm, to 11.2 ± 2.0 cm, and then to 8.7 ± 1.2 cm, respectively. Most of the involution is complete by 3 to 4 weeks; by the seventh postpartum week, the uterus has returned to its baseline size.

The technique of scanning is important, particularly in the early postpartum period. During this time the uterus is large, "spongy," and very easily compressed. Even slight transducer pressure can change the uterine size, and therefore careful scanning with a small-headed transducer is necessary. Additionally, the uterus is so large that it expands out of the pelvis into the abdomen,

Table 17-2	Postpartum uterine size: increase in uterine length in the early (mean, 1.4 days) and middle (mean, 2.7 weeks) postpartum periods caused by increasing parity	
	Sagittal dimensions in cm (± SD)	
Parity	**Early**	**Middle**
1	19.1 (1.7)	10.4 (0.4)
2	19.7 (2.1)	10.9 (0.3)
3	20.7 (2.0)	11.4 (0.4)
4	21.6 (1.8)	11.9 (0.6)

From Wachsberg RH et al: Real-time ultrasonographic analysis of the normal postpartum uterus: technique, variability, and measurements, *J Ultrasound Med* 13:215, 1994.
SD, standard deviation.

forming an angle over the sacral promontory. To measure uterine length in the first 2 postpartum weeks, an unusual but reproducible technique is needed. This consists of two long-axis measurements taken along the endometrial canal, one from the fundus to the angle and the other from the angle to the cervix, and then these are totaled (Fig. 17-11, *A*). The width and anteroposterior dimensions are not consistent in the early postpartum period because of the spontaneous uterine contractions that occur. By 3 to 4 weeks, the uterus has decreased enough in size that its length can be measured in the usual way (Fig. 17-11, *B*).

The length of the uterus is influenced by only one factor—the number of previous pregnancies (the woman's parity). This is only an issue in the early and middle (up to 3 to 4 weeks) postpartum periods (Table 17-2). No other factors, not even infant birth weight and breast-feeding, affect uterine size or the timing of its involution.

Sonographically the normal postpartum endometrium appears thin, typically less than 15 mm and often less than 10 mm. Thickening is not normal, and, if found, retained products or infection, or both, should be considered.

PREMENSTRUAL AND POSTMENOPAUSAL NORMAL FINDINGS

The premenstrual period commences at birth and continues until the time of menses. Initially the neonatal uterus is affected by maternal hormones. It remains slightly prominent for several weeks after birth (although no size is known) and has the shape of a fertile uterus, with the body and fundus larger than the cervix.

After the hormone effects dissipate, the fundus involutes, leaving a prominent cervix (Fig. 17-12). The uterus is then small but enlarges as the fertile years approach (Table 17-3). The endometrial stripe is typically not identified but can infrequently be seen as a very thin hyperechoic stripe.

Menopause is defined as beginning 1 year after the cessation of menses. The postmenopausal uterus progressively atrophies and decreases to its prepubertal size by 15 to 20 postmenopausal years. The body and fundus, however, remain more prominent than the cervix. The endometrial stripe is normally either thin and hyperechoic or not identified. If imaged, it is always normal when 4 mm or less in thickness and is usually normal up to a thickness of 7 mm. With hormone replacement therapy (primarily estrogens), the uterus and endometrium do not involute appreciably and may have a premenopausal appearance.

There are transitional periods between the premenstrual and fertile years and between the fertile and postmenopausal years. These transitions last an unpredictable number of years but usually occur between 9 to 13 years of age and last for 5 to 10 years after the cessation of menstrual periods, respectively. During these times the uterine size, shape, and endometrial shape are intermediate in appearance.

ENDOMETRIAL ABNORMALITIES

Two questions should be considered when evaluating any endometrial abnormality: (1) What period of female life, that is, premenstrual, fertile, or, postmenopausal is the patient in? and (2) Is the abnormality an unusually thick endometrium or is it a collection that is spreading the endometrial canal?

An abnormality is very uncommon during the premenstrual years. If present, it is almost always a collection within the vaginal canal, caused by vaginal (colpos) obstruction. Occasionally there is additional proximal obstruction of the uterus (metrocolpos). In the neonate mucosal secretions or fluid collects behind a vaginal atresia or an imperforate hymen (Fig. 17-13). Later in premenstrual life, near the time of menses, blood can accumulate behind an imperforate hymen. Surgical repair commonly causes the uterus and vagina to return to normal.

In the fertile years almost all abnormalities are related to pregnancy, either intrauterine or extrauterine, and almost all are detected in the first trimester (Fig. 17-14). The appearance of an intrauterine gestational sac, both normal and abnormal, is described in Chapter 9. In an ectopic pregnancy, a pseudogestational sac may be present. This is discussed in Chapters 9 and 19.

After miscarriages (spontaneous abortions), retained products of conception (POCs) assume varied appear-

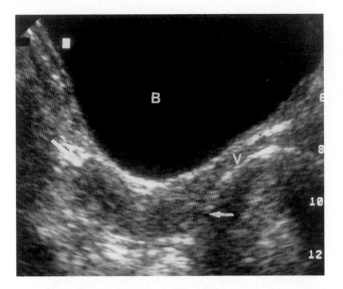

Fig. 17-12 Premenstrual uterus. Transabdominal sagittal image of the uterus in a 9-year-old girl shows the cervix to be more prominent than the body and fundus. The fundus is denoted by a large arrow and the cervix by a small arrow. *V*, vagina; *B*, urinary bladder.

Table 17-3 Normal uterine and cervical dimensions in pediatric (premenstrual) age groups

Age	Length (cm), mean (± SD)	AP dimension of corpus (cm), mean (± SD)	AP dimension of cervix (cm), mean (± SD)
2-7 years	3.3 (0.4)	0.7 (0.2)	0.8 (0.2)
8 years	3.6 (0.7)	0.9 (0.3)	0.8 (0.2)
9 years	3.7 (0.4)	1.0 (0.3)	0.9 (0.2)
10 years	4.0 (0.6)	1.3 (0.5)	1.1 (0.3)
11 years	4.2 (0.5)	1.3 (0.3)	1.1 (0.3)
12 years	5.4 (0.8)	1.7 (0.5)	1.4 (0.5)
13 years	5.4 (1.1)	1.6 (0.5)	1.5 (0.2)

From Orsini LF et al: Pelvic organs in premenarchal girls: real-time ultrasonography, *Radiology* 153:113-116, 1984.
AP, anteroposterior; *SD*, standard deviation.

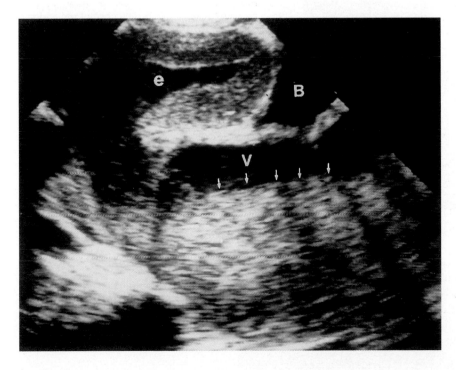

Fig. 17-13 Hydrometrocolpos with mucosal secretions secondary to vaginal atresia in a neonate. Transabdominal sagittal image of the uterus shows a markedly distended vagina *(V)* with a fluid-debris level *(arrows)* and a distended endometrial canal *(e)*. *B*, urinary bladder.

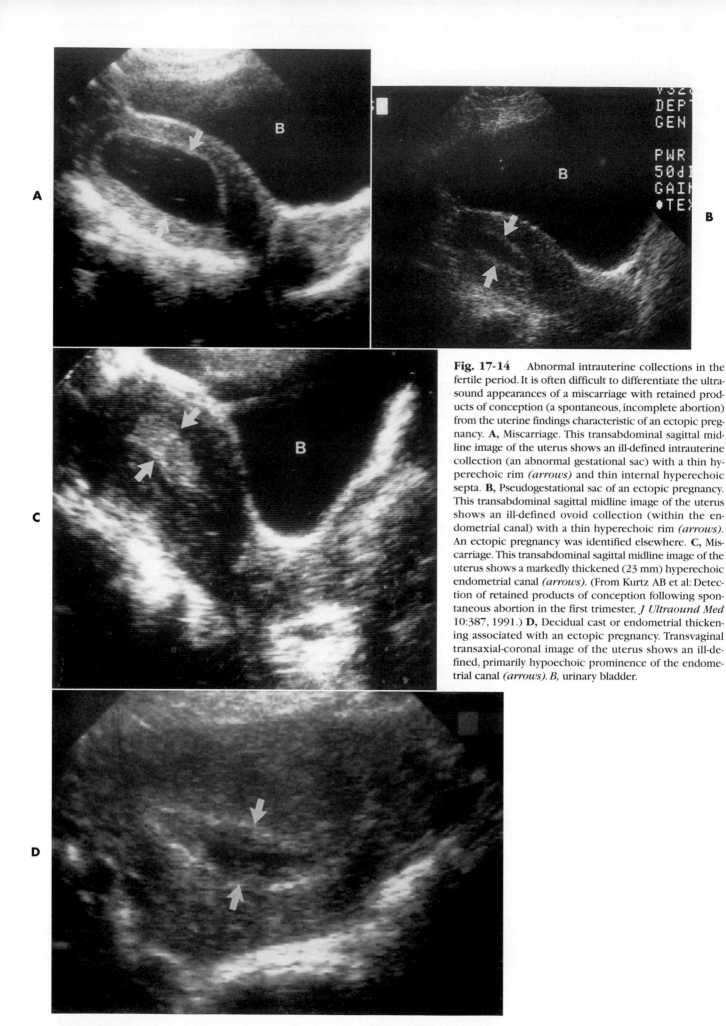

Fig. 17-14 Abnormal intrauterine collections in the fertile period. It is often difficult to differentiate the ultrasound appearances of a miscarriage with retained products of conception (a spontaneous, incomplete abortion) from the uterine findings characteristic of an ectopic pregnancy. **A,** Miscarriage. This transabdominal sagittal midline image of the uterus shows an ill-defined intrauterine collection (an abnormal gestational sac) with a thin hyperechoic rim *(arrows)* and thin internal hyperechoic septa. **B,** Pseudogestational sac of an ectopic pregnancy. This transabdominal sagittal midline image of the uterus shows an ill-defined ovoid collection (within the endometrial canal) with a thin hyperechoic rim *(arrows)*. An ectopic pregnancy was identified elsewhere. **C,** Miscarriage. This transabdominal sagittal midline image of the uterus shows a markedly thickened (23 mm) hyperechoic endometrial canal *(arrows)*. (From Kurtz AB et al: Detection of retained products of conception following spontaneous abortion in the first trimester, *J Ultraound Med* 10:387, 1991.) **D,** Decidual cast or endometrial thickening associated with an ectopic pregnancy. Transvaginal transaxial-coronal image of the uterus shows an ill-defined, primarily hypoechoic prominence of the endometrial canal *(arrows). B,* urinary bladder.

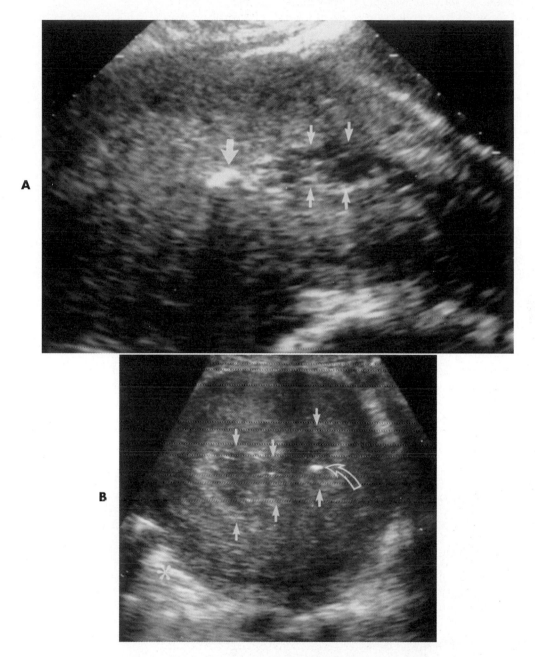

Fig. 17-15   Postpartum scans of the uterus obtained within 1 week of delivery. **A,** Normal appearance. This transabdominal sagittal image of the uterus identifies a moderately thin endometrial canal (14 mm) with one focus of gas *(large arrow),* which is seen as a large (1-cm) hyperechoic area with sharp distal acoustic shadowing in the upper body. Toward the lower uterine segment, a slightly hypoechoic endometrial canal is identified *(small arrows).* **B,** Endometritis in a patient with severe uterine tenderness and fever. This transabdominal transaxial image shows a markedly distended endometrial canal *(arrows).* There is at least one small focus of gas *(curved open arrow)* without distal acoustic shadowing. Note that the focus is as bright as bowel gas (*) adjacent to the uterus.

ances. It is important to detect them because persistent POCs can lead to uterine infection, the formation of synechiae, and metaplasia. The ultrasound appearances of POC are a gestational sac (with or without a nonliving embryo), a round to ovoid fluid collection, and a thickened hyperechoic endometrial stripe of more than 5 mm (Fig 17-14, *A* and *C*). A thinner endometrial stripe of less than 5 mm, particularly when it is less than 2 mm, favors only retained blood.

The postpartum uterus is not routinely studied. However, a pelvic ultrasound may be needed in the event of unexplained fever or pelvic pain. The primary concern is endometritis, which is typically diagnosed on clinical grounds. The ultrasound appearance of gas in the endometrial canal is a supportive finding. In general, however, bright endometrial reflectors (gas) with either a "dirty" or "clean" shadow can be seen in 15% of clinically normal postpartum women in the first 3 to 4 postpartum weeks (Fig. 17-15). If the focus of gas is small, a discrete shadow may not be detected. It is still likely to be gas if its brightness is equal to that of gas in adjacent loops of bowel.

Periuterine abnormalities may also be confused with endometritis in the postpartum period. An ovarian vein thrombus, which almost always occurs on the right side, can be detected by computed tomography (CT) and occasionally by ultrasound. Hematomas can accumulate after either a vaginal or cesarean delivery. Hematomas can be detected in the anterior abdominal wall or in a bladder flap after a cesarean section. A bladder flap hematoma arises between the urinary bladder (initially dissected away from the uterus) and the uterus, if reattached. Hematomas are typically hypoechoic collections (Fig. 17-16). If secondarily infected, their appearance may not change unless gas is present.

In the postmenopausal years a thickened endometrium or fluid collection in the endometrial canal (provided the woman is not on hormone replacement therapy) is a well-established sign of endometrial malignancy, in some series found in as many as 90% of the patients. The differential diagnosis for a hyperechoic endometrial thickening of 8 mm or more typically includes hyperplasia and polyps (Fig. 17-17). A uniformly thickened endometrium more likely signifies glandular hyperplasia; focal thickening more typically represents cancer or polyps. However, this distinction is not absolute. Perhaps disruption of the junctional zone (more consistently seen with MRI) may be an important sign because it would be expected only in the setting of invasive cancer. Rarely a fibroid may be submucosal and disrupt the junctional zone and endometrial complex (Fig. 17-18), or may prolapse into the endometrial canal, both causing focal endometrial thickening. Fibroids are usually hypoechoic and therefore not often confused with the hyperechoic processes just described.

TV ultrasound with the instillation of water into the endometrial canal, is called hysterosonography (see Figs. 17-17 and 17-18). This technique may have future impact on the diagnosis of endometrial and submucosal abnormalities, especially when focal, in both the fertile and postmenopausal years. Using a technique called endolu-

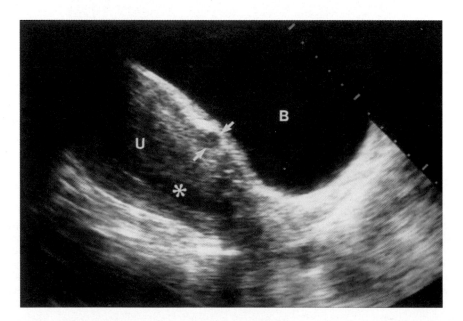

Fig. 17-16   Bladder-flap hematoma in a woman 1 week after cesarean section. This transabdominal sagittal image of the uterus *(U)* shows a small amount of fluid (*) within the endometrial canal. A small hypoechoic hematoma *(arrows)* is identified between the uterus and the distended urinary bladder *(B)*.

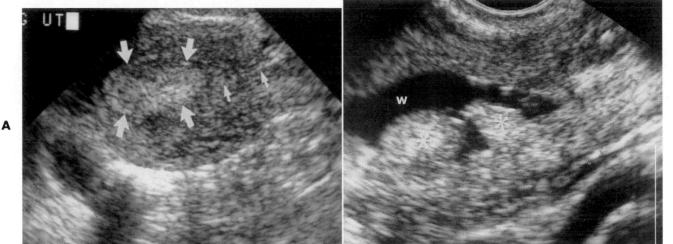

Fig. 17-17   Endometrial polyps. Transvaginal study in a postmenopausal woman, first without and then with the instillation of water into the endometrial canal (hysterosonogram). **A,** Sagittal image of the uterus shows focal hyperechoic thickening of the endometrial canal in the upper body and fundus *(large arrows)*. Small arrows show the normally thin endometrial complex in the lower uterine segment. **B,** After the instillation of water *(w)* into the endometrial canal, two discrete hyperechoic polyps (*) are detected.

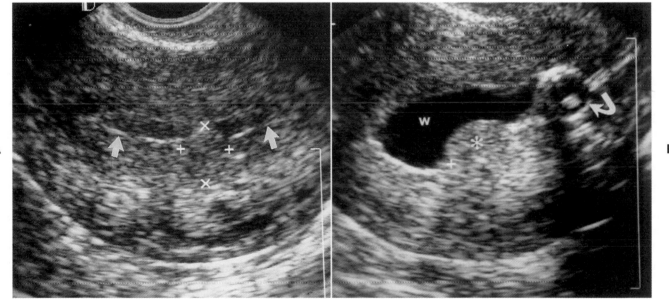

Fig. 17-18   Submucosal fibroid. Transvaginal study in a 40-year-old woman, first without and then with the instillation of water into the endometrial canal (hysterosonogram). **A,** Sagittal image of the uterus shows the thin endometrial canal *(arrows)* distorted by a small hypoechoic mass (+ and ×). **B,** After the instillation of water *(w)* into the endometrial canal, the smooth margin of the submucosal fibroid (+ along its margin and * in the middle) is better seen. A curved arrow denotes the bulbous tip of the catheter inserted into the uterus before the procedure.

minal sonography with a transducer connected to the end of a catheter, the endometrial canal can be imaged better in selected cases.

A postmenopausal endometrial canal collection is never a normal finding. Even when cervical stenosis is noted clinically, an obstructing malignant tumor (not always identified) may be either endometrial or cervical cancer. The endometrial collections range in echogenicity from hypoechoic to hyperechoic and can have a number of etiologies (serous, mucin, or blood) (Fig. 17-19). They can also be secondarily infected (in which case they are termed a *pyometria*); if this goes undiagnosed, serious consequences including uterine rupture can result.

There may be a role for Doppler in the evaluation of suspected malignant growths. Some observers have found that endometrial cancers exhibit abnormal arterial waveforms, either together with an elevated peak systole or with an unusually high diastolic flow. These Doppler abnormalities are thought to be signs of tumor invasion and neovascularity. However, the findings are not always present and their sensitivity and positive predictive values have not yet been established.

INTRAUTERINE DEVICES

The use of intrauterine devices (IUDs) has declined because they are only moderately effective as a contraceptive and do not protect against gynecologic infections. Sometimes they are even responsible for causing infections. Nevertheless, their ultrasound appearances are nevertheless important because IUDs are still prescribed in selected instances or have been in place for many years.

In a woman who is known to have an IUD, the most common clinical problem is to determine whether the IUD is still in situ or whether it has been expelled spontaneously. This is particularly pertinent when the string from the IUD is no longer identified in the vagina. A woman with an IUD may also be studied when she has unexplained pelvic pain and IUD perforation or secondary pelvic inflammatory disease is suspected on clinical grounds or when pregnancy is suspected (either intrauterine or extrauterine).

Ultrasound can determine whether an IUD is present within the uterus and is normally in the midline position within the endometrial canal, equidistant from the uterine margins (Fig. 17-20). Only when fibroids are present does an off-center position still favor the IUD position within the canal.

The sonographic appearance of an IUD is related to its shape and the material it is made of—plastic or metal (copper), or both. Most IUDs are now shaped like a "7" or a T. Previous shapes included an S configuration. The IUD

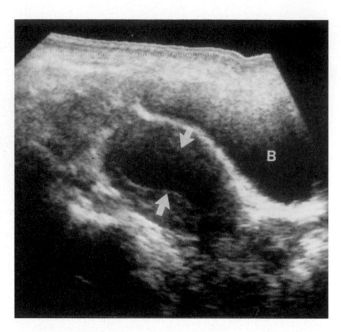

Fig. 17-19   Pyometra secondary to cervical cancer in a postmenopausal woman. Transabdominal sagittal midline image of the uterus shows the endometrial canal distended with fluid *(arrows)*. Although the patient had clinical evidence of cervical stenosis, a biopsy specimen obtained through the stenosis revealed cervical cancer. The fluid was drained and found to be infected. *B,* urinary bladder.

materials are easily differentiated. Plastic is seen as two parallel lines of equal intensity (called an *entrance-and-exit echo*). Metal, which is usually wound around the plastic, is seen as a single bright line with a posterior reverberation artifact consisting of multiple repeating lines of lessening intensity that fade into the posterior soft tissues. A sharp shadow is created by both materials, but only in the short axis of the IUD. This is related to the breaking of the Z axis of the ultrasound beam.

When ultrasound does not detect an IUD, this is usually a sign of unrecognized expulsion, but it can also indicate that the IUD has perforated the myometrium. The signs of perforation can vary from an unexplained obliquely positioned IUD to indefinite visualization. By distorting the IUD position, fibroids can mimic the appearance of partial perforation (Fig. 17-21, *A*). Bright adjacent bowel gas can mimic (or mask) the appearance of complete perforation. It is therefore difficult to diagnose perforation. If the ultrasound findings are normal but there is still clinical concern that the IUD has perforated the myometrium, anteroposterior pelvic radiography or CT may be needed to determine whether the radiopaque IUD is present within the pelvis but outside the uterus.

If a woman with an IUD has pelvic pain, the area around the uterus needs to be assessed to determine whether she has pelvic inflammatory disease (Fig. 17-21, *B*). Dilated fallopian tubes (usually hydrosalpinx) and related abscesses are discussed in Chapter 18.

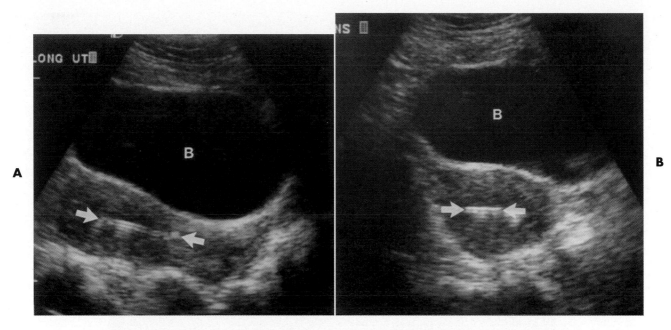

Fig. 17-20   An intrauterine device (copper "7") that is normally positioned in the center of the uterus, in the expected position of the endometrial canal. **A,** Transabdominal image of the uterus shows a well-defined hyperechoic reflector within the endometrial canal *(arrows)* with a distal reverberation artifact. This is consistent with the long copper-wound arm. **B,** Transabdominal transaxial image shows two discrete hyperechoic lines *(arrows)* that represent the short plastic arm of the device. *B,* urinary bladder.

On occasion a pregnancy occurs despite the "protection" of the IUD. If it is an intrauterine pregnancy, an ultrasound examination is needed to identify the gestational sac and determine whether the IUD is still present (Fig. 17-21, *C*). Even if present, the IUD is not of clinical concern because it is in a different anatomic space from that of the pregnancy unless its string remains within the vagina. Then an ascending infection may occur and the IUD must be removed. Removal is best accomplished transcervically under ultrasound guidance and is most successful (without causing pregnancy loss) when the IUD is adjacent to or below the sac. When it is above the sac, the sac is considerably distorted during removal and miscarriage is more likely. Because the incidence of an extrauterine pregnancy is increased in women with IUDs, though the reason for this is not fully understood, the possibility of an ectopic pregnancy must be considered whenever the pregnancy test results are positive but no intrauterine gestation is seen.

FIBROIDS (LEIOMYOMAS)

Fibroids are the most common myometrial abnormality. They are benign soft-tissue tumors that more frequently affect women in certain racial groups, particularly blacks, and women of advancing age. However, fibroids can develop in all women and at all ages. Fibroids can be solitary or multiple, small or large, and located anywhere, from completely within the myometrium, to exophytic, to prolapsing into the endometrial canal. Fibroids usually continue to grow until menopause; afterward they often involute. Rarely sarcomas may develop within the myometrium, either de novo or secondary to fibroid degeneration.

The most common sonographic appearance of a fibroid is a hypoechoic, solid mass (Fig. 17-22, *A*). However, the echogenicity can vary from heterogeneous to hyperechoic, sometimes within the same mass. Fibroids can also calcify and necrose, thus further complicating the sonographic appearance. Because fibroids are solid masses (unless they are necrotic), they absorb sound and cause some degree of acoustic shadowing.

It is not always possible to differentiate a single large fibroid from a close grouping of multiple smaller fibroids (Fig. 17-22, *B*). Usually this distinction is not important unless a uterine-sparing myomectomy is being contemplated. Then MRI is of value to better define the extent of the fibroid (or fibroids) and to determine how much normal uninvolved uterus remains.

The clinical symptoms and the appearance of the fibroids depend on their position, size, and number. The symptoms are usually most pronounced when the fibroids are submucosal or prolapse into the endometrial canal (see Fig. 17-18). Pain and vaginal bleeding are then common, often unrelated to the menstrual cycles. If a fibroid is exophytic, it can torse and necrose and cause pain.

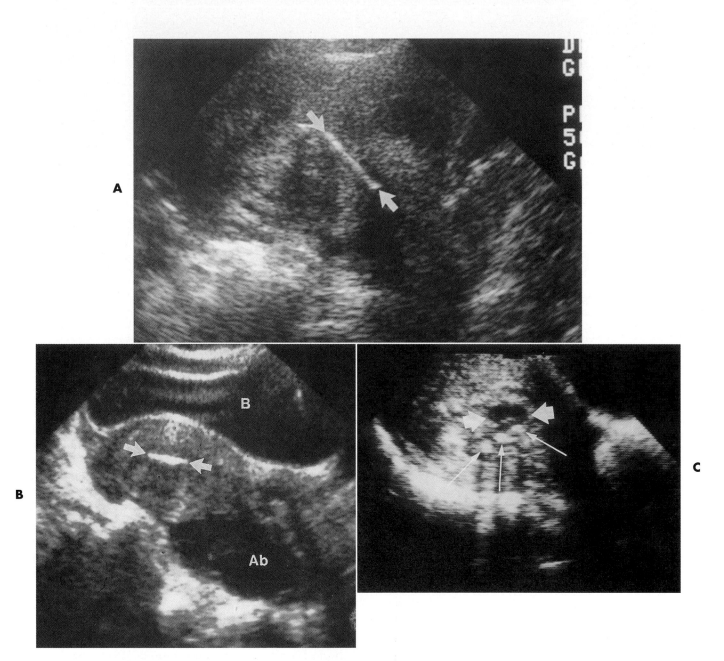

Fig. 17-21   Intrauterine devices—problems with position and complications. **A,** Distortion by fibroids. This transabdominal sagittal image of the uterus identifies the long arm of the copper "7" *(arrows).* Because the uterus is markedly distorted by multiple fibroids, its exact position relative to the
endometrial canal cannot be established. **B,** Pelvic inflammatory disease with an abscess *(Ab).* This
transabdominal sagittal image of the uterus shows the long arm of an intrauterine device *(arrows)*
that is well positioned within the middle of the uterus. A large hypoechoic collection is seen posteriorly. *B,* urinary bladder. **C,** Failed contraception with an intrauterine device (a Lippes loop) in place.
This transabdominal sagittal image of the uterus shows a well-defined gestational sac *(short arrows)*
with a living embryo. Adjacent to the sac are three hyperechoic plastic coils of a Lippes loop *(long
thin arrows).*

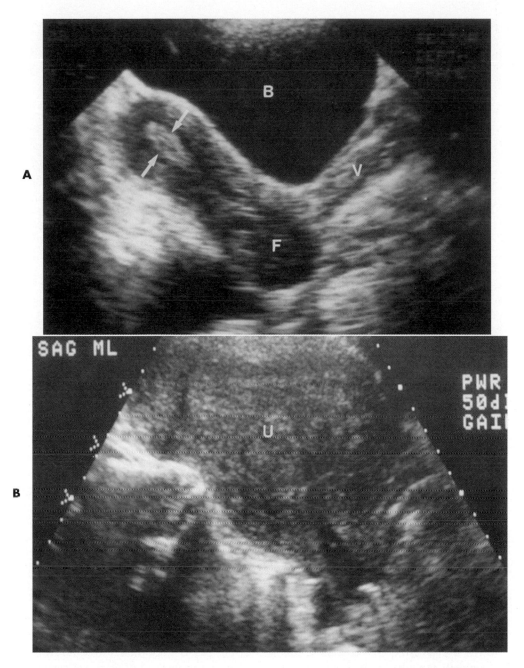

Fig. 17-22   Leiomyomas (fibroids) of the uterus. **A,** Transabdominal sagittal image of the uterus shows a normal-appearing body and fundus with a prominent hyperechoic endometrial stripe *(arrows)*. The cervical region is distorted by a hypoechoic, solid fibroid *(F)*. *B,* urinary bladder; *V,* vagina. **B,** Transabdominal sagittal image of the uterus *(U)* shows a completely distorted uterine shape and echogenicity caused by multiple heterogeneous, solid fibroids. The endometrial canal cannot be identified.

Most fibroids develop in the middle of the myometrium. They may, however, cause a bulge in the uterine contour and distort the junctional zone. Distortion of the uterine contour, even when the uterine echogenicity is normal, makes fibroids (usually small ones) likely. An enlarged uterus that exhibits abnormal echogenicity but

shows no discrete mass is often a sign of diffuse leiomyomatosis (Fig. 17-23).

As previously described, a normal retroverted or retroflexed uterus is normally more globular in shape and attenuates more of the ultrasound beam than an anteverted uterus. It may initially give the impression of a sin-

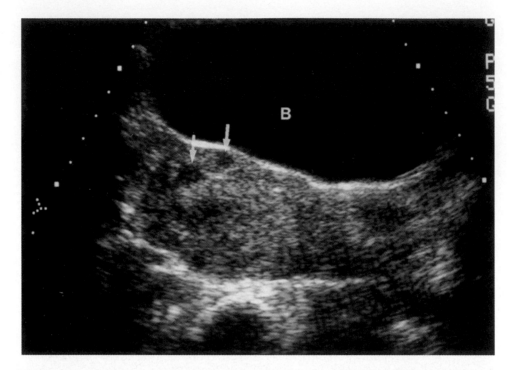

Fig. 17-23   Diffuse uterine leiomyomas. This transabdominal sagittal image of the uterus shows a totally distorted hyperechoic uterus. Two discrete, small hypoechoic fibroids are identified *(arrows)*. Note the irregularity of the margin of the uterus with the urinary bladder *(B)*. Although the uterus still grossly maintains its normal shape, it is enlarged and the endometrial complex and the junctional zone are lost.

gle large hypoechoic fibroid. Increasing the ultrasound gain and perhaps TV scanning can usually show the uterus to be normal.

Fibroids may calcify, sometimes heavily (Fig. 17-24). These calcifications are usually clumpy and, when numerous, confluent. They have a typical sonographic appearance consisting of well-defined hyperechoic areas with sharp acoustic shadowing. The calcifications can often be identified within the confines of the fibroid but are occasionally the only presenting sign of a fibroid. If the calcifications become extensive, they may completely obscure the uterus and a pelvic radiograph is then needed to establish the diagnosis of a myomatous uterus.

Fibroids may necrose, often causing unusual sonographic appearances. If the appearance is very atypical or if the mass is unusually large, especially when associated with ascites, a sarcoma should be considered. This distinction is otherwise not possible. The differentiation of a fibroid from an endometrial carcinoma is usually straightforward unless the endometrial carcinoma has extensively invaded the myometrium.

Adenomyosis is the uterine form of endometriosis and is discussed further in Chapter 18. It is pathologically the extension of endometrial rests (usually microscopic) into the myometrium. Adenomyosis typically causes pain, particularly around the time of menstruation, and can be identified by MRI and occasionally by ultrasound, primar-

ily by the finding of a distorted junctional zone and often a distorted myometrium. Ultrasound studies show the junctional zone to be lost and replaced by multiple small hypoechoic, solid masses (<10 to 15 mm in diameter) that give a "moth-eaten" appearance to the myometrium (Fig. 17-25). This is similar to the appearance of multiple small fibroids. It is claimed that MRI can consistently differentiate these two processes, but currently there is little pathologic evidence to confirm this claim.

When fibroids cause the uterus to enlarge, the ovaries are displaced from their normal position, usually into the upper pelvis–abdomen. Infrequently the ovaries may become fixed in the cul-de-sac. Although the ovaries continue to lie adjacent to the enlarged uterus, distortion of the uterine contour often makes it difficult to identify the ovary (unless typical follicles are present). However, it is at least possible to survey the area around the uterus to rule out the existence of an extrauterine mass, typically a cystic or complex abnormality.

Fibroids can present clinically, sonographically, or both for the first time during pregnancy (Fig. 17-26). Although their development is not caused by the pregnancy, their growth is often accelerated at this time. If the fibroid is in a critical uterine position, that is, in the lower uterine segment or below the placental attachment, it should be carefully monitored to determine whether it could cause problems at delivery (dystocia) or during fetal growth.

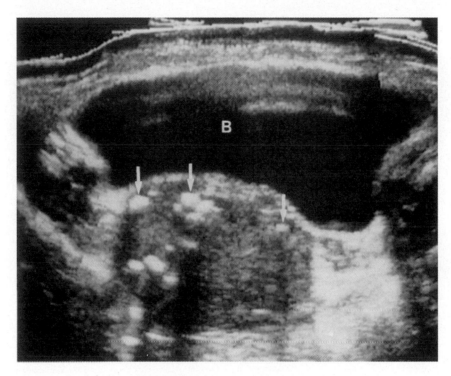

Fig. 17-24   Leiomyomatous uterus with calcifications. This transabdominal transaxial image shows an enlarged, distorted uterus. In addition to its heterogeneous echogenicity, there are multiple discrete hyperechoic foci with sharp distal acoustic shadowing (three denoted by arrows) consistent with calcifications. *B,* urinary bladder.

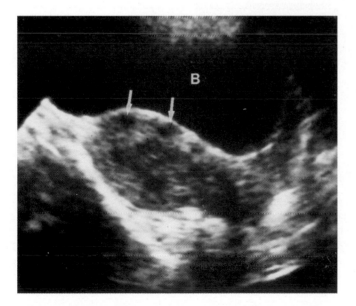

Fig. 17-25   Adenomyosis of the uterus. Transabdominal sagittal image of the uterus shows complete distortion by multiple small hypoechoic, solid areas (two denoted by arrows). Although these could be small fibroids, this pattern is occasionally seen in the intrauterine form of endometriosis. *B,* urinary bladder.

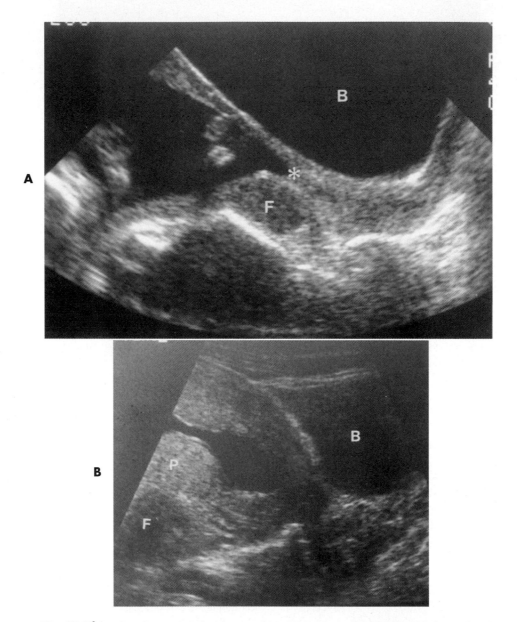

Fig. 17-26 Fibroids associated with second-trimester pregnancies. **A,** Transabdominal sagittal image of the lower uterine segment shows a small hypoechoic, solid fibroid *(F)* distorting the lower uterine segment adjacent to the internal cervical os (*). **B,** Transabdominal sagittal scan through the lower uterine segment shows a large solid fibroid *(F)* posterior to and displacing the placenta *(P)* anteriorly. *B,* urinary bladder.

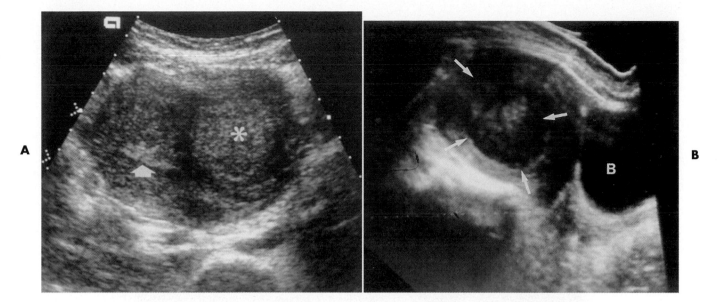

Fig. 17-27 Fibroids mimicking the appearance of uterine duplication and endometrial canal obstruction. **A,** Transabdominal transaxial image of the uterus shows what initially appears to be a duplicated "squared-off" uterus. The uterus, however, is displaced toward the right with its endometrial canal identified *(arrow)*. Toward the left, extending into the broad ligament, is a hyperechoic fibroid (*). **B,** Transabdominal sagittal midline image of the uterus shows what initially appears to be an obstructed uterus. Instead a large fibroid with a necrotic center *(arrow)* is present. *B,* urinary bladder.

FIBROIDS—THE PELVIC MIMICKER

Although the sonographic appearance of fibroids is usually straightforward, it may mimic that of other pelvic conditions, both normal and abnormal, in less than 5% of the cases. Fibroids can assume the appearance of uterine variants, uterine abnormalities, pregnancy-related conditions, IUD perforation, and adnexal masses.

Fibroids can mimic the appearance of uterine duplication and obstruction (Fig. 17-27). If a fibroid extends directly lateral to the body of the uterus, usually into the broad ligament, it may have the approximate shape and size of a second uterine horn. If necrotic, a large fibroid may look like a fluid collection in an obstructed uterus. If multiple and small, fibroids may mimic the appearance of adenomyosis (as previously stated).

Atypical fibroid appearances may mimic pregnancy-related conditions or distort their appearance, primarily in the first trimester (Fig. 17-28). Multiple fibroids can surround a small gestational sac. A fibroid may also necrose such that the necrotic center looks like a gestational sac. If the fibroids are large and very hyperechoic, they can occasionally mimic the appearance of a hydatidiform mole. A fibroid that calcifies along its rim may be mistaken for the calvarium of a fetal head. Fibroids may so distort the position of a single normal gestational sac that the sac appears to be at the edge of or outside the uterus, then falsely appearing in an ectopic position.

An IUD is expected to be in the middle of the uterus, within the endometrial canal. As already stated, fibroids can distort the canal, making it appear partially perforated into the uterine wall (see Fig. 17-21, *A*).

When fibroids are primarily subserosal or exophytic, they can mimic the appearance of adnexal masses (Figs. 17-29 and 17-30, *A*). These appearances may be so atypical that the diagnosis of fibroids is not considered unless other more typical appearing fibroids are present. On occasion when a pedunculated fibroid can be palpated, it can be observed to move but never away from the uterus. Fibroids can mimic the appearances of dermoids, endometriomas, cystadenomas, hemorrhagic cysts, and even ovarian malignant tumors (Fig. 17-30, *B*). Conversely, very infrequently a solid ovarian mass may mimic the appearance of a fibroid (Fig. 17-31).

Even pelvic Doppler findings may be misleading. Some fibroids, similar to the some ovarian cancers, have an arterial waveform showing high diastolic flow (see Fig. 17-29). This finding is discussed further in Chapter 18.

When the diagnosis of a fibroid is uncertain, TV scanning may be helpful. Although not always able to image the entire uterus (especially when the uterus is enlarged), TV imaging may show that there are additional more typical appearing fibroids and even identify the connection of an exophytic fibroid to the uterus.

On occasion a woman is found to have a large, solid pelvoabdominal mass (Fig. 17-32). If the uterus is not detected and the mass has no other site of origin, a fibroid should be considered.

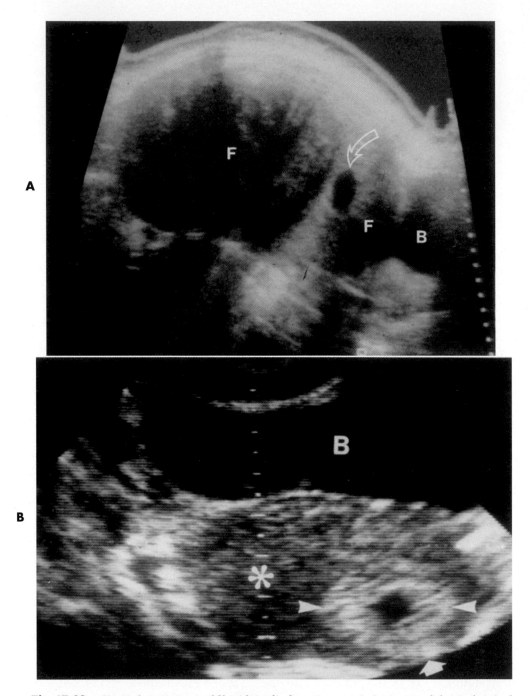

Fig. 17-28   Unusual appearance of fibroids in the first trimester. **A,** Static transabdominal sagittal midline image shows marked distortion and enlargement of the uterus caused by multiple hypoechoic, solid fibroids *(F)*. An intrauterine gestational sac *(curved open arrow)* is identified. No normal uterine tissue can be seen. **B,** Transabdominal transaxial image of the uterus shows a gestational sac *(arrowheads)* that a large fibroid (*) has caused to deviate markedly to the left. There is still a thin margin of myometrium *(arrow)* surrounding the intrauterine sac. *B,* urinary bladder.

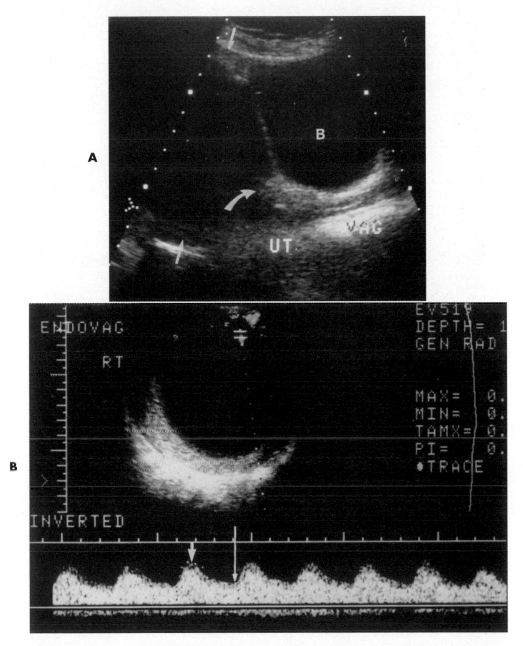

Fig. 17-29   Necrotic exophytic fibroid mimicking the appearance of ovarian cancer in a post-menopausal patient. **A,** Transabdominal sagittal image shows a small uterus *(UT)*. Its fundus appears to end at the curved arrow, and more superiorly a large cystic mass *(arrow)* is identified. *B,* urinary bladder; *VAG,* vagina. **B,** Split-image study of the necrotic fibroid, the upper image showing the Doppler cursor placed in the wall of the mass and the lower image its arterial Doppler waveform. Diastolic flow is prominent, with end-diastole *(long arrow)* more than half peak systole *(short arrow)*, falsely suggestive of malignant neovascularity.

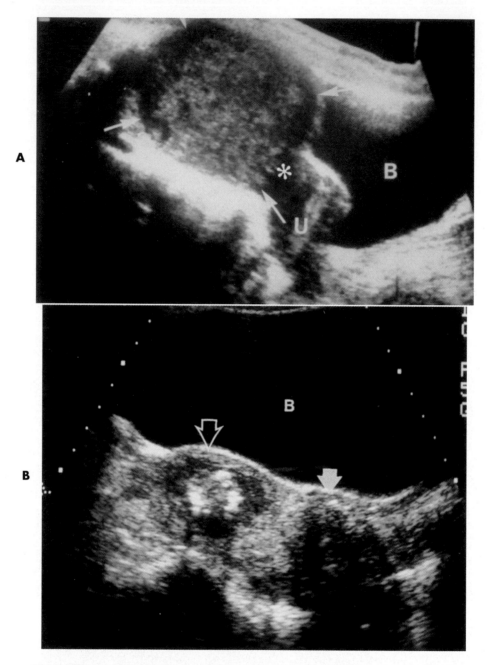

Fig. 17-30   Fibroids mimicking the appearance of adnexal masses. **A,** Subserosal-exophytic fibroid. This transabdominal sagittal midline image of the pelvis shows the uterus *(U)* with an adjacent large hyperechoic mass *(arrows)*. This fibroid was initially thought to be an adnexal mass but is connected to the uterus by a thin stalk of myometrium (*). (From Baltarowich OH et al: Pitfalls in the sonographic diagnosis of uterine fibroids, *AJR* 151:725, 1988.) **B,** Calcified fibroid. This transabdominal sagittal midline image of the pelvis shows two abnormalities. The lower one, toward the right, is a hypoechoic solid area with moderate acoustic shadowing *(solid arrow)*. The upper one *(open arrow)* is a hypoechoic, well-circumscribed mass with central calcifications, initially thought to be a dermoid. However, because a normal uterus could not be identified, these were correctly diagnosed as fibroids. *B,* urinary bladder.

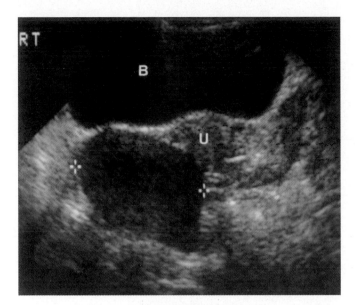

Fig. 17-31   Ovarian fibroma mimicking the appearance of a fibroid. Transabdominal transaxial image of the pelvis shows a large hypoechoic solid mass (+) to the right of the uterus *(U)*. Although its sonographic appearance is typical of a fibroid and although subserosal-exophytic fibroids can originate from the uterine margin, this is instead a benign, solid ovarian mass. *B,* urinary bladder.

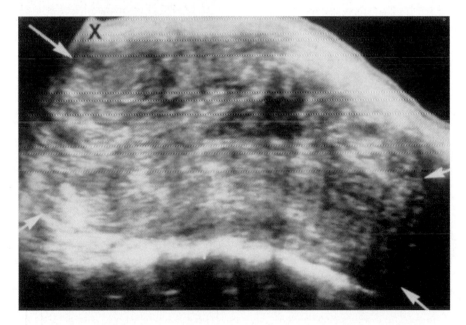

Fig. 17-32   Huge leiomyomatous uterus in a postmenopausal woman, presenting as a large hard abdominal mass. Static sagittal midline image from the pubic symphysis (on the right) to the xiphoid process *(X)* shows a massive solid, heterogeneous mass *(arrows)* completely filling the pelvis and abdomen. This mass did not arise from any abdominal organ. No uterus could be identified. (From Baltarowich OH et al: Pitfalls in the sonographic diagnosis of uterine fibroids, *AJR* 151:725, 1988.)

Key Features

Two ultrasound techniques are used in the pelvis: the transabdominal study performed through a full bladder and a transvaginal examination performed with the bladder empty. The transabdominal study can obtain an overview of pelvic structures. The transvaginal scan is able to show structures in greater detail but is limited in terms of the movement of the transducer and in its depth of field.

On any initial examination, the transabdominal scan should be performed, with transvaginal scanning done when indicated. It may only be necessary to use the more diagnostic technique on a follow-up examination.

There is an angle to the ultrasound beam as it exits from the transvaginal probe. This must be taken into account when imaging pelvic structures both in the sagittal plane and in the transaxial-coronal plane.

In the fertile years the uterus should be evaluated for the following: its position and size, the endometrial echogenicity and thickness, the junctional zone, and the myometrial echogenicity.

In the estrogen or proliferative phase the endometrium has either a uniformly hyperechoic or a striated appearance and is 8 mm or less thick. In the progesterone or secretory phase, the endometrium continues to thicken (up to 15 mm) and is uniformly hyperechoic.

In the fertile years the normal size of the uterus has no upper limits, provided all uterine layers and its echogenicity are normal.

The uterus is normally anteverted. When retroverted, the uterus assumes a more globular shape, occasionally mimicking the appearance of a fibroid.

It is important to differentiate uterine flexion from version, particularly if the woman is to undergo evacuation of the endometrial canal.

Congenital uterine anomalies are usually not detected by ultrasound. On occasion ultrasound can detect two uterine horns or the renal finding (ptosis or agenesis) that suggests a uterine anomaly. Transvaginal ultrasound may better define these abnormalities.

The postpartum uterus involutes rapidly, occurring mostly during the first 3 to 4 weeks. The uterus returns to normal by the seventh week. The postpartum uterus can be reliably measured in its long axis.

The postpartum endometrium is usually thin, typically or less than 15 mm thickness. The existence of retained products is likely if it is thicker. If gas is detected in the first 4 weeks, it is usually a normal finding unless it is associated with the physical findings of endometritis.

After the neonatal period the premenstrual uterus is small, enlarging until the time of puberty. The cervix is larger than the body and fundus, and the endometrial canal is usually not identified.

The postmenopausal uterus (in the absence of hormone replacement therapy) progressively involutes and by 15 to 20 postmenopausal years reaches a size similar to that of a premenopausal uterus, except that the fundus and body remain larger. The endometrial stripe either is not identified or is hyperechoic and thin but is always normal if 4 mm or greater and probably normal up to 7 mm in thickness.

When an abnormality of the endometrium is encountered, two questions need to be answered: (1) Is the patient in the premenstrual, fertile, or postmenopausal periods? and (2) Is the abnormality an unusually thick endometrium or is it a collection within the endometrial canal?

Abnormalities of the endometrium in the premenstrual period are almost always related to a vaginal obstruction. In the fertile years they are almost always related to pregnancies and the abnormality is either a thickened endometrium or a collection. In the postmenopausal years a thickened endometrium and obstruction are relatively highly associated with endometrial or cervical cancer.

In a woman who is known to have an intrauterine device, scans are performed primarily to determine whether the device is still in place and well positioned within the uterus. Additionally, evidence of associated pelvic inflammatory disease (fallopian tube abnormalities or an abscess) and pregnancy (intrauterine or extrauterine) can be sought. It is difficult, and often impossible, to identify perforation.

A typical fibroid is a hypoechoic, solid mass that is positioned within the myometrium. However, there is tremendous variability in its echogenicity, size, number, and position.

Often when an enlarged myomatous uterus is identifed, the ovaries cannot be clearly defined. It may only be possible to evaluate the surrounding area to rule out the presence of an extrauterine mass.

During pregnancy fibroids may become evident and often enlarge. If critically placed, such as in the lower uterine segment, they should be closely watched.

Fibroids are the great pelvic mimicker. In less than 5% of the cases they may assume the appearance of a number of pelvic conditions: uterine variants, uterine abnormalities, pregnancy-related conditions, IUD perforation, and adnexal masses. An early intrauterine pregnancy may be so displaced by the fibroid as to appear in an ectopic position.

Sarcomas (either de novo or secondary to fibroid degeneration), adenomyosis, and occasionally endometrial carcinoma (if extensive) may need to be differentiated from fibroids.

When a solid pelvic mass, but not a site of origin, is identified, a fibroid should be one of the abnormalities considered.

SUGGESTED READINGS

Baker ME, Bowie JD, Killam AP: Sonography of post-cesarean-section bladder-flap hematoma, *AJR* 144:757, 1985.

Baltarowich OH: *Female pelvic organ measurements*. In Goldberg BB, Kurtz AB, editors: *Atlas of ultrasound measurements*. Chicago, 1990, Year Book Medical Publishers.

Baltarowich OH et al: Pitfalls in the sonographic diagnosis of uterine fibroids, *AJR* 151:725, 1988.

Breckenridge JW et al: Postmenopausal uterine fluid collection: indicator of carcinoma, *AJR* 139:529, 1982.

Carter JR et al: Gray scale and color flow Doppler characterization of uterine tumors, *J Ultrasound Med* 13:835, 1994.

Cicinelli E et al: Transabdominal sonohysterography, transvaginal sonography, and hysteroscopy in the evaluation of submucous myomas, *Obstet Gynecol* 85:42, 1995.

Dubinsky TJ et al: Transvaginal hysterosonography in the evaluation of small endoluminal masses, *J Ultrasound Med* 14:1, 1995.

DuBose TJ et al: Sonography of arcuate uterine blood vessels, *J Ultrasound Med* 4:229, 1985.

Goldberg BB et al: Endoluminal gynecologic ultrasound: preliminary results, *J Ultrasound Med* 10:583, 1991.

Haynor DR et al: Changing appearance of the normal uterus during the menstrual cycle: MR studies, *Radiology* 161:459, 1986.

Kupfer MC et al: Transvaginal sonographic evaluation of endometrial polyps, *J Ultrasound Med* 13:535, 1994.

Kurtz AB et al: Detection of retained products of conception following spontaneous abortion in the first trimester, *J Ultrasound Med* 10:387, 1991.

Langlois PL: The size of the normal uterus, *J Reprod Med* 4:221, 1970.

Mitchell DG et al: Zones of the uterus: discrepancy between US and MR images, *Radiology* 174:827, 1990.

Najarian KE, Kurtz AB: New observations in the sonographic evaluation of intrauterine contraceptive devices, *J Ultrasound Med* 5:205, 1986.

Orsini LF et al: Pelvic organs in premenarchal girls: real-time ultrasonography, *Radiology* 153:113, 1984.

Pellerito JS et al: Diagnosis of uterine anomalies: relative accuracy of MR imaging, endovaginal sonography, and hysterosalpingography, *Radiology* 183:795, 1992.

Shalev J et al: Continuous sonographic monitoring of IUD extraction during pregnancy: preliminary report, *AJR* 139:521, 1982.

Siedler D et al: Uterine adenomyosis. A difficult sonographic diagnosis, *J Ultrasound Med* 6:345, 1987.

Strobelt N et al: Natural history of uterine leiomyomas in pregnancy, *J Ultrasound Med* 13:399, 1994.

Thickman D et al: Sonographic assessment of the endometrium in patients undergoing in vitro fertilization, *J Ultrasound Med* 5:197, 1986.

Togashi K et al: Adenomyosis: diagnosis with MR imaging, *Radiology* 166:111, 1988.

Tongson T, Pongnarisorn C, Mahanuphap P: Use of vaginosonographic measurements of endometrial thickness in the identification of abnormal endometrium in peri- and postmenopausal bleeding, *J Clin Ultrasound* 22:479, 1994.

Varner RE et al: Transvaginal sonography of the endometrium in postmenopausal women, *Obstet Gynecol* 78:195, 1991.

Wachsberg RH, Kurtz AB: Gas within the endometrial cavity at postpartum US: a normal finding after spontaneous vaginal delivery, *Radiology* 183:431, 1992.

Wachsberg RH et al: Real-time ultrasonographic analysis of the normal postpartum uterus: technique, variability, and measurements, *J Ultrasound Med* 13:215, 1994.

18

Adnexa

Ovarian Position
Normal Ovaries in the Fertile Period
Fertility Medications
Normal Ovaries in the Premenstrual (Pediatric) and Postmenopausal Periods
TA versus TV Scanning
Functioning and Nonfunctioning Ovarian Cysts
Complex Cysts
Cystic Teratoma (Dermoid)
Endometriosis
Pelvic Inflammatory Disease
Ovarian Torsion
Ovarian Malignancy

For a Key Features summary see p. 413.

The adnexa contains many structures. Each has an ovary, its mesosalpinx, a fallopian tube, a broad ligament, and uterine and ovarian blood vessels.

Sonographically (and clinically) only the ovaries are detected consistently. The normal nondilated fallopian tubes are not identified, although thin hypoechoic soft-tissue bands, containing the tubes, can often be imaged adjacent to the lateral margins of the uterine fundus. The mesosalpinges and broad ligaments are not seen, even when abnormal. Although normal-caliber uterine and ovarian arteries and veins are not identified distinctly, their Doppler flow can be detected along the lateral uterine margins and adjacent to the ovaries.

OVARIAN POSITION

The ovaries are the only truly intraperitoneal adnexal structures. Their position, however, is not always constant (Fig. 18-1). They are usually found directly lateral to the body of the uterus in shallow depressions called the *ovarian fossae*. These fossae are bordered laterally and ante-

riorly by the external iliac blood vessels and bordered posteriorly by the ureter and internal iliac (hypogastric) blood vessels. When the uterus is deviated toward the right or left (a normal variant), the ovary on that side is usually displaced superiorly, taking a position lateral to the uterine fundus. When the uterus is tilted posteriorly, the ovaries follow and appear as "ears" at the top of the uterine fundus (Fig. 18-1, *D*).

With uterine enlargement (including pregnancy), the ovaries are displaced, typically to a more superior and lateral position. After a myomectomy and after delivery the ovaries often remain in their new position, seldom returning to the ovarian fossae. On occasion an ovary (either normal or abnormal) becomes fixed in the cul-de-sac (Fig. 18-1, *E*). After hysterectomy the ovaries move caudally, typically assuming a position more medial and directly superior to the vaginal cuff.

NORMAL OVARIES IN THE FERTILE PERIOD

The fertile (ovulating) woman is usually 14 to 50 years of age and has normal menstrual cycles. During these cycles the ovaries often vary in size because of the changing number and size of its follicles (functional cysts). The ovary is classically *ovoid* (not round) and it has a low-level, uniform echogenicity and a thin hyperechoic rim (Fig. 18-1). Its maximum dimensions in young nulliparous women are smaller than those in older parous women (Table 18-1).

Many observers think that ovarian size should be expressed as a volume. Using three perpendicular (orthogonal) measurements, the volume is calculated by the prolated ellipse equation: length × width × anteroposterior dimension × 0.5. This formula yields maximum volumes of 6.0 and 15.0 cc for nulliparous and parous women, respectively (Table 18-1). With multiple follicles (which can-

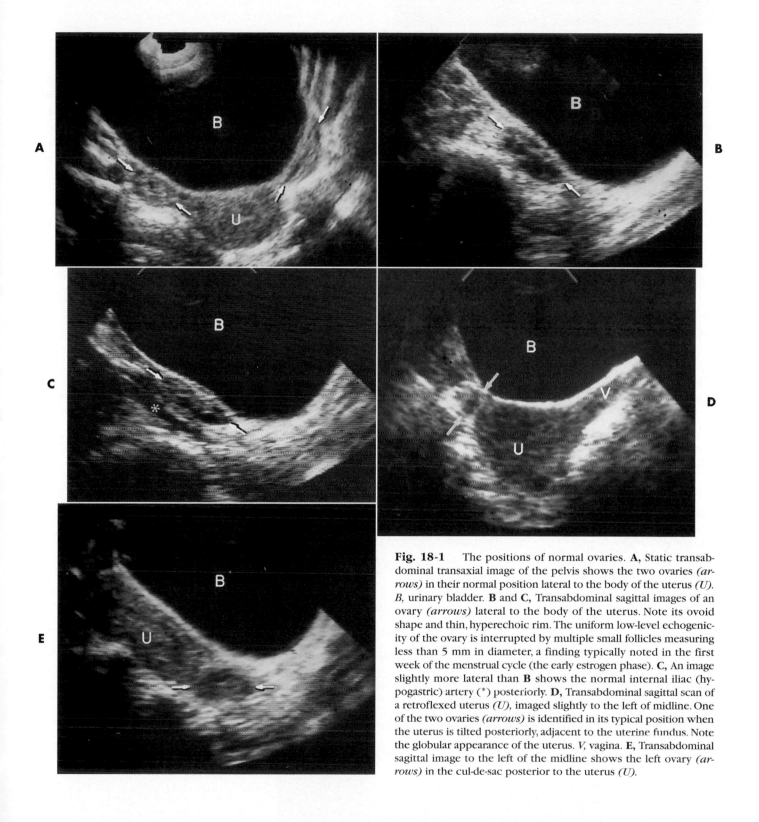

Fig. 18-1   The positions of normal ovaries. **A,** Static transabdominal transaxial image of the pelvis shows the two ovaries *(arrows)* in their normal position lateral to the body of the uterus *(U)*. *B,* urinary bladder. **B** and **C,** Transabdominal sagittal images of an ovary *(arrows)* lateral to the body of the uterus. Note its ovoid shape and thin, hyperechoic rim. The uniform low-level echogenicity of the ovary is interrupted by multiple small follicles measuring less than 5 mm in diameter, a finding typically noted in the first week of the menstrual cycle (the early estrogen phase). **C,** An image slightly more lateral than **B** shows the normal internal iliac (hypogastric) artery (*) posteriorly. **D,** Transabdominal sagittal scan of a retroflexed uterus *(U)*, imaged slightly to the left of midline. One of the two ovaries *(arrows)* is identified in its typical position when the uterus is tilted posteriorly, adjacent to the uterine fundus. Note the globular appearance of the uterus. *V,* vagina. **E,** Transabdominal sagittal image to the left of the midline shows the left ovary *(arrows)* in the cul-de-sac posterior to the uterus *(U)*.

Table 18-1	Approximate top normal ovarian linear dimensions and volumes during the fertile (ovulatory) years	
Patient category	**Dimensions (L × W × AP)***	**Volume†**
Young adult, nulliparous	3 × 2 × 2	6
Adult, parous	5 × 3 × 2	15

From Baltarowich OH: *Female pelvic organ measurements.* In Goldberg BB, Kurtz AB, editors: *Atlas of ultrasound measurements,* Chicago, 1990, Year Book Medical Publishers.
*The three perpendicular orthogonal diameters in centimeters: *L,* length; *W,* width; *AP,* anteroposterior.
†Volume calculated by the prolated ellipse equation in cubic centimeters: L × W × AP × 0.5.

not be separated from the ovarian stroma when measurements are needed), the dimensions can be larger. If the remaining ovarian tissue appears normal, ovarian volumes may be normal, even when they exceed 20 cc.

There is no statistically significant difference in the size of the right and left ovaries. Their volumes, however, may be discrepant by as much as 14 cc.

The ovaries in the normally fertile woman go through cycles lasting approximately 28 days (Figs. 18-1, *B*, and 18-2). These cycles can be divided into the time before ovulation (the estrogen phase) and the time afterward (the progesterone phase). In the estrogen phase at the time of menstruation, the ovaries are at their smallest and contain follicles that are either too small to be detected or less than 5 mm in diameter. By day 10 in the cycle one

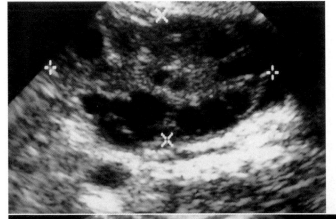

A

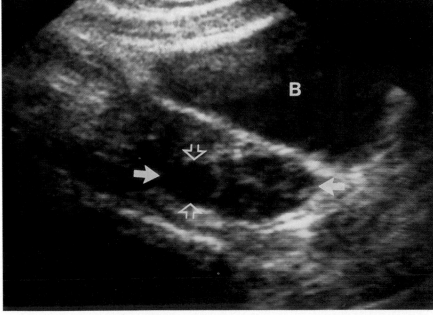

B

Fig. 18-2   Normal ovaries in the estrogen phase in different women. **A,** Day 10. This transvaginal sagittal image of the ovary (+ and *x*) shows multiple follicles less than 10 mm in diameter. **B,** Day 12. Transabdominal sagittal image of the ovary *(closed arrows)* shows a dominant follicle with a diameter of 18 mm *(open arrows)* at its superior margin.

follicle typically begins to dominate and increases to 15 mm, with other follicles, usually bilateral ones, remaining less than 10 mm. By midcycle this largest follicle attains a size of 20 to 25 mm and is then considered mature. A small hyperechoic, soft-tissue area can occasionally be identified on its inner margin. This is the cumulus oophorus and contains the egg or ovum.

The luteinizing hormone surge at midcycle causes the mature follicle to rupture and release its egg. All the other follicles begin to shrink in the progesterone phase. The ruptured follicle loses its fluid, rapidly shrinks, and becomes a corpus luteum. Its small amount of fluid can often be detected in the cul-de-sac. On occasion the ruptured follicle bleeds internally and reexpands, even becoming large enough to present as a mass (Fig. 18-3). This mass, termed a *hemorrhagic cyst*, usually resolves within one to two menstrual cycles. It is discussed further in the section on complicated cysts. By the end of the progesterone phase, as menstruation begins, all the follicles have involuted and the cycle starts again.

FERTILITY MEDICATIONS

Fertility medicines such as clomiphene citrate (Clomid) "overdrive" the ovaries, forcing the maturation of many of their follicles. With successful treatment it is not uncommon for the ovaries to show multiple follicles of 20 mm or more in diameter by midcycle. The role of ultrasound is to identify and measure these follicles. If the follicles are of this appropriate size, then the woman can be stimulated with luteinizing hormone or the follicles can be harvested by cyst aspiration.

Infrequently the ovaries can be so stimulated that the ovarian hyperstimulation syndrome (OHS) develops. OHS is often caused by increasing doses of medication. It can, however, be idiopathic, occurring in one cycle but not in the preceding or subsequent cycle (even with the same dose of medication). OHS is a clinical syndrome in which both ovaries become so enlarged with multiple follicles that they are easily palpable (Fig. 18-4). The ovaries may each measure more than 20 cm in maximum length. The follicles leak fluid across their walls, causing transudative ascites and even pleural effusions. If a woman with OHS becomes pregnant, the hyperstimulation may persist and even worsen. The pregnant woman may suffer considerable hemodilution and electrolyte disturbances and require prolonged care or hospitalization during her pregnancy. The condition can even be life-threatening.

Ultrasound can easily detect these hyperstimulated ovaries, even before they become clinically obvious. Before gross enlargement the ovaries are already slightly enlarged and yet are completely replaced by follicles (Fig. 18-5). When no identifiable ovarian tissue remains, luteinizing hormone stimulation and pregnancy induction should be avoided until the ovaries revert to normal.

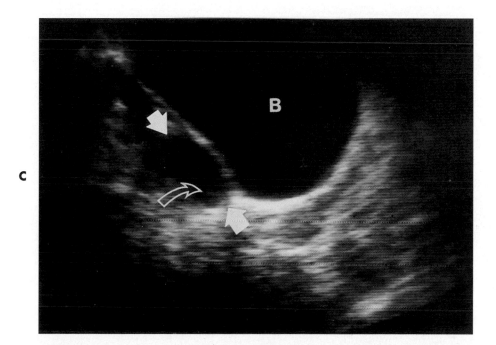

Fig. 18-2, cont'd. C, Midcycle image of a mature 25-mm follicle *(closed arrows)* with the cumulus oophorus *(curved open arrow)* at its lower margin. *B,* urinary bladder.

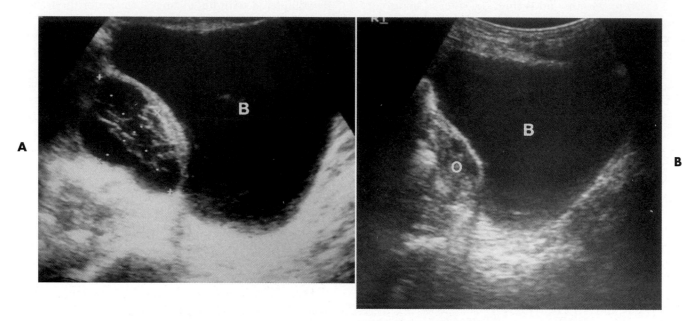

Fig. 18-3   Transabdominal sagittal images of the left adnexa showing a hemorrhagic cyst with resolution. **A,** The initial image shows an ovoid, complex mass (+ and *x*) with cystic areas, septations, and good-through transmission. **B,** Two menstrual cycles later this has completely resolved and only a normal left ovary *(O)* is identified. *B,* urinary bladder.

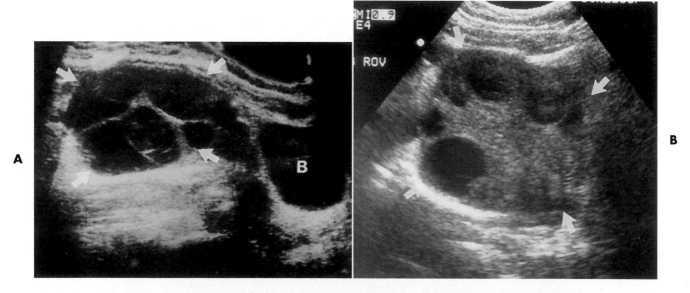

Fig. 18-4   Transabdominal images of enlarged palpable ovaries *(arrows)* in two different patients with clinically evident ovarian hyperstimulation syndrome. **A,** Sagittal image of an ovary showing almost total distortion by enlarged cysts. *B,* urinary bladder. **B,** Sagittal image of an ovary in another woman showing both enlarged cysts and hyperechoic stroma *(arrows).* The other ovary was similarly affected in both women.

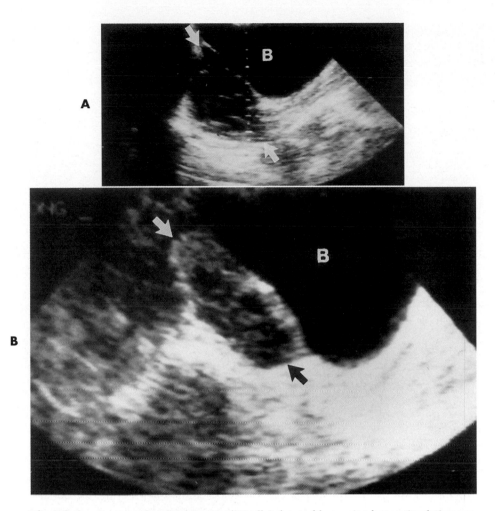

Fig. 18-5   Sonographically (but not clinically) detectable ovarian hyperstimulation syndrome. **A,** Transabdominal sagittal image of the left ovary *(arrow)* in a woman taking fertility medication shows a 6 × 4-cm multicystic structure. No normal ovarian tissue is identified. **B,** Two months after cessation of the medication, the same ovary *(arrows)* has returned to normal and normal small follicles can be identified. *B,* urinary bladder.

Table 18-2	Normal ovarian volumes in pediatric (premenstrual) age groups	
Pediatric groups	**Age**	**Volume (cc), mean (±1 SD)**
Neonatal	≤6 wk	<1.0
Infancy	6 wk-2 yr	≤1.0
Early childhood	2-8 yr	0.9 (0.3)
Late childhood	9 yr	2.0 (0.8)
	10 yr	2.2 (0.7)
	11 yr	2.5 (1.3)
	12 yr	3.8 (1.4)
	13 yr	4.2 (2.3)
Puberty	13-14 yr	4.1 (3.0)

From Baltarowich OH: *Female pelvic organ measurements.* In Goldberg BB, Kurtz AB, editors: *Atlas of ultrasound measurements,* Chicago, 1990, Year Book Medical Publishers.
1 SD, 1 standard deviation.

NORMAL OVARIES IN THE PREMENSTRUAL (PEDIATRIC) AND POSTMENOPAUSAL PERIODS

In the premenstrual period (before puberty), the ovaries are relatively quiescent. Nevertheless, size changes (calculated as volumes) can be divided into four groups: neonatal (≤6 weeks), infancy (6 weeks to 2 years), early childhood (2 to 8 years), and late childhood (9 to 13 years) (Table 18-2). Ovaries less than 1 cc cannot be identified and are therefore not detected until some time in early childhood (between 2 and 8 years of age). More rapid growth begins by 8 years of age, with doubling of the ovarian volume between 8 and 9 years of age and then again between 9 and 13 years of age as puberty approaches.

Table 18-3   Approximate mean ovarian volumes in normal fertile (premenopausal) and postmenopausal women by age groups*

Age groups (yr)	Approximate mean ovarian volume (cc)
40-44	7.9
45-49	6.8
50-54	4.8
55-59	3.4
60-64	2.7
65-69	1.9
70+	1.0

Adapted from Andolf E et al: Ultrasound measurement of the ovarian volume, *Acta Obstet Gynecol Scand* 66:387, 1987.

*This study does not separate premenopausal and postmenopausal women in any age group. The older age groups, however, would be expected to have increasing numbers of postmenopausal women.

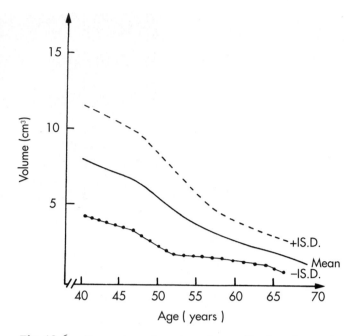

Fig. 18-6   Comparison of ovarian volume with advancing age in women more than 40 years old, a combined group of premenopausal and postmenopausal women. The ovarian volumes, calculated by a prolated ellipse formula, are displayed as a mean and 1 standard deviation *(1 S.D.)*. Note the steady decrease in volume with age. (Adapted from Andolf E et al: *Acta Obstet Gynecol Scand* 66:387, 1987.

The ovaries in the premenstrual period may contain follicles, and many ovaries having a polycystic appearance. True follicles occur in all pediatric age groups, most measuring between 4 to 8 mm (range, 1-15 mm).

Menopause is most commonly defined as commencing 1 year after the complete cessation of menses. Initially postmenopausal ovaries remain unchanged from their premenopausal (fertile) volumes (Table 18-3). They then steadily atrophy and by age 70 are no greater than 1 cc in volume. The size of a postmenopausal ovary is considered abnormal (even without a mass) if it exceeds the upper limits of normal or if it is twice the size of the other ovary (even if both are still within normal limits) (Fig. 18-6). Atrophy is prevented in women receiving hormone replacement therapy, and the ovaries then remain relatively unchanged from their size during the fertile years.

Follicles in postmenopausal ovaries may continue to develop in approximately one third of women. Most of these (80%) either disappear or regress. In the other 20%, new follicles are seen to form on follow-up studies. These cysts are simple, have no internal echoes, and are usually less than 3.5 cm in their longest axis. Infrequently they may measure up to 5 cm.

It may be difficult to detect postmenopausal ovaries. Although in the literature authors state that *one* or *both* postmenopausal ovaries can be identified in approximately 80% to 90% of women (whether studied transabdominally or transvaginally), this still means that numerous ovaries can be missed (Fig. 18-7). This is particularly a problem in elderly women who are more likely to have atrophic ovaries without follicles. There are additional cases in which the structure identified as the ovary is not confirmed at surgery or laparoscopy. Therefore their true incidence is not known but may be considerably lower than 80%. Some examiners have stated, however, that, when ovaries are not visualized by either the transab-

dominal (TA) or transvaginal (TV) technique, normal physical examination findings rule out an abnormality. This argument is fraught with potential error because ultrasound can detect subtle size or echogenicity changes, both possible early signs of a malignant lesion, which physical examination cannot detect.

TA VERSUS TV SCANNING

Sonographically the technique for evaluating the adnexa is the same for both the TA study performed through the distended urinary bladder and the TV examination performed with the bladder empty. After the long axis of the uterus is identified, parallel scans are obtained laterally to image the long axis of the adnexa and identify the ovaries. Transaxial-coronal views of the adnexa are then obtained.

Two issues with regard to TV scanning discussed in Chapter 17 must be reemphasized here. First, the TV transducer beam usually exits from the probe at an angle. Although this is excellent for evaluating anteverted structures in the long axis, it can cause difficulties in imaging ovaries that are positioned posteriorly. The left adnexa can be similarly difficult to image when the probe is turned toward the right in the transaxial-coronal plane. In both cases it may be necessary to turn the probe a full 180 degrees. Second, there is no contraindication to the use of the TV technique in evaluating the adnexa. The transducer

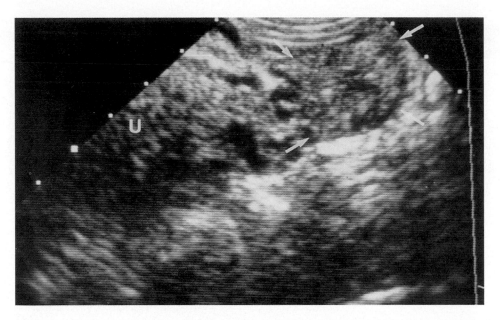

Fig. 18-7   This transvaginal transaxial-coronal view of the left ovary *(arrows)* in a postmenopausal woman shows an ovoid structure. Without follicles, the ovary is difficult to distinguish from the adjacent soft tissues. *U,* uterus.

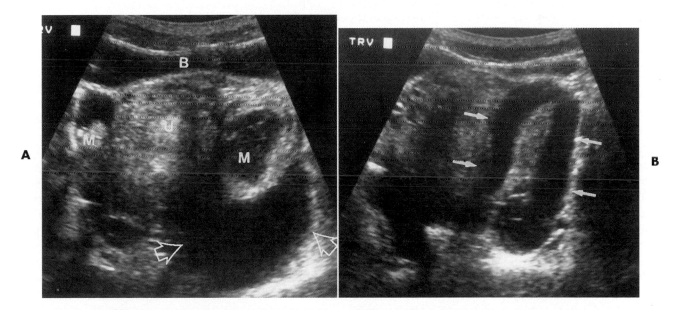

Fig. 18-8   Comparison of transabdominal and transvaginal techniques in identifying adnexal abnormalities. The hydrosalpinx is only detected transvaginally. **A,** Transabdominal transaxial image of the pelvis shows two large complex masses *(M)* lateral to the uterus *(U)*. There is also fluid in the cul-de-sac *(open arrows)* posterior to the left adnexal mass. *B,* urinary bladder. **B,** Transvaginal transaxial-coronal image of the left adnexal "mass" shows it to be a dilated, anechoic tubular structure *(arrows)* without blood flow.

is typically placed only halfway into the vagina, and there is no undue pressure on the adnexal regions.

Both the TA and TV techniques have been evaluated in terms of their ability to image the adnexa to determine which is better for identifying an abnormality, analyzing its ultrasound characteristics, and determining its site of origin. In general TV ultrasound has been found to be su-

perior for identifying and characterizing an abnormality; both are equal in their ability to determine its site of origin (Figs. 18-8 and 18-9).

It is therefore recommended that TA scanning be performed first in a patient who has not undergone a previous study. This allows visualization of the entire pelvic area. If the TA study findings are deemed completely nor-

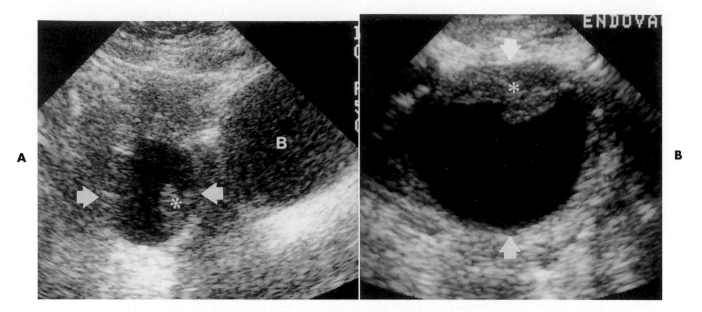

Fig. 18-9   Comparison of transabdominal and transvaginal techniques in evaluating an adnexal abnormality. This is a hemorrhagic cyst. Although it is better seen transvaginally, both techniques correctly identify its site of origin. **A,** Transabdominal sagittal image of the left adnexa in a very obese woman. The image quality is markedly degraded, and there are false echoes everywhere, even within the urinary bladder *(B)*. A cystic ovarian mass *(arrows)* with internal echoes is also seen, and an additional hyperechoic area (*) is noted along one margin. **B,** Transvaginal transaxial-coronal image of the cystic mass *(arrows)* shows a somewhat thick-walled cyst that is anechoic except for the same focal hyperechoic area (*).

mal or a well-defined anomaly and its site of origin are detected, it is often possible to stop the examination. However, the TV study should also be performed when findings are uncertain or when patients have normal findings but are at high risk for abnormalities (for example, a woman with normal ovaries but with a strong family history of ovarian cancer). It has not been shown that the TV examination should be performed instead of the TA study. In fact, in patients with large abnormalities, very distorted anatomic features, and abnormalities more than 6 cm from the TV probe, the TV study may miss the findings or the TV findings may be misinterpreted in the absence of a TA study. On a subsequent study, however, it is often appropriate to use only TV scanning because the pelvic anatomic characteristics or abnormality is then known.

FUNCTIONING AND NONFUNCTIONING OVARIAN CYSTS

Functioning cysts (follicles) are affected by the cyclic hormonal changes that occur during the menstrual cycle. These cysts are benign and usually 25 mm or less in diameter. They may rarely, however, attain a diameter of up to 40 mm. Because they are under hormonal influence,

all follicles should regress by the beginning of the next menstrual cycle.

Most follicles do not need to be reexamined. However, if their appearance (e.g., with internal echoes) or size is unusual, a follow-up study should not be performed until the start of the next menstrual cycle or the one after that. There is no well-defined interval in premenopausal (fertile) women who have had either a hysterectomy or who have very irregular menstrual periods, and 6 weeks is often taken as an arbitrary waiting period between examinations in both these and all postmenopausal women.

If a cyst persists and either does not change or increases in size, it is then considered nonfunctioning (not under hormonal influence). Most are still benign and usually either ovarian or paraovarian in origin. In the differential diagnosis, a cystic neoplasm (usually cystadenoma) and an endometrioma must be considered; a dermoid and nongynecologic masses are less likely. In general, if the cyst is simple (i.e., anechoic and smooth walled with good distal acoustic enhancement) and less than 5 cm in its longest axis, it is almost always benign (Fig. 18-10). Nevertheless, it should be checked with at least one additional study. If it is 5 cm or more, the likelihood of malignancy increases and surgical removal is usually indicated.

Multiple small, nonfunctioning cysts may be present in

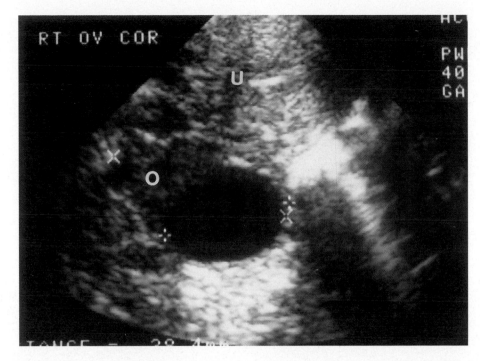

Fig. 18-10 Postmenopausal ovary with a simple benign cyst. Transvaginal transaxial-coronal image of the right ovary *(x)* shows a 28-mm cyst (+) that meets all the criteria for a simple cyst: anechoic, smooth and thin walled, and good through-transmission. The remainder of the ovarian tissue *(O)* is normal. *U,* uterus.

polycystic ovaries. These ovaries are typically round (not oval) and have a bright, somewhat thick hyperechoic capsule (Fig. 18-11). This appearance is often (but not always) identified in infertile women and may be part of the Stein-Leventhal syndrome, which includes obesity and hirsutism. The cysts are typically less than 5 mm in diameter and usually line up just inside the capsule in a "string-of-pearls" configuration. In the past, women with this syndrome could only be treated by wedge resection of the fibrous capsule, thus allowing the release of developing follicles. Now, advances in fertility treatment have made this diagnosis less important because these women are only treated with medication.

COMPLEX CYSTS

A complex cyst has some but not all of the properties of a simple cyst. A cyst is considered complex if it has irregular or thickened walls, internal echoes, or septations (Figs. 18-3, 18-9, and 18-12). Almost always good through-transmission is maintained. If lost, the mass is likely solid.

A hemorrhagic cyst (either functioning or nonfunctioning), endometrioma, dermoid, abscess, ovarian torsion, and cystic neoplasm (benign and malignant) must be considered in the differential diagnosis of a complex

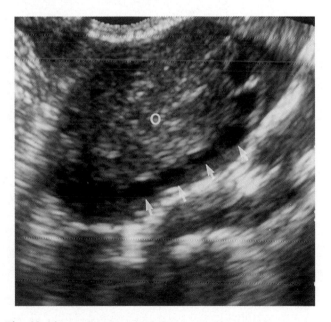

Fig. 18-11 Polycystic ovary. Transvaginal transaxial-coronal image of the right ovary *(O)* shows it to be rounded and have a somewhat thickened rim. Multiple very small follicles (<5 mm) line up just inside the capsule *(arrows).* The other ovary has a similar appearance.

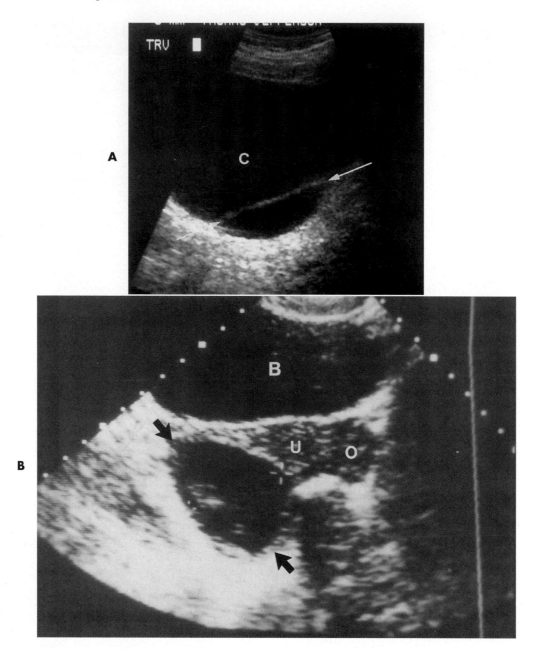

Fig. 18-12   Complex cystic ovarian masses. **A,** Transabdominal transaxial image of a left ovarian cyst (C) with one thin septation *(arrows)*. **B,** Hemorrhagic cyst. This transabdominal transaxial image of the pelvis shows a normal uterus *(U)* and left ovary *(O)*. A large complex, oval mass *(arrows and +)* is seen in the right adnexal region. It has somewhat thickened walls and internal echoes. Note the good through-transmission. *B,* urinary bladder.

cyst. Less commonly a nongynecologic complex cyst (e.g., a mesenteric cyst) may be seen in the pelvis. Necrotic fibroids rarely present as a cystic mass.

The possibility of malignancy needs to be considered when a complex cystic mass is detected. These cystic masses should be analyzed in terms of the degree of wall thickening, the structure of their inner wall, the presence and thickness of septa, and their echogenicity. Recently this analysis has been quantitated (Table 18-4). As might be expected, the more abnormal and numerous the ul-

trasound properties, the greater the likelihood of malignancy (Fig. 18-13). The complementary use of Doppler is discussed later (in the section on ovarian malignancy). At present its findings are not specific enough to be included in a quantitated analysis.

Hemorrhagic cysts exhibit widely variable patterns and may mimic the appearance of a number of other adnexal masses from the standpoint of both size and echogenicity. The most typical pattern is a 2- to 3-cm, uniformly hyperechoic mass that can look like a cystic

Table 18-4   Scoring system for the evaluation of adnexal masses, either ovarian or extrauterine masses (if of uncertain origin)*

Variables	Mass evaluation	Variables	Mass evaluation
Wall thickness (mm)		Septa (mm)	
Thin (≤3 mm)	1	No septa	1
Thick (>3 mm)	2	Thin (≤3 mm)	2
Not applicable, mostly solid	3	Thick (>3 mm)	3
Inner wall structure		Echogenicity	
Smooth	1	Anechoic	1
Irregularities	2	Low echogenicity	2
Papillary projections >3 mm	3	Low echogenicity with hyperechoic core	3
Not applicable, mostly solid	4	Mixed echogenicity	4
		Hyperechoic	5

Adapted from Sassone AM et al: Transvaginal sonographic characterization of ovarian disease: evaluation of a new scoring system to predict ovarian malignancy, *Obstet Gynecol* 78:70, 1991.

*To calculate the total score, add up the individual scores for all four variables (minimum score = 4; maximum score = 15). Benign = 4. The higher the number >5, the more likely malignant.

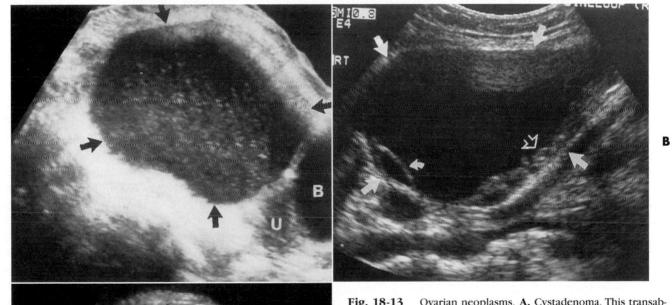

Fig. 18-13 Ovarian neoplasms. **A,** Cystadenoma. This transabdominal sagittal midline image shows a large mass *(arrows)* with multiple internal echoes and good through-transmission that is above and separate from the uterus *(U). B,* urinary bladder. **B,** Papillary cystadenocarcinoma. This transabdominal sagittal image of the right adnexa shows an ovoid complex mass that is primarily anechoic *(arrows).* A slightly thickened septation *(curved arrow)* and multiple intraluminal papillary projections (one denoted by an open arrow) are seen. The through-transmission is poor, a finding indicating the presence of a solid mass. **C,** Ovarian carcinoma. This transabdominal oblique image of the left adnexa shows a large ovoid, complex mass *(arrows)* with a markedly thickened wall (*), markedly thickened septations, and two irregular cysts (+ and *x*). Although there is good through-transmission, the rest of the sonographic findings indicate malignancy.

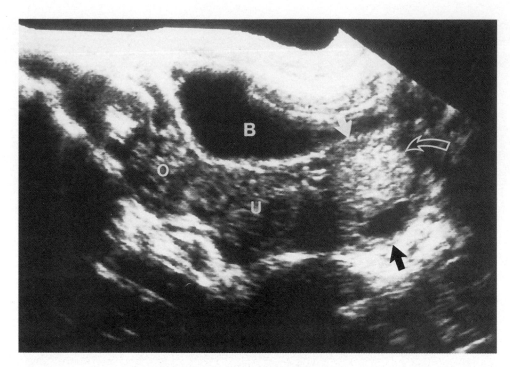

Fig. 18-14   Left ovarian hemorrhagic cyst. Transabdominal transaxial image of the pelvis shows the uterus *(U)* and right ovary *(O)* to be normal. The left ovary *(closed arrows)* has a simple cyst posteriorly (near the black arrow) and a large, uniformly hyperechoic mass *(curved open arrow)* in its middle; the latter is a hemorrhagic cyst. Note the excellent through-transmission. *B,* urinary bladder.

teratoma (Fig. 18-14). In many (but not all) cases these two entities can be differentiated because most hemorrhagic cysts have good through-transmission; most dermoids do not (Fig. 18-15, *A*). Hemorrhagic cysts, however, can be of any size (up to 15 cm) and echogenicity at presentation. Unless malignancy is strongly indicated by clinical or ultrasound criteria, or both, it is often prudent to wait one to two menstrual cycles before rendering this diagnosis. A hemorrhagic cyst will characteristically decrease markedly in size and often completely resolve.

CYSTIC TERATOMA (DERMOID)

Cystic teratomas or dermoids account for 10% to 15% of all ovarian neoplasms. They are benign ovarian tumors and are bilateral in 10% of cases. Dermoids are composed of mature epithelial elements, a combination of skin, hair, desquamated epithelium, and teeth. These masses do not contain fat (an endothelial element). The lucency that is sometimes detected on radiographs is due to the presence of pure sebum, a fluid of lipid density.

Dermoids are present from birth. Because of slow growth, they are typically detected in young women in the second and third decades of life. Dermoids are usually relatively soft masses and on physical examination may be difficult to palpate. They are therefore frequently

either missed or their size is underestimated. If large, a dermoid may torse, then presenting with acute abdominal pain.

Dermoids can range widely in size and echogenicity (Figs. 18-15 and 18-16). Depending on the extent and admixture of their epithelial elements, the ultrasound patterns can vary markedly, even within a single mass. There are, however, some typical patterns. The two "classic" dermoid appearances are the "tip of the iceberg" sign, caused by absorption of most of the ultrasound beam at the top of the mass (because of the multiple interfaces), and the "dermoid plug" sign, which has the appearance of hyperechoic, rounded areas within a hypoechoic mass. It is important to recognize the "tip of the iceberg" sign, if present, because it usually helps in differentiating a typical dermoid from a typical hemorrhagic cyst (see Figs. 18-14 and 18-15, *A*).

Other less commonly seen characteristic appearances are the "target" (or "bull's eye" sign), consisting of a hyperechoic center and a hypoechoic rim, and thick calcifications, that is, teeth that can be confirmed by a pelvic radiograph or a computed tomographic (CT) scan (see Fig. 18-16, *A* and *B*). Rarely a lipid-fluid level can be identified within the mass, which moves when the patient is moved (see Fig. 18-16, *C*). Very rarely, dermoids can be almost completely anechoic; this is encountered most commonly in adolescent girls (see Fig. 18-16, *D*).

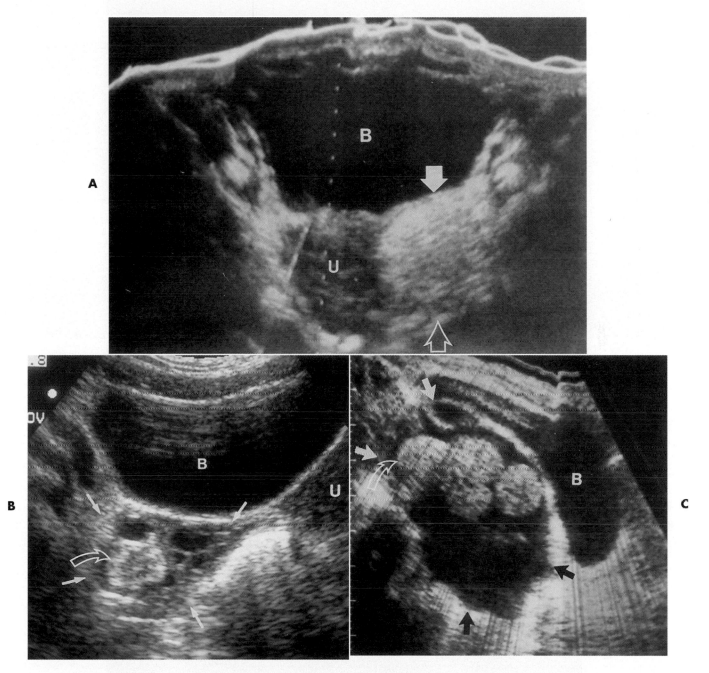

Fig. 18-15   "Classic" appearances of dermoids. **A,** "Tip of the iceberg" sign. This static transabdominal transaxial image of the pelvis shows a markedly hyperechoic mass in the left adnexa. There is marked echogenicity at its anterior border *(closed arrow),* which decreases toward the bottom arrow *(open arrow).* This is caused by weakening of the ultrasound beam (attenuation) as the sound traverses the mass. Compare this with the hemorrhagic cyst shown in Fig. 18-14. *B,* urinary bladder; *U,* uterus. **B,** Mimicker of a hemorrhagic cyst. This transaxial image of the right ovary *(closed arrows)* shows multiple follicles with one hyperechoic mass that is slightly inhomogeneous *(curved open arrow).* This was initially thought to be a hemorrhagic cyst. Follow-up study done 2 months later showed it to have grown slightly. **C,** "Dermoid plug" sign. This static transabdominal image of the right adnexa shows a primarily hypoechoic mass *(closed arrows)* with multiple internal hyperechoic, rounded, ball-like areas (one denoted by a curved open arrow).

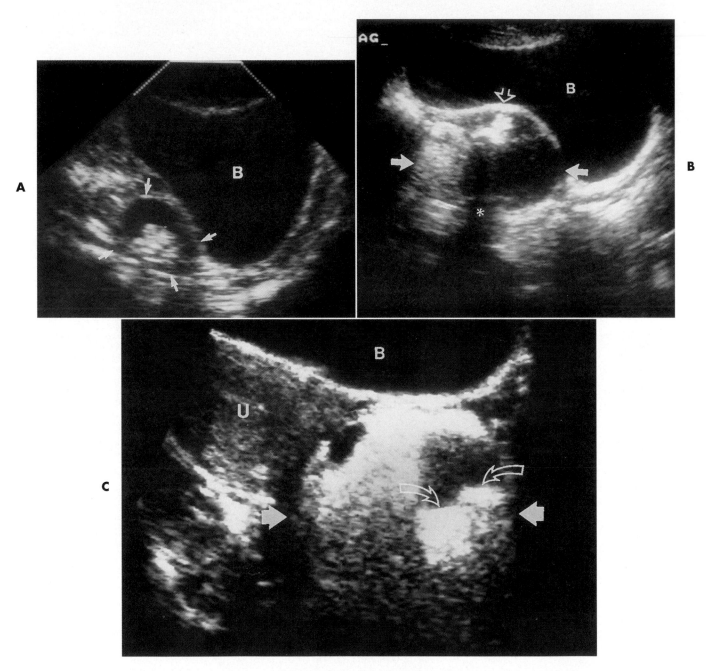

Fig. 18-16 Other dermoid appearances, all scanned transabdominally. **A,** The "target" sign. This sagittal image of the left adnexa shows a primarily anechoic mass with a hyperechoic center *(arrows)*. *B,* urinary bladder. **B,** Sagittal image of the right adnexa shows an ovoid mass *(closed arrows)* of mixed echogenicity, ranging from anechoic to hyperechoic. At its anterior border *(open arrow)* there is a hyperechoic area of calcification with sharp distal acoustic shadowing (*). **C,** Transaxial image of the left adnexa shows a large mass of markedly different echogenicities *(closed arrows)*. The mass has two lipid-fluid levels *(open curved arrows)*. *U,* uterus.

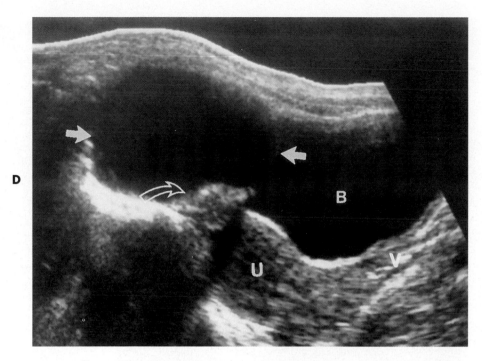

Fig. 18-16, cont'd.   D, Sagittal midline image in a young girl shows a primarily anechoic mass *(closed arrows)* with one hyperechoic area exhibiting some shadowing *(curved open arrow).* The mass is separate from the uterus *(U). V,* vagina.

A dermoid is often removed in an attempt to save what remains of the ovary. Surgical removal should, however, be delayed 1 or 2 months if a hemorrhagic cyst is a reasonable diagnostic alternative.

ENDOMETRIOSIS

Endometriosis is the presence of endometrial glands or stroma, or both, in abnormal locations. There are two forms. The more common one occurs outside of the uterus and is generally referred to as *endometriosis.* More specifically it is the *external* or *indirect* form. This external form is usually confined to adnexal structures but may be widely distributed and vary in extent from small foci to widespread sheets of tissue to focal masses (endometriomas). The second form, adenomyosis, is the less common one. Called the *internal* or *direct form,* it remains within the uterus, invading the junctional zone and myometrium.

Both forms of endometriosis may occur in any menstruating female. Classically the presenting symptoms of endometriosis are a triad of infertility, dysmenorrhea, and dyspareunia. However, this triad is only present in 10% of patients. Symptoms depend on the location of lesions. Patients can be asymptomatic if the condition is confined to the ovaries or suffer severe pain if it is widespread, with symptoms varying between these two extremes depending on the extent of the process. Usually the most severe symptoms are associated with adenomyosis. Although typically associated with infertility, an endometrioma may even be identified in a pregnant patient.

The success of ultrasound in identifying and confirming the clinical diagnosis of endometriosis is variable. It is rarely detected sonographically if the process is extrauterine unless it presents as an endometrioma. These masses may be multiple. The echogenicity and size of endometriomas often vary from cystic to complex to solid and from less than 1 cm to more than 10 cm (Fig. 18-17). The masses are the result of multiple episodes of bleeding. As a general rule the more unusual or varied the echogenicity and the more ovoid or irregular its contour, the more likely the mass is an endometrioma. Inflammation (abscess), trophoblastic tissue (ectopic pregnancy), and occasionally dermoids can, however, exhibit a similar appearance.

The lesions in adenomyosis (the intrauterine form) are typically microscopic and detected only by pathologic studies. However, adenomyosis may present sonographically (and on magnetic resonance imaging [MRI]) with distortion of the junctional zone and extension into the myometrium. Ultrasound can occasionally show a "moth-eaten" appearance; this consists of small hypoechoic, round, indistinct masses that range up to 10 to 15 mm in diameter. It may be difficult to differentiate them from multiple small fibroids, and this is discussed further in Chapter 17.

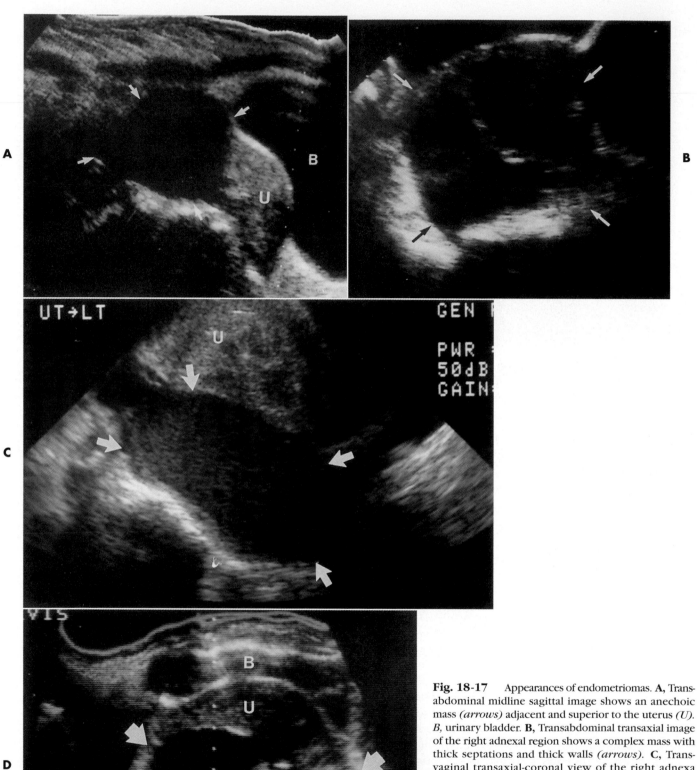

Fig. 18-17   Appearances of endometriomas. **A,** Transabdominal midline sagittal image shows an anechoic mass *(arrows)* adjacent and superior to the uterus *(U)*. *B,* urinary bladder. **B,** Transabdominal transaxial image of the right adnexal region shows a complex mass with thick septations and thick walls *(arrows)*. **C,** Transvaginal transaxial-coronal view of the right adnexa shows an ovoid, uniformly hyperechoic mass *(arrows)* posterior to and to the right of the uterus *(U)*. **D,** Transabdominal transaxial image of the pelvis shows a large irregular mass of mixed echogenicity *(arrows)* posterior and to the left of the uterus *(U)*. *B,* urinary bladder.

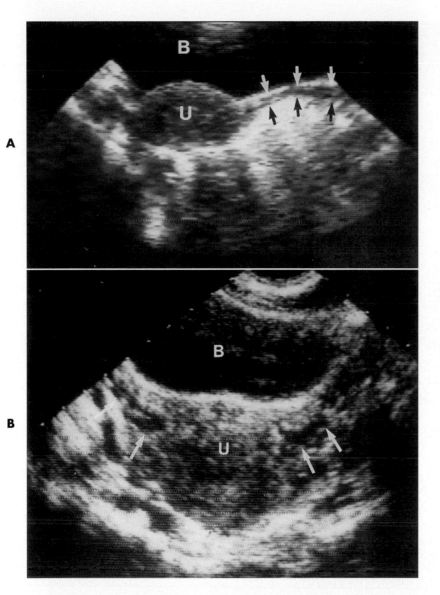

Fig. 18-18   Normal versus abnormal fallopian tube. **A,** Normal appearance. This transabdominal transaxial image of the uterus *(U)* and left adnexa shows a hypoechoic band *(arrows)* extending laterally from the fundus of the uterus. Note that this area is not anechoic. **B,** Hydrosalpinx. This transabdominal transaxial image of the uterus *(U)* shows anechoic tubular structures extending bilaterally from the lateral margins of the uterine fundus *(arrows)*. These areas were not shown to have blood flow on color-Doppler analysis. *B,* urinary bladder.

PELVIC INFLAMMATORY DISEASE

In the acute phase of pelvic inflammatory disease (PID), salpingitis and less commonly endometritis are obvious clinically. It is rare for an ultrasound examination to be necessary. When the process is more chronic, however, particularly in patients who have responded inappropriately to antibiotics, an ultrasound study may be needed to evaluate for persistent disease. PID always involves the fallopian tubes, and fluid in the cul-de-sac and masses (abscesses) should be sought.

Sonographically, normal fallopian tubes cannot be identified. Sometimes a normal thin (5-mm), hypoechoic soft-tissue band originating from the uterine fundus can be imaged in a transaxial-coronal view (Fig. 18-18, *A*). If dis-

tinct tubular structures are seen instead, hydrosalpinx (dilated tube) is diagnosed (see Figs. 18-8 and 18-18, *B*). Almost always, if one tube is dilated, the disease is bilateral (even if it is not appreciated sonographically). Although contrast-enhanced salpingography is the definitive test, ultrasound appears accurate in identifying the pathologic process, particularly when performed transvaginally. Occasionally prominent blood vessels may be present in the adnexa. Although these may initially be misinterpreted as a hydrosalpinx, color or pulsed Doppler can rule this out by detecting blood flow.

A hydrosalpinx may be subtle, only several millimeters in diameter, or it may be massive, as much as 5 to 6 cm in diameter, and very tortuous. It can then be mistaken for a large cystic mass. If the dilated tube has internal echoes,

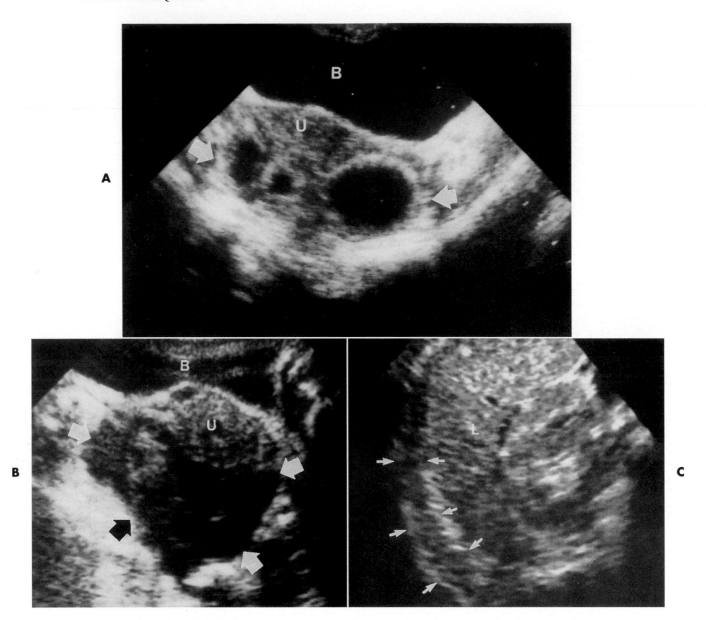

Fig. 18-19 Sequelae of pelvic inflammatory disease. **A,** Pyosalpinx. This transabdominal transaxial image of the pelvis shows complex areas *(arrows)* lateral and posterior to the uterus *(U)*. These areas have thick hyperechoic walls and some internal echoes. *B,* urinary bladder. **B,** Abscess. This transabdominal transaxial image of the pelvis shows a large, irregular complex mass of mixed echogenicity *(arrows)* posterior to and to the right of the uterus *(U)*. *B,* urinary bladder. **C,** Fitz-Hugh-Curtis syndrome. This transaxial, right upper quadrant image shows a perihepatic hypoechoic collection between the liver *(L)* and the right ribs *(arrows)*.

very infrequently with a fluid-debris level, the tube is usually infected and this is called a *pyosalpinx* (Fig. 18-19, *A*). A tortuous pyosalpinx can appear as a complex mass; TV ultrasound can usually detect the tubular nature of this abnormal fallopian tube.

When a hydrosalpinx is identified (even one dilated tube), the likelihood of recurrent infection and ectopic pregnancy increases. In addition to detecting a pyosalpinx, TV ultrasound can reveal the existence of intraperi-

toneal fluid in the cul-de-sac and abscesses. Abscesses are typically hypoechoic masses, often with some internal echogenicity, and usually with relatively good through-transmission (Fig. 18-19, *B*). Their walls are ill defined and sometimes thick, and their shapes vary from irregular to ovoid to round; they may be numerous.

If the pregnancy test result is positive, any adnexal mass (except a simple cyst) should be considered suspicious for an ectopic pregnancy. A concomitant ectopic

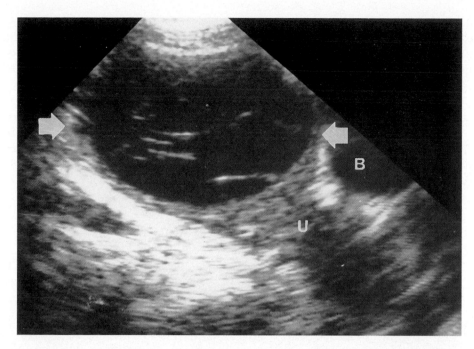

Fig. 18-20   Ovarian torsion in a woman with worsening pelvic pain. This transabdominal sagittal midline image of the pelvis shows a large, thick-walled complex mass *(arrows)* with internal septations. It is adjacent and superior to the uterus *(U)*. Pathologically this area was found to contain the necrotic and hemorrhagic fallopian tube and ovary, without evidence of a "lead" ovarian mass. *B*, urinary bladder.

pregnancy is possible even if there is an intrauterine pregnancy. Primarily because of partially treated PID, the incidence of a heterotopic pregnancy is now estimated at 1 in 7000 pregnancies.

Infrequently, particularly in patients with PID resulting from gonorrhea, a pelvic infection may ascend up the right flank, causing a perihepatic inflammation. The pain from this may mimic liver, gallbladder, and even right renal pain. Perihepatic inflammation can be detected sonographically by scanning along the liver margin and identifying a hypoechoic rim between the liver and the adjacent ribs. This is called the *Fitz-Hugh-Curtis syndrome* and is typically caused by an ascending gonorrhea infection (Fig. 18-19, *C*).

OVARIAN TORSION

Ovarian torsion is an unusual but serious problem because it accounts for 3% of gynecologic operative emergencies. Torsion typically involves not only the ovary but also its fallopian tube. It is most common in women during the fertile years and occurs during pregnancy in 20% of the cases. Torsion may, however, present at any time in female life from childhood to the postmenopausal period. Occasionally the lead point is an ovarian mass. Once torsion has occurred, there is a 10% chance of torsion occurring on the other side.

Acute, severe unilateral pain is typically the presenting

symptom in patients with torsion. Intermittent pain may precede the acute pain by weeks. Sonographically a mass of hemorrhagic or necrotic tissue, or both, is often detected. Masses are large (>4 cm in diameter) (Fig. 18-20). They vary in appearance from cystic to solid and from relatively anechoic to markedly hyperechoic. Although there may be a lead mass, it is often mixed in with the necrosis and hemorrhage and not appreciated.

The differentiation of torsion from other adnexal masses is often not possible unless it is strongly suspected on clinical grounds. Doppler evaluation, particularly color-Doppler, may be of value if it can accurately show lack of detectable flow in the mass. However, adnexal flow is often found to be asymmetric, particularly during normal menstrual cycles, and the lack of flow (or decreased flow) may at times be normal. In addition, some adnexal masses do not have a detectable Doppler flow.

OVARIAN MALIGNANCY

Ovarian cancer can present as either a complex cystic or a solid mass and is more likely to be cystic by a ratio of 3:1. As much as 20% are bilateral. Endometriosis, ovarian torsion, PID, and all benign ovarian neoplasms (e.g., dermoids and fibromas) must be considered in the differential diagnosis. Rarely an exophytic fibroid or a nongynecologic mass may also appear in the adnexa. Unless obvious additional pelvic and abdominal abnormalities exist, such as complex ascites and adenopathy, malignancy cannot be diagnosed but only included in the list of possibilities. Of these, endometriosis appears to be the most common mimicker of cancer, both clinically and sonographically.

Ovarian cancer is often detected by a combination of physical examination, laboratory, and imaging findings, almost always ultrasound but sometimes CT or MRI. Sixty percent of the cases occur in women between 40 and 60 years of age, encompassing both fertile and postmenopausal women. The other 40% of the cases occur earlier and later, from early in the third decade to the end of the ninth decade. Ovarian malignancy is a "silent" cancer, commonly not detected until it is advanced, either having spread beyond the capsule but still within the pelvis (stage II) or into the abdomen (stage III) in 50% of the women by the time of initial detection. Physical examination findings are variable, ranging from almost "normal" to slightly enlarged, firm, irregular ovaries to pelvic masses. Ascites and omental masses may also be palpated. The blood chemistry test CA 125 has been disappointing in its ability to detect ovarian cancer. It is plagued by many false-positive and false-negative results, and elevated levels are found in only 50% of patients with stage III ovarian cancer. If a baseline level is known, however, such as

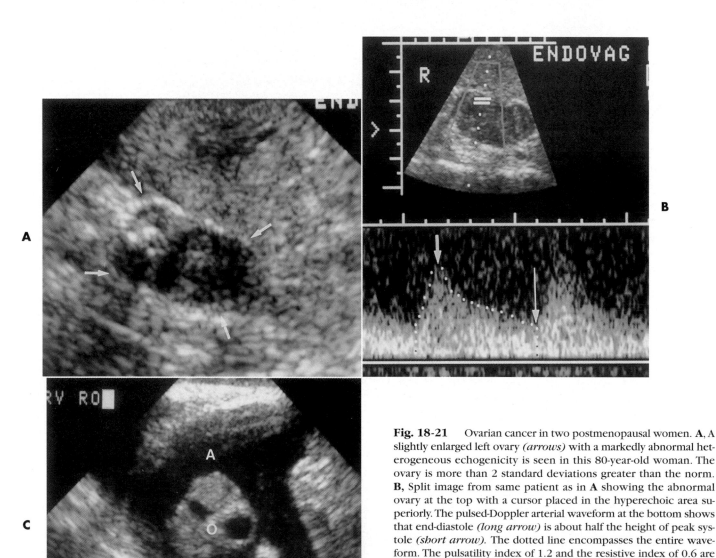

Fig. 18-21   Ovarian cancer in two postmenopausal women. **A,** A slightly enlarged left ovary *(arrows)* with a markedly abnormal heterogeneous echogenicity is seen in this 80-year-old woman. The ovary is more than 2 standard deviations greater than the norm. **B,** Split image from same patient as in **A** showing the abnormal ovary at the top with a cursor placed in the hyperechoic area superiorly. The pulsed-Doppler arterial waveform at the bottom shows that end-diastole *(long arrow)* is about half the height of peak systole *(short arrow).* The dotted line encompasses the entire waveform. The pulsatility index of 1.2 and the resistive index of 0.6 are in the indeterminate range. **C,** A rounded right ovary *(O)* with two small cysts is identified in this 73-year-old woman. The ovary measures at the upper limits of normal and is unusually round. There is ascites *(A)* surrounding the ovary, indicating probable cancer spread outside the ovary.

in patients who have undergone resection of primary ovarian cancer, then an elevated follow-up level has greater significance.

TA and TV ultrasound are of value in detecting ovarian abnormalities. As previously stated, ultrasound can determine ovarian size and echogenicity. It can identify masses and further show them to be cystic, complex, or solid. The ovaries are often identified in menstruating women. Their location, size, typical ovoid appearance, and follicles allow for easy detection. In the postmenopausal period, the ovaries become atrophic, quite frequently do not have follicles, and can be difficult to identify. Only women receiving hormone replacement therapy continue to have normal-sized ovaries. Abnormal ovaries, defined as more than 2 standard deviations above the norm (for the woman's age), as twice the size of the other, or as showing abnormal echogenicity, are suggestive of malignancy (Fig. 18-21).

Most ovarian cancers are detected as masses. In general the size of the mass, the age of the patient, and the ultrasound characteristics of the mass relate directly to its potential for being malignant. Masses less than 5 cm in their longest axis are much more likely to be benign; masses more than 10 cm are much more likely to be malignant; the malignant potential in intermediately sized masses is intermediate. A postmenopausal study conducted by Rulin and Preston showed that the incidence of malignancy in patients with masses less than 5 cm, 5 to 10 cm, and more than 10 cm in diameter increased from 3% to 11% to 64%, respectively. These incidences might have been lower if premenopausal masses had been included. Increasing age also correlates with an increased incidence of malignancy. In the same postmenopausal study, the incidence of masses more likely to be malignant was found to increase steadily with each decade, from 24% (between the ages 50 and 60 years) to more than 60% (after the age of 80). Finally, the ultrasound characteristics of the mass are important. Unilocular or thinly septated cysts are more likely to be benign. Multilocular, thickly septated masses and masses with solid nodules are more likely to be malignant (Table 18-4); (Figs. 18-13 and 18-22).

Metastatic disease to the ovaries may mimic the appearance of primary ovarian abnormalities. These cancers arise from other pelvic organs and from the upper gastrointestinal tract. Krukenberg's tumors are "drop" metastases to the ovaries, primarily from the stomach (Fig. 18-23). They can also arise from the breast, pancreas, and gallbladder. These masses are typically solid. Cystic metastatic masses appear to result more commonly from rectosigmoid colon cancers. When the ovaries are involved, all of these malignant lesions are often widespread, with metastasis to the peritoneum (including ascites) and to the mesentery. These malignant masses therefore usually mimic the behavior of stage III primary ovarian cancer. To further complicate the diagnosis, the incidence of

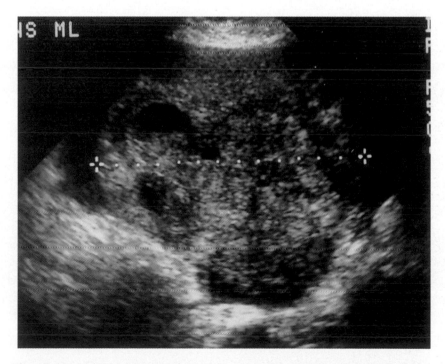

Fig. 18-22   Large solid ovarian cancer. This transabdominal transaxial image shows a large solid mass (+ and *dotted line*) filling the pelvis in a woman who has had a hysterectomy. The other ovary could not be identified.

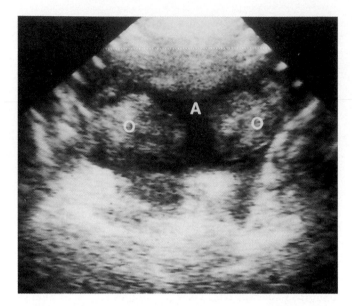

Fig. 18-23 Ovarian metastatic masses from a primary malignant tumor of the stomach (Krukenberg's tumor). This transabdominal transaxial image of the pelvis shows enlarged, prominent, rounded ovaries *(O)* surrounded by ascites *(A)*. There was already widespread metastatic disease in the abdomen.

ovarian cancer is increased in women who have had breast and colon cancer.

Although ultrasound is able to identify masses and analyze their sonographic characteristics, it is not always possible for it to distinguish benign from malignant lesions. Doppler has been studied to determine if it can detect the neovascularity of malignant masses. Color-Doppler is used to survey large areas of tissue and identify areas of flow. Pulsed-Doppler is then performed to obtain and analyze its arterial component, if detected (Fig. 18-24). At present only the solid and complex soft-tissue areas of the abnormal ovary or mass have been evaluated. The surrounding soft tissues, their feeding blood vessels, and normal ovaries have not. Care must be taken to sample from the margins of the abnormal ovary or mass; if its walls are too thin to ensure that a correct sample volume is obtained, Doppler should not be performed.

A Doppler arterial waveform has a systolic and a diastolic component. Two Doppler indices have been evaluated. The pulsatility index (PI) is the peak systolic pressure minus the end-diastolic pressure over the mean area under the curve. The resistive index (RI) is the peak systolic pressure minus the end-diastolic pressure over the peak systolic pressure. Although both indices have different cut-off values, both evaluate the relative amount of diastolic to systolic flow. In general the more the diastolic

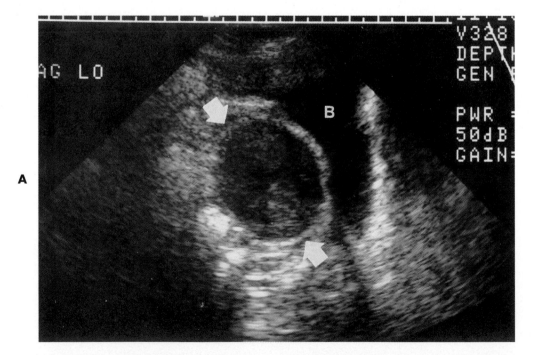

Fig. 18-24 Doppler comparison of benign versus malignant adnexal abnormalities. **A** and **B,** Ovarian cancer. **A,** Transabdominal sagittal image of the left adnexa shows a large ovoid mass *(arrows)* with somewhat thickened walls and multiple internal echoes. *B,* urinary bladder.

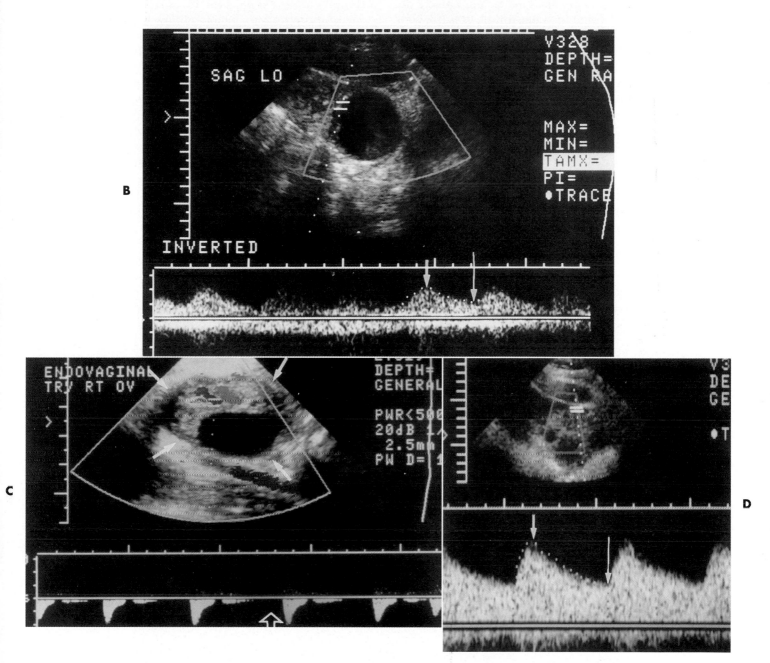

Fig. 18-24, cont'd. **B,** A split image. The top image shows the mass with a cursor on the thickened wall. The bottom image shows a pulsed-Doppler arterial velocity waveform with peak systole *(short arrow)* and end-diastole *(large arrow).* The area under the velocity waveform is denoted by a dotted line. Note that end-diastole is more than half peak systole. Both index values are in the malignant range; the pulsatility index is 0.7 and the resistive index is 0.2. **C,** Dermoid. Split image showing a thick-walled ovarian mass *(arrows)* at the top with the Doppler cursor in its soft-tissue portion. On the bottom, the Doppler arterial velocity waveform shows peak systole but no end-diastole *(open arrow).* The values of both the resistive and pulsatility indices are therefore markedly elevated and in the benign range. **D,** Abscess. This split image shows a large soft-tissue mass in the right adnexa with a Doppler cursor in its wall. On the bottom the Doppler arterial waveform is in the malignant range; the pulsatility index is 0.8 and the resistive index is 0.3. *Short arrow,* peak systole; *long arrow,* end diastole; *dotted line,* area under the velocity waveform.

flow, the more likely is neovascularity present and therefore the more likely is the mass malignant. The cut-off value for the PI is 1.0 and the value for the RI is 0.4, with malignancy indicated below and benignity above these values. Other abnormalities may, however, have low indices, thus mimicking cancer. These abnormalities include inflammatory masses, active endocrine tumors, and trophoblastic disease (ectopic pregnancies). In addition, many index values are borderline, making differentiation impossible (see Fig. 18-21, *B*).

A mass showing a complete absence of or very little diastolic flow (very elevated RI and PI values) is almost always benign. A diastolic notch (in early diastole) may also be a sign of benignity. This notch, caused by arterial rebound, indicates the presence of a normal smooth muscle wall. Neovascular vessels do not have this smooth muscle and therefore do not have this notch. However, this finding is not often noted and its absence has no diagnostic value.

In the fertile years (menstrual and perimenstrual), the PI and RI values vary considerably during each menstrual cycle. Because the lowest adnexal flow is present during the first 7 days (the index values are at their highest), a Doppler study should only be performed in this first week. Afterward, variable blood flow to the ovaries, particularly to the dominant ovary, complicates the analysis.

Screening for ovarian cancer has been suggested. However, there are many problems with this. For screening to be adequate, women need to be divided into two groups: those at such low risk that a "safe" interval between studies can be established and those at higher risk who require more immediate attention. This division is not possible at present. A very large multiyear study needs to be performed, and it is estimated by some that this should consist of up to 100,000 women who are studied for as much as 10 years. Currently no more than 5000 women have been evaluated for up to 3 years. Additionally, at best only 80% of postmenopausal ovaries can now be identified sonographically. More fundamentally, the doubling time of ovarian cancer is not known; without this information the appropriate reexamination interval cannot be established. Because of all these basic flaws, screening for ovarian cancer is not now a serious scientific consideration.

Key Features

The ovaries are most commonly found lateral to the body of the uterus. They are readily displaced, usually to a more superior position, by any change in uterine position, by a uterine mass, or by a pregnancy.

The size of the ovary is most often expressed as a volume, calculated from a prolated ellipse formula: length × width × anteroposterior dimension × 0.5.

In the fertile (ovulating) women the ovaries are typically ovoid, have a low-level echogenicity, and have a thin, hyperechoic rim. Because of the continually developing follicles (functioning cysts), their appearance changes throughout each menstrual cycle.

There is no true upper limit of normal for ovarian size during the fertile years, provided (aside from follicles) the ovarian tissue is uniformly normal in echogenicity.

By midcycle the dominant follicle is usually between 20 and 25 mm in diameter. It may rarely approach 40 mm. All follicles resolve by the next menstrual cycle.

In the premenstrual (pediatric) years, the ovaries begin to enlarge from early childhood on, accelerating toward the time of puberty. Follicles can be seen at any time and are usually 4 to 8 mm in diameter.

In the postmenopausal period (in the absence of hormone replacement therapy), the ovaries steadily shrink. Follicles can normally be identified in up to 30% of women.

Nonfunctioning cysts (those not under hormonal influence) are usually benign and are either ovarian or paraovarian in origin. However, a cystic neoplasm cannot be excluded, and the likelihood of malignancy increases when the mass is more than 5 cm in diameter.

Fertility medications commonly stimulate the ovaries to produce multiple follicles that are larger than 20 mm in diameter. When the follicles become so numerous that they involve all of the ovarian tissue, the possibility of an early ovarian hyperstimulation syndrome must be considered and such medication discontinued.

Both transabdominal and transvaginal techniques are thought to be equal in their ability to identify the site of origin of an abnormality. Transvaginal ultrasound is superior in identifying and characterizing an abnormality.

Transabdominal scanning should be the initial study in a woman undergoing an ultrasound examination for the first time, with a transvaginal examination performed if needed. The transvaginal study may be used exclusively for a subsequent evaluation, if indicated.

The differential diagnosis of complicated cysts includes numerous possibilities. Of these, hemorrhagic cysts are a mimicker of many adnexal masses. Unless malignancy is strongly suspected, a follow-up study should be performed, usually in 4 to 6 weeks. A marked decrease in or resolution of a mass confirms its hemorrhagic nature.

Cystic teratomas (dermoids) are benign masses of varied size and echogenicity, typically found in young women. The most "classic" patterns are the "tip of the iceberg" sign, the "dermoid plug" sign, the "target" sign, and a lipid-fluid level. A dermoid is also diagnosed if sharp shadowing can be identified and a radiograph shows a tooth.

Endometriosis occurs in two forms: adenomyosis of the uterus and endometriosis of the adnexa.

In most cases endometriosis is diagnosed on clinical grounds and cannot be detected by ultrasound. When identified, it presents as adnexal mass or masses (endometriomas) of variable echogenicity, shape, and size.

Adenomyosis (probably better detected by MRI) can initially appear as multiple small, hypoechoic areas that distort the junctional zone and sometimes the myometrium. It can sonographically mimic the appearance of small fibroids.

In the setting of chronic pelvic inflammatory disease, ultrasound is used to try and identify a dilated fallopian tube (hydrosalpinx or pyosalpinx), abscesses, and intraperitoneal fluid.

Ovarian torsion is an unusual problem but accounts for 3% of gynecologic emergencies. In the context of acute pain or intermittent, cyclic worsening pain, an adnexal mass may be a torsion. Doppler at present has only limited value in identifying the condition.

Ovarian cancers are either complex cystic masses or solid masses and occur in a ratio of 3:1. Malignancy is suspected when the mass is more than 5 cm in its long axis, if the woman is of advanced age, and when there are prominent soft-tissue components.

Metastatic disease to the ovary can mimic primary ovarian abnormalities.

Doppler evaluation of the mass, not of the surrounding area, has been shown to be of limited use. If the arterial waveforms show no diastolic flow (i.e., high resistance), these masses are almost always benign. The possibility of ovarian malignancy increases for masses or abnormal ovaries showing increased diastolic flow (low resistance). There are, however, other diagnostic considerations in this setting.

Doppler has not yet been proved to be of any value either in evaluating the surrounding tissues, the feeding vessels to ovaries, or masses, or in evaluating normal ovaries.

SUGGESTED READINGS

Andolf E, Jørgensen C: A prospective comparison of transabdominal and transvaginal ultrasound with surgical findings in gynecologic disease, *J Ultrasound Med* 9:71, 1990.

Andolf E et al: Ultrasound measurement of the ovarian volume, *Acta Obstet Gynecol Scand* 66:387, 1987.

Baltarowich OH: *Female pelvic organ measurements.* In Goldberg BB, Kurtz AB, editors: *Atlas of ultrasound measurements,* Chicago, 1990, Year Book Medical Publishers.

Baltarowich OK et al: The spectrum of sonographic findings in hemorrhagic ovarian cysts, *AJR* 148:901, 1987.

Barloon TJ et al: Predictive value of normal endovaginal sonography in excluding disease of the female genital organs and adnexa, *J Ultrasound Med* 13:395, 1994.

Bromley B, Goodman H, Benacerraf BR: Comparison between sonographic morphology and Doppler waveform for the diagnosis of ovarian malignancy, *Obstet Gynecol* 83:434, 1994.

Brown DL et al: Ovarian masses: can benign and malignant lesions be differentiated with color and pulse Doppler US, *Radiology* 190:333, 1994.

Campbell S et al: Transabdominal ultrasound screening for early ovarian cancer, *Br Med J* 299:1363, 1989.

Cohen HL, Tice HM, Mandel FS: Ovarian volumes measured by US: bigger than we think, *Radiology* 177:189, 1990.

Fleischer AC, Gordon AN, Entman SS: Transabdominal and transvaginal sonography of pelvic masses, *Ultrasound Med Biol* 15:529, 1989.

Fleischer AC et al: Assessment of ovarian tumor vascularity with transvaginal color Doppler sonography, *J Ultrasound Med* 10:563, 1991.

Granberg S, Wikland M: A comparison between ultrasound and gynecologic examination for detection of enlarged ovaries in a group of women at risk for ovarian carcinoma, *J Ultrasound Med* 7:59, 1988.

Guttman PH Jr: In search of the elusive benign cystic ovarian teratoma: application of the ultrasound "tip of the iceberg" sign, *J Clin Ultrasound* 5:403, 1977.

Hamper UM et al: Transvaginal color Doppler sonography of adnexal masses: differences in blood flow impedance in benign and malignant lesions, *AJR* 160:1225, 1993.

Helvie MA, Silver TM: Ovarian torsion: sonographic evaluation, *J Clin Ultrasound* 17:327, 1989.

Jain KA: Prospective evaluation of adnexal masses with endovaginal gray-scale and duplex and color Doppler US: correlation with pathologic findings, *Radiology* 191:63, 1994.

Leibman AJ, Kruse B, McSweeney MB: Transvaginal sonography: comparison with transabdominal sonography in the diagnosis of pelvic masses, *AJR* 151:98, 1988.

Levine D et al: Simple adnexal cysts: the natural history in postmenopausal women, *Radiology* 184:653, 1992.

Ritchie WGM: Sonographic evaluation of normal and induced ovulation, *Radiology* 161:1, 1986.

Rosado WM Jr et al: Adnexal torsion: diagnosis by using Doppler sonography, *AJR* 159:1251, 1992.

Rulin MC, Preston AL: Adnexal masses in postmenopausal women, *Obstet Gynecol* 70:578, 1987.

Salem S, White LM, Lai J: Doppler sonography of adnexal masses: the predictive value of the pulsatility index in benign and malignant disease, *AJR* 163:1147, 1994.

Sassone AM et al: Transvaginal sonographic characterization of ovarian disease: evaluation of a new scoring system to predict ovarian malignancy, *Obstet Gynecol* 78:70, 1991.

Sheth S et al: The variable sonographic appearances of ovarian teratomas: correlation with CT, *AJR* 151:331, 1988.

Steer CV et al: Transvaginal colour flow imaging of the uterine arteries during the ovarian and menstrual cycles, *Hum Reprod* 5:391, 1990.

Taylor KJW, Schwartz PE: Screening for early ovarian cancer, *Radiology* 192:1, 1994.

Tessler FN et al: Endovaginal sonographic diagnosis of dilated fallopian tubes, *AJR* 153:523, 1989.

Yeh H-C, Futterweit W, Thornton JC: Polycystic ovarian disease: US features in 104 patients, *Radiology* 163:111, 1987.

CHAPTER 19

Ectopic Pregnancy

Definitions
Intrauterine Findings
Extrauterine Findings
The Use of Doppler

For a Key Features summary, see p. 430.

For a Key Features summary, see p. 430.

The incidence of ectopic pregnancies has risen considerably in the United States from 4.5 per 1000 total pregnancies in 1970 to 14.3 in 1986. In absolute terms this represents a rise of from 17,800 ectopic pregnancies in 1970 to more than 70,000 by 1986! There is some indication, however, that this number may finally be leveling off.

There is also a well-documented incidence of death resulting from ectopic pregnancies, mostly related to blood loss. Although this death rate has substantially decreased, from 3.6 per 1000 ectopic pregnancies in 1970 to 0.5 per 1000 in 1986, the numbers are nevertheless disturbing. Because ectopic pregnancies occur in relatively young women, often without other health problems, death can be avoided.

The presenting signs and symptoms of an ectopic pregnancy are not always typical. Only approximately 60% of women have a history of a missed menstrual period. The classic triad of irregular menstrual bleeding, abdominal or pelvic pain, and a palpated tender adnexal mass is not always present. In fact, a mass may not be detected. However, certain groups of women are at particularly high risk: (1) those with abnormal fallopian tubes as the result of previous infection (salpingitis), developmental defects, or prior tubal reconstructive surgery; (2) those with normal fallopian tubes but who have an intrauterine device, who are taking ovulation-inducing agents, who are treated by in vitro fertilization–embryo transfer, or who suffer from delayed ovulation or tubal transport; and (3) those who have a history of prior ectopic pregnancies.

The new pregnancy tests, which are performed on both urine and blood samples, are highly accurate. The tests are an immunoassay of the beta-subunit of the human chorionic gonadotropin (βhCG). The urine tests (usually a monoclonal-enzyme–linked assay) are not, as yet, as sensitive as the serum radioimmunologic tests. The serum tests can detect concentrations as low as 1 to 2 IU/L and can also be quantitated. These levels are important in anticipating when normal intrauterine findings should be present.

An additional serum test, one that determines the progesterone level, has been proposed as a method of discriminating between a normal and an abnormal intrauterine pregnancy (IUP). Unfortunately, the value that distinguishes between the two (with a normal level higher) has not proved 100% certain. Furthermore, this method does not permit an abnormal IUP to be differentiated from an ectopic pregnancy.

The βhCG levels normally rise throughout the first trimester. A single quantitative level (above a discriminatory level) is accurate for diagnosing an IUP, usually a normal but occasionally an abnormal pregnancy. When below this level, a single absolute value is greatly limited, with the differential diagnosis among a normal early IUP, an abnormal IUP, and an ectopic pregnancy. It is typical for an ectopic pregnancy never to exceed this discriminatory threshold.

If serial quantitative βhCG levels are obtained, there is an expected normal IUP doubling time. In general the βhCG level is expected to double every 2 days, slightly faster before 7 weeks (1.4 days) and slightly slower thereafter (3.4 days). The doubling time can be abnormally slow in the settings of an abnormal IUP and an ectopic pregnancy. Both can also be manifested by a declining βhCG level, although a rapid decrease is more typical of an abnormal IUP.

There is more than one measurement standard for serum βhCG levels. There are two tests and two reported concentration values. The most commonly used test is the International Reference Preparation (IRP), reported in international units per liter. There is also a Second International Standard (2nd IS), which is approximately half as pure and usually is also reported in international units per liter. The value yielded by the purer IRP is approximately twice the value yielded by the 2nd IS. For example, 2 IU/L (IRP) = 1 IU/L (2nd IS). There will soon be a third serum βhCG test that is expected to be equivalent to the IRP. Finally, some laboratories report their results in nanograms per milliliter. As a rough guide, 1 ng/ml = 10 to 12 IU/L (IRP).

DEFINITIONS

An ectopic pregnancy is defined as the implantation of a fertilized ovum outside the endometrial lining of the uterus. Ectopic pregnancies are most common in the fallopian tubes (95% to 97%), usually in the ampullar or isthmus regions. However, ectopic implantation can occur anywhere in the tube, from the fimbriated end (near the ovary) to the interstitial portion (as it enters the muscular wall of the uterus). Adnexal ectopic pregnancies sometimes occur outside the fallopian tube: within the ovary (<1%), between the leaves of the broad ligament, and on the intraperitoneal surface (approximately 0.03%), which is the rarest form and called an abdominal pregnancy. It is often not possible to predict the exact anatomic position of an adnexal pregnancy prior to surgery.

Within the uterus, ectopic pregnancies can occur in the cornual region of the uterine fundus (<5%) and in the cervix (0.1%). Cervical pregnancies are very low uterine implantations located in the endocervical canal at or below the internal cervical os. They have increased in frequency because of the use of in vitro fertilization, with transcervical insertion of fertilized ova.

Because of the small diameter of most of the fallopian tube, particularly the isthmus and interstitial regions, these ectopic pregnancies frequently cause early signs and symptoms. Conversely, pregnancies outside the tube, particularly in the expandable muscular cornual portion of the uterus and in the abdomen, may present later, even in the second and rarely in the third trimester. The onset of symptoms can vary in women with cervical pregnancies.

A heterotopic pregnancy is a concomitant intrauterine and extrauterine pregnancy. Although it was initially rare, with an incidence of 1 in 30,000 births, it has become more common: it now occurs in 1 in 7000 pregnancies, with an approximate range of 1 in 4000 to 1 in 8000 pregnancies. This increased incidence appears to be related to the presence of partially damaged fallopian tubes (a causative factor for many ectopic pregnancies) and to the use of assisted reproductive techniques.

INTRAUTERINE FINDINGS

In a patient whose pregnancy test result is positive, the differential possibilities are a normal IUP, an abnormal IUP (miscarriage), or an ectopic pregnancy. The clinical symptoms and physical findings may indicate a specific diagnosis. However, as previously stated, the signs and symptoms of an ectopic pregnancy can be nonspecific or at times misleading. In addition, on occasion there is more than one type of abnormality present. For example, a patient with a normal IUP may have a palpable ovarian cyst, an adnexal mass, or an ectopic pregnancy.

Normal pelvic ultrasound findings (when the pregnancy test result is positive) do not have any diagnostic value, except that then an ectopic pregnancy is more likely. Even equivocal intrauterine findings mandate closer patient surveillance. Conversely, abnormal ultrasound findings (intrauterine and extrauterine) can be very helpful and are often diagnostic.

When the pregnancy test result is positive, the primary value of ultrasound is its ability to identify an IUP. Specifically, the intrauterine identification of a gestational sac, an embryo, and occasionally a yolk sac proves the presence of an IUP. The further detection of normal characteristics, in particular an embryo with heart motion, confirms the presence of a normal IUP. First-trimester intrauterine landmarks (i.e., gestational sac, embryo, and yolk sac) and normal gestational sac measurements and crown-rump lengths are discussed in Chapter 9.

It has been shown that, when the βhCG level is at or above a certain concentration, an intrauterine gestational sac should be detected by ultrasound. The normal results are different for transabdominal (TA) and transvaginal (TV) imaging, with TV identification occurring when the concentrations are lower because of its superior resolution and near-field focusing capability. Although the exact levels have not been established, the following are approximate IUP values. The gestational sac should be imaged by TV scanning when it is 1000 IU/L and by TA scanning when it is 6500 IU/L. Furthermore, the identification of the yolk sac and the living embryo within the intrauterine gestational sac should normally be identified by TV imaging when the βhCG is 7200 and 10,000 IU/L, respectively. Because of the expected fast doubling time of the βhCG levels, a wait of 2 to 4 days is often clinically appropriate when findings are borderline or equivocal.

The sonographic diagnosis of a normal IUP can frequently be made transabdominally (Fig. 19-1, A). If, however, appropriate intrauterine landmarks cannot be detected or the findings are equivocal, a TV examination should then be performed (Fig. 19-1, B and C). Both techniques can show the normal gestational sac to have a relatively well defined hyperechoic rim that is at least 2 mm thick. This hyperechoic rim is interrupted along approx-

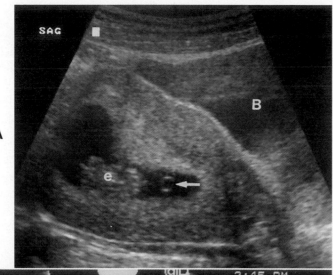

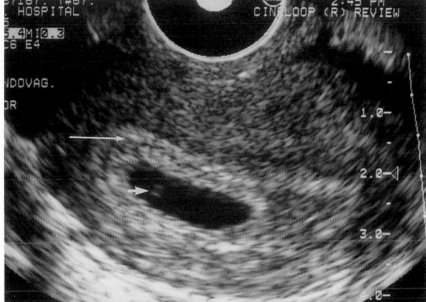

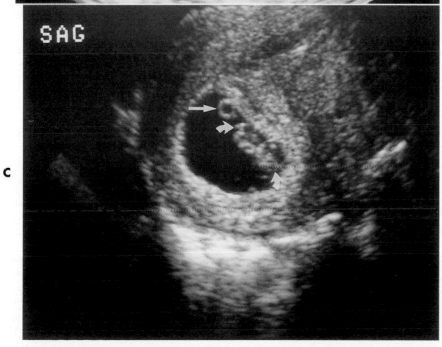

Fig. 19-1 Normal intrauterine pregnancies. **A,** Transabdominal sagittal image of the uterus in a 7.5-week pregnancy shows a well-defined gestational sac. Within the sac is an embryo *(e)* showing heart motion and a yolk sac *(arrow). B,* urinary bladder. **B,** Transvaginal coronal-transaxial image of the uterus in a 5-week pregnancy shows a gestational sac with a well-defined hyperechoic rim. The rim is interrupted by a hypoechoic line *(long arrow),* thus creating the double decidual sac sign of a normal intrauterine pregnancy. A yolk sac *(small arrow)* is identified within the sac. **C,** Transvaginal sagittal image of the uterus in a 6.5-week pregnancy shows a well-defined gestational sac with a living embryo *(curved arrows)* and a yolk sac *(straight arrow).*

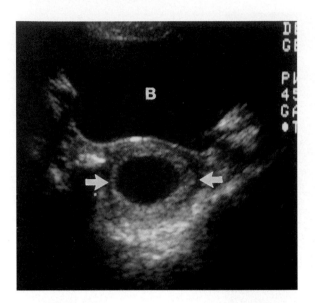

Fig. 19-2 Abnormal intrauterine pregnancy at 9 weeks. This transabdominal transaxial image shows a well-defined gestational sac surrounded by a normal hyperechoic rim *(arrows)*. No embryo is identified. Because the sac has a mean diameter of 38 mm, it should not be "empty." *B*, urinary bladder.

imately half of its margin by a thin hypoechoic line. This is called the *double decidual sac* (DDS) sign (discussed in Chapter 9). Although the DDS sign strongly supports the likelihood of a normal IUP, its absence does not completely rule it out. A normal very early gestational sac can be identified within the thickened decidua, adjacent to but not involving the endometrial canal. This is called the *intradecidual sign* and is also discussed in Chapter 9.

The presence of the DDS sign helps predict the presence of a normally developing intrauterine gestation (Fig. 19-1, *B*). It is a most important finding during the interval between the identification of the gestational sac and the detection of the embryo. TA scanning routinely detects the gestational sac by 5 menstrual weeks when the mean gestational sac diameter (MGSD) is 10 mm or more. The embryo is not routinely seen until 6.5 weeks when the MGSD is 27 mm or more. It is this interval MGSD of between 10 and 27 mm that is most important. TV scanning detects the gestational sac earlier, by 4 to 4.5 weeks, when the MGSD is approximately 2 mm. The embryo is also identified earlier, by 5.5 weeks, when the MGSD is 12 mm (sometimes earlier). Therefore the most important interval MGSD for the TV scanning is between 2 and 12 mm. The yolk sac may also be helpful. It has been identified slightly earlier than the embryo at MGSDs of 20 mm on TA studies and 8 mm on TV studies.

An intrauterine collection surrounded by a hyperechoic rim but without the DDS sign is more likely abnormal, either an abnormal gestational sac or a pseudogestational sac of an ectopic pregnancy (Figs. 19-2 and 19-3). The pseudogestational sac is caused by a collection of either fluid or hyperechoic material (termed a *decidual cast*) that is distending the endometrial canal. On occasion the hyperechoic material blends in with the hyperechoic rim. It then looks like (and probably is) thickened endometrium (Fig. 19-4).

A pseudogestational sac occurs in approximately 5%

of ectopic pregnancies. It is not always possible to differentiate it from the abnormal sac of an abnormal IUP. However, an abnormal IUP sac is more likely round or oval with a fairly well preserved hyperechoic rim; a pseudogestational "sac," on the other hand, is more likely to be irregular in shape and elongated because it conforms to the endometrial canal (see Fig. 19-3, *C*). Hyperechoic endometrial thickening can be either retained products of conception or can be caused by the hormonal effects of an ectopic pregnancy. These cannot often be differentiated sonographically.

Some ectopic pregnancies may initially (and falsely) look like normal IUPs, and some IUPs may initially (and falsely) look like extrauterine pregnancies. The ectopic pregnancies within the cornual portion of the uterine fundus and within the cervix are both easily identified as pregnancies but may be difficult to appreciate in an ectopic location. A cornual pregnancy is eccentrically positioned within the fundus (Fig. 19-5). A careful examination can reveal the absence of myometrium surrounding a portion of the gestational sac. This can be particularly apparent if the sac abuts on the distended urinary bladder. A cervical pregnancy needs to be differentiated from a low but normal uterine pregnancy and from a miscarriage in progress. The distinction is often possible, although the key landmark, the internal cervical os, is not clearly identified in the first trimester.

Conversely, a normal IUP may be mistaken for an ectopic pregnancy. Sometimes in a retroverted or retroflexed uterus with its globular shape, only a thin rim of myometrium appears to separate the gestational sac from its margin. A myomatous uterus can be so distorted as to displace the gestational sac so that it appears either at the margin of or beyond the boundaries of the uterus. In almost all instances, if myometrium (no matter how thin) can be identified surrounding the gestational sac, the sac is intrauterine. If uncertainty exists, however, TV scan

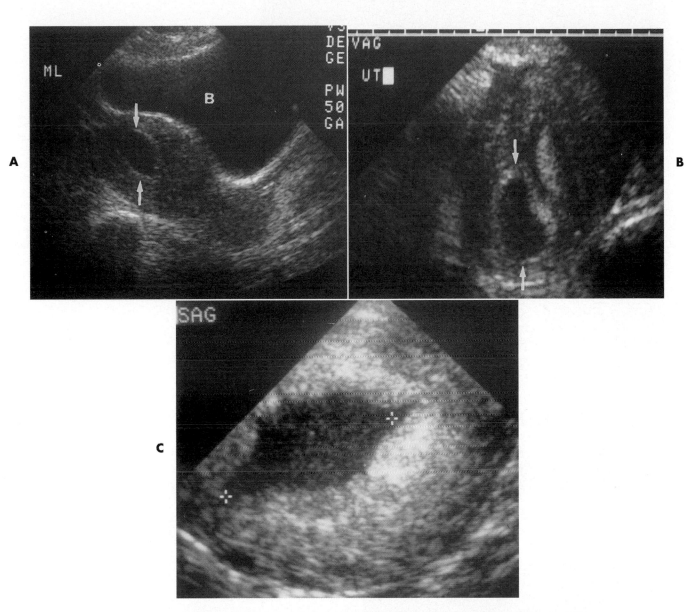

Fig. 19-3   Pseudogestational sacs of ectopic pregnancies. Transabdominal **(A)** and transvaginal **(B)** sagittal images of the same pseudogestational sac showing an intrauterine hypoechoic collection surrounded by a thin hyperechoic rim *(arrows)*. The average diameter of this collection is 30 mm. The appearance of this collection cannot be definitively differentiated from that of an abnormal intrauterine pregnancy. *B,* urinary bladder. **C,** Transvaginal sagittal image of the uterus in another patient shows a hyperechoic collection. It is pointed at both ends (+), conforms to the endometrial canal, and is sometimes called a *decidual crest.*

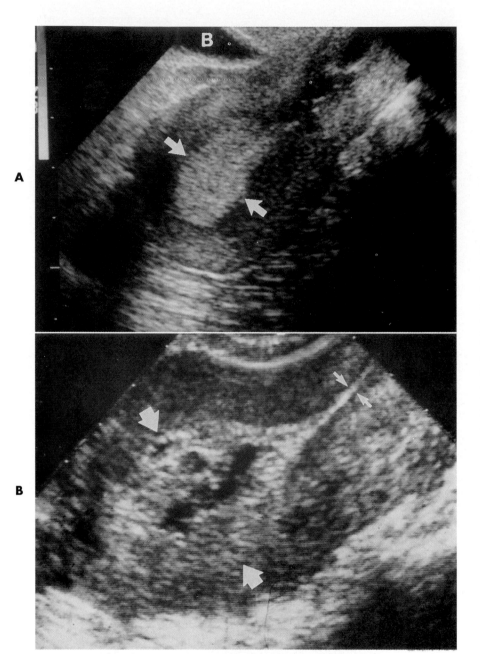

Fig. 19-4 Thickened endometrium caused by ectopic pregnancies. These appearances cannot be differentiated from the endometrial thickening secondary to retained products. **A,** Transvaginal sagittal image of the uterus shows a markedly hyperechoic, thickened endometrium *(arrows)*. A minimally distended urinary bladder *(B)* is seen. **B,** Transvaginal sagittal image of the uterus in another patient shows a markedly and focally thickened, heterogeneous endometrium in the upper body and fundus *(large arrows)*. The endometrium in the cervix and lower uterine segment is of normal thickness *(small arrows)*.

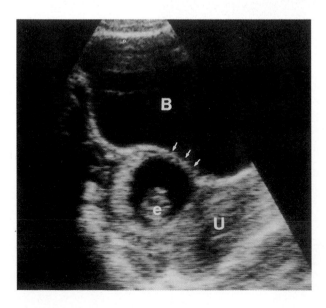

Fig. 19-5 Cornual ectopic pregnancy at 8 weeks. This transabdominal sagittal image of the uterus *(U)* shows a well-defined gestational sac with a living embryo *(e)*. The sac is eccentrically positioned and only partially within the uterus. Along its surface where it abuts on the distended urinary bladder *(B),* the margin is very thin and does not have a surrounding myometrium *(arrows).*

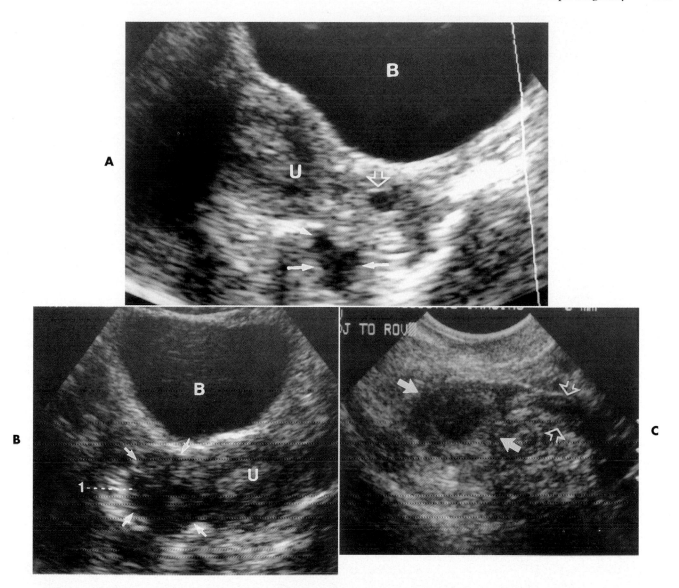

Fig. 19-6   Comparison of transabdominal and transvaginal ultrasound images in a woman with a positive pregnancy test result. **A,** Transabdominal sagittal image of the uterus *(U)* shows no evidence of an intrauterine pregnancy. A mild amount of fluid *(arrows)* is detected within the cul-de-sac. *Open arrow,* nabothian cyst (a normal variant); *B,* urinary bladder. **B,** Transabdominal transaxial image of the uterus *(U)* and the right adnexa *(arrows).* The right adnexa is ill-defined and there is the suggestion of a minimal anechoic center along dotted line *1. B,* urinary bladder. **C,** Transvaginal transaxial-coronal view of the right adnexa (closed arrows) through the plane of section *1* in **B** shows the tubal ring characteristic of an ectopic pregnancy that has no definable internal structures. Open arrows denote a slightly dilated right fallopian tube (hydrosalpinx). Both are adjacent to a normal right ovary (not shown).

ning can often confirm the presence of surrounding myometrium.

EXTRAUTERINE FINDINGS

Extrauterine findings are not always observed in ectopic pregnancies. In fact, the adnexa appear normal in a third of ectopic pregnancies. When the pregnancy test re-

sult is positive, the only finding that rules out the presence of an ectopic pregnancy is the detection of an IUP, except in the rare instance of a concomitant extrauterine pregnancy. If an IUP is not detected by either TV or TA scanning, the likelihood of an ectopic pregnancy is then increased.

TV scanning is often better at detecting subtle abnormalities than is TA scanning (Figs. 19-6 to 19-8). However, TA scanning is important for giving an initial overview of

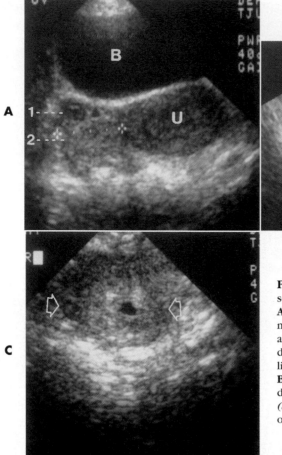

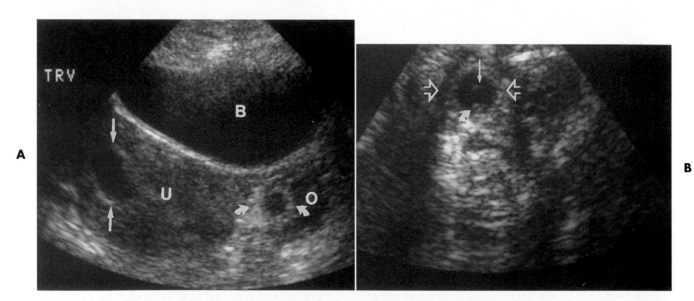

Fig. 19-7 Comparison of transabdominal and transvaginal ultrasound images in a woman with a positive pregnancy test result. **A,** Transabdominal transaxial image of the uterus *(U)* and right adnexa *(+)*. The right adnexa is somewhat irregular and ill-defined, and two areas are noted: a smaller hypoechoic anterior area along dotted line *1* and a larger hyperechoic posterior area along dotted line *2*. There was no intrauterine pregnancy. *B,* urinary bladder. **B** and **C** are transvaginal transaxial-coronal images obtained along dotted lines *1* and *2* in **A,** respectively. **B** shows the normal ovary *(arrows)* and **C** shows the tubal ring *(open arrows)* characteristic of an ectopic pregnancy.

Fig. 19-8 Comparison of transabdominal and transvaginal ultrasound images in a woman with a positive pregnancy test result. **A,** Transabdominal transaxial image of the uterus *(U)* and left ovary *(O)*. Within the uterus is an eccentrically placed, poorly defined collection *(straight arrows)*, a pseudogestational sac. Within the left adnexal region, between the uterus and ovary, is a tubal ring *(curved arrows)* with ill-defined internal echoes. *B,* urinary bladder. **B,** Transvaginal sagittal image through the area of the tubal ring *(open arrows)* identifies intragestational landmarks, an embryo with heart motion *(curved arrow)* and a yolk sac *(long arrow)*. These confirm the presence of an ectopic pregnancy.

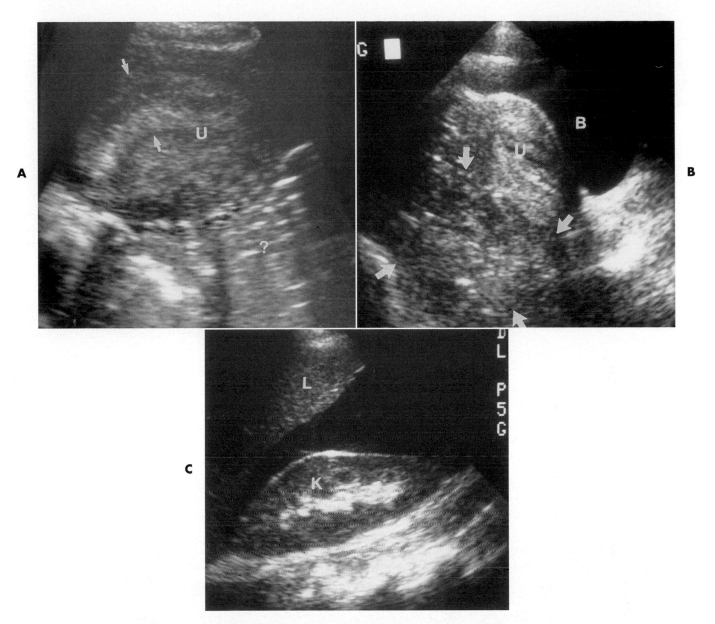

Fig. 19-9   The value of the transabdominal study in a woman with a positive pregnancy test result. **A,** This initial transvaginal sagittal study of the uterus *(U)* shows a markedly hyperechoic, thickened decidual cast or endometrium *(arrows)*. No intrauterine pregnancy is detected. Posterior to the uterus is an ill-defined area *(?)* that was thought to be normal nonperistalsing bowel. **B,** Transabdominal midline image of the uterus *(U)*, scanned through a distended urinary bladder *(B)*, confirms the absence of an intrauterine pregnancy. The large hyperechoic area posterior to the uterus *(arrows)* is pushing the uterus anteriorly. It is trophoblastic tissue and hemorrhage stemming from a ruptured ectopic pregnancy. **C,** Transabdominal sagittal scan of the right upper quadrant shows anechoic fluid (hemoperitoneum) between the liver *(L)* and right kidney *(K)* secondary to the ruptured ectopic pregnancy.

the pelvis and abdomen and should be performed even when the urinary bladder is empty (Fig. 19-9). If the TA study clearly identifies an IUP and normal adnexa, the study can usually be stopped. If not, a TV study should always be performed.

When the pregnancy test result is positive and there is no evidence of an IUP, adnexal findings assume great importance. In general, except for the detection of a simple cyst, any adnexal abnormality could be an ectopic pregnancy. These abnormalities are divided into four categories (Table 19-1). The most definitive is a living extrauterine pregnancy, that is, an embryo with heart motion, detected within a typical gestational sac outside the uterus. This can be identified by both TA and TV

Table 19-1 **The diagnosis of ectopic pregnancies based on ultrasound adnexal findings***

Ultrasound findings	Positive predictive value
Extrauterine embryo with positive heart motion	100%
Adnexal mass containing a yolk sac or nonliving embryo	100%
"Tubal" or "adnexal" ring surrounding a fluid collection	95%
Complex or solid adnexal mass (*no* embryo, yolk sac, or tubal ring)	92%

Adapted from Brown DL, Doubilet PM: Transvaginal sonography for diagnosing ectopic pregnancy: positivity criteria and performance characteristics, *J Ultrasound Med* 13:259, 1994.
*All patients had a positive pregnancy test result and no evidence of an intrauterine pregnancy.

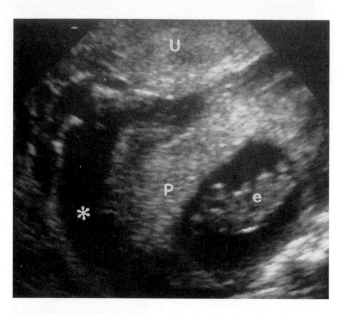

Fig. 19-10   Abdominal pregnancy at 9 weeks. This transvaginal sagittal image of the uterus *(U)* and cul-de-sac shows a well-defined extrauterine embryo *(e)* and adjacent placenta *(P)*. There was no well-defined sac. Ascites surrounds the edge of the placenta (*). The size of the ectopic pregnancy and the poorly defined margins (with ascites) indicate an abdominal (intraperitoneal) location.

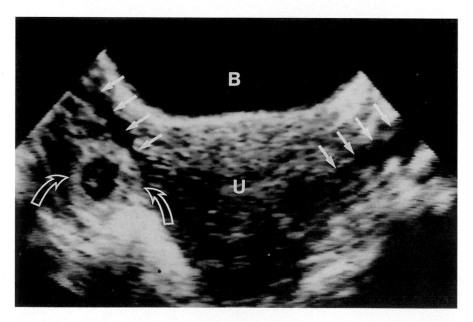

Fig. 19-11   Ectopic pregnancy secondary to pelvic inflammatory disease. In a young woman who had a positive pregnancy test result and previously treated pelvic inflammatory disease, a transabdominal transaxial view of the uterus *(U)* shows no evidence of an intrauterine pregnancy. Dilated fallopian tubes, called *hydrosalpinges (straight arrows)*, are identified bilaterally as they enter the uterine fundus. A well-defined extrauterine gestational sac with a hyperechoic rim is identified in the right adnexa *(curved open arrows)*. Within the sac is a nonliving embryo. *B,* urinary bladder.

scanning and is diagnostic for an ectopic pregnancy (Figs. 19-8 and 19-10). It is estimated that a living extrauterine pregnancy is detected by 15% of TA and 30% of TV studies. The positive predictive value (PPV) of this finding is 100%. The PPV of an adnexal mass (not a well-defined gestational sac) containing either a yolk sac or nonliving embryo is also 100% (Figs. 19-11 and 19-12).

A tubal ring (also called an *adnexal ring, "bagel" sign,* and other monikers) is a mass with a hyperechoic rim surrounding extrauterine fluid. The rim is probably trophoblastic tissue. No embryo or yolk sac is identified (see Figs. 19-6 and 19-7). Finally, an adnexal mass can have a nonspecific appearance, either complex or solid. It can have any shape, from round to oval to irregular. If the ectopic pregnancy has ruptured, the mass can be very irregular because it conforms to its available space (Figs. 19-9 and 19-13). The tubal ring sign and the appearance of the mass are less specific findings and have PPVs of 92% to 95%, respectively.

An additional and most likely equally important finding (in a woman with a positive pregnancy test result) is the amount of intraperitoneal fluid detected and its internal echogenicity. A small amount or "sliver" of fluid in the cul-de-sac can sometimes be seen in normal pregnancies (Figs. 19-6 and 19-14). A larger amount of intraperitoneal fluid in the cul-de-sac, especially if it extends into the flanks and upper abdomen, must be considered abnormal. Although there is no quantitated amount, if the volume of fluid is judged subjectively to be moderate to large, the likelihood of an ectopic pregnancy is considerably increased (see Figs. 19-9, 19-10, and 19-13). Internal echoes within the fluid (probably the result of hemorrhage), though a nonspecific finding, are also associated with an ectopic pregnancy.

A combination of these extrauterine findings further increases the likelihood of an ectopic pregnancy when the pregnancy test result is positive. A noncystic adnexal mass with a moderate to large amount of amniotic fluid has been found to be a highly specific and accurate (at 100%) sign of an ectopic pregnancy. Even if there is a normal IUP, if any of the adnexal findings just discussed are observed, the probability of a concomitant extrauterine pregnancy is greatly increased (Fig. 19-15).

All of the sonographic findings characteristic of an ectopic pregnancy, aside from the identification of an extrauterine embryo with heart motion, can be mimicked by other abnormalities. Endometriomas, pelvic inflammatory disease without or with abscess formation, and even dermoids on occasion exhibit some of the appearances described (Fig. 19-16). For this reason the βhCG level is critical in establishing the diagnosis of an ectopic pregnancy. If the pregnancy test result is negative or the results are pending, these other abnormalities should also be considered. In addition, pelvic inflammatory disease causes the fallopian tubes to be abnormal. If abnormal fallopian tubes are found or there is a known clinical history of pelvic inflammatory disease, or both exist, this raises the level of suspicion for an ectopic pregnancy.

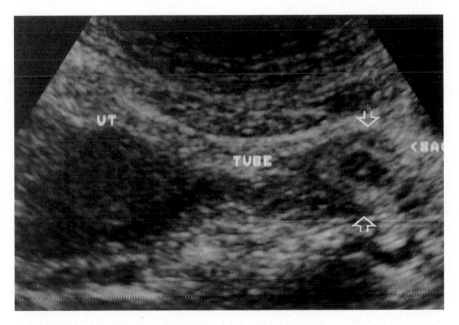

Fig. 19-12   Left adnexal tubal pregnancy. The uterus *(UT)* in a woman with a positive pregnancy test result shows no evidence of an intrauterine pregnancy. The area of the left fallopian tube *(TUBE)* is prominent but does not have the anechoic tubular appearance of a hydrosalpinx. Within the tube, however, is a well-defined extrauterine gestational sac *(open arrows* and *SAC).* Ill-defined structures were identified within the extrauterine gestational sac, suggestive of a nonliving embryo and a yolk sac.

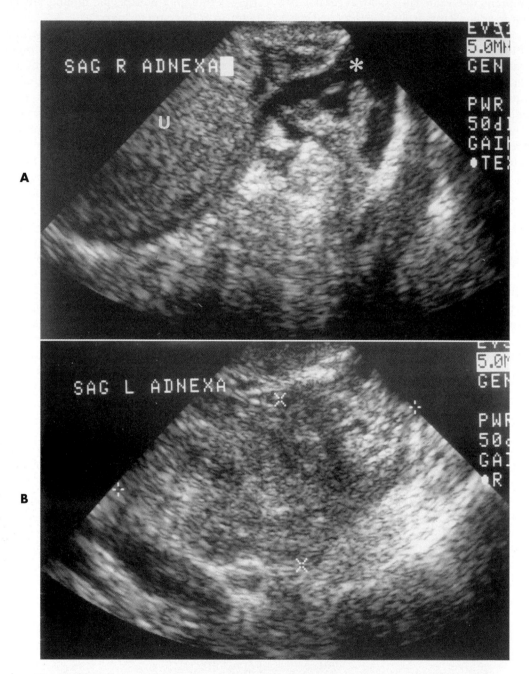

Fig. 19-13   Ectopic pregnancy in a woman with a positive pregnancy test result whose last menstrual period had occurred 8 weeks earlier. There was no evidence of an intrauterine pregnancy (images not shown), and therefore transvaginal sagittal images of the right and left adnexal regions were obtained. **A,** In the right adnexa at the edge of the uterus *(U),* there is a mild to moderate amount of cul-de-sac fluid (*). The right ovary could not be identified. **B,** A large, irregular, ill-defined mass of heterogeneous echogenicity (+ and *x*) is found in the left adnexa, consistent with a ruptured ectopic pregnancy. The left ovary could not be detected.

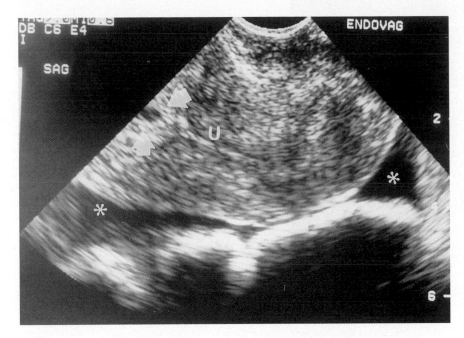

Fig. 19-14 Normal cul-de-sac fluid in the first trimester. This transvaginal sagittal image of the lower two thirds of the uterus *(U)* shows the edge of a normal intrauterine gestational sac *(arrows)*. Behind the uterus is a small amount of intraperitoneal fluid (*). This can be a normal finding but occasionally warrants a follow-up examination. In this case the fluid resolved spontaneously.

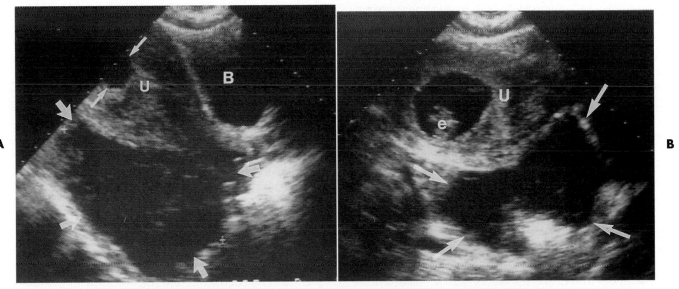

Fig. 19-15 Heterotopic pregnancy, a concomitant intrauterine and extrauterine pregnancy. **A,** Transabdominal sagittal midline view of the uterus *(U)* shows part of a normal intrauterine gestational sac *(small arrows)*. A large, irregular, primarily anechoic fluid collection is identified within the cul-de-sac, which shows multiple small hyperechoic internal echoes *(large arrows)*. *B,* urinary bladder. **B,** Transabdominal transaxial image through the upper part of the uterus *(U)* shows a normal intrauterine gestational sac with a well-defined living embryo *(e)*. Posteriorly, within the cul-de-sac, is the same large complex fluid collection *(arrows)*.

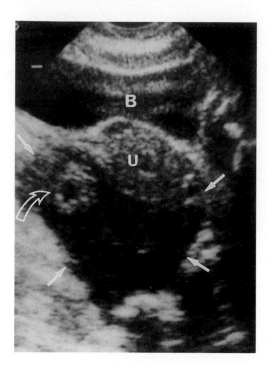

Fig. 19-16 Partially treated pelvic inflammatory disease in a woman with a negative pregnancy test result. This transabdominal transaxial view shows a grossly normal uterus *(U)*. Behind the uterus is an ill-defined complex collection *(straight arrows)* that fills the cul-de-sac and extends into the right adnexa where there is the suggestion of a tubal ring *(open curved arrow)* characteristic of an ectopic pregnancy. However, the pregnancy test result was negative, and this area proved to be part of a large abscess. *B,* urinary bladder.

THE USE OF DOPPLER

Both color- and pulsed-Doppler waveform analysis have been used to evaluate pregnancies. Color-Doppler can survey a large amount of tissue and find arterial signals; pulsed-Doppler can then obtain an arterial waveform. The trophoblastic tissue that surrounds a pregnancy, whether intrauterine or extrauterine, commonly has a low-resistance (high-diastolic) arterial waveform. This is not a diagnostic pattern for trophoblastic tissue and has also been seen in the settings of ovarian cancer (malignant neovascularity), endocrine-active tumors, and inflammation.

The intrauterine trophoblastic reaction of the gestational sac (the hyperechoic rim) of an IUP can be detected by the finding of an arterial waveform with an elevated diastolic flow. This finding should in theory differentiate an IUP from the pseudogestational sac of an ectopic pregnancy, but it is of value only in those cases in which only the gestational sac (not its yolk sac and embryo) is identified. Even then, more Doppler evaluation is needed because the trophoblastic tissues of all normal and abnormal intrauterine gestational sacs may not have this low-resistance waveform. The specificity of this sign is not known, particularly in the context of abnormal IUPs.

It has been suggested that this high-diastolic arterial pattern of trophoblastic tissue in the adnexa can be of value, perhaps identifying the existence of an ectopic pregnancy. However, problems can arise in the Doppler evaluation of the adnexa. There are multiple arteries (both uterine and ovarian) under the influence of a woman's menstrual cycles. During each cycle these arteries normally fluctuate in the amount of their diastolic flow, in particular that going to the ovary on the dominant side for that cycle. The amount going to a corpus luteum is also increased. Therefore the low-resistance, high-diastolic flow pattern may be completely normal in either adnexa. Additionally, certain masses (e.g., endometriomas, abscesses, and dermoids) that are unrelated to an ectopic pregnancy may have an elevated diastolic flow. Therefore Doppler adnexal findings are not diagnostic in a woman whose pregnancy test result is positive but is not found to have an IUP; they can only help confirm the presence of an ectopic pregnancy when an adnexal abnormality is identified (Fig. 19-17).

It has also been suggested that the same low-resistance arterial waveforms can be used to *detect* an ectopic pregnancy even when no adnexal abnormality is observed sonographically. This is an intriguing concept, but one that requires further study.

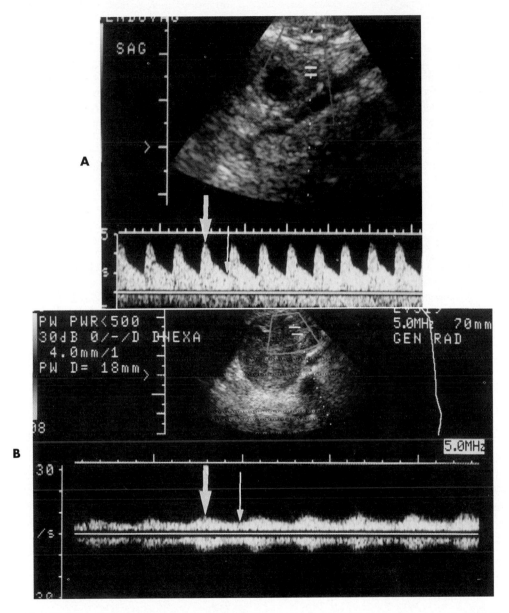

Fig. 19-17   Doppler arterial spectral waveforms in two cases of ectopic pregnancies. **A,** Split image showing the transvaginal image of an adnexal tubal ring at the top. The Doppler sample is taken from the edge of the tubal ring. On the bottom the Doppler arterial waveform shows a relatively small amount of diastolic flow (end-diastole is denoted by a long thin arrow) compared with the systolic flow (peak systole is denoted by a large thick arrow). This waveform is nonspecific. **B,** Split image showing the transvaginal image of a large hyperechoic adnexal mass at the top with the Doppler sample taken from its edge. On the bottom the Doppler arterial waveform is seen to have a relatively large amount of diastolic flow (end-diastole is denoted by a long thin arrow) compared with the systolic flow (peak systole is denoted by a large thick arrow). This pattern is more typical for trophoblastic tissue but can be seen in other conditions.

Key Features

The incidence of ectopic pregnancies has steadily increased in the United States over the past two decades. Although the death rate has fallen, it is still a serious health problem.

The presentation of ectopic pregnancy is variable, often not typical. Certain high-risk patients should be carefully evaluated: those with abnormal fallopian tubes, those with a history of ectopic pregnancy, those with an intrauterine device, those taking fertility medication, and those undergoing in vitro fertilization.

The new pregnancy tests that measure the level of the beta-subunit of the human chorionic gonadotropin (βhCG) in urine and serum are highly accurate. The serum test is more sensitive and can be quantitated.

There are certain βhCG levels (discriminatory levels) above which specific intrauterine landmarks are routinely detected by ultrasound. The serum βhCG levels also normally double approximately every 2 days in the first trimester.

The βhCG level in a woman with an ectopic pregnancy rarely rises above the expected discriminatory level. The doubling time is either unusually slow or slowly decreases.

There are two serum βhCG tests. The First International Reference Preparation (IRP) is purer and more widely used. The βhCG value yielded by the IRP is approximately twice that yielded by the Second International Standard. The values are usually given in international units per liter.

An ectopic pregnancy is defined as the implantation of a fertilized ovum outside the endometrial lining. Most are in the fallopian tube, but they can be in many other adnexal positions, including the abdomen (on the peritoneal surface). The exact position of an adnexal ectopic pregnancy is seldom accurately predicted before surgical intervention.

Ectopic pregnancies can occur in two places within the uterus: in the cornual portion of the fundus and in the cervix.

A heterotopic pregnancy, which is a concomitant intrauterine and extrauterine pregnancy, now occurs in approximately 1 in 7000 pregnancies.

In a patient who has a positive pregnancy test result, the differential possibilities are a normal intrauterine, an abnormal intrauterine, and an ectopic pregnancy.

In a woman with a positive pregnancy test result, normal ultrasound findings, particularly when the examination is performed transvaginally, do not rule out the presence of an ectopic pregnancy and actually increases the likelihood of an ectopic pregnancy.

A pseudogestational sac occurs in approximately 5% of ectopic pregnancies. This is caused either by a collection of fluid or a decidual cast within the endometrial canal or by a thickened endometrium. Occasionally it is possible to differentiate it from an abnormal intrauterine gestational sac.

An ectopic pregnancy *within* the cornual portion of the uterus or within the cervix can initially (falsely) appear to be a normal intrauterine pregnancy.

In a retroverted uterus or in a uterus with multiple fibroids, an intrauterine sac may be displaced to the margin of the uterus and falsely appear in an ectopic position. If myometrium can be shown to encompass the sac, the pregnancy is intrauterine.

Transvaginal scanning has been shown to be better for detecting subtle abnormalities, either within the uterus or adnexa. If the transabdominal study shows the intrauterine findings characteristic of a normal pregnancy, the examination can most likely be stopped. However, a transvaginal scan should always be performed in a woman with a positive pregnancy test result and equivocal or normal transabdominal ultrasound findings.

There are five adnexal findings that (in a woman with a positive pregnancy test result) have high positive predictive values in establishing the diagnosis of an ectopic pregnancy: (1) a normal gestational sac in an ectopic location, (2) an adnexal mass containing either a yolk sac or a nonliving embryo, (3) a tubal ring appearing as an empty gestational sac, (4) a complex or solid adnexal mass, and (5) a moderate to a large amount of intraperitoneal fluid, particularly with internal echoes.

When significant extrauterine findings are encountered in the context of an intrauterine pregnancy, the likelihood of a concomitant ectopic pregnancy is increased.

Doppler waveform analysis is currently used in the evaluation of intrauterine and extrauterine pregnancies only as a confirmatory test.

SUGGESTED READINGS

Bree RL et al: Transvaginal sonography in the evaluation of normal early pregnancy: correlation with HCG level, *AJR* 153:75, 1989.

Brown DL, Doubilet PM: Transvaginal sonography for diagnosing ectopic pregnancy: positivity criteria and performance characteristics, *J Ultrasound Med* 13:259, 1994.

Cacciatore B, Stenman UK, Ylöstalo P: Comparison of abdominal and vaginal sonography in suspected ectopic pregnancy, *Obstet Gynecol* 73:770, 1989.

Dashefsky SM et al: Suspected ectopic pregnancy: endovaginal and transvesical US, *Radiology* 169:181, 1988.

Dillon EH, Feyock AL, Taylor KJW: Pseudogestational sacs: Doppler US differentiation from normal or abnormal intrauterine pregnancies, *Radiology* 176:359, 1990.

Dorfman SF: Deaths from ectopic pregnancy, United States: 1979 to 1980, *Obstet Gynecol* 62:334, 1983.

Filly RA: Ectopic pregnancy: the role of sonography, *Radiology* 162:661, 1987.

Frates MC et al: Cervical ectopic pregnancy: results of conservative treatment, *Radiology* 191:773, 1994.

Frates MC et al: Tubal rupture in patients with ectopic pregnancy: diagnosis with transvaginal US, *Radiology* 191:769, 1994.

Holman JF, Tyrey EL, Hammond CB: A contemporary approach to suspected ectopic pregnancy with use of quantitative and qualitative assays for the β-subunit of human chorionic gonadotropin and sonography, *Am J Obstet Gynecol* 150:151, 1984.

Kadar N, Romero R: Abnormal pregnancy: early diagnosis by US and serum chorionic gonadotropin levels [letter], *Radiology* 161:854, 1986.

Lawson HW et al: Ectopic pregnancy in the United States, 1970-1986, *MMWR CDC Surveill Summ* 83(SS-2):1, 1989.

Mahony BS, Filly RA, Nyberg DA, Callen PW: Sonographic evaluation of ectopic pregnancy, *J Ultrasound Med* 4:221, 1985.

Marks WM, Filly RA, Callen PW, Laing FC: The decidual cast of ectopic pregnancy: a confusing ultrasonographic appearance, *Radiology* 133:451, 1979.

Nyberg DA et al: Extrauterine findings of ectopic pregnancy at transvaginal US: importance of echogenic fluid, *Radiology* 178:823, 1991.

Nyberg DA et al: Endovaginal sonographic evaluation of ectopic pregnancy: a prospective study, *AJR* 149:1181, 1987.

Parvey HR, Maklad N: Pitfalls in the transvaginal sonographic diagnosis of ectopic pregnancy, *J Ultrasound Med* 3:139, 1993.

Pittaway DE, Reish RL, Wentz AC: Doubling times of human chorionic gonadotropin increase in early viable intrauterine pregnancies, *Am J Obstet Gynecol* 152:299, 1985.

Romero R et al: Diagnosis of ectopic pregnancy: value of the discriminatory human chorionic gonadotropin zone, *Obstet Gynecol* 66:357, 1985.

Rubin GL et al: Ectopic pregnancy in the United States, *JAMA* 249:1725, 1983.

Russell SA, Filly RA, Damato N: Sonographic diagnosis of ectopic pregnancy with endovaginal probes: what really has changed?, *J Ultrasound Med* 3:145, 1993.

Taylor KJW et al: Ectopic pregnancy: duplex Doppler evaluation, *Radiology* 173:93, 1989.

Weinstein L et al: Ectopic pregnancy: a new surgical epidemic, *Obstet Gynecol* 61:698, 1983.

SUPERFICIAL PARTS AND VASCULAR SYSTEM

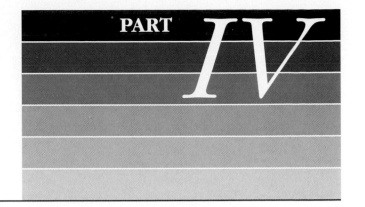

PART *IV*

Scrotum
Thyroid
Parathyroid
Musculoskeletal System
Appendix
Prostate

For a Key Features summary see p. 462.

SCROTUM

Sonography is the primary method used to image the scrotum. The normal testicles appear as homogeneous ovoid organs that are symmetric bilaterally. The seminiferous tubules converge to form the rete testis, which is located at the testicular mediastinum. The mediastinum itself appears as a peripherally located, elongated hyperechoic structure (Fig. 20-1). The rete testes drain out of the testes into the efferent ductules, which subsequently drain into the tubules that form the epididymal head. The head of the epididymis is triangular with rounded edges and its echogenicity is similar to that of the testis (Fig. 20-2). It rests directly on the upper pole of the testis and should be seen in almost all men. It continues inferiorly with the body and tail of the epididymis, which are isoechoic or hypoechoic to the testis (Fig. 20-3). The body and tail of the epididymis are more difficult to identify than the head, but with practice, they can usually be seen along the anterolateral or posterolateral aspect of the testis.

Unlike other organs, the major arteries of the testis are located peripherally and are called *capsular arteries*. They supply blood to the testicular parenchyma by means of branches called *centripetal arteries*. The centripetal arteries enter the testis and travel toward the mediastinum (Fig. 20-4 [see color insert, Plate 29]). As they approach the mediastinum, they branch into recurrent rami that curve away from the mediastinum. In approximately 50% of testes, one or more major branches of the testicular artery enter the testis through the mediastinum (Fig. 20-4). These transmediastinal arteries are often large enough to be seen by gray-scale sonography. The veins of the testis drain through the mediastinum and through the capsule of the testis. They are more difficult to visualize than the arteries, but with improved Doppler sensitivity and power-Doppler techniques, they are being seen more frequently. (See Table 20-1 for a summary of the characteristics of normal testes.)

One of the major roles of sonography is the evaluation of scrotal masses, and the most important determination is whether the mass is inside or outside the testis. The vast majority of extratesticular masses are benign, but the majority of intratesticular masses are malignant. In addition to location, it is also important to determine whether the mass is cystic or solid (Table 20-2). Overall the most common scrotal mass is the spermatocele. These are cystic lesions that form in the head of the epididymis and are filled with spermatozoa-containing fluid (Fig. 20-5). Epididymal cysts may also form in the epididymal head as well as the body and tail. They contain serous fluid and are anechoic and indistinguishable from spermatoceles. Both are benign lesions that rarely produce symptoms other than those related to the mass effect.

Intratesticular cysts are less common than spermatoceles or epididymal cysts. Nonetheless, they have been reported to be found in as many as 10% of testicular sonograms (Fig. 20-6). They are most common in elderly patients and are typically located near the mediastinum of the testis. If they are simple appearing on ultrasound studies and are nonpalpable, they can be ignored. However, if they are multiseptated, contain intraluminal internal echogenicity, exhibit solid components, or have a thick wall, then a cystic tumor such as a teratoma is a possibility. Lesions such as this should be removed. There is also evidence that cystic lesions which are palpable are much

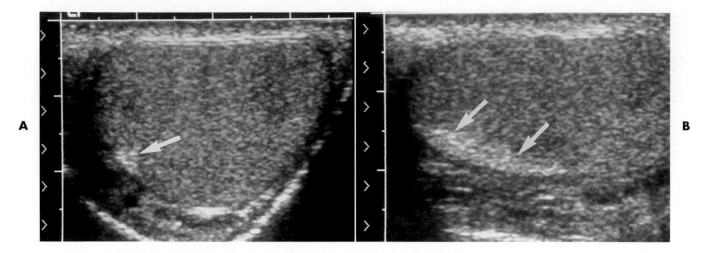

Fig. 20-1 Normal testis. **A,** Transverse view of the right testis demonstrates normal homogeneous echogenicity throughout the testicular parenchyma, with the exception of a small, peripherally located, hyperechoic structure representing the mediastinum *(arrow)*. **B,** Longitudinal view again demonstrates normal homogeneous echogenicity of the testicular parenchyma. On the longitudinal view the mediastinum is seen as an elongated region of increased echogenicity *(arrows)*.

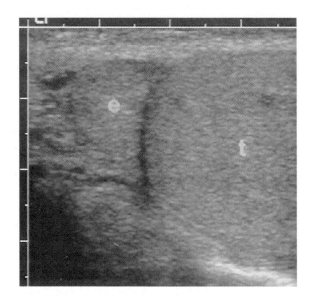

Fig. 20-2 Normal epididymal head. Longitudinal view of the upper pole of the testis *(t)* and epididymal head *(e)* demonstrates similar echogenicity of these two structures and the typical caplike appearance of the epididymal head.

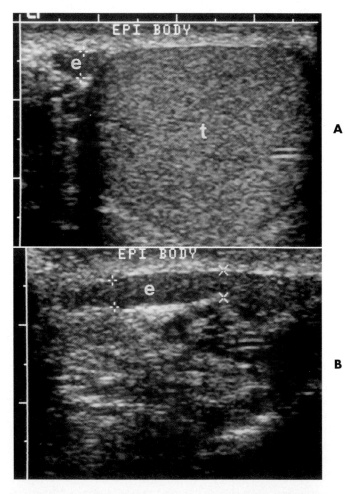

Fig. 20-3 Normal epididymal body. **A,** Transverse view of the right scrotum demonstrates a normal testis *(t)* and a cross-sectional view of the body of the epididymis *(e)*. Notice that the epididymal body is slightly less echogenic than the testis. **B,** Longitudinal view shows the elongated nature of the body of the epididymis *(e)*.

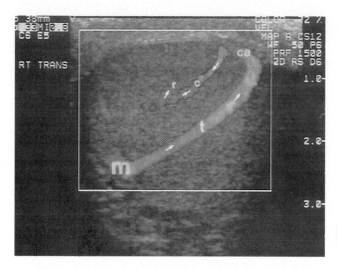

Fig. 20-4   Normal testicular arteries. Transverse Doppler view of the testis shows a transmediastinal artery *(t)* passing through the mediastinum *(m)* and continuing to the opposite side of the testis, where it becomes a capsular artery *(ca)*. The capsular artery then supplies a centripetal artery *(c)* that enters the testicular parenchyma and heads toward the mediastinum. Before reaching the mediastinum the centripetal artery branches into a recurrent rami *(r)*. Arrows indicate the direction of blood flow (see color insert, Plate 29).

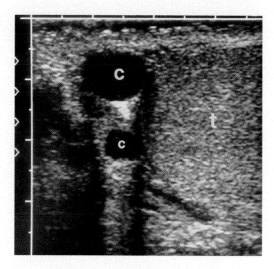

Fig. 20-5   Spermatoceles. Longitudinal view of the scrotum demonstrates the upper pole of the testis *(t)* and two cysts *(c)* in the expected location of the epididymal head. This is a typical appearance of spermatoceles. They vary in size, and when they are large, the normal epididymal head becomes difficult to identify.

Table 20-1   Characteristics of a normal testis

Characteristic	Appearance
Echogenicity	Medium level
Texture	Homogeneous
Surface	Smooth
Vascularity	Largest vessels on surface
Size	16-20 ml

Table 20-2   Scrotal lesions versus chance of malignancy

Sonographic characteristic	Chance of malignancy
EXTRATESTICULAR	Very low
INTRATESTICULAR	
Solid, palpable	High
Solid, nonpalpable	Intermediate
Complex cystic, palpable	High
Complex cystic, nonpalpable	Intermediate
Simple cystic, palpable	Low
Simple cystic, nonpalpable	Very low

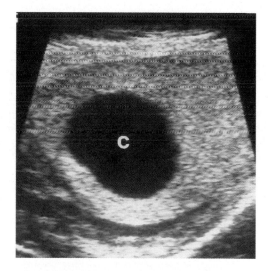

Fig. 20-6   Testicular cyst. Longitudinal view of the testis demonstrates a cyst *(c)* within the parenchyma. The walls are smooth and well defined, and there is increased through-transmission deep to the cyst. Provided this is a nonpalpable lesion, no further evaluation is required.

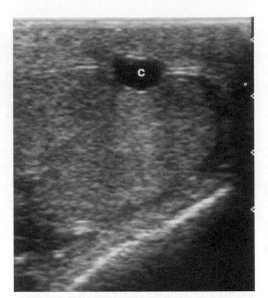

Fig. 20-7 Tunica albugenia cyst. Transverse view of the testis demonstrates a small cyst *(c)* centered on the tunica albuginea. Despite its firmness on physical examination, this satisfies all the sonographic criteria for a simple cyst and does not need to be evaluated further.

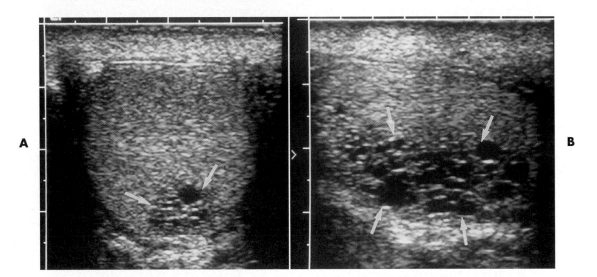

A B

Fig. 20-8 Tubular ectasia of the rete testes. **A,** Transverse view of the testis demonstrates a multicystic-appearing region posteriorly *(arrows)*. On this single image, a cystic neoplasm would be a consideration. **B,** Longitudinal view demonstrates the elongated nature of this multicystic region *(arrows)*. This sonographic appearance, shape, and position in the expected location of the mediastinum are all virtually diagnostic of tubular ectasia of the rete testes, which is a benign condition requiring no further evaluation.

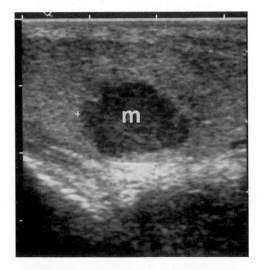

Fig. 20-9 Seminoma. Longitudinal view of the testis demonstrates a solid hypoechoic homogeneous mass *(m)*, a finding consistent with the appearance of a testicular tumor. The sonographic appearance is most suggestive of a seminoma, and this was confirmed after orchiectomy.

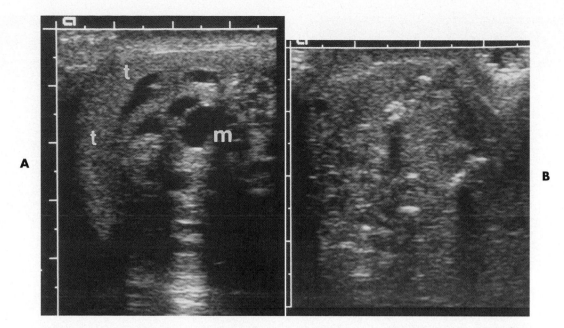

Fig. 20-10   Mixed–germ cell tumor. **A,** Transverse view of the testis demonstrates some minimal normal testicular parenchyma *(t)* draped around a complex mass *(m)* composed of both solid and cystic elements. **B,** Transverse view through another area of the testicular mass demonstrates multiple, shadowing, hyperechoic foci, a finding consistent with the appearance of calcifications within the mass. The sonographic characteristics are consistent with those of a mixed–germ cell tumor. A lesion composed of teratomatous elements, embryonal cell elements, and yolk sac elements was identified histologically after orchiectomy.

more likely to be malignant and should be removed, provided they truly arise from testicular parenchyma. On the other hand, cysts that arise from the tunica albugenia frequently are very firm and easily palpable. Despite their firmness, if they satisfy the sonographic criteria for a simple cyst, they can also be ignored (Fig. 20-7).

Tubular ectasia of the rete testis can also produce tiny cystic-appearing changes in the mediastinum. This is usually bilateral, although it can be quite asymmetric and in a minority of cases can be unilateral. It is often associated with spermatoceles and with intratesticular cysts. Sonographically it has the appearance of multiple small cystic or tubular spaces that replace and enlarge the mediastinum (Fig. 20-8). This is a very characteristic appearance and should not be mistaken for a testicular tumor.

Solid lesions in the testis are likely to be malignant tumors, especially if they are palpable. Most testicular tumors are germ cell in origin, and they are the most common malignant neoplasm in young adult men. The most common germ cell tumor is a seminoma, and mixed–germ cell tumors are the next most common. Seminomas typically are homogeneous and hypoechoic (Fig. 20-9) until they become large, at which point they may become heterogeneous. They are highly sensitive to irradiation and carry a good prognosis. Teratomas are usually complex cystic tumors that often include calcifica-

tion (Fig. 20-10). In adults they are considered malignant even when they appear mature histologically. Their behavior in children is benign. Embryonal cell carcinoma and choriocarcinoma generally occur in the setting of mixed–germ cell tumors, and they assume a variety of appearances (Fig. 20-10). Non–germ cell tumors account for 5% to 10% of testicular tumors. The most common are Leydig and Sertoli cell tumors (Fig. 20-11). Although benign, these stromal tumors can produce hormonal changes, and they are always removed because they cannot be distinguished from germ cell tumors. They appear as solid masses, and their echogenicity ranges from hypoechoic to hyperechoic. Epidermoid cysts are also benign tumors similar to teratomas, but they contain only ectodermal derivatives. Their sonographic appearance is variable, but classically they appear as a cyst or mass with a hyperechoic, calcified wall (Fig. 20-12).

It was initially hoped that color-Doppler imaging might serve as a potential means of distinguishing the different types of tumors, but unfortunately, the color-Doppler findings are more dependent on the size of the lesion than on its histologic nature. Lesions larger than 1.5 cm tend to be hypervascular (Fig. 20-13 [see color insert, Plate 30]), and smaller lesions tend to be hypovascular.

In addition to primary testicular tumors, the testes may be the site of metastatic disease. This usually appears as a

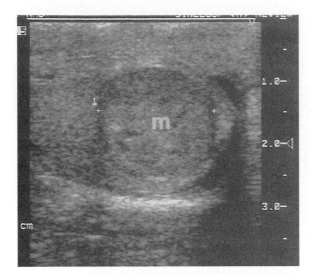

Fig. 20-11 Leydig cell tumor. Longitudinal view of the testis demonstrates a focal hypoechoic testicular mass *(m)*. The sonographic appearance overlaps with that of malignant germ cell tumors of the testis; however, this was proved surgically to represent a benign Leydig cell tumor.

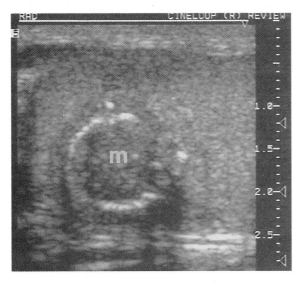

Fig. 20-12 Epidermoid cyst. Longitudinal view of the testis demonstrates a mass *(m)* with a hyperechoic, partially shadowing rim. This is the classic appearance of an epidermoid cyst with peripheral calcification. Because neoplasm cannot be excluded in cases such as this, surgery was performed and the diagnosis of an epidermoid cyst was confirmed.

focal testicular mass or masses with a variable echogenicity (Fig. 20-14 [for Fig. 20-14, *B,* see color insert, Plate 31]). In elderly patients metastatic disease is more common than primary germ cell tumors. The testes are also a sanctuary for lymphoma and leukemia in that the testes may be involved when the patient's disease is in apparent remission elsewhere in the body. Lymphoma and

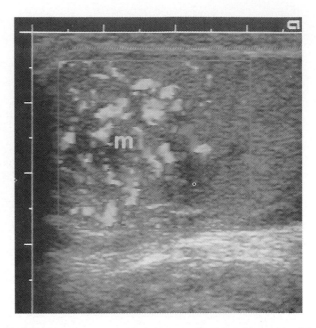

Fig. 20-13 Tumor vascularity. Longitudinal Doppler view of the testis shows a hypervascular mass *(m)* in the upper pole. This corresponded to a mass exhibiting mixed echogenicity on gray-scale studies and to a palpable lesion found on physical examination. Orchiectomy confirmed a mixed germ cell tumor (see color insert, Plate 30).

leukemia can both appear either as focal unilateral or bilateral hypoechoic masses or as diffuse testicular infiltration (Fig. 20-15). When the testes are diffusely infiltrated bilaterally, the decreased echogenicity may be difficult to appreciate if the testes are involved symmetrically. In such cases color-Doppler imaging can be helpful in detecting an abnormality because the testis will be hypervascular. Magnetic resonance imaging can also be useful for further evaluation because the signal characteristics will be obviously abnormal.

Sonography is highly sensitive (95% to 100%) in detecting testicular tumors. In fact, an important role of sonography is to detect nonpalpable lesions in young adult men with metastatic disease from an unknown primary (Fig. 20-16). The specificity of ultrasound varies depending on the referral patterns. There are numerous lesions that can simulate testis tumors (Box 20-1). These include infarcts, focal orchitis (Fig. 20-17), focal atrophy, hematomas (Fig. 20-18), and abscesses. In many cases the patient's history is useful in suggesting the correct diagnosis. The physical examination is also very important because most palpable intratesticular lesions are tumors and most of the nonpalpable lesions larger than 1 cm in diameter are not tumors. Lesions smaller than 1 cm may be nonpalpable tumors or benign lesions.

Solid lesions outside the testis are almost always benign. The most common tumor of the epididymis is the adenomatoid tumor. It is a rare benign lesion that varies in

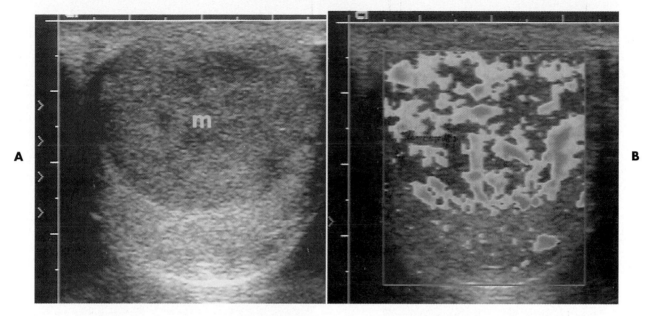

Fig. 20-14   Metastatic disease to the testis. **A,** Transverse view of the testis demonstrates a hypo-echoic mass *(m)*. **B,** Transverse power-Doppler view shows intense hypervascularity of this mass. This patient had a history of rhabdomyosarcoma. The sonographic and Doppler characteristics are consistent with those of either a primary testicular tumor or metastasis to the testis. Orchiectomy confirmed the presence of rhabdomyosarcoma metastatic to the testis (see color insert, Plate 34).

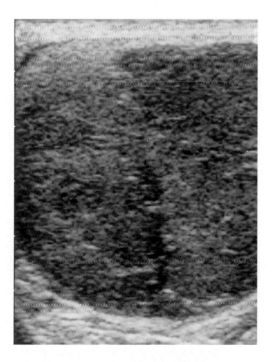

Fig. 20-15   Testicular lymphoma. Transverse view of the testis showed enlargement and diffuse inhomogeneity. This testis was also found to be firm and nontender on physical examination. This combination of findings in a patient with a history of lymphoma is strongly suggestive of testicular involvement. This was confirmed by testicular biopsy findings.

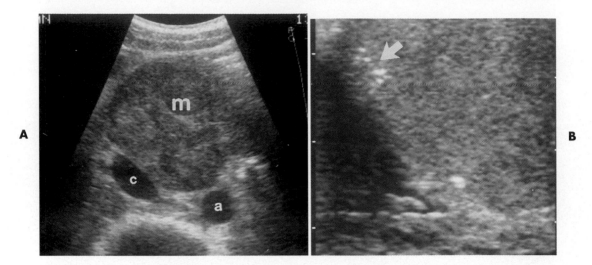

Fig. 20-16 Occult testicular tumor in a patient with retroperitoneal metastases. **A,** Transverse view of the abdomen in a patient who presented with back pain and a palpable abdominal mass demonstrates a large retroperitoneal mass *(m)* that is positioned anterior to the inferior vena cava *(c)* and aorta *(a)*. In a young man such as this, metastatic testicular carcinoma should always be considered a potential cause of retroperitoneal adenopathy. **B,** Transverse view of the testis demonstrates a cluster of microcalcifications in the peripheral aspect of the testicular parenchyma *(arrow)*. An orchiectomy was performed, and a burned-out testicular tumor consisting of scar tissue was identified histologically together with foci of intratubular germ cell neoplasia.

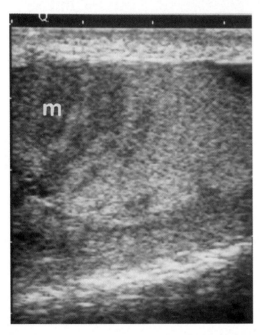

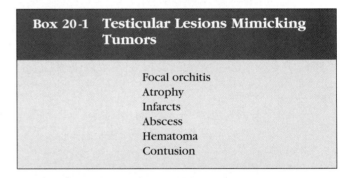

Box 20-1	Testicular Lesions Mimicking Tumors
	Focal orchitis
	Atrophy
	Infarcts
	Abscess
	Hematoma
	Contusion

Fig. 20-17 Focal orchitis. Longitudinal view of the testis demonstrates a focal, poorly marginated region of decreased echogenicity simulating a mass *(m)* in the upper pole of the testis. This was noted to be markedly hypervascular on color-Doppler ultrasound studies. On physical examination it was found to be extremely tender but nonpalpable. Antibiotic therapy was started and the patient's symptoms resolved. This was presumed to represent focal orchitis. Ideally a repeat ultrasound study should be done in patients with lesions such as this to confirm interval resolution after antibiotic therapy is completed.

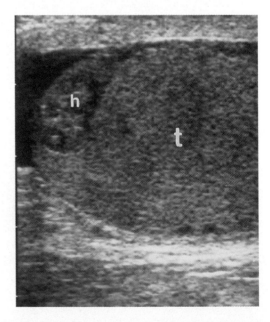

Fig. 20-18 Testicular hematoma. Longitudinal view of the testis *(t)* in a patient who sustained scrotal trauma shows a peripherally located, inhomogeneous, slightly hypoechoic mass *(h)*. Because of the possibility of testicular rupture, surgery was performed and a subcapsular hematoma was found.

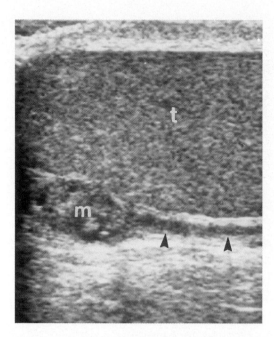

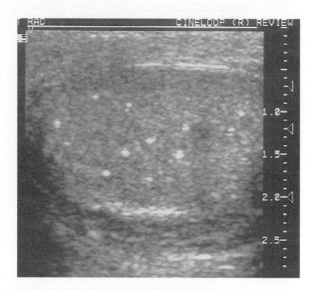

Fig. 20-19   Sperm cell granuloma. Longitudinal view of the scrotum in a patient after vasectomy demonstrates a normal testis *(t)*. The body of the epididymis *(arrowheads)* is seen posterior to the testis, and a focal inhomogeneous solid mass *(m)* is seen arising from the epididymal body. Given the patient's history, this was thought to be most consistent with the characteristics of a sperm cell granuloma. A benign adenomatoid tumor of the epididymis was also considered. No further evaluation was recommended other than regular clinical follow up.

Fig. 20-20   Microlithiasis. Longitudinal view shows multiple, nonshadowing, bright reflectors throughout the testis consistent with the appearance of microlithiasis. No tumor was identified sonographically, and this patient is now being observed sonographically until the risk of microlithiasis is better understood.

its ultrasound appearance. Chronic inflammatory masses and sperm cell granulomas are also solid lesions that can occur outside the testis (Fig. 20-19).

Testicular microlithiasis is a condition in which laminated concretions form in the lumen of the seminiferous tubules. On sonography they appear as tiny, nonshadowing, bright reflectors in the testicular parenchyma (Fig. 20-20). Microlithiasis has been reported to occur in association with numerous conditions, the most important of which is testicular tumors. Approximately 40% of the patients with microlithiasis will have a testicular germ cell tumor detected sonographically at the time of their initial ultrasound examination (Fig. 20-21). This alarmingly high association raises the question whether patients with microlithiasis but no tumor at presentation are predisposed to having a tumor develop in the future. Anecdotal experience suggests this may be true. However, the only longitudinal study performed to date showed that in none of the 20 patients with microlithiasis whose testes were otherwise normal on the basis of initial sonographic imaging did tumors eventually develop during the 1 to 6 years of follow-up. Therefore the risk, if real, is probably quite low. Until more information is gathered, it is currently recommended that patients with microlithiasis undergo ultrasound examinations at

yearly intervals to determine whether testicular tumors have developed. The risk of intratubular germ cell neoplasia (the equivalent of carcinoma in situ of the testis) developing in the contralateral testis of patients who initially present with a testicular tumor in one testis and microlithiasis in the contralateral testis is clearly increased. Therefore a biopsy of the contralateral testis is necessary to obtain tissue for histologic study. This is usually done at the time orchiectomy is performed for removal of the ipsilateral tumor (Fig. 20-21).

In addition to evaluating scrotal masses, ultrasound is helpful in the work-up of patients with acute scrotal pain and swelling. In the adult patient population, this primarily involves differentiating testicular torsion from inflammatory conditions such as epididymitis. Testicular torsion occurs as the result of the faulty attachment of the testis to the scrotal wall. The most common anatomic anomaly producing this faulty attachment is the bell-clapper deformity. It consists of a tunica vaginalis that completely surrounds the testis, causing the testis to be attached only to the spermatic cord and otherwise freely suspended in the scrotal sac like the clapper in a bell. The first hemodynamic consequence of testicular torsion is venous obstruction, followed rapidly by obstruction of arterial inflow and testicular ischemia. The viability of the testis

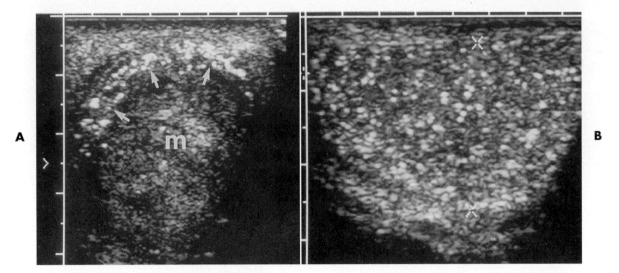

Fig. 20-21   Microlithiasis associated with testicular tumor. **A,** Transverse view of the right testis demonstrates an inhomogeneous mass *(m)* replacing most of the testicular parenchyma. A small amount of testicular tissue *(arrows)* is seen draped around the anterior aspect of the mass. Multiple punctate, nonshadowing, hyperechoic foci are seen in the testicular parenchyma, a finding consistent with the appearance of microlithiasis. A right orchiectomy was performed and a mixed–germ cell tumor of the right testis was found. **B,** Transverse view of the left testis demonstrates multiple hyperechoic foci scattered diffusely throughout the testicular parenchyma, a finding consistent with the appearance of diffuse microlithiasis. No abnormal masses were seen in this testis. At the time of surgery for the right testis, biopsy specimens from the left testis were found to demonstrate intratubular germ cell neoplasia.

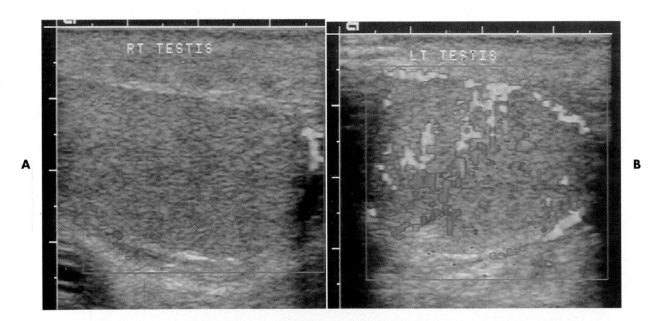

Fig. 20-22   Testicular ischemia. **A,** Longitudinal Doppler view of the right testis obtained in a patient after a gunshot wound to the right groin shows almost no detectable intratesticular blood flow, a finding consistent with the appearance of ischemia. The gray-scale appearance of this testis is normal, which strongly suggests that the testis is viable despite being ischemic. **B,** For comparison, this longitudinal view of the left testis shows normal, readily detectable intratesticular blood flow (see color insert, Plate 32).

depends on the duration of the torsion as well as the number of twists of the spermatic cord. Infarction can occur as soon as 4 hours after the appearance of symptoms. However, if the degree of torsion is low (180 to 360 degrees), the testes can remain viable for more than 24 hours. In general urologists try to operate before the symptoms have lasted for 6 hours.

Gray-scale ultrasound is not valuable in diagnosing torsion because it may not identify abnormalities. Nonspecific abnormalities that sometimes occur include decreased testicular echogenicity, testicular swelling, and reactive hydroceles. Fortunately color-Doppler imaging is an effective way to detect testicular ischemia because it can show absent or asymmetrically decreased testicular vascularity (Fig. 20-22 [see color insert, Plate 32]). In adults color-Doppler imaging is as good or slightly better than scintigraphy in the diagnosis of testicular torsion. Given its speed, low cost, lack of radiation, and better depiction of scrotal anatomy, color-Doppler imaging is generally the preferred way to evaluate these patients. However, in a given practice the preferred test should probably be the one that can be performed the most rapidly.

Ultrasound can also provide useful information about testicular viability in patients with torsion identified by color-Doppler imaging. If the testis is normal on gray-scale analysis, then it is very likely viable regardless of the duration of symptoms (Fig. 20-22). If the testis is hypoechoic or inhomogeneous, it is very likely nonviable (Fig. 20-23) [for Fig. 20-23, *B, C,* and *D,* see Plate 33]).

Although color-Doppler imaging is quite good at evaluating patients with suspected testicular torsion, false-positive and false-negative results can occur. A false-positive finding means that the patient will undergo surgery, which he would have anyway if the ultrasound had not been performed. False-negative findings are more of a problem because most of these patients will then go on to suffer infarction of the testis. False-negative findings can occur when the torsion is intermittent, low grade, or spontaneously resolves. No technique that relies on blood flow determinations can establish the diagnosis if the blood flow is not decreased when the examination is performed.

Scrotal inflammatory disease usually involves the epididymis initially and spreads from there to the testis, scrotal sac, or scrotal wall. The hallmark of epididymitis on

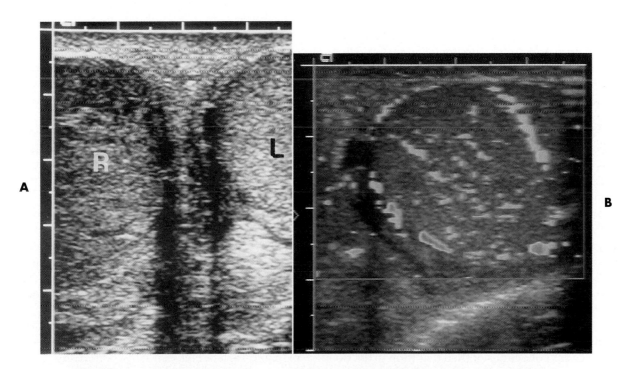

Fig. 20-23 Testicular torsion with nonviable testis. **A,** Transverse gray-scale sonogram of the scrotum obtained in a patient with right testicular pain of 48 hours' duration. The right testis *(R)* is enlarged and hypoechoic compared with the normal left testis *(L).* The differential diagnosis based on this gray-scale appearance includes testicular torsion, orchitis, and tumor infiltration. Clinical information and the use of Doppler techniques are required to distinguish among these possibilities. **B,** Transverse power-Doppler image of the asymptomatic testis demonstrates normal homogeneous echogenicity and readily detectable intratesticular blood flow.

Continued.

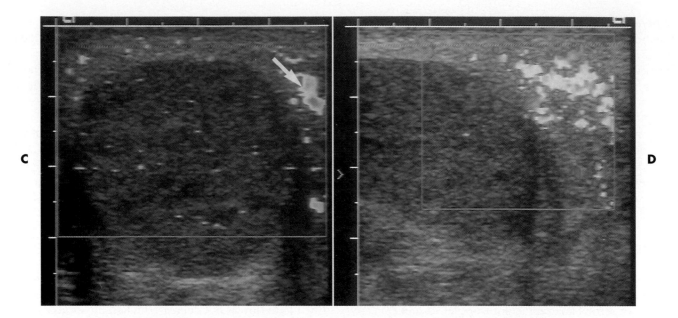

Fig. 20-23, cont'd. **C,** Transverse power-Doppler image of the symptomatic testis demonstrates minimal color noise throughout the image but no true intratesticular flow. A peritesticular vessel *(arrow)* is identified. **D,** Oblique Doppler view of the symptomatic testis shows no detectable intratesticular blood flow but increased peritesticular flow. This occurs because of the inflammatory response in the scrotal wall of patients with a testicular infarct. A torsed and infarcted testis was confirmed at scrotal exploration (see color insert, Plate 33).

gray-scale studies is enlargement and decreased echogenicity of the epididymis. Involvement of the epididymis may be diffuse but also is frequently focal (Fig. 20-24 [see color insert, Plate 34]). Color-Doppler imaging is valuable when the gray-scale findings are equivocal or normal because it can detect inflammatory hyperemia as increased epididymal vascularity.

Orchitis usually occurs in conjunction with epididymitis. Isolated orchitis is less common and generally is viral in nature (i.e., mumps). Testicular enlargement, decreased echogenicity, and hypervascularity are all typical findings. As with epididymitis, hypervascularity may be the only abnormal finding, so color-Doppler is more sensitive in the diagnosis of orchitis than is gray-scale sonography alone (Fig. 20-25 [see color insert, Plate 35]). Orchitis is much less frequently focal than is epididymitis. In such cases it can be difficult to distinguish a hypoechoic hypervascular tumor from focal orchitis (see Fig. 20-17). Clues to look for that make orchitis more likely include the finding of pain and tenderness without a palpable mass on physical examination and the sonographic finding of associated involvement of the epididymis (Table 20-3).

Hydroceles are collections of fluid that form in the potential space of the tunica vaginalis. Most hydroceles are idiopathic, but they are also commonly associated with underlying pathologic conditions such as scrotal inflammatory processes, testicular torsion, and testicular tumors. They usually occur in the anterior aspect of the scrotum and displace the testis posteriorly (Fig. 20-26). Chronic hydroceles can acquire cholesterol crystals in the fluid that may appear as mobile low-level reflectors. In addition to hydroceles, pyoceles and hematoceles can produce fluid collections in the scrotal sac. They appear as complex collections, often in conjunction with scrotal wall hyperemia (Fig. 20-27 [see color insert, Plate 36]). They should be suspected on the basis of the combined clinical and sonographic features.

Varicoceles are dilated peritesticular veins that form as the result of incompetent valves in the spermatic veins. The left spermatic vein drains into the left renal vein and the right spermatic vein drains into the inferior vena cava. Because the left renal vein is compressed by the superior mesenteric artery, the pressure on the left side is higher than that on the right, and this presumably explains why 85% of the varicoceles are on the left. Most of the remaining 15% are bilateral. It is so unusual to have an isolated right-sided varicocele that compression of the right spermatic vein by retroperitoneal masses should be considered whenever one is detected.

Varicoceles generally do not cause pain or discomfort until they become quite large. However, even small nonpalpable varicoceles can cause infertility. Therefore a search for varicoceles is important in the evaluation of an infertile couple. Gray-scale sonography depicts varicoceles as dilated, tortuous, tubular channels in the peritesticular tissues. The upper limits of normal for the caliber of scrotal veins has been reported as both 2 and 3 mm. At rest, the blood flow in varicoceles is usually

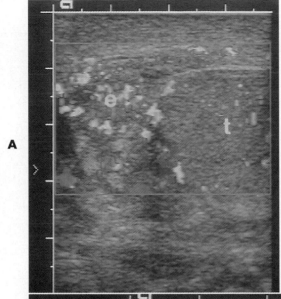

A

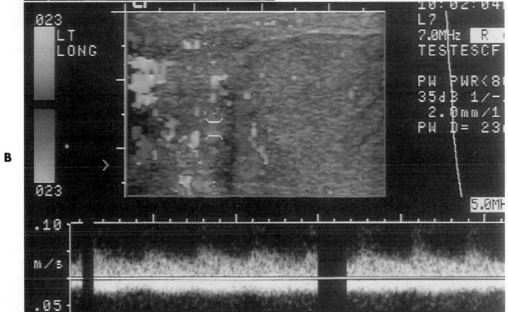

B

Fig. 20-24 Epididymitis. **A,** Longitudinal Doppler view shows the upper pole of the testis *(t)* and a hypervascular epididymal head *(e)*. **B,** A similar view and a pulsed-Doppler waveform shows readily detectable arterial and venous flow in the epididymal head (see color insert, Plate 34).

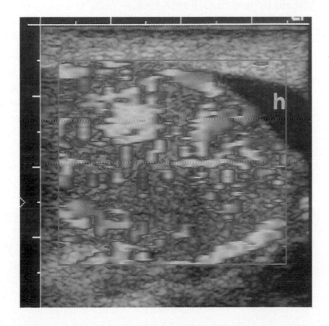

Fig. 20-25 Orchitis. Longitudinal view of the testis shows diffuse hypervascularity. In this patient the testis was normal in size and echogenicity. A small reactive hydrocele *(h)* is present (see color insert, Plate 35).

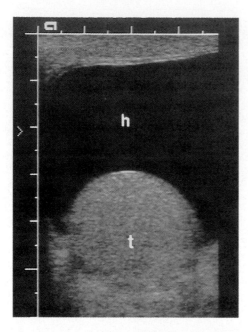

Fig. 20-26   Hydrocele. Transverse image of the scrotum demonstrates hydrocele fluid *(h)* anterior to the testis *(t)*. This is a typical appearance of and location for a large hydrocele.

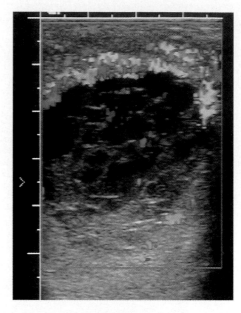

Fig. 20-27   Pyocele. Transverse Doppler view of the inferior aspect of the scrotum shows a complex fluid collection in the scrotal sac with surrounding hypervascularity of the scrotal wall (see color insert, Plate 36).

Table 20-3 Causes of an enlarged hypoechoic testis		
Abnormality	Blood flow	Physical examination finding
Orchitis	↑	Tender
Torsion	↓	Tender
Lymphoma	↑	Nontender
Diffuse seminoma	↑	Nontender

too slow for it to be detected with color-Doppler studies. However, when the patient performs a Valsalva maneuver, this causes the incompetent valves in the spermatic vein to allow blood to flow rapidly and retrograde into the pampiniform plexus, and this is detectable on color-Doppler studies (Fig. 20-28 [see color insert, Plate 37]). In most patients this Valsalva maneuver–induced flow augmentation is readily detectable when the patient is supine. If the examination findings are normal with the patient supine, then the study should be repeated with the patient upright because the increased hydrostatic pressure may then accentuate the varicocele's appearance.

THYROID

The thyroid gland is readily imaged with sonography. The normal thyroid is homogeneous and hyperechoic compared with the appearance of the overlying sternocleidomastoid and strap muscles. The left and right lobes are positioned between the trachea and the common carotid arteries and are connected across the midline by the thin thyroid isthmus (Fig. 20-29). The normal thyroid lobe should measure less than 4 cm long, less than 2 cm wide, and less than 2.5 cm thick. The thyroid isthmus should be less than 3 mm thick.

The ability of sonography to image the thyroid is similar to its ability to image the scrotum, in that it is extremely sensitive in detecting both benign and malignant tumors and nodules. Unfortunately, however, the findings are extremely nonspecific. Because of this, sonography should not be used as a means of characterizing lesions in the thyroid. Rather the proper indications for thyroid sonography are:

1. To identify nonpalpable tumors in patients with metastatic disease from an unknown primary
2. To screen patients who are at risk for the development of thyroid malignancies (patients who have undergone neck irradiation)
3. To determine if a palpable nodule is inside or outside the thyroid

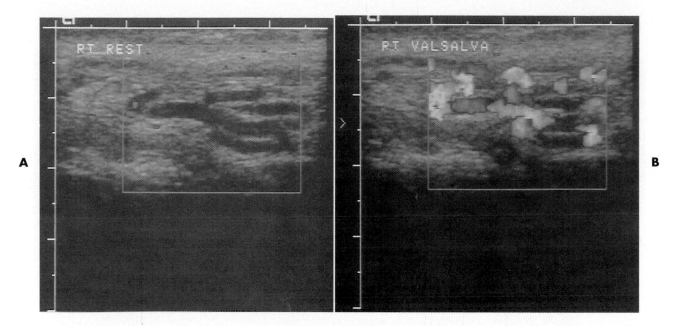

Fig. 20-28 Varicocele. **A,** Doppler image of the scrotum obtained with the patient at rest demonstrates mildly dilated tortuous tubular structures. Despite low-flow settings, blood flow in these vessels is too slow to be detected at rest. **B,** Similar image obtained with the patient performing a Valsalva maneuver demonstrates easily detectable blood flow within these dilated peritesticular veins (see color insert, Plate 37).

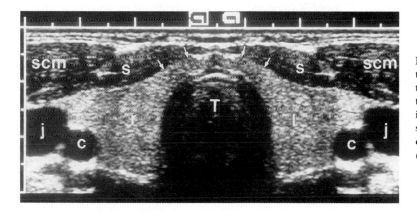

Fig. 20-29 Normal thyroid. Dual transverse image of the right *(r)* and left *(l)* lobes of the thyroid demonstrates the normal homogeneous echogenicity and relative size of the thyroid. The thyroid isthmus *(arrows)* is seen extending across the midline anterior to the trachea *(T)*. Other structures visualized on this scan include the common carotid artery *(c)*, internal jugular vein *(j)*, strap muscle *(s)*, and sternocleidomastoid muscle *(scm)*.

4. To look for recurrent disease in the neck of patients who have previously been treated for thyroid cancer
5. To guide biopsies of nonpalpable lesions in the thyroid or to guide biopsies when previous biopsies of a palpable nodule have been nondiagnostic (Fig. 20-30)

The primary difficulty with thyroid sonography is that benign nodules are extremely common and cannot be distinguished from thyroid cancer, which is relatively rare by comparison. Therefore it is always difficult to know what to do when nodules are detected with sonography. It has been shown that, when multiple nodules are detected by scintigraphy, the risk of cancer is less than 1%, but the risk ranges from 15% to 25% if a single cold nodule is found. However, the benign implications of the scintigraphic finding of multinodularity do not apply to such sonographic findings. Sonography is so much more sensitive than scintigraphy in detecting nodules that it is common for it to reveal a cancer coexisting with another visible benign or malignant nodule, or nodules. In addition, approximately 20% of the papillary thyroid cancers are multifocal, and sonography is much more likely to identify these multiple sites than is scintigraphy (Fig. 20-31).

There are certain statistical trends that apply to sonographic findings that are occasionally useful in the evalu-

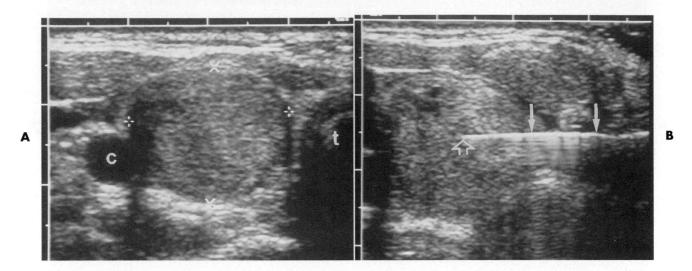

Fig. 20-30   Fine-needle aspiration biopsy of a thyroid nodule. **A,** Transverse view of the right lobe of the thyroid demonstrates a round nodule *(cursors)* replacing all of the normal thyroid parenchyma at this level. Also seen is the common carotid artery *(c)* and the trachea *(t).* **B,** Similar image obtained during ultrasound-guided fine-needle aspiration. The echogenic needle *(arrows)* is seen with its tip *(open arrow)* positioned in the middle of the lesion. Cytologic studies revealed the existence of changes consistent with the characteristics of adenomatous hyperplasia.

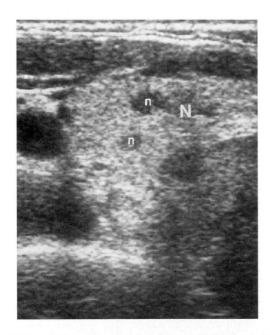

Fig. 20-31   Multifocal papillary carcinoma of the thyroid. Transverse view of the right lobe of the thyroid demonstrates one slightly hypoechoic, poorly marginated nodule *(N)* as well as two other smaller hypoechoic nodules *(n).* Fine-needle aspiration was performed and the findings showed papillary carcinoma. Multiple areas of papillary carcinoma were found at subsequent thyroidectomy.

Table 20-4   Thyroid nodules

Ultrasound feature	Benign	Malignant
INTERNAL CONTENTS		
Solid	I	I
Cystic	P	—
Mixed	P	—
ECHOGENICITY		
Hypo	I	I
Iso	I	I
Hyper	P	—
MARGIN		
Well defined	P	—
Ill defined	—	P
HALO		
Thin/uniform	P	—
Thick/incomplete	I	I
CALCIFICATION		
Peripheral	P	—
Large	I	I
Small	—	P

Modified from James EM, Charboneau JW, Hay ID: *The thyroid.* In Rumak CM, Wilson SR, Charboneau JW, editors: Diagnostic ultrasound, St. Louis, 1991, Mosby–Year Book.
I, Indeterminate; *P,* probable.

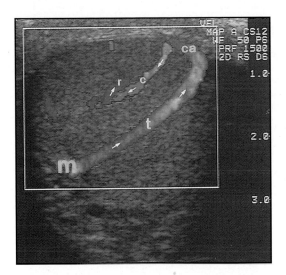

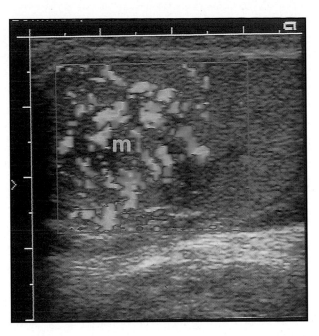

Plate 29 Normal testicular arteries. Transverse color-Doppler view of the testis shows a transmediastinal artery *(t)* passing through the mediastinum *(m)* and continuing to the opposite side of the testis, where it becomes a capsular artery *(ca)*. The capsular artery then supplies a centripetal artery *(c)* that enters the testicular parenchyma and heads toward the mediastinum. Before reaching the mediastinum the centripetal artery branches into a recurrent rami *(r)*. Arrows indicate the direction of blood flow (see also Fig. 20-4).

Plate 30 Tumor vascularity. Longitudinal color-Doppler view of the testis shows a hypervascular mass *(m)* in the upper pole. This corresponded to a mass exhibiting mixed echogenicity on gray-scale studies and to a palpable lesion found on physical examination. Orchiectomy confirmed a mixed germ cell tumor (see also Fig. 20-13).

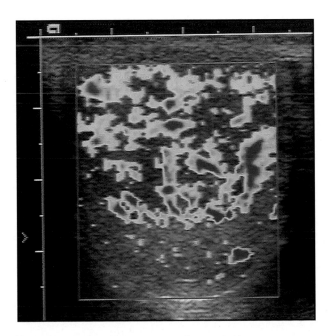

Plate 31 Metastatic disease to the testis. Transverse power-Doppler view shows intense hypervascularity of this mass. This patient had a history of rhabdomyosarcoma. The sonographic and Doppler characteristics are consistent with those of either a primary testicular tumor or metastasis to the testis. Orchiectomy confirmed the presence of rhabdomyosarcoma metastatic to the testis (see also Fig. 20-14, *B*).

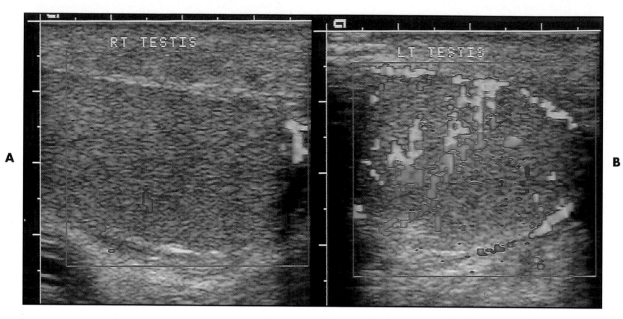

Plate 32 Testicular ischemia. **A,** Longitudinal color-Doppler view of the right testis obtained in a patient after a gunshot wound to the right groin shows almost no detectable intratesticular blood flow, a finding consistent with the appearance of ischemia. The gray-scale appearance of this testis is normal, which strongly suggests that the testis is viable despite being ischemic. **B,** For comparison, this longitudinal view of the left testis shows normal, readily detectable intratesticular blood flow (see also Fig. 20-22).

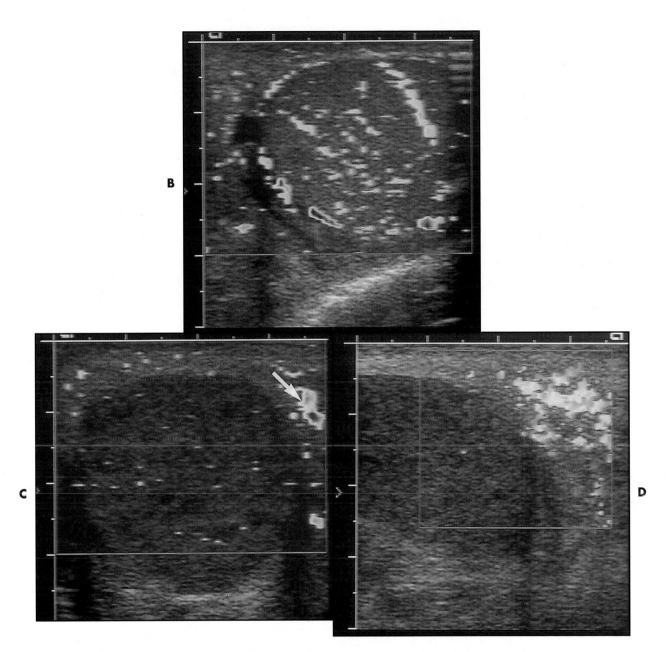

Plate 33 Testicular torsion with nonviable testis. **B,** Transverse power-Doppler image of an asymptomatic testis demonstrates normal homogeneous echogenicity and readily detectable intratesticular blood flow. **C,** Transverse power-Doppler image of the symptomatic testis demonstrates minimal color noise throughout the image but no true intratesticular flow. A peritesticular vessel *(arrow)* is identified. **D,** Oblique color-Doppler view of the symptomatic testis shows no detectable intratesticular blood flow but increased peritesticular flow. This occurs because of the inflammatory response in the scrotal wall of patients with a testicular infarct. A torsed and infarcted testis was confirmed at scrotal exploration (see also Fig. 20-23, *B*, C, and *D*).

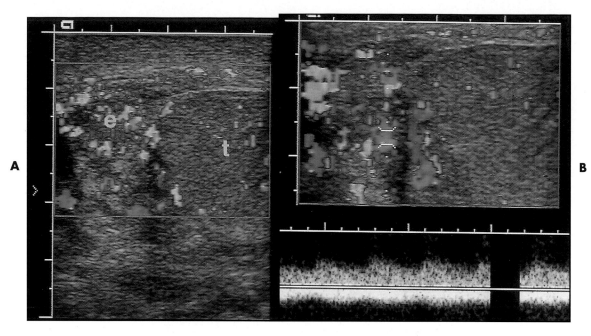

Plate 34 Epididymitis. **A,** Longitudinal color-Doppler view shows the upper pole of the testis *(t)* and a hypervascular epididymal head *(e)*. **B,** A similar view and a pulsed-Doppler waveform shows readily detectable arterial and venous flow in the epididymal head (see also Fig. 20-24).

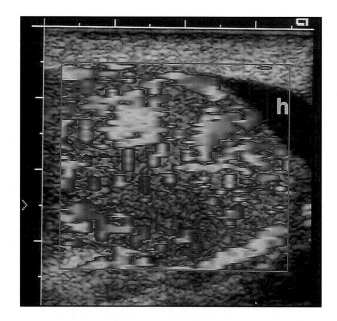

Plate 35 Orchitis. Longitudinal view of the testis shows diffuse hypervascularity. In this patient the testis was normal in size and echogenicity. A small reactive hydrocele *(h)* is present (see also Fig. 20-25).

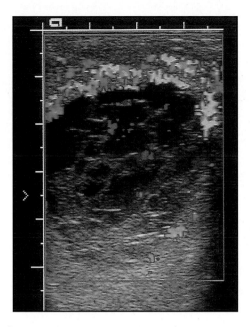

Plate 36 Pyocele. Transverse color-Doppler view of the inferior aspect of the scrotum shows a complex fluid collection in the scrotal sac with surrounding hypervascularity of the scrotal wall (see also Fig. 20-27).

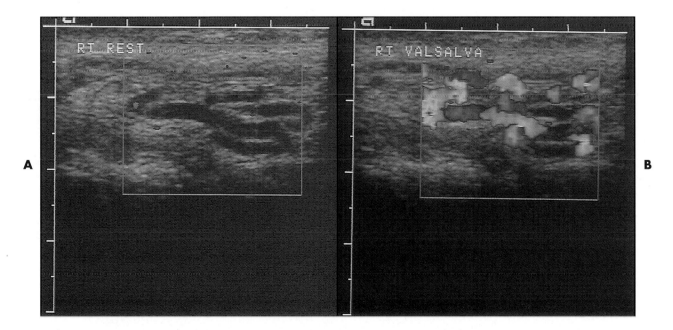

Plate 37 Varicocele. **A,** Color-Doppler image of the scrotum obtained with the patient at rest demonstrates mildly dilated tortuous tubular structures. Despite low-flow settings, blood flow in these vessels is too slow to be detected at rest. **B,** Similar image obtained with the patient performing a Valsalva maneuver demonstrates easily detectable blood flow within these dilated peritesticular veins (see also Fig. 20-28).

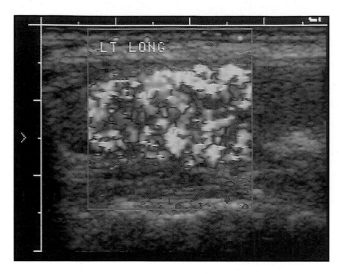

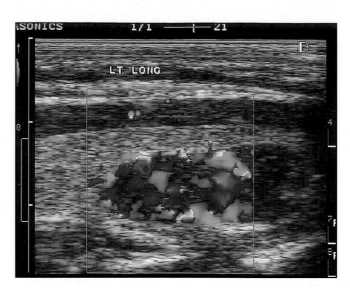

Plate 38 Grave's disease. Longitudinal view through the left lobe of the thyroid demonstrates marked hypervascularity within the thyroid parenchyma. This patient's thyroid gland was found to be enlarged and hypoechoic on gray-scale sonography (see also Fig. 20-36).

Plate 39 Parathyroid adenoma. Color-Doppler image demonstrates marked hypervascularity of a mass. The gray-scale findings are typical of those for a large parathyroid adenoma. This was subsequently confirmed surgically (see also Fig. 20-37, *B*).

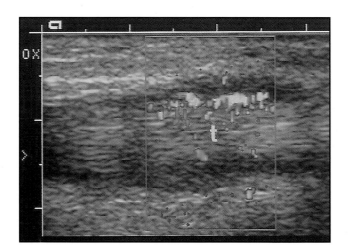

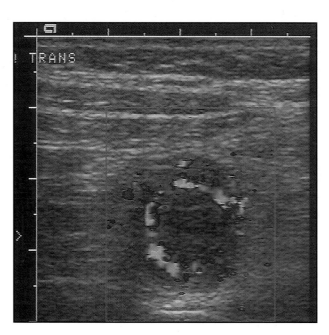

Plate 40 Posterior tibial tendinitis. Longitudinal color-Doppler view of the inframalleolar portion of the posterior tibial tendon *(t)* shows fluid around the tendon sheath and associated hypervascularity, findings consistent with the appearance of tendinitis. Results of tenography subsequently confirmed the diagnosis of tenosynovitis. Injection of the tendon sheath with a mixture of anesthetics and steroids resulted in complete pain relief (see also Fig. 20-45).

Plate 41 Appendicitis. Color-Doppler image demonstrates peripheral hypervascularity, a finding consistent with the appearance of inflammatory hyperemia. Appendicitis was confirmed surgically (see also Fig. 20-50, *B*).

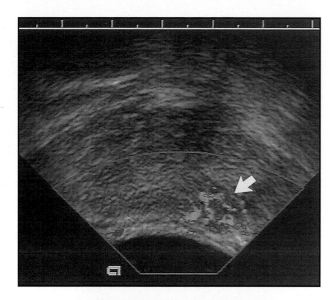

Plate 42 Hypervascular prostate cancer. Transverse color-Doppler view of the prostate demonstrates a focal nodular region of increased vascularity in the left peripheral zone *(arrow)*. Biopsy findings proved this to be prostate carcinoma (see also Fig. 20-56).

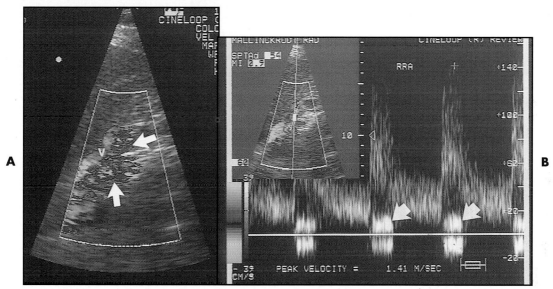

Plate 43 Color-Doppler appearance of tissue vibration. **A,** Color-Doppler view of the right renal artery in a patient with fibromuscular dysplasia shows random red and blue assignment in the tissues around the renal artery *(arrows)*. This arises from the vibrating tissue interfaces in the perivascular soft tissues. The normal renal vein *(v)* is seen anterior to the renal artery. **B,** Pulsed-Doppler waveform from the renal artery shows the arterial waveform as expected, but also shows a low-magnitude, but strong, bidirectional systolic signal *(arrow)* below the arterial waveform. This secondary signal arises from red blood cell and vessel wall vibration (see also Fig. 21-3).

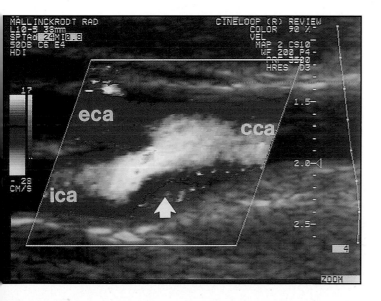

Plate 44 Normal flow reversal in the carotid bulb. Longitudinal color-Doppler image of the carotid bifurcation shows the common carotid artery *(cca)*, internal carotid artery *(ica)*, and external carotid artery *(eca)*. A focal region of flow reversal manifested as a blue assignment *(arrow)* is seen in the carotid bulb. This is a normal expected finding and should not be confused with flow turbulence or other flow abnormality. Notice that in this image the internal carotid is deep to the external carotid because the transducer was positioned anteriorly on the neck. A contrasting view obtained from a posterior approach is shown in Fig. 21-12 (see also Fig. 21-10).

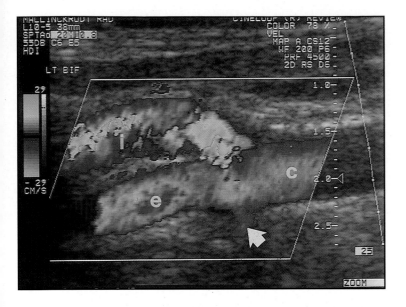

Plate 45 Differentiation between the internal carotid artery and external carotid artery. Longitudinal color-Doppler image of the distal common carotid artery *(c)* and carotid bifurcation obtained from a posterolateral approach shows the internal carotid *(i)* as the vessel that is most superficial. The external carotid *(e)* is seen in the deeper aspect of the field of view. A branch vessel *(arrow)* is seen arising from the origin of the external carotid (see also Fig. 21-12).

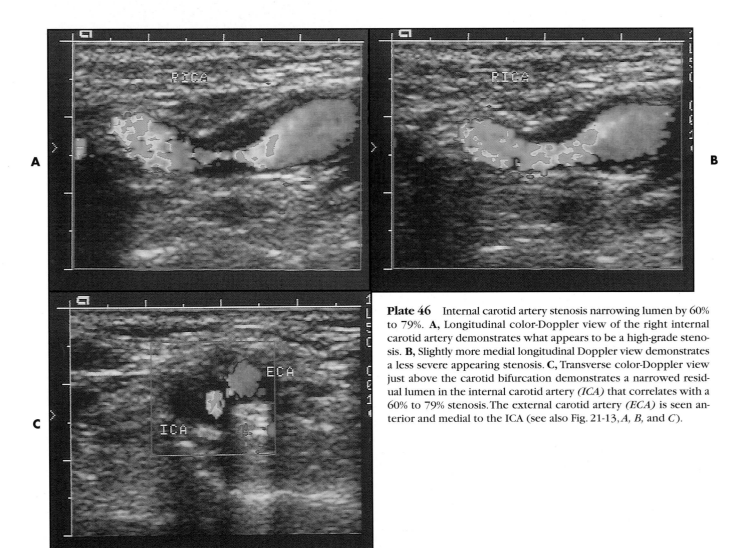

Plate 46 Internal carotid artery stenosis narrowing lumen by 60% to 79%. **A,** Longitudinal color-Doppler view of the right internal carotid artery demonstrates what appears to be a high-grade stenosis. **B,** Slightly more medial longitudinal Doppler view demonstrates a less severe appearing stenosis. **C,** Transverse color-Doppler view just above the carotid bifurcation demonstrates a narrowed residual lumen in the internal carotid artery *(ICA)* that correlates with a 60% to 79% stenosis. The external carotid artery *(ECA)* is seen anterior and medial to the ICA (see also Fig. 21-13, *A, B,* and *C*).

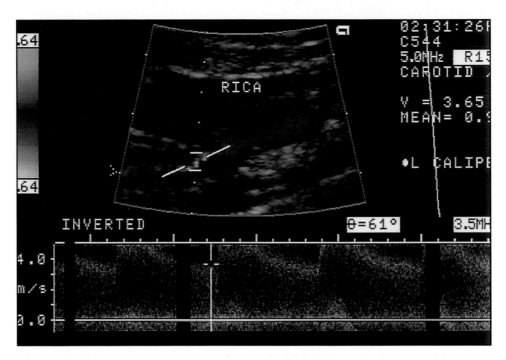

Plate 47 Severe carotid artery stenosis. Longitudinal color-Doppler image and pulsed-Doppler waveform demonstrate marked narrowing of the proximal internal carotid artery. The pulsed-Doppler waveform shows aliasing of the systolic peak, thus precluding accurate systolic velocity measurements. However, the end-diastolic velocity has been measured to be 365 cm/sec, which correlates with a stenosis causing a greater than 80% diameter reduction (see also Fig. 21-14).

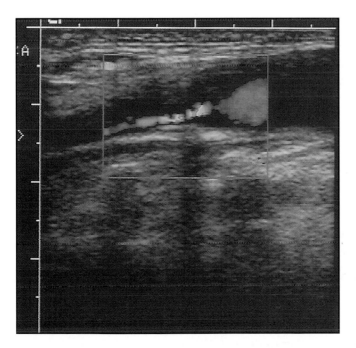

Plate 48 High-grade carotid stenosis with normal flow velocities. Color-Doppler image of the internal carotid artery demonstrates an extremely narrowed residual lumen producing the Doppler equivalent of an angiographic "string" sign. The plaque producing this stenosis is extremely hypoechoic and was not detectable on grayscale imaging (see also Fig. 21-15, *B*).

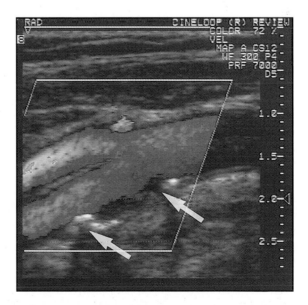

Plate 49 Stenosis of the internal carotid artery causing a less than 50% narrowing. Longitudinal color-Doppler image of the carotid bifurcation demonstrates partially calcified and noncalcified plaque *(arrows)* in the region of the carotid bulb and the origin of the internal carotid artery. Note that the flow reversal normally seen in the carotid bulb is not present (see also Fig. 21-17, *B*).

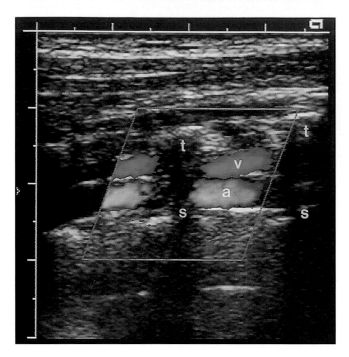

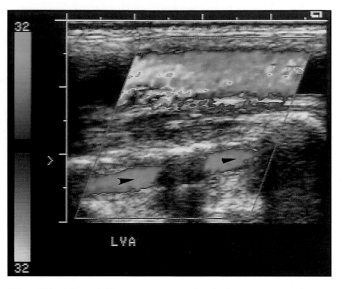

Plate 50 Normal vertebral artery and vein. Longitudinal Doppler image demonstrates the vertebral artery *(a)* and overlying vertebral vein *(v)*. Transverse processes of the cervical spine *(t)* and associated shadows *(s)* preclude visualization of the entire vertebral vessels. The vertebral vein is seen unusually well in this person (see also Fig. 21-22).

Plate 51 Three different patients with subclavian steal syndrome. Longitudinal color-Doppler view of the left neck shows flow in the common carotid artery directed superiorly *(red)*. Flow in the vertebral artery is directed inferiorly *(blue)*. Flow direction is indicated by the arrows (see also Fig. 21-23, *A*).

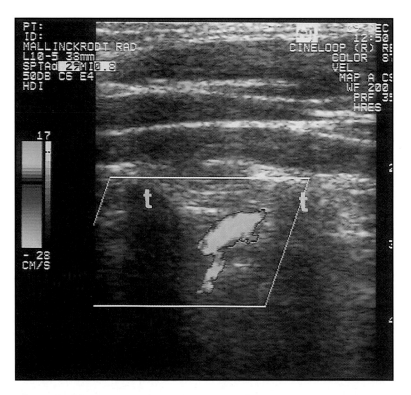

Plate 52 Vertebral vein mimicking reversal of flow in the vertebral artery. Longitudinal color-Doppler view of the neck between the transverse processes *(t)* demonstrates a vessel with flow directed inferiorly in the neck. Based solely on the color-Doppler appearance, this could represent reversal of flow in the vertebral artery (see also Fig. 21-24, *A*).

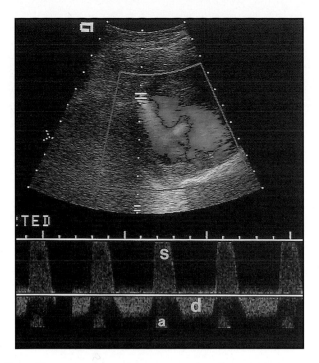

Plate 53 Large pseudoaneurysm. Longitudinal color-Doppler view shows a swirling pattern of internal flow in the center of a large mass, a finding consistent with the appearance of luminal flow in a pseudoaneurysm. Pulsed-Doppler waveform from the pseudoaneurysm neck shows a to-and-fro flow pattern at the aneurysm neck. Antegrade flow into the aneurysm occurs during systole *(s)* and is displayed above the baseline. Reversed flow out of the aneurysm occurs during diastole *(d)* and is displayed below the baseline. Aliasing of the systolic peak *(a)* results in wrap-around of the systolic signal to below the baseline (see also Fig. 21-25, *B*).

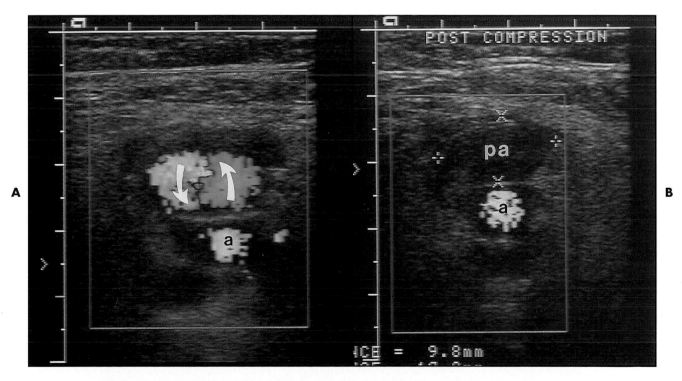

Plate 54 Ultrasound-directed obliteration of a pseudoaneurysm. **A,** Transverse color-Doppler image of the groin demonstrates the common femoral artery *(a)* and a more superficially positioned pseudoaneurysm with a swirling intraluminal blood flow *(curved arrows)*. **B,** After two successive 10-minute compressions at the level of the pseudoaneurysm neck and one 20-minute compression at this level, repeat scans showed flow in the common femoral artery *(a)* but no flow in the pseudoaneurysm *(pa)* (see also Fig. 21-26).

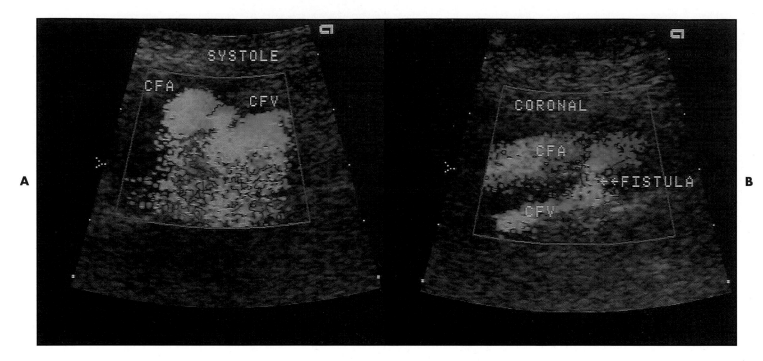

Plate 55 Arteriovenous fistula. **A,** Transverse view of the right groin obtained during peak systole demonstrates flow in the common femoral artery *(CFA)* and common femoral vein *(CFV)*. Extensive random red and blue assignment produced by perivascular soft tissue vibration is seen deep to these vessels. This indicates turbulent blood flow, and in a postcatheterization patient this is strong evidence of an arteriovenous fistula. **B,** Semicoronal view of the common femoral artery *(CFA)* and common femoral vein *(CFV)* demonstrates the site of fistulous connection between these two vessels (see also Fig. 21-27).

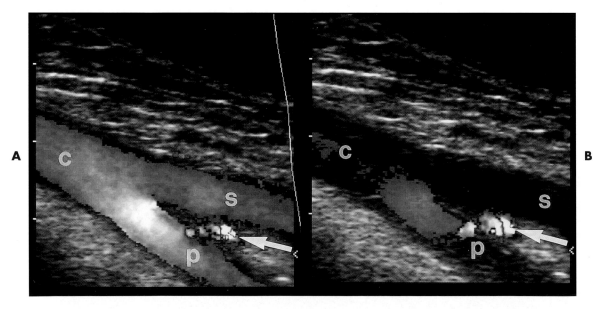

Plate 56 Arteriovenous fistula. **A,** Longitudinal view of the femoral bifurcation obtained in peak systole demonstrates antegrade flow in the common femoral artery *(c)*, superficial femoral artery *(s)*, and profunda femoral artery *(p)*. A small branch vein *(arrow)* is seen between the superficial and profunda femoral arteries. **B,** Similar longitudinal color-Doppler image obtained at end-diastole demonstrates normal absence of detectable flow in the common femoral artery and superficial femoral artery but maintained flow in the origin of the profunda femoral artery to the level of the small branch vein (see also Fig. 21-28, *A* and *B*).

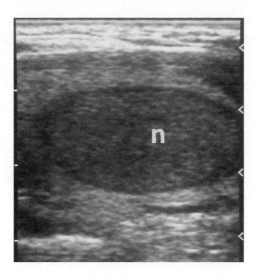

Fig. 20-32   Benign thyroid adenoma. Longitudinal view of the thyroid demonstrates a well-defined nodule *(n)* with a uniform concentric hypocchoic rim. This is the classic sonographic appearance of a thyroid adenoma. This is only rarely seen in thyroid carcinoma.

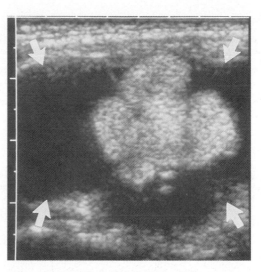

Fig. 20-33   Benign adenomatous hyperplasia. Longitudinal view of the thyroid demonstrates a large, predominantly cystic mass *(arrows)* with a cauliflower-shaped solid internal component. Fine-needle aspiration revealed adenomatous hyperplasia. Cystic lesions with solid components or solid lesions with cystic components are usually benign.

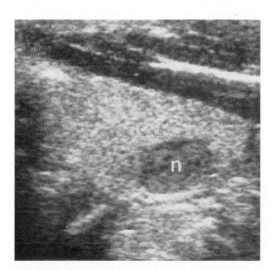

Fig. 20-34   Medullary carcinoma of the thyroid. Longitudinal view of the thyroid demonstrates a hypoechoic nodule *(n)*. This patient presented with an elevated carcinoembryonic antigen level, and sonography was performed to search for an occult malignancy. After identification of this nodule, fine-needle aspiration was performed and the findings confirmed the presence of medullary carcinoma.

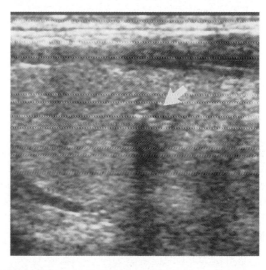

Fig. 20-35   Thyroid carcinoma with microcalcifications. Longitudinal view of the thyroid demonstrates a poorly defined hypoechoic nodule *(arrow)* in the lower pole. Several small bright reflectors are seen within the nodule, a finding consistent with the appearance of microcalcifications. Although this cluster of microcalcifications is producing an acoustic shadow, individual microcalcifications generally do not cause shadows.

ation of nodules, even though they cannot be used for making definitive diagnoses (Table 20-4). Characteristics that increase the likelihood of a nodule being benign include a uniform well-defined, hypoechoic rim (Fig. 20-32), cystic components (Fig. 20-33), peripheral eggshell calcification, or an echogenicity greater than that of ad-

jacent normal thyroid. On the other hand, thyroid cancer is typically hypoechoic and has poorly defined margins (Fig. 20-34). One feature that should prompt particular concern is microcalcifications, because these are more predictive of cancer than is any other sonographic finding (Fig. 20-35).

Diffuse disease of the thyroid is generally not evaluated with sonography. Nonetheless, certain conditions are encountered occasionally. Grave's disease appears as an enlarged homogeneous hypoechoic gland on gray-scale studies. On color-Doppler studies it is typically associated with an intense hypervascularity that has been called the "thyroid inferno" (Fig. 20-36 [see color insert, Plate 38]). Thyroiditis tends to have a more inhomogeneous and less enlarged appearance compared with that of Grave's disease, but may also appear quite hypervascular. Hashimoto's thyroiditis typically appears heterogeneous and hypoechoic and may exhibit a micronodular pattern.

PARATHYROID

There are four parathyroid glands. The paired superior glands arise embryologically with the thyroid and are usually located behind the middle aspect of the thyroid gland. The paired inferior glands arise with the thymus and are usually located behind the inferior aspect of the thyroid. It is very difficult or impossible for sonography to visualize normal parathyroid glands. Approximately 3% of parathyroid glands are ectopic. Ectopic inferior glands

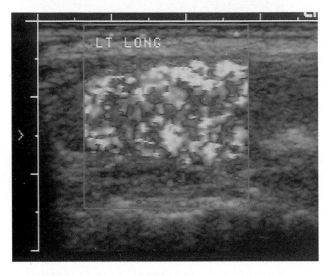

Fig. 20-36   Grave's disease. Longitudinal view through the left lobe of the thyroid demonstrates marked hypervascularity within the thyroid parenchyma. This patient's thyroid gland was found to be enlarged and hypoechoic on gray-scale sonography (see color insert, Plate 38).

Box 20-2   Locations of Ectopic Parathyroids

Thoracic inlet/superior mediastinum
Tracheoesophageal groove
Carotid sheath
Intrathyroidal

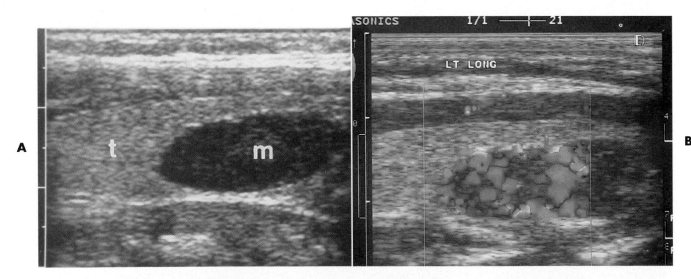

Fig. 20-37   Parathyroid adenoma. **A,** Longitudinal gray-scale image of the neck demonstrates the lower pole of the thyroid gland *(t)* and a hypoechoic, ovoid mass *(m)* adjacent to the thyroid. **B,** Corresponding Doppler image in the same patient demonstrates marked hypervascularity of this mass. The gray-scale findings are typical of those for a large parathyroid adenoma. This was subsequently confirmed surgically (see color insert, Plate 39).

tend to migrate, at least partially, with the thymus into the inferior neck or the anterior superior mediastinum. Ectopic superior glands tend to be displaced posteriorly in the groove between the trachea and esophagus or in the posterior superior mediastinum. (See Box 20-2 for a list of the locations of ectopic parathyroids.)

Sonography is an excellent means of localizing enlarged parathyroid glands in patients with primary hyperparathyroidism. Any parathyroid gland that can be seen sonographically should be assumed to be abnormally enlarged. Whether sonography or any other imaging method should be used in routine cases is debatable. Many would argue that the only localization required preoperatively is to "localize" a good endocrine surgeon to perform the procedure. The success of a skilled surgeon in identifying abnormal parathyroid glands is as high as that of any imaging study. Sonography is more valuable when a less-experienced surgeon is performing the procedure because preoperative localization can then result in a decrease in the operating room time and in the failure rate. Sonography and other imaging methods are clearly valuable in patients whose hyperparathyroidism persists or recurs after parathyroid surgery. In such cases reexploration of the neck is hampered by the presence of scar tissue and surgical localization of parathyroid adenomas can then be very challenging. Preoperative knowledge of the site of the adenoma greatly simplifies the operation and is welcome information to even experienced and skilled surgeons.

Primary hyperparathyroidism is caused by a single adenoma in 80% to 90% of the patients. The rest are caused by hyperplasia of all four glands or multiple adenomas. Parathyroid carcinoma is a rare cause of primary hyper-

parathyroidism. Parathyroid adenomas are typically ovoid masses and have their long axis in the vertical dimension. They are usually homogeneous and hypoechoic on gray-scale studies and hypervascular on color-Doppler images (Fig. 20-37 [for Fig. 20-37, *B,* see color insert, Plate 39]). If a typical adenoma is not seen adjacent to the thyroid, then the most common ectopic sites should be scanned. The superior mediastinum can be visualized by angling the transducer inferiorly from a suprasternal approach. Using a high-frequency sector transducer, it is possible to see to the level of the thymus in many patients. The retrotracheal region and the tracheoesophageal groove can be visualized by having patients turn their head to the contralateral side and scanning from a lateral approach with the transducer angled medially. The carotid sheath should be scanned from the bifurcation to the base of the neck because ectopic glands can occur anywhere along the sheath (Fig. 20-38). Finally, the thyroid itself should be scanned because intrathyroidal parathyroid adenomas do occur and can simulate other thyroid lesions.

The sensitivity of ultrasound in localizing parathyroid adenomas is 80%. False-negative findings can occur when the glands are ectopic, only minimally enlarged, or adjacent to an enlarged multinodular thyroid. False-positive findings can result from the misinterpretation of cervical lymph nodes (Fig. 20-39), thyroid nodules, and the misinterpretation of normal anatomic structures such as the esophagus and the longus colli muscle (Fig. 20-40). The esophagus and longus colli muscle can be distinguished from parathyroid nodules on longitudinal scans by showing that they elongate over the course of many centimeters. Having the patient swallow water can also help in the definitive identification of the esophagus.

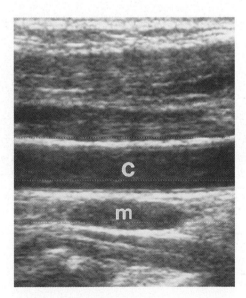

Fig. 20-38 Ectopic parathyroid adenoma within the carotid sheath. Longitudinal view of the neck demonstrates the common carotid artery *(c)* and a hypoechoic, ovoid mass *(m)* immediately deep to the carotid. This patient had undergone prior failed neck exploration to search for the cause of primary hyperparathyroidism and was being reimaged before repeat operation.

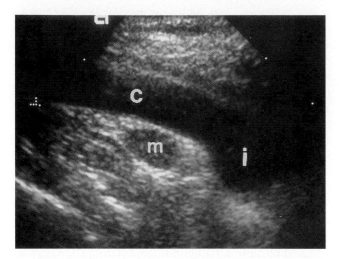

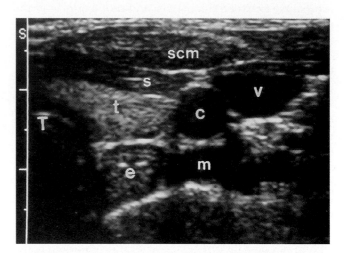

Fig. 20-39   False-positive ultrasound finding in a patient with hyperparathyroidism. Longitudinal view of the base of the right neck demonstrates the origin of the common carotid artery *(c)* and the innominate artery *(i)*. An ovoid, hypoechoic mass *(m)* with a diameter of less than 1 cm is seen underneath the common carotid. This patient had undergone a failed neck exploration to search for the source of primary hyperparathyroidism and was being reimaged before repeat operation. This mass identified sonographically was shown at surgery to represent a lymph node. A 3-cm parathyroid adenoma was identified more inferiorly in the mediastinum.

Fig. 20-40   Normal esophagus and longus colli muscles simulating parathyroid nodules. Transverse view of the left neck demonstrates multiple normal structures, including the trachea *(T)*, thyroid *(t)*, common carotid artery *(c)*, internal jugular vein *(v)*, strap muscle *(s)*, and the sternocleidomastoid muscle *(scm)*. A portion of the esophagus *(e)* is seen posterior to the thyroid and posterolateral to the trachea. It has the typical appearance of a bowellike structure with a hypoechoic peripheral muscular layer. The longus colli muscle *(m)* is seen posterior to the common carotid artery. Like most muscular tissue, it is quite hypoechoic.

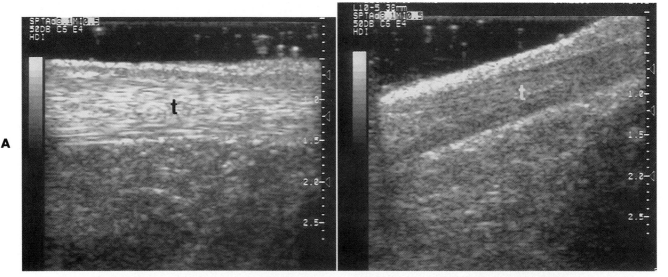

Fig. 20-41   Normal tendon. **A,** Longitudinal view of the Achilles tendon *(t)* with the tendon oriented perpendicular to the direction of the sound demonstrates the typical internal architecture, consisting of multiple, parallel, linear, hyperechoic reflectors. These represent the internal tendon fibers. **B,** Longitudinal view with the tendon oriented at an angle to the sound beam demonstrates loss of the typical internal architecture and conversion from a hyperechoic to a hypoechoic appearance.

MUSCULOSKELETAL SYSTEM

Sonography of the musculoskeletal system is gaining acceptance because of its low cost, ready availability, and comparative accuracy. Because of the architecture and geometry of tendons and muscles, they are well demonstrated sonographically. Tendons are composed of multiple parallel fibers that are strong reflectors of sound

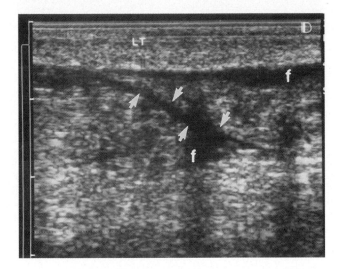

Fig. 20-42   Complete Achilles tendon tear. Longitudinal view of the Achilles tendon demonstrates complete disruption *(arrows)* of the tendon with some overlap of fragments. Also note the fluid *(f)* representing peritendinous and intratendinous hematoma. The normal tendon architecture is also completely disrupted.

when they are oriented nearly perpendicular to the sound beam. In this orientation tendons appear as bright bands containing multiple linear internal reflectors (Fig. 20-41). When tendons are imaged at less than 90 degrees, they appear hypoechoic. Most of the large tendons in the body are straight and relatively easy to scan. Muscles appear hypoechoic regardless of their relative orientation to the sound beam. They contain bright linear reflectors arising from the internal fibrous septations between different muscle bundles.

The main indication for performing muscle and tendon sonography is to determine whether trauma has resulted in a tear or hematoma. Tendon tears typically appear as complete (Fig. 20-42) or partial (Fig. 20-43) hypoechoic disruptions in the otherwise normal echogenic pattern of the tendon. Associated hematomas may form and produce adjacent fluid collections in the soft tissues (Fig. 20-44). Inflammatory responses are common in the acute and subacute settings, and these can be detected as hyperemia on color-Doppler imaging (Fig. 20-45 [see color insert, Plate 40]).

The greatest amount of work in musculoskeletal sonography has focused on imaging of the rotator cuff. This is somewhat paradoxical because the rotator cuff is more difficult to examine sonographically than the other large tendons of the body. Nevertheless, sonography can be very accurate (>90% sensitivity and specificity) in distinguishing normal from torn rotator cuffs. The normal rotator cuff is similar to other tendons, but because it is curved, it does not appear as homogeneously hyper-

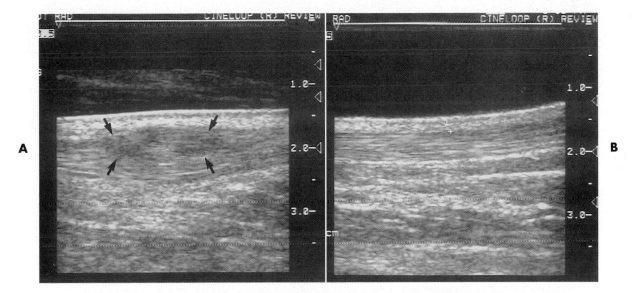

Fig. 20-43   Partial Achilles tendon tear. **A,** Longitudinal view of the left Achilles tendon in a runner suffering from pain and swelling shows a focal defect *(arrows)* in the superficial aspect of the tendon. Normal tendon architecture is seen superior, inferior, and deep to this partial tear. **B,** Similar view of the right Achilles tendon shows normal tendon architecture throughout.

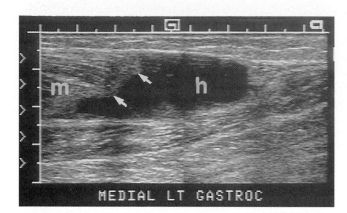

Fig. 20-44   Muscle rupture and hematoma. Longitudinal view of the medial gastrocnemius muscle *(m)* shows the retracted edge of the torn proximal muscle *(arrows)* and a liquefied hematoma *(h)* at the site of the tear.

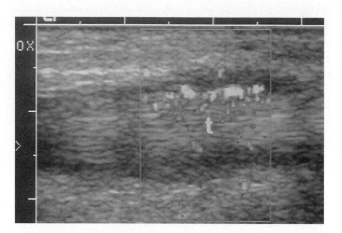

Fig. 20-45   Posterior tibial tendinitis. Longitudinal Doppler view of the inframalleolar portion of the posterior tibial tendon *(t)* shows fluid around the tendon sheath and associated hypervascularity, findings consistent with the appearance of tendinitis. Results of tenography subsequently confirmed the diagnosis of tenosynovitis. Injection of the tendon sheath with a mixture of anesthetics and steroids resulted in complete pain relief (see color insert, Plate 40).

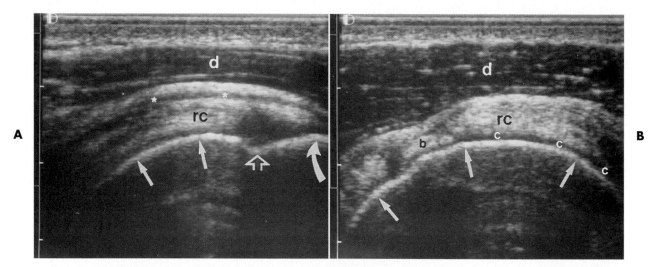

Fig. 20-46   Normal rotator cuff **A,** Longitudinal view of the shoulder demonstrates the greater tuberosity *(curved arrow),* the anatomic neck of the humeral head *(open arrow),* and the humeral head itself *(arrows).* The rotator cuff *(rc)* is a 5-mm-thick band of tissue immediately overlying the humeral head. It appears echogenic in some areas but hypoechoic in others because of the relative orientation of the tendon fibers to the sound beam. The hypoechoic layer immediately above the rotator cuff *(*)* represents the subdeltoid space where the subdeltoid bursa is located. The deltoid muscle *(d)* is seen overlying the rotator cuff. **B,** Transverse view of the rotator cuff again demonstrates the humeral head *(arrows).* The intraarticular portion of the biceps tendon *(b)* is seen as an ovoid, echogenic structure. Immediately posterior to the biceps tendon is the supraspinatus portion of the rotator cuff *(rc).* The hypoechoic tissue between the humeral head and the rotator cuff is articular cartilage *(c).* The deltoid muscle *(d)* overlies the rotator cuff.

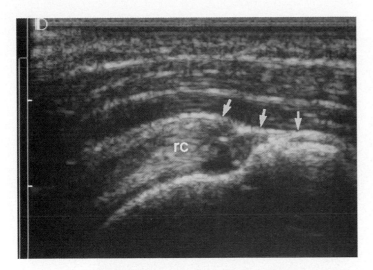

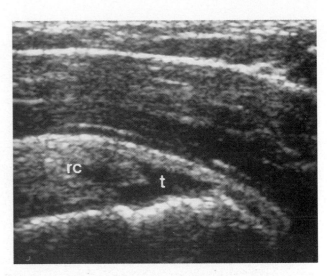

Fig. 20-47   Rotator cuff tear. Longitudinal view of the rotator cuff demonstrates absence of rotator cuff tissue overlying the greater tuberosity. The deltoid muscle has become opposed to the bone in this region, producing a concave interface *(arrows)* in the expected location of the rotator cuff insertion. Normal rotator cuff tissue *(rc)* is seen more proximally overlying the humeral head.

Fig. 20-48   Rotator cuff tear. Longitudinal view of the rotator cuff demonstrates a fluid-filled tear *(t)* at the insertion site of the cuff. Normal proximal rotator cuff tissue *(rc)* is seen adjacent to the tear.

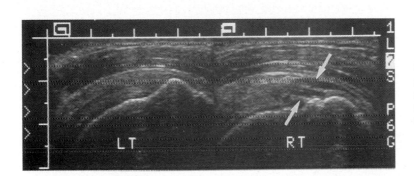

Fig. 20-49   Torn right rotator cuff compared with a normal left rotator cuff. Dual longitudinal images of the left and right rotator cuffs demonstrate normal findings on the left side, but an irregular, somewhat complex tear *(arrows)* at the insertion of the rotator cuff on the right side.

echoic as other tendons. Generally, there are segments that appear hypoechoic because they are not oriented at 90 degrees to the sound beam (Fig. 20-46), and these segments should not be misinterpreted as tears. The major signs of tears are a focal loss of tendon substance (Fig. 20-47), focal fluid-filled defects in the tendon (Fig. 20-48), and complete nonvisualization of the rotator cuff. Comparison of the images of the symptomatic and asymptomatic shoulders can often increase diagnostic confidence when the findings are subtle (Fig. 20-49). Frequently there will be fluid in the subdeltoid bursa and the biceps tendon sheath on the affected side.

APPENDIX

Sonography has assumed an important role in the evaluation of patients with right lower quadrant pain who exhibit less than classical clinical characteristics of acute appendicitis. The accuracy of sonography in the diagnosis

of acute appendicitis ranges from 85% to 95%. Therefore the risk of needlessly performing a laparotomy can be reduced by carrying out sonography preoperatively in patients with clinically indeterminate findings. In addition, alternative diagnoses can be established, particularly in young women in whom pelvic disorders can commonly mimic appendicitis.

The normal appendix is a blind-ended tubular structure that connects to the cecum and measures less than 6 mm in diameter. In most persons it is not possible to see the normal appendix. An inflamed appendix is nonperistaltic, noncompressible, and more than 6 mm in diameter (Fig. 20-50 [for Fig. 20-50, *B,* see color insert, Plate 41]). Associated findings in the setting of acute appendicitis include visualization of an appendicolith as an echogenic shadowing structure and inflamed periappendiceal fat as echogenic material surrounding the appendix, as well as the detection of hyperemia as increased vascularity on color-Doppler studies. Perforation should be considered when periappendiceal fluid collections are present. To lo-

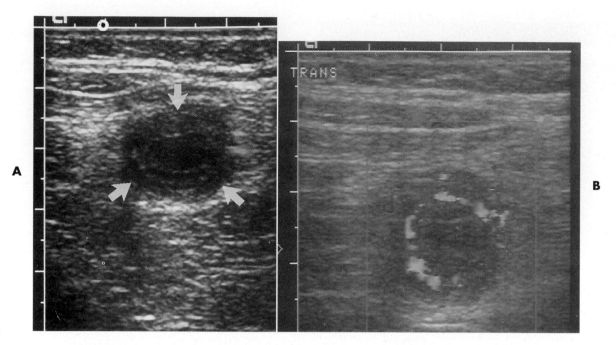

Fig. 20-50   Appendicitis. **A,** Transverse view of the right lower quadrant demonstrates a dilated appendix with thickened walls *(arrows).* **B,** Doppler image demonstrates peripheral hypervascularity, a finding consistent with the appearance of inflammatory hyperemia. Appendicitis was confirmed surgically (see color insert, Plate 41).

calize an inflamed appendix sonographically, it is very useful to have the patient point to the area of maximal pain and scan directly over this area. Graded compression is also critical to eliminate overlying bowel gas.

PROSTATE

Prostate cancer is the most common malignant tumor and is the second most common cause of cancer-related mortality in men. It is most common in blacks, less common in whites, and uncommon in Asians. As many as 50% of men in their 50s and 80% of men in their 80s will have at least microscopic foci of prostate cancer. Despite the relatively ubiquitous nature of prostate cancer in elderly men, there is only a 5% to 10% chance of their exhibiting symptoms from the disease. Therefore most of these cancers are clinically occult.

The prostate is composed of four zones. In the normal gland, the peripheral zone is the largest. It is located posteriorly and extends to both lateral margins (Fig. 20-51). It becomes thicker in the apex (inferior aspect of the gland) and thinner in the base (superior aspect of the gland). Approximately 70% of the cases of prostate cancer occur in the peripheral zone. The central zone is the next largest zone and is positioned immediately deep to the peripheral zone. It is located predominantly in the base (Fig. 20-

51). Five percent of the cases of cancer are located in the central zone. The transitional zone is located in the periurethral region between the base and apex. It is the smallest zone in the normal gland, but because benign prostatic hypertrophy arises in the transitional zone, it is rarely seen in its normal state. Twenty percent of the cases of cancer occur in the transitional zone. The anterior aspect of the prostate is composed of nonglandular tissue and is called the *fibromuscular stroma.* The seminal vesicles are bilateral symmetric structures situated immediately above the prostate. They are bulbous laterally and taper medially (Fig. 20-51). (See Table 20-5 for a summary of the characteristics of prostate cancer.)

The primary role of transrectal sonography is to guide prostate biopsies. With modern transducers it is very easy to direct core biopsy needles into a specified area of the prostate. When focal lesions are visualized sonographically or palpated on rectal examinations, they should be sampled and random biopsies of at least all four quadrants should be obtained. These random biopsy specimens are very important because cancer is found in up to 20% of such cases. If the prostate-specific antigen (PSA) level is elevated, then random biopsy specimens should be obtained even when there are no focal lesions.

It was originally hoped that transrectal sonography would be capable of detecting prostate carcinoma with a sensitivity high enough for it to serve as a screening test.

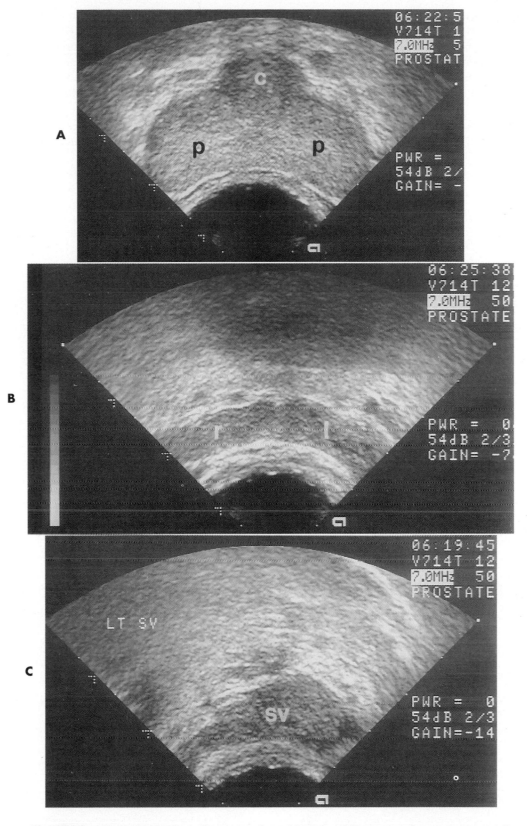

Fig. 20-51   Normal prostate. **A,** Transverse view of the base of the prostate demonstrates a small, relatively hypoechoic central zone *(c)* anteriorly. The larger, more hyperechoic peripheral zone *(p)* is positioned posteriorly and laterally. In this normal gland the peripheral zone accounts for most of the prostatic tissue. **B,** Transverse view just superior to the base of the prostate demonstrates the medial aspect of the left *(l)* and right *(r)* seminal vesicles. **C,** Transverse view slightly superior to and angled toward the left demonstrates the left seminal vesicle *(sv)* and its bulbous lateral configuration.

Unfortunately, its sensitivity is only 60% to 70%. In addition, the specificity of sonography is not such that a focal lesion of any type can be assumed to be a cancer. Therefore there is very little reason to perform prostate sonography without performing prostate biopsies at the same time.

The sonographic appearance of prostate cancer varies, but 70% are hypoechoic with respect to the peripheral zone (Fig. 20-52). The remainder are hyperechoic (Fig. 20-53) or mixed. Cancer may appear either as a discrete nodule or as an infiltrative hypoechoic region (Fig. 20-54). Cystic cancer is very rare. Although the classic appearance of prostate cancer is that of a hypoechoic nodule in the peripheral zone, only 20% to 30% of such nodules are actually cancers. The rest are benign conditions such as prostatitis, atrophy, fibrosis, infarct, and benign prostatic hyperplasia (Fig 20-55). Most prostate cancers appear hypervascular on color-Doppler analysis (Fig. 20-56 [see color insert, Plate 42]), and in a limited number of cases the hypervascularity is detectable even when a focal nodule is not seen on gray-scale studies.

The American Cancer Society currently recommends that screening for prostate cancer consist of both the digital rectal examination and determination of the PSA level. This should be started at age 50, unless the patient is at high risk (African American or strong family history). The PSA level is considered normal if it is 0 to 4 ng/ml, borderline if it is 4 to 10 ng/ml, and abnormal if it exceeds 10 ng/ml. Besides prostate cancer, benign prostatic hy-

Table 20-5 Characteristics of prostate cancer	
Characteristic	**Frequency (%)**
LOCATION	
Peripheral zone	75%
Central zone	5%
Transitional zone	20%
ECHOGENICITY	
Hypoechoic	70%
Hyperechoic/mixed	30%

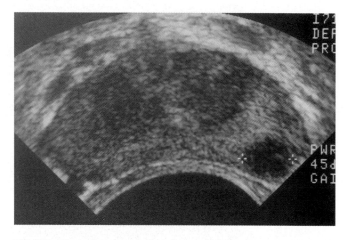

Fig. 20-52 Typical prostate carcinoma. Transverse view of the prostate demonstrates a focal, hypoechoic peripheral nodule *(cursors)* in the left side of the gland.

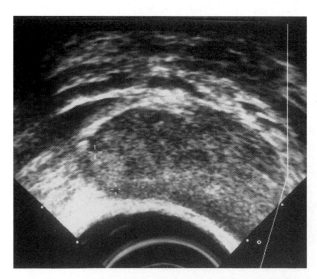

Fig. 20-53 Hyperechoic prostate cancer. Transverse view of the right lateral aspect of the prostate demonstrates a hyperechoic nodule *(cursors)*. Biopsy findings proved this to be prostate carcinoma.

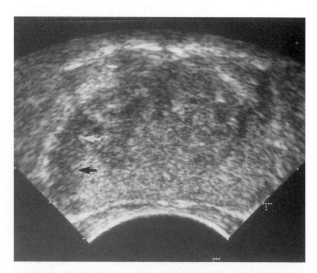

Fig. 20-54 Infiltrative prostate cancer. Transverse view of the mid-gland demonstrates a poorly marginated and irregularly shaped hypoechoic region in the right peripheral zone *(arrows)*.

pertrophy (BPH), prostatitis, and prostate infarcts can also cause the PSA level to be elevated. On the other hand, not all patients with prostate cancer have abnormal PSA levels. Additional factors that are helpful in determining the significance of the PSA value are the age of the patient, the degree of BPH, and the rate of change from one determination to the next. Elevated or borderline levels are more worrisome in young men, men without significant BPH, and men who have had previously normal levels.

BPH involves the transitional zone and produces enlargement, inhomogeneity, calcification, and occasionally cystic changes (see Fig. 20-55). These changes make it very difficult to detect cancer when it occurs in this zone.

Prostatic cysts are occasionally encountered and can occur from a variety of causes. Cysts that arise in or near the midline of the prostatic base include utricle cysts, müllerian duct cysts, and ejaculatory duct cysts (Fig. 20-57). They are difficult to differentiate with sonography alone, although ultrasound-guided aspiration of the cyst will reveal spermatozoa only in ejaculatory duct cysts. Cysts of the seminal vesicles may be congenital and associated with other genitourinary tract anomalies such as renal agenesis, or they may arise as the result of obstruction of the seminal vesicle. Retention cysts can occur anywhere in the prostate. Cystic changes can also occur in the settings of prostatitis and BPH.

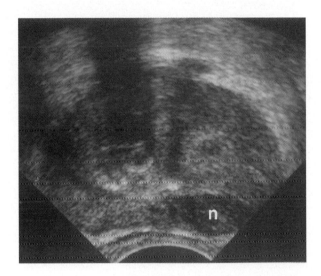

Fig. 20-55   Benign prostatic nodule. Transverse view at the midlevel of the prostate demonstrates a hypoechoic nodule *(n)* in the left peripheral zone. Biopsy specimens showed no evidence of malignancy in this region.

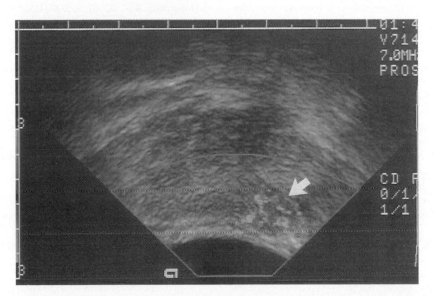

Fig. 20-56   Hypervascular prostate cancer. Transverse Doppler view of the prostate demonstrates a focal nodular region of increased vascularity in the left peripheral zone *(arrow)*. Biopsy findings proved this to be prostate carcinoma (see color insert, Plate 42).

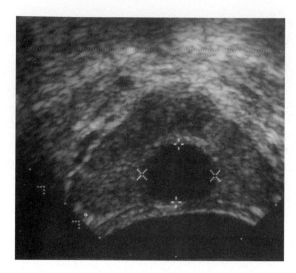

Fig. 20-57   Midline prostatic cyst. Transverse view of the base of the prostate demonstrates a midline cyst *(cursors)*. This likely represents a prostatic utricle cyst, müllerian duct cyst, or ejaculatory duct cyst. This was palpated on physical examination, but was causing no symptoms and was therefore not evaluated further.

SUGGESTED READINGS

Akerstrom G, Malmaeus J, Bergstrom R: Surgical anatomy of human parathyroid glands, *Surgery* 95:14, 1984.

Atkinson GO Jr et al: The normal and abnormal scrotum in children: evaluation with color Doppler sonography, *AJR* 158: 613, 1992.

Borushok KF et al: Sonographic diagnosis of perforation in patients with acute appendicitis, *AJR* 154:275, 1990.

Brander A et al: Thyroid gland: ultrasound screening in middle-aged women with no previous thyroid disease, *Radiology* 173:507, 1989.

Brown DL et al: Cystic testicular mass caused by dilated rete testis: sonographic findings in 31 cases, *AJR* 158:1257, 1992.

Burks DD et al: Suspected testicular torsion and ischemia: evaluation with color Doppler sonography, *Radiology* 175:815, 1990.

Cass AS, Cass BP, Veeraraghavan K: Immediate exploration of the unilateral acute scrotum in young male subjects, *J Urol* 124:829, 1980.

Catalona WJ et al: Measurement of prostate-specific antigen in serum as a screening test for prostate cancer, *N Engl J Med* 324:1156, 1991.

Dubin L, Amelar RD: Varicocele, *Urol Clin North Am* 5:563, 1978.

Dyke CH, Toi A, Sweet JM. Value of random US-guided transrectal prostate biopsy, *Radiology* 176:345, 1990.

Fournier GR Jr et al: High resolution scrotal ultrasonography: a highly sensitive but nonspecific diagnostic technique, *J Urol* 134:490, 1985.

Gooding GA, Leonhardt W, Stein R: Testicular cysts: US findings, *Radiology* 163:537, 1987.

Graif M et al: Parathyroid sonography: diagnostic accuracy related to shape, location and texture of the gland, *Br J Radiol* 60:439, 1987.

Hamm B, Fobbe F, Loy V: Testicular cysts: differentiation with US and clinical findings, *Radiology* 168:19, 1988.

Hamper UM et al: Cystic lesions of the prostate gland: a sonographic-pathologic correlation, *J Ultrasound Med* 9:395, 1990.

Horstman WG, Middleton WD, Melson GL: Scrotal inflammatory disease: color Doppler US findings, *Radiology* 179:55, 1991.

Horstman WG et al: Testicular tumors: findings with color Doppler US, *Radiology* 185:733, 1992.

Horstman WG et al: Color Doppler US of the scrotum, *Radiographics* 11:941, 1991.

James EM, Charboneau JW, Hay ID: *The thyroid.* In Rumack CM, Wilson SR, Charboneau JW, editors: Diagnostic ultrasound, St. Louis, 1991, Mosby–Year Book.

Jeffrey RB Jr, Jain KA, Nghiem HV: Pictorial essay. Sonographic diagnosis of acute appendicitis: interpretive pitfalls, *AJR* 162: 55, 1994.

Jeffrey RB Jr, Laing FC, Townsend RR: Acute appendicitis: sonographic criteria based on 250 cases, *Radiology* 167:327, 1988.

Katz JF et al: Thyroid nodules: sonographic-pathologic correlation, *Radiology* 151:741, 1984.

Lee F Jr, Bronson JP, Lee F, et al: Nonpalpable cancer of the prostate: assessment with transrectal US, *Radiology* 178:197, 1991.

Lerner RM et al: Color Doppler US in the evaluation of acute scrotal disease, *Radiology* 176:355, 1990.

Leung ML, Gooding GA, Williams RD: High-resolution sonography of scrotal contents in asymptomatic subjects, *AJR* 143:161, 1984.

Marsman JW: Clinical versus subclinical varicocele: venographic findings and improvement of fertility after embolization, *Radiology* 155:635, 1985.

Middleton WD, Bell MW: Analysis of intratesticular arterial anatomy with emphasis on transmediastinal arteries, *Radiology* 189:157, 1993.

Middleton WD, Melson GL: Testicular ischemia: color Doppler sonographic findings in five patients, *AJR* 152:1237, 1989.

Middleton WD, Thorne DA, Melson GL: Color Doppler ultrasound of the normal testis, *AJR* 152:293, 1989.

Middleton WD et al: Acute scrotal disorders: prospective comparison of color Doppler US and testicular scintigraphy, *Radiology* 177:177, 1990.

Miller DL et al: Localization of parathyroid adenomas in patients who have undergone surgery. Part I. Noninvasive imaging methods, *Radiology* 162:133, 1987.

Nghiem HT et al: Cystic lesions of the prostate, *Radiographics* 10:635, 1990.

Phillips G, Kumari-Subaiya S, Sawitsky A: Ultrasonic evaluation of the scrotum in lymphoproliferative disease, *J Ultrasound Med* 6:169, 1987.

Puylaert JB: Acute appendicitis: US evaluation using graded compression, *Radiology* 158:355, 1986.

Puylaert JB et al: A prospective study of ultrasonography in the diagnosis of appendicitis, *N Engl J Med* 317:666, 1987.

Ralls PW et al: Color-flow Doppler sonography in Graves disease: "thyroid inferno," *AJR* 150:781, 1988.

Randel SB et al: Parathyroid variants: ultrasound evaluation, *Radiology* 165:191, 1987.

Reading CC: *The parathyroid.* In Rumack CM, Wilson SR, Charboneau JW, editors: Diagnostic ultrasound, St. Louis, 1991, Mosby–Year Book.

Reading CC et al: Postoperative parathyroid high-frequency sonography: evaluation of persistent or recurrent hyperparathyroidism, *AJR* 144:399, 1985.

Rifkin MD et al: Comparison of magnetic resonance imaging and ultrasonography in staging early prostate cancer. Results of a multi-institutional cooperative trial, *N Engl J Med* 323:621, 1990.

Rifkin MD, McGlynn ET, Choi H: Echogenicity of prostate cancer correlated with histologic grade and stromal fibrosis: endorectal US studies, *Radiology* 170:549, 1989.

Rioux M: Sonographic detection of the normal and abnormal appendix, *AJR* 158:773, 1992.

Rojeski MT, Gharib H: Nodular thyroid disease: evaluation and management, *N Engl J Med* 313:428, 1985.

Schwerk WB, Schwerk WN, Rodeck G: Testicular tumors: prospective analysis of real-time US patterns and abdominal staging, *Radiology* 164:369, 1987.

Silverberg E: Cancer in young adults (ages 15 to 34), *CA Cancer J Clin* 32:32, 1982.

Steinfeld AD: Testicular germ cell tumors: review of contemporary evaluation and management, *Radiology* 175:603, 1990.

Tackett RE et al: High resolution sonography in diagnosing testicular neoplasms: clinical significance of false positive scans, *J Urol* 135:494, 1986.

Williamson RC: Torsion of the testis and allied conditions, *Br J Surg* 63:465, 1976.

Vascular System

For a Key Features summary see p. 487.

GENERAL CHARACTERISTICS

Many of the vascular characteristics pertinent to specific organs have been described in the preceding chapters. Several general principles are also useful to remember, however. All parenchymal organs (e.g., brain, kidney, liver, spleen, and testis) have a low resistance to arterial flow. Therefore they have similar-appearing Doppler waveforms with broad systolic peaks and well-maintained diastolic flow throughout the cardiac cycle (Fig. 21-1, *A*). The extremities, on the other hand, have a high resistance to arterial flow. The classic appearance of an extremity arterial waveform is triphasic, with a narrow antegrade systolic peak, a brief early diastolic retrograde peak, and a final antegrade diastolic peak that is variable in duration (Fig. 21-2). During exercise arterial waveforms in the extremities convert to a low-resistance pattern. Intestinal arteries such as the superior and inferior mesenteric arteries and their branches behave like extremity vessels, with high-resistance waveforms during fasting and low-resistance waveforms after meals.

In most large superficial arteries (carotids and femorals), the Doppler waveform shows a clear space between the arterial signal and the baseline. This is referred to as the *spectral window* (see Fig. 21-1, *A*). It occurs because the Doppler sample volume only includes red blood cells traveling in a uniform direction (along the long axis of the vessel) and, at any point in time, traveling at a narrow range of velocities. When blood flow becomes turbulent, red blood cells travel at a greater range of velocities and travel in a variety of nonaxial directions within the vessel. This produces a wider range of frequency shifts at any given point in time that causes the spectral window to fill in, a process referred to as *spectral broadening*. Before the advent of color-Doppler imaging, spectral broadening was used as a clue to the existence of underlying arterial stenosis. Unfortunately, many technical factors such as high Doppler gain, high power settings, and large sample volumes can also cause spectral broadening (see Fig. 21-1, *B*). In addition, it is normal to see spectral broadening in small vessels. For these reasons, and because color-Doppler imaging is superior in detecting stenotic vessels, spectral broadening is not now given as much attention as it used to be.

Another sign of turbulent flow is vibrating tissues. This occurs because turbulence occasionally causes pressure fluctuations in the vessel lumen that produce vessel wall vibration. When the vessel wall vibration is significant, the tissues around the vessel may start to vibrate. This is what causes the bruit that can be heard with a stethoscope or the thrill that can be felt on palpation. It also can be detected on Doppler analysis because the vibrating tissue interfaces produce a Doppler frequency shift just as other moving reflectors do. On waveform analysis, the frequency shifts are found to be low (because the motion is slow) and are displayed symmetrically above and below the baseline (because the vibratory motion goes both toward and away from the transducer). The abnormal signal can be obtained both from the perivascular tissues and from the lumen of the vessel itself (Fig. 21-3 [see color insert, Plate 43]).

Whenever the outflow of blood from an organ or structure is interrupted, the pattern of arterial flow is altered. With complete obstruction to outflow, arterial inflow may still occur by way of the supplying artery, but it produces only a narrow antegrade systolic peak. The blood that enters the organ during systole must exit by way of the supplying artery during diastole. This

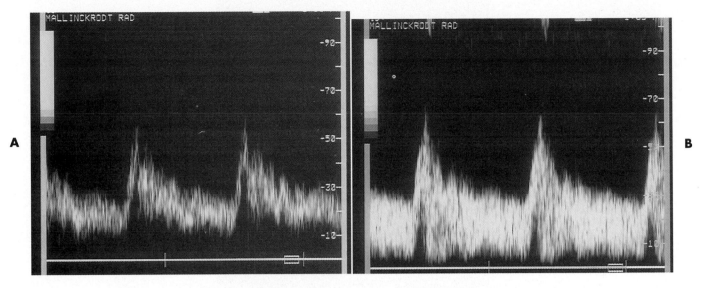

Fig. 21-1   Low-resistance arterial waveform. **A,** Pulsed-Doppler waveform shows a broad systolic peak and well-maintained diastolic flow throughout the cardiac cycle. This is typical of an artery that supplies a parenchymal organ. There is also a relatively clear window under the arterial envelope. **B,** Waveform from the same vessel obtained with a larger Doppler sample volume size (5 mm as opposed to 1 mm in **A**) and a higher Doppler gain setting. These changes in the technical aspects have caused the clear window to be filled in so that it simulates spectral broadening.

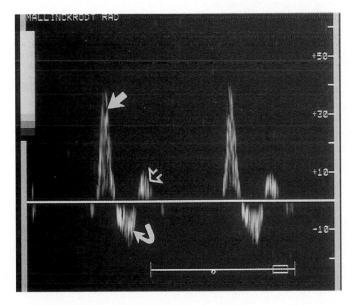

Fig. 21-2   High-resistance triphasic arterial waveform. Pulsed-Doppler waveform shows a short antegrade systolic pulse *(arrow),* followed by a short reversed early diastolic pulse *(curved arrow),* followed by a final short antegrade pulse *(open arrow).*

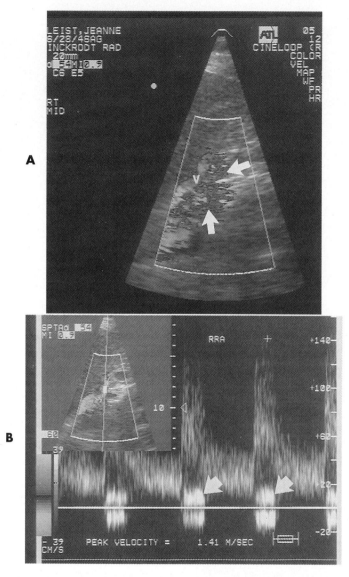

Fig. 21-3   Doppler appearance of tissue vibration. **A,** Doppler view of the right renal artery in a patient with fibromuscular dysplasia shows random red and blue assignment in the tissues around the renal artery *(arrows).* This arises from the vibrating tissue interfaces in the perivascular soft tissues. The normal renal vein *(v)* is seen anterior to the renal artery. **B,** Pulsed-Doppler waveform from the renal artery shows the arterial waveform as expected, but also shows a low-magnitude, but strong, bidirectional systolic signal *(arrow)* below the arterial waveform. This secondary signal arises from red blood cell and vessel wall vibration (see color insert, Plate 43).

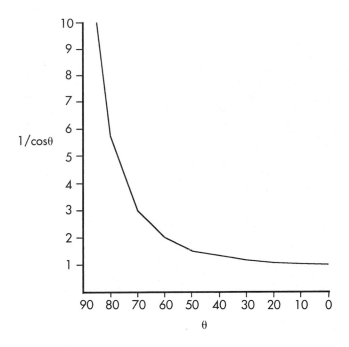

Fig. 21-4   Graph showing the Doppler angle (θ) on the horizontal axis and 1/cosθ on the vertical axis. Note that small differences in the Doppler angle cause little change in 1/cosθ between 0 and 60 degrees. On the other hand, when the Doppler angle is greater than 60 degrees, small differences in the angle produce large changes in 1/cosθ.

phenomena produces pandiastolic flow reversal and is sometimes referred to as the *to-and-fro pattern*. It was illustrated in Chapter 4 in a patient with renal vein thrombosis (see Fig. 4-79), but it applies to other organs as well. As shown later in this chapter, this pattern is also seen at the neck of pseudoaneurysms.

A number of measurements are used to analyze arterial waveforms. The most common measurement is the arterial velocity. This can be done by converting the frequency shift information contained in the Doppler waveform into velocity information. The basic Doppler equation is:

$$Fd = Ft \times V \times (1/C) \times \cos\theta \times 2,$$

where:

- Fd = Doppler frequency shift
- Ft = Transmitted frequency
- V = Blood flow velocity
- C = Speed of sound
- θ = The Doppler angle (the angle between the direction of sound and the direction of blood flow)

This equation can be solved for velocity, as follows:

$$V = Fd \times (1/Ft) \times (C/2) \times (1/\cos\theta).$$

From this equation it is apparent that the velocity is proportional to the Doppler frequency shift. Thus higher-frequency shifts indicate higher velocities. The velocity is also proportional to the inverse of the cosθ. Fig. 21-4 shows the value of 1/cosθ with respect to θ. This graph indicates that there is little change in 1/cosθ between angles of 0 and 60 degrees. However, at angles greater than 60 degrees there is a great change in 1/cosθ for minimal changes in θ. Because of this, minimal uncertainties in the Doppler angle (which are unavoidable) will produce large errors in velocity calculations when the angle is greater than 60 degrees but minimal errors when the angle is less than 60 degrees (Fig. 21-5). For this reason, one should always attempt to image a vessel so that the Doppler angle is less than 60 degrees if velocity calculations are being obtained.

Another common measurement is the resistive index *(RI)*, defined as:

$$RI = 1 - (D/S) = (S - D)/S,$$

where *D* is the end-diastolic velocity (or frequency shift) and *S* is the peak systolic velocity (or frequency shift) (Fig. 21-6). The resistive index goes up when the resistance to flow goes up. When there is no diastolic flow, the resistive index is 1. Parenchymal organs normally have a resistive index of less than 0.7. Because the calculation

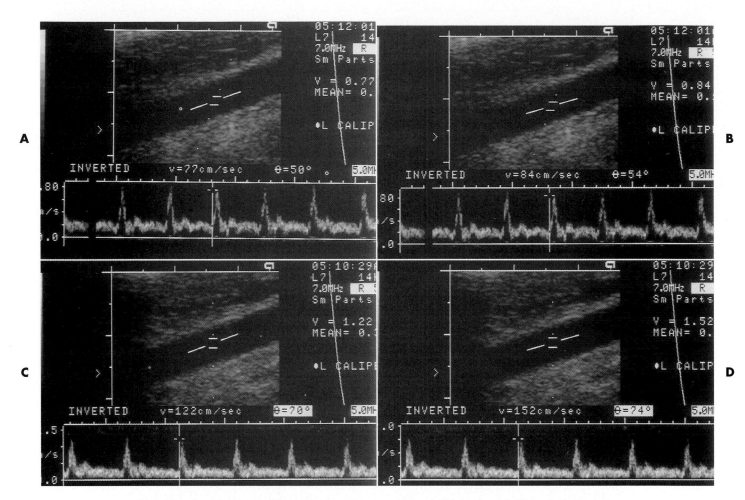

Fig. 21-5 Effect of Doppler angle on velocity measurements. **A,** In this image a waveform has been obtained from a normal common carotid at a Doppler angle of approximately 50 to 54 degrees. When the angle indicator (i.e., the white line oriented parallel to the long axis of the vessel) is set at 50 degrees, the calculated peak systolic velocity is 77 cm/sec. **B,** This is the same image and waveform as in **A,** but in this case the Doppler angle indicator has been set at 54 degrees and the calculated velocity is 84 cm/sec. In analyzing the vessel and the Doppler angle indicator, it is not possible to determine if the true angle is 50 or 54 degrees or something in between. However, because the Doppler angle is less than 60 degrees, the difference in the calculated velocity is minimal (7 cm/sec) despite the 4-degree uncertainty in the angle. **C,** In this image the Doppler beam has been steered so that the same common carotid is being sampled at a Doppler angle of between 70 and 74 degrees. When the angle indicator is set at 70 degrees, the calculated velocity is 122 cm/sec. **D,** This is the same image and waveform as in **C,** but in this case the Doppler angle indicator has been set at 74 degrees. This results in a calculated velocity of 152 cm/sec. This shows the significant variations in the estimated velocity (in this case 30 cm/sec) caused by minimal uncertainties in the actual Doppler angle when the Doppler angle is greater than 60 degrees.

depends only on the ratio of systolic-to-diastolic flow, it is independent of the Doppler angle.

Another common measurement is the pulsatility index *(PI)*, defined as:

$$PI = (S - D)/M,$$

where M is the mean flow velocity throughout the cardiac cycle (Fig. 21-7). The pulsatility index is probably a truer indication of vascular resistance than the resistive index, but because it is more difficult to measure, it has not gained widespread use.

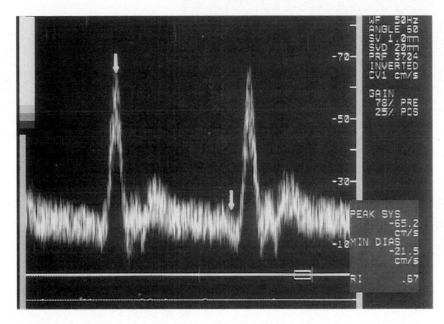

Fig. 21-6   Resistive index measurement. Determination of peak systolic and end-diastolic velocity *(arrows)* is all that is required for the calculation of a resistive index. The value is then computed by built-in software and displayed on the monitor. In this case the systolic velocity, diastolic velocity, and resistive index are 65.2 cm/sec, 21.5 cm/sec, and 0.67, respectively.

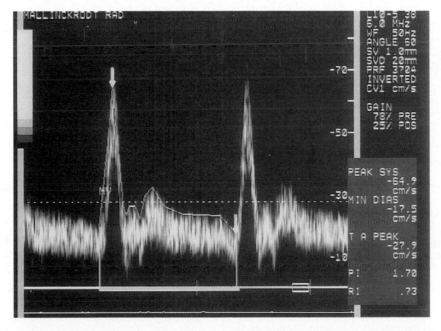

Fig. 21-7   Pulsatility index measurement. Determination of peak systolic, end-diastolic, and a time-average mean velocity is required for the calculation of a pulsatility index. In this case the respective values are 64.9 cm/sec, 17.5 cm/sec, 27.9 cm/sec, and 1.70.

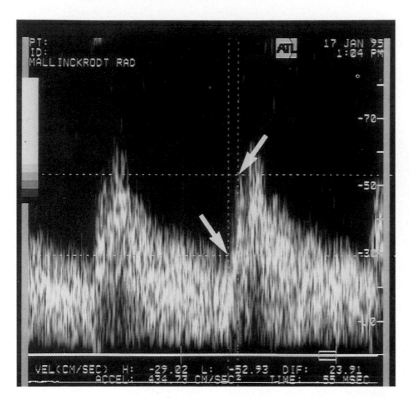

Fig. 21-8   Systolic acceleration measurement. Crosshairs have been placed at the beginning of systole and at the end of the rapid systolic upstroke *(arrows)*. Based on the position of these crosshairs, the change in velocity over the change in time can be calculated in order to obtain the systolic acceleration. In this case the result was 434.73 cm/sec^2.

In addition to these measurements of vascular resistance, measurements of systolic upstroke are also becoming more widely used as a means of detecting proximal arterial stenosis. The early systolic acceleration is the measurement that is in most widespread use. It is obtained by measuring the slope (change in velocity/change in time) of the early systolic upstroke (Fig. 21-8). Unlike the resistive index and pulsatility index, systolic acceleration requires the determination of an absolute difference in velocities, and thus must be calculated from an angle-corrected velocity waveform.

CAROTIDS

Doppler sonography of the carotids has matured in the past decade into a well-established noninvasive test for detecting, quantitating, and monitoring carotid stenoses. Analysis relies on the combined information furnished by gray-scale images, pulsed-Doppler waveforms, and color-Doppler imaging. Using all three techniques together, the sensitivity and specificity exceed 90% in the detection of stenosis causing a greater than 50% diameter narrowing.

A carotid Doppler study should be viewed as a screening test to identify patients with atherosclerotic plaques and to determine the severity of the plaque in order to decide which patients need to undergo more invasive tests. The North American Symptomatic Carotid Endarterectomy Trial has shown that patients who are symptomatic and have a stenosis of 70% or greater can benefit from carotid endarterectomy. Therefore patients

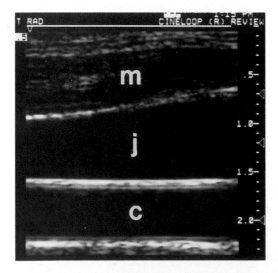

Fig. 21-9   Gray-scale appearance of the normal common carotid artery. Longitudinal view of the neck demonstrates the sternocleidomastoid muscle *(m)*, internal jugular vein *(j)*, and common carotid artery *(c)*. Note that the wall of the common carotid artery consists of a bright linear reflection off of the intimal surface and a hypoechoic layer immediately underneath the intimal reflection. Using the jugular vein as a window often provides an excellent view of the wall of the common carotid artery.

with an estimated stenosis of 70% or greater shown by Doppler studies should then undergo angiography for the further evaluation of their carotids. Symptomatic patients with less severe stenosis do better with medical management and under most circumstances do not need angiographic studies. What the proper management of asymptomatic patients with carotid stenosis should be is the subject of current ongoing studies.

The normal carotid wall appears hypoechoic on grayscale studies. The reflection from the interface between the luminal surface of the wall and the blood within the lumen produces an inner bright line along the carotid wall. This sonographic morphology of the carotid wall is easily seen in most common carotid arteries (CCAs) (Fig. 21-9), but may be difficult to demonstrate in the internal (ICA) and external (ECA) carotid arteries. Flow patterns in the carotid artery have been analyzed with color-Doppler analysis, and these studies have consistently shown a region of flow reversal in the carotid bulb where the normal vessel expands (Fig. 21-10 [see color insert, Plate 44]). This is an expected finding and should not be equated with disturbed or abnormal flow. In fact, the absence of flow reversal in the bulb may be a sign of an early atherosclerotic plaque.

The ICA supplies brain tissue. Like other parenchymal organs, the brain has a low resistance to arterial inflow; therefore waveforms from the ICA have broad systolic peaks and well-maintained diastolic flow throughout the cardiac cycle (Fig. 21-11, *A*). The ECA supplies the scalp

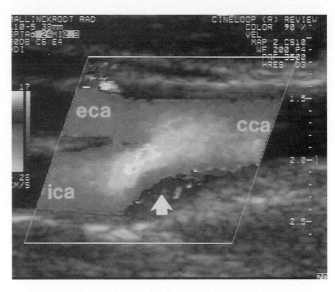

Fig. 21-10   Normal flow reversal in the carotid bulb. Longitudinal Doppler image of the carotid bifurcation shows the common carotid artery *(cca),* internal carotid artery *(ica),* and external carotid artery *(eca).* A focal region of flow reversal manifested as a blue assignment *(arrow)* is seen in the carotid bulb. This is a normal expected finding and should not be confused with flow turbulence or other flow abnormality. Notice that in this image the internal carotid is deep to the external carotid because the transducer was positioned anteriorly on the neck. A contrasting view obtained from a posterior approach is shown in Fig. 21-12 (see color insert, Plate 44).

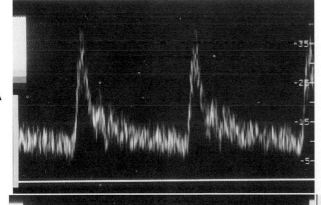

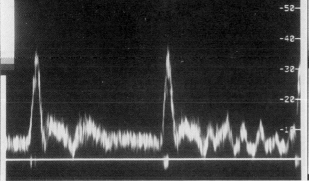

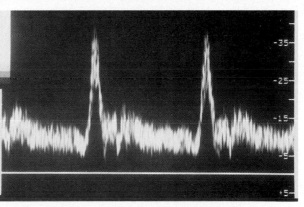

Fig. 21-11   Normal carotid hemodynamic characteristics. **A,** Pulsed-Doppler waveform from the internal carotid artery demonstrates a relatively broad systolic peak with a gradual down-slope into the diastolic portion of the cardiac cycle. Persistent high levels of diastolic flow are seen throughout the cardiac cycle. **B,** Pulsed-Doppler waveform from the external carotid artery demonstrates a high resistance–type profile with less diastolic flow than that seen in the internal carotid artery. Also note the pulses in the diastolic portion of the second waveform. These were produced by tapping on the superficial temporal artery. **C,** Pulsed-Doppler waveform from the common carotid artery demonstrates a pattern intermediate between that of the internal carotid and that of the external carotid.

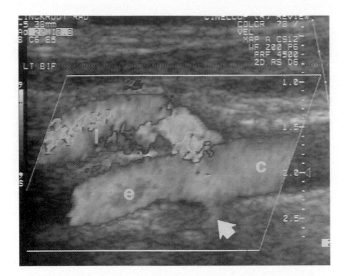

Fig. 21-12 Differentiation between the internal carotid artery and external carotid artery. Longitudinal Doppler image of the distal common carotid artery *(c)* and carotid bifurcation obtained from a posterolateral approach shows the internal carotid *(i)* as the vessel that is most superficial. The external carotid *(e)* is seen in the deeper aspect of the field of view. A branch vessel *(arrow)* is seen arising from the origin of the external carotid (see color insert, Plate 45).

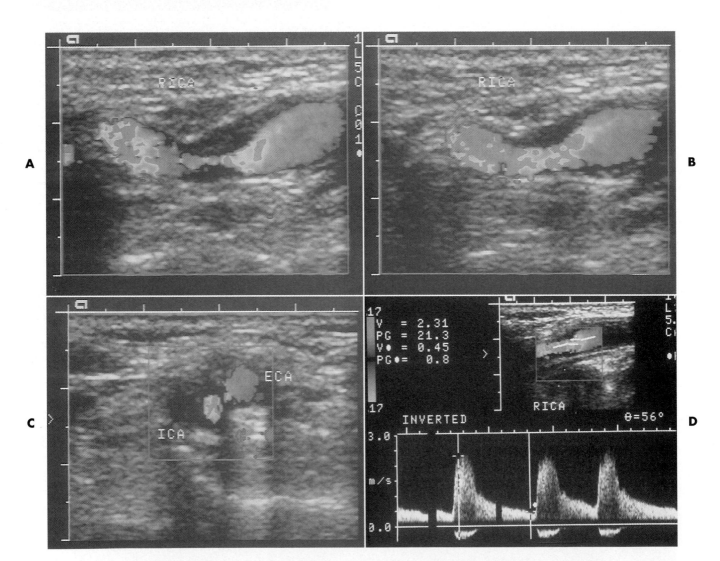

Fig. 21-13 Internal carotid artery stenosis narrowing lumen by 60% to 79%. **A,** Longitudinal Doppler view of the right internal carotid artery demonstrates what appears to be a high-grade stenosis. **B,** Slightly more medial longitudinal Doppler view demonstrates a less severe appearing stenosis. **C,** Transverse color-Doppler view just above the carotid bifurcation demonstrates a narrowed residual lumen in the internal carotid artery *(ICA)* that correlates with a 60% to 79% stenosis. The external carotid artery *(ECA)* is seen anterior and medial to the ICA (see color insert, Plate 46). **D,** Pulsed-Doppler waveform from the area of stenosis reveals peak systolic and end-diastolic flow velocities of 231 and 45 cm/sec, respectively. These correlate with an estimated stenotic narrowing of 60% to 79%.

and face, both of which have a high resistance to arterial inflow. This results in a high-resistance arterial waveform with narrow systolic peaks and decreased or absent diastolic flow (Fig. 21-11, *B*). In addition to the differences in the waveforms, the ECA can be distinguished from the ICA on the basis of its more anterior and medial position, its smaller size, and its branch vessels (Fig. 21-12 [see color insert, Plate 45]). A maneuver that can also assist in distinguishing these vessels is tapping the superficial temporal artery (located immediately anterior to the ear). Because this vessel is a branch of the ECA, pulsations produced by the tapping are transmitted into the ECA and appear on the waveform (see Fig. 21-11, *B*). The CCA has characteristics of both the ICA and ECA, but because 70% to 80% of its flow goes to the ICA, the CCA waveform tends to mirror the waveform in the ICA more than the waveform in the ECA (see Fig. 21-11, *C*). (See Table 21-1 for a summary of the differences between ICAs and ECAs.)

Lesions producing greater than 50% diameter reduction are considered hemodynamically significant because they produce a decrease in flow volume. Stenoses producing greater than 50% diameter narrowing also produce elevated flow velocities that can be detected by

measuring the arterial waveforms. A number of criteria have been developed for estimating the degree of carotid stenosis (Table 21-2). Those most commonly used include peak systolic flow velocity, end-diastolic flow velocity, and the ratio of peak systolic velocity in the ICA to the peak systolic velocity in the ipsilateral CCA. The ICA/CCA systolic velocity ratio is theoretically helpful in situations in which the baseline velocities either are increased (such as in a contralateral carotid occlusion) or are decreased (such as in patients with low cardiac output).

As expected, the ICA systolic velocity and the ICA/CCA velocity ratio progressively increase as the degree of ICA stenosis worsens (Figs. 21-13 [for Figs. 2-13, *A*, *B*, and *C*, see color insert, Plate 46] and 21-14 [see color insert, Plate 47]). However, there is a point in the very high grade stenoses when the velocity starts to drop back down into the normal range (Fig. 21-15, *A*). In such cases a high-grade stenosis is generally evident on color-Doppler imaging (Fig. 21-15, *B* [see color insert, Plate 48]), and despite normal velocities, the pulsed-Doppler waveform appears distorted and abnormal.

Total occlusion of the ICA causes a lack of detectable ICA flow on pulsed-Doppler and color-Doppler studies. When no flow is detected in the ICA, the vessel is very likely occluded. However, it is also possible that an extremely tight stenosis can diminish flow so much that it becomes impossible to detect with Doppler imaging. Therefore most experts would recommend angiography be performed to further evaluate such patients because a very tight stenosis represents a surgical lesion, but a complete occlusion does not. A secondary sign of ICA occlusion is the "externalization" of the CCA waveform (Fig. 21-16). This occurs because all of the CCA flow goes into the ECA.

Lesions that produce a less than 50% diameter narrowing are difficult to detect and quantitate with pulsed-Doppler waveform analysis (Fig. 21-17, *A*). In the vast majority of instances these low-grade lesions are easily detected with a combination of gray-scale and color-

---

Table 21-1   Differences between the internal and external carotids

Characteristic	Internal carotid artery	External carotid artery
Location	Posterior/lateral	Anterior/medial
Size	Larger	Smaller
Branches	No	Yes
Waveform	Low resistance	High resistance
Temporal tap	No	Yes

Table 21-2   Diagnostic Doppler criteria for carotid artery disease

Diameter stenosis (%)	Peak systolic velocity (cm/sec)	Peak diastolic velocity (cm/sec)	Systolic velocity ratio (ICA/CCA)	Diastolic velocity ratio (ICA/CCA)
0	<110	<40	<1.8	<2.4
1-39	<110	<40	<1.8	<2.4
40-59	<130	40	<1.8	<2.4
60-79	>130	>40	>1.8	>2.4
80-99	>250	>100	>3.7	>5.5
100 (occlusion)	N/A	N/A	N/A	N/A

Modified from Bluth EI et al: Carotid duplex sonography: a multicenter recommendation for standardized imaging and Doppler criteria, *Radiographics* 8:487-506, 1988.
CCA, Common carotid artery; *ICA,* internal carotid artery; *N/A,* not applicable.

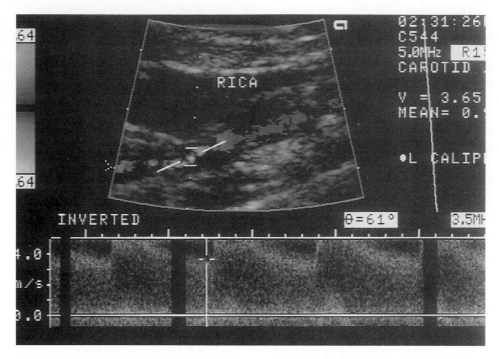

Fig. 21-14   Severe carotid artery stenosis. Longitudinal color-Doppler image and pulsed-Doppler waveform demonstrate marked narrowing of the proximal internal carotid artery. The pulsed-Doppler waveform shows aliasing of the systolic peak, thus precluding accurate systolic velocity measurements. However, the end-diastolic velocity has been measured to be 365 cm/sec, which correlates with a stenosis causing a greater than 80% diameter reduction (see color insert, Plate 47).

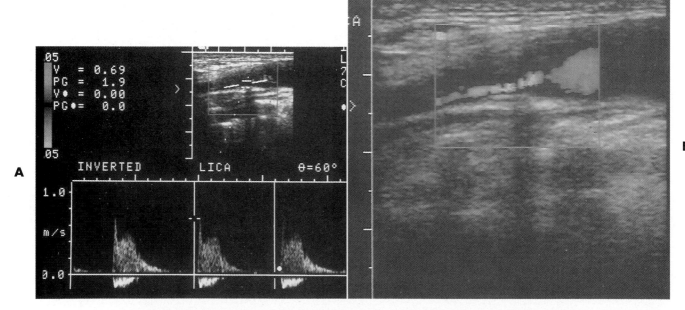

Fig. 21-15   High-grade carotid stenosis with normal flow velocities. **A,** Pulsed-Doppler waveform from the internal carotid artery shows a normal peak systolic velocity of 69 cm/sec. However, the waveform is very abnormal for an internal carotid artery, with complete absence of end-diastolic flow. **B,** Doppler image of the internal carotid artery demonstrates an extremely narrowed residual lumen producing the Doppler equivalent of an angiographic "string" sign. The plaque producing this stenosis is extremely hypoechoic and was not detectable on gray-scale imaging (see color insert, Plate 48).

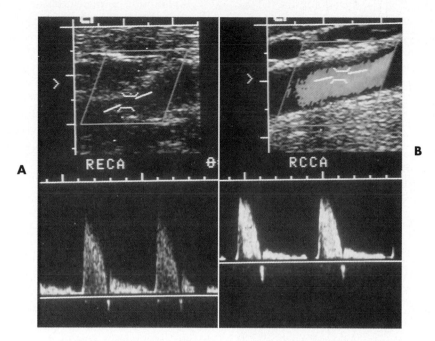

Fig. 21-16   Complete occlusion of the internal carotid artery with "externalization" of the common carotid artery. **A,** Pulsed-Doppler waveform from the external carotid artery shows a typical high-resistance appearance. **B,** A high-resistance waveform from the common carotid artery almost identical to that seen in the external carotid. This is strong evidence of a high-grade stenosis or, more likely, a complete occlusion of the internal carotid artery.

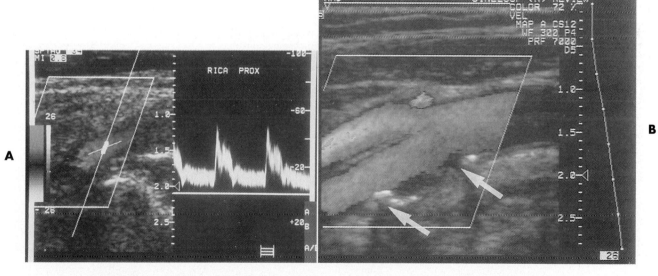

Fig. 21-17   Stenosis of the internal carotid artery causing a less than 50% narrowing. **A,** Pulsed-Doppler waveform from the proximal right internal carotid artery demonstrates a normal-appearing waveform with a normal peak systolic flow velocity of approximately 50 cm/sec. This case illustrates the inability of Doppler waveform analysis to detect stenosis producing a less than 50% narrowing. **B,** Longitudinal Doppler image of the carotid bifurcation demonstrates partially calcified and noncalcified plaque *(arrows)* in the region of the carotid bulb and the origin of the internal carotid artery. Note that the flow reversal normally seen in the carotid bulb is not present (see color insert, Plate 49).

Doppler sonography (Fig. 21-17, *B* [see color insert, Plate 49]). Highly echogenic or calcified lesions are shown well with gray-scale sonography (Fig. 21-18), but hypoechoic plaques are visualized much better as a defect in the flow lumen on color-Doppler sonography (Figs. 21-15 and 21-19).

In addition to measuring velocities, it is also possible to roughly estimate the degree of stenosis on the basis of the information furnished by longitudinally oriented gray-scale and color-Doppler images. However, because plaque is rarely concentric, the degree of stenosis can be both overestimated and underestimated on longitudinal images (see Fig. 21-13, *A* and *B*). In real-time analysis, it is often possible to scan back and forth through the lumen of the vessel and to thereby form a visual impression of the degree of luminal narrowing. Transverse views are also quite helpful in gauging the degree of stenosis, although it is often more difficult to define the outer wall of the carotid on transverse views (see Fig. 21-13, *C*).

In addition to using gray-scale sonography to detect and quantitate stenosis, there is also some interest in using it to evaluate plaque morphology. Study findings have suggested that a homogeneous plaque tends to be stable over time. On the other hand, inhomogeneity and hypoechoic defects (Fig. 21-20) correlate with the presence of intraplaque hemorrhage, and these plaques tend to break down and produce emboli and clinical symptoms. Despite encouraging results in some studies, the analysis of plaque morphology remains a subjective and controversial method and is not widely accepted as a valuable means of directing patient management.

The detection of plaque ulceration is difficult but possible with gray-scale and color-Doppler sonography (Fig. 21-21). Although many ulcers are missed, when a well-defined crater is detected, it should be reported because this may explain symptoms arising from a hemodynamically insignificant lesion.

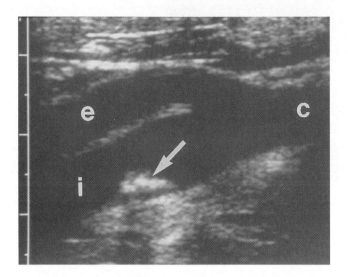

Fig. 21-18   Calcified plaque. Longitudinal gray-scale image of the carotid bifurcation demonstrates a shadowing, echogenic, calcified plaque *(arrow)* at the origin of the internal carotid artery *(i)*. Also seen are the external carotid artery *(e)* and common carotid artery *(c)*.

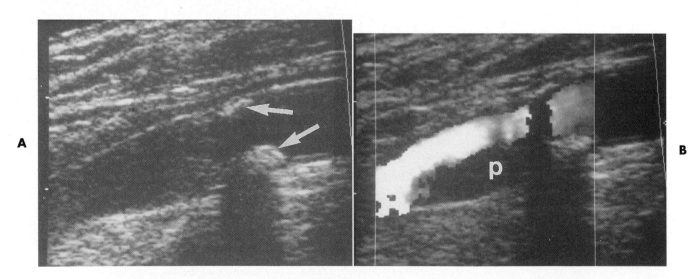

Fig. 21-19   Hypoechoic plaque. **A,** Longitudinal gray-scale view of the proximal internal carotid artery demonstrates calcified plaque along the near and far walls *(arrows)*. Low-level echoes fill the lumen of the internal carotid artery, and it is impossible to determine whether noncalcified plaque is present distally. **B,** Black-and-white reproduction of a color-Doppler image of the same area as shown in **A** demonstrates blood flow in the superficial aspect of the internal carotid artery and a very hypoechoic plaque *(p)* in the deep aspect of the internal carotid.

The vertebral arteries should also be evaluated routinely. The vertebral arteries are best seen as they travel between the transverse processes of the cervical spine (Fig. 21-22 [see color insert, Plate 50]). Shadowing from the transverse processes results in only segmental visualization of the vertebral arteries, which makes it difficult to

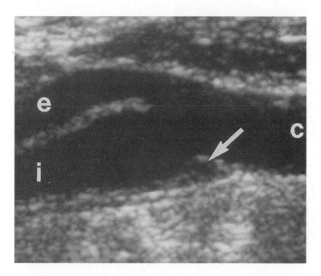

Fig. 21-20   Plaque inhomogeneity. Longitudinal gray-scale view of the carotid bifurcation demonstrates a combined hypoechoic and anechoic region *(arrow)* within a small plaque at the carotid bulb. This is likely due to intraplaque hemorrhage. *i,* Internal carotid; *e,* external carotid; *c,* common carotid.

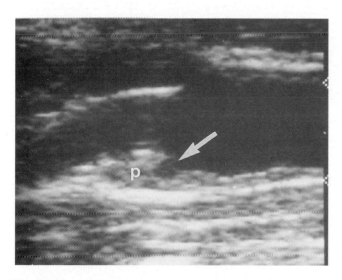

Fig. 21-21   Plaque ulceration. Longitudinal view of the carotid bulb demonstrates a hyperechoic, noncalcified plaque *(p).* A hypoechoic defect *(arrow)* is seen in the proximal portion of the plaque. This defect filled with blood flow on color-Doppler sonography and its appearance is consistent with that of an ulcer crater.

identify vertebral arterial stenotic lesions. However, it is possible to determine the patency of the vertebral arteries and the direction of flow in the vertebral arteries. Reversed flow in a vertebral artery indicates a stenosis or occlusion at the origin of the subclavian or innominate artery (Fig. 21-23 [for Fig. 21-23, *A,* see color insert, Plate 51]). In this setting flow to the ipsilateral upper extremity is maintained by means of antegrade flow in the contralateral carotid and vertebral artery, with cross flow in the circle of Willis and retrograde flow in the ipsilateral vertebral artery. One potential pitfall in the detection of retrograde vertebral arterial flow is the possibility of misconstruing a vertebral vein (which normally has flow directed caudally) to represent a vertebral artery with reversed flow (Fig. 21-24 [for Fig. 21-24, *A,* see color insert, Plate 52]). Doppler waveform analysis of the vessel in question should help to prevent this potential diagnostic error.

THE GROIN

Doppler analysis is frequently requested when focal swelling or a new bruit develops in a patient who has undergone femoral catheterization. The major causes include hematomas, pseudoaneurysms, and arteriovenous

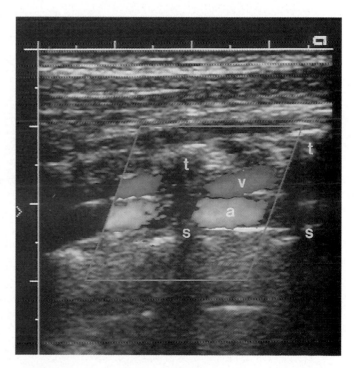

Fig. 21-22   Normal vertebral artery and vein. Longitudinal Doppler image demonstrates the vertebral artery *(a)* and overlying vertebral vein *(v).* Transverse processes of the cervical spine *(t)* and associated shadows *(s)* preclude visualization of the entire vertebral vessels. The vertebral vein is seen unusually well in this person (see color insert, Plate 50).

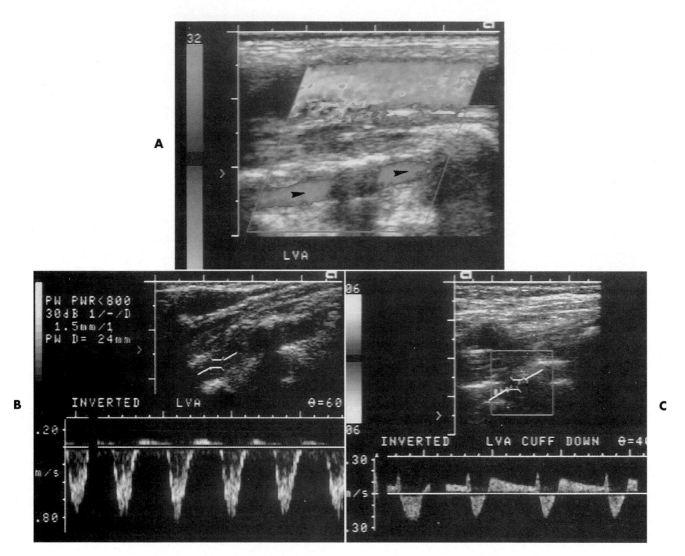

Fig. 21-23   Three different patients with subclavian steal syndrome. **A,** Longitudinal Doppler view of the left neck shows flow in the common carotid artery directed superiorly. Flow in the vertebral artery is directed inferiorly. Flow direction is indicated by the arrows (see color insert, Plate 51). **B,** Pulsed Doppler waveform from another patient shows almost complete reversal of flow (below the Doppler baseline) in the left vertebral artery. Minimal antegrade diastolic flow (above the Doppler baseline) likely represents diastolic rebound from the left upper extremity into the vertebral artery. **C,** Pulsed Doppler waveform from a third patient shows slight systolic flow reversal (below the Doppler baseline) but significant antegrade flow (above the Doppler baseline) during diastole. The prominent antegrade diastolic flow in this case must arise from subclavian flow and indicates that the subclavian artery is not completely occluded but just significantly stenosed.

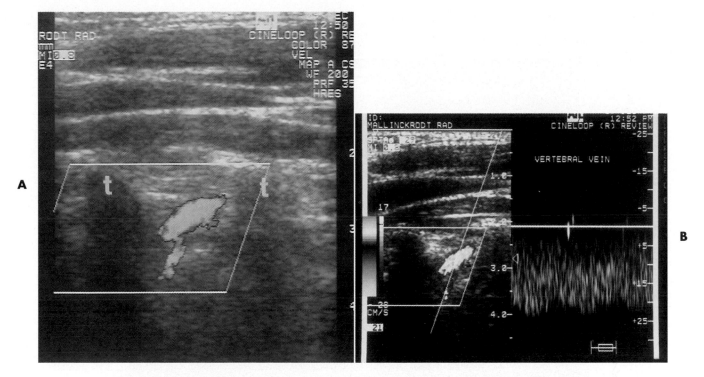

Fig. 21-24   Vertebral vein mimicking reversal of flow in the vertebral artery. **A,** Longitudinal Doppler view of the neck between the transverse processes *(t)* demonstrates a vessel with flow directed inferiorly in the neck. Based solely on the Doppler appearance, this could represent reversal of flow in the vertebral artery (see color insert, Plate 52). **B,** Pulsed-Doppler waveform from this vessel confirms venous flow characteristics consistent with those of a normal vertebral vein. In this case the vertebral vein is seen particularly well because of obstruction or aplasia of the vertebral artery.

Box 21-1   Characteristics of Pseudoaneurysms
Swirling luminal flow
Variable amounts of mural thrombus
Often multiple loculations
To-and-fro flow at aneurysm neck

fistulas. As mentioned in previous chapters, hematomas can assume a variety of appearances, depending on their age. They range from solid-appearing masses to complex fluid collections to more simple-appearing fluid collections as clot lysis and liquefaction progress. In some persons, extensive local hemorrhage can occur without there being sonographic evidence of a discrete fluid collection. This can probably happen when there is an infiltrative type of hemorrhage or when imaging is done during the phase when the hemorrhage is isoechoic to surrounding tissues.

Pseudoaneurysms can be distinguished from hematomas by the finding of internal blood flow within the pseu-doaneurysm lumen (Box 21-1). Typically blood flow in a pseudoaneurysm assumes a swirling pattern, with flow directed toward the transducer in half of the lumen and flow directed away from the transducer in the other half of the lumen (Fig. 21-25). In some cases the internal flow patterns are more complex than this. Pseudoaneurysms are actually hematomas that have maintained some communication with the arterial lumen by means of the puncture site. Therefore they vary in the amount of clot and the extent of patent lumen. In addition, they often have multiple communicating components, perhaps stemming from separate episodes of bleeding and rebleeding. A characteristic waveform that is often obtained in the setting of pseudoaneurysms arises at the pseudoaneurysm neck. Because blood flow into the pseudoaneurysm lumen goes in one direction during systole and exits the pseudoaneurysm in the opposite direction during diastole, the resultant waveform shows a to-and-fro pattern (Fig. 21-25, *B* [see color insert, Plate 53]).

In addition to identifying pseudoaneurysms, sonography can be a useful aid in guiding and monitoring attempts at the ablation of these vascular lesions. By localizing the pseudoaneurysm neck, sonography can precisely guide where compression should be applied. As com-

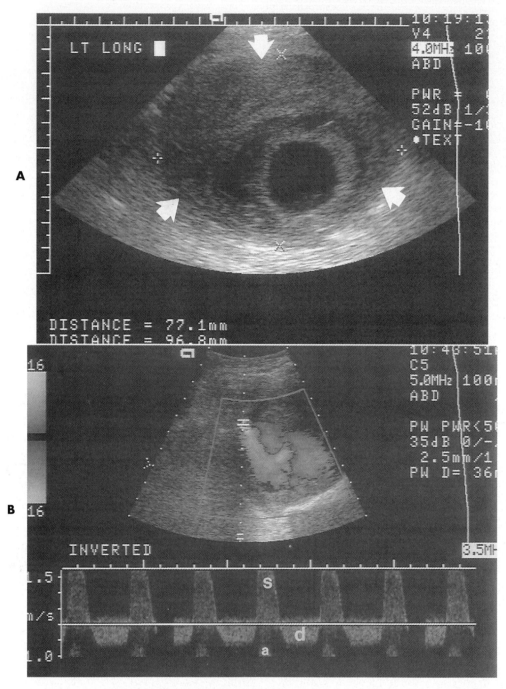

Fig. 21-25   Large pseudoaneurysm. **A,** Transverse view of the groin shows a large mass *(arrows)* with a small circular anechoic center. Although the appearance is suggestive of a pseudoaneurysm, a hematoma could also have this appearance. **B,** Longitudinal color-Doppler view shows a swirling pattern of internal flow in the center of the mass, a finding consistent with the appearance of luminal flow in a pseudoaneurysm. Pulsed-Doppler waveform from the pseudoaneurysm neck shows a to-and-fro flow pattern at the aneurysm neck. Antegrade flow into the aneurysm occurs during systole *(s)* and is displayed above the baseline. Reversed flow out of the aneurysm occurs during diastole *(d)* and is displayed below the baseline. Aliasing of the systolic peak *(a)* results in wrap-around of the systolic signal to below the baseline (see color insert, Plate 53).

pression is applied, color-Doppler imaging can determine when adequate pressure has been applied to obliterate flow in the pseudoaneurysm lumen. The success of ultrasound-guided compression of pseudoaneurysms varies. In general, the likelihood of successfully obliterating acute and subacute pseudoaneurysms with narrow necks is high (Fig. 21-26 [see color insert, Plate 54]). The chance of successfully obliterating more chronic pseudoaneurysms or those with wider necks is less. It is also important to reverse anticoagulation to improve the chances of success.

Arteriovenous (A-V) fistulas are suspected when a bruit becomes audible in a patient after femoral catheterization. They may coexist with pseudoaneurysms. Grayscale sonography rarely reveals any detectable abnormalities in patients with isolated A-V fistulas. The hemodynamic changes that occur, however, are generally readily detected with Doppler analysis (Box 21-2). In many patients high-velocity flow at the site of an A-V communication results in turbulence and focal perivascular tissue vibration. As mentioned earlier, this can produce a dramatic color-Doppler display of random red and blue pixels in the perivascular soft tissues (Fig. 21-27 [see color insert, Plate 55]). Another hemodynamic consequence of an A-V fistula is decreased resistance to flow in the artery supplying the fistula. This is manifested as higher diastolic flow velocities and persistent forward flow throughout the cardiac cycle (Fig. 21-28 [for Figs. 21-28, *A* and *B,* see color insert, Plate 56]). This pandiastolic antegrade flow contrasts with the normally absent or reversed diastolic flow that occurs in most peripheral arteries. Finally, direct arterial inflow into the vein produces turbulent flow in the venous lumen and often produces an arterialized venous waveform or a turbulent waveform. All of these hemodynamic changes are quite focal and can generally only be detected within 1 to 2 cm of the actual site of communication.

Box 21-2   Characteristics of Arteriovenous Fistulas

No abnormalities on gray-scale studies
Localized perivascular tissue vibration
Localized low-resistance arterial flow
Localized turbulent or arterialized venous flow

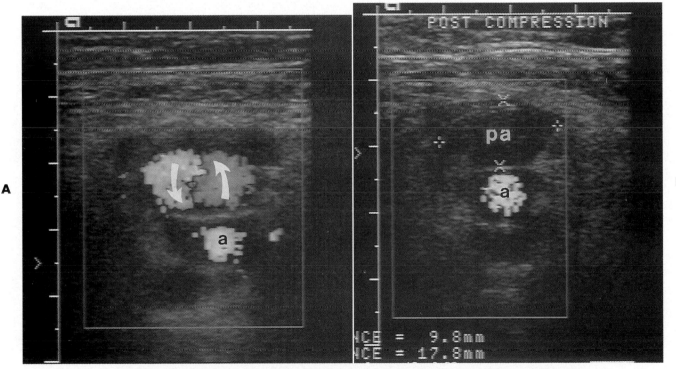

Fig. 21-26   Ultrasound-directed obliteration of a pseudoaneurysm. **A,** Transverse Doppler image of the groin demonstrates the common femoral artery *(a)* and a more superficially positioned pseudoaneurysm with a swirling intraluminal blood flow *(curved arrows)*. **B,** After two successive 10-minute compressions at the level of the pseudoaneurysm neck and one 20-minute compression at this level, repeat scans showed flow in the common femoral artery *(a)* but no flow in the pseudoaneurysm *(pa)* (see color insert, Plate 54).

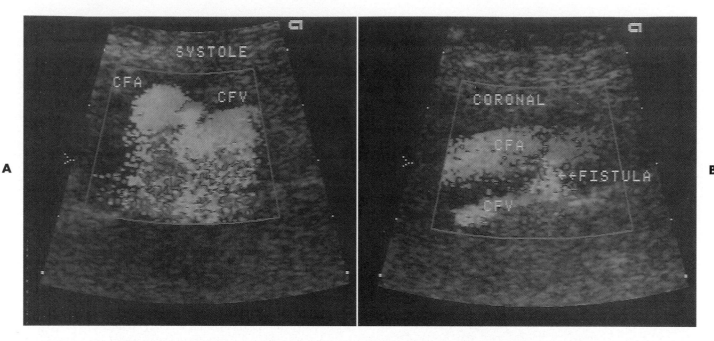

Fig. 21-27   Arteriovenous fistula. **A,** Transverse view of the right groin obtained during peak systole demonstrates flow in the common femoral artery *(CFA)* and common femoral vein *(CFV).* Extensive random red and blue assignment produced by perivascular soft tissue vibration is seen deep to these vessels. This indicates turbulent blood flow, and in a postcatheterization patient this is strong evidence of an arteriovenous fistula. **B,** Semicoronal view of the common femoral artery *(CFA)* and common femoral vein *(CFV)* demonstrates the site of fistulous connection between these two vessels (see color insert, Plate 55).

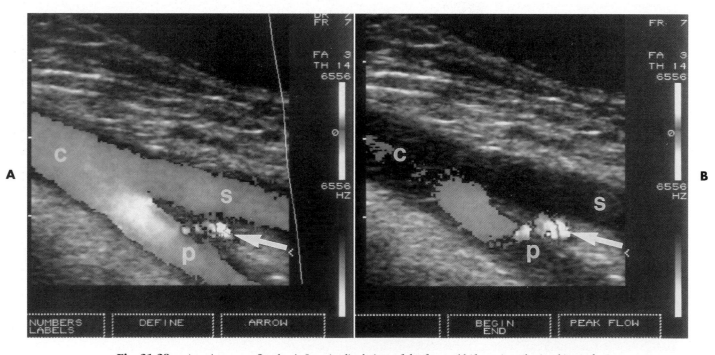

Fig. 21-28   Arteriovenous fistula. **A,** Longitudinal view of the femoral bifurcation obtained in peak systole demonstrates antegrade flow in the common femoral artery *(c),* superficial femoral artery *(s),* and profunda femoral artery *(p).* A small branch vein *(arrow)* is seen between the superficial and profunda femoral arteries. **B,** Similar longitudinal Doppler image obtained at end-diastole demonstrates normal absence of detectable flow in the common femoral artery and superficial femoral artery but maintained flow in the origin of the profunda femoral artery to the level of the small branch vein (see color insert, Plate 56).

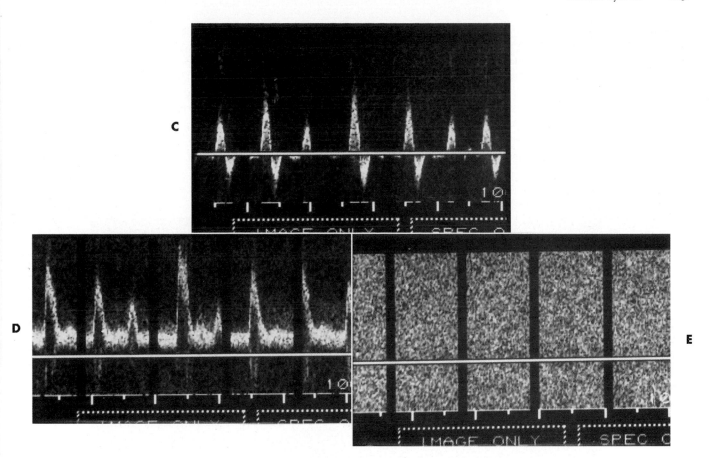

Fig. 21-28, cont'd.   **C,** Pulsed-Doppler waveform from the superficial femoral artery demonstrates a high-resistance pattern with diastolic flow reversal. The variations in systolic peaks are due to a cardiac arrhythmia. **D,** Pulsed-Doppler waveform from the origin of the profunda femoral artery demonstrates persistent antegrade diastolic flow throughout the cardiac cycle. **E,** Pulsed-Doppler waveform from the small branch vein identified between the superficial and profunda femoral arteries demonstrates an extremely high velocity and highly turbulent pattern with no recognizable systolic or diastolic component. This signal could be misinterpreted as noise, but the signal was obtained using identical Doppler controls as those used in the superficial and profunda femoral arteries. The distorted signal reflects the presence of high flow velocities, flow turbulence, and aliasing of the Doppler signal.

Box 21-3	Characteristics of Deep Vein Thrombosis

ALWAYS PRESENT

Noncompressible lumen

SOMETIMES PRESENT

Echogenic filling defect
Venous enlargement
No detectable flow
Loss of flow augmentation
Loss of phasicity

EXTREMITY VEINS

Sonography has now become the method of choice in the initial evaluation of patients with suspected deep vein thrombosis (Box 21-3). Under normal circumstances the veins of the extremities are easily compressible (Fig. 21-29). Vein compressibility can usually be assessed with little difficulty by gray-scale sonography. Color-Doppler sonography is useful in identifying veins that are deeply situated in obese individuals. On color-Doppler studies, the entire lumen of the vein should be seen to contain blood flow. Pulsed-Doppler waveforms from extremity veins should demonstrate spontaneous flow that varies with respiration. In some instances it is necessary to slow down the pulsed-Doppler sweep speed in order to display respiratory phasicity in patients who have a low respiratory rate. Venous flow should also be augmented when the distal extremity is compressed.

Acute deep venous thrombosis can appear as a hypoechoic filling defect within the anechoic lumen of the vein. However, in many persons artifactual echoes are present within the venous lumen and the detection of filling defects on gray-scale studies is not possible. In addition, venous thrombosis can appear extremely hypoechoic and occasionally even anechoic. In such cases gray-scale imaging alone is not helpful. However, when it is combined with compression maneuvers, it can be an extremely reliable means of detecting venous thrombosis (Figs. 21-30 and 21-31). When there is thrombus in the vein lumen, it is not then possible to completely com-

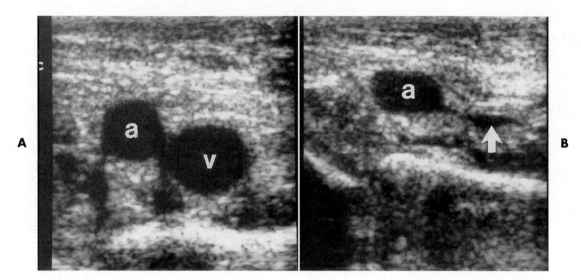

Fig. 21-29   Normal venous compressibility. **A,** Transverse view of the right groin demonstrates the common femoral artery *(a)* and common femoral vein *(v)*. This image is obtained without compression. **B,** Transverse view of the groin obtained with compression demonstrates obliteration of the venous lumen *(arrow)* with persistence of the arterial lumen *(a)*.

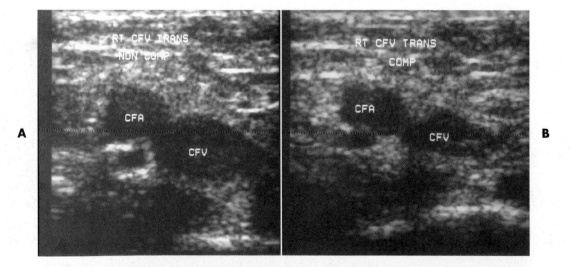

Fig. 21-30   Common femoral vein thrombosis. **A,** Transverse view of the right common femoral vessels without compression demonstrates the common femoral vein *(CFV)* adjacent to the common femoral artery *(CFA)*. **B,** Transverse view with compression shows only partial compressibility of the common femoral vein secondary to venous thrombosis.

press the vein. Therefore the primary criterion used for diagnosing deep venous thrombosis is the inability to compress the vein. This is best detected on transverse views of the vein while pressure is applied with the transducer.

In the femoropopliteal system, the deep venous system can be followed from the common femoral vein down the medial aspect of the thigh and then along the posterior aspect of the knee in the popliteal fossa. Compression should be applied every few centimeters to exclude fo-

cal thrombosis. It is quite easy to visualize venous compression in the region of the common femoral vein. The compressibility of the superficial femoral vein is most easily assessed by positioning the transducer such that the superficial femoral artery is oriented directly over the superficial femoral vein. This is accomplished by placing the transducer in an anteromedial location in the proximal thigh, in a medial location in the midthigh, and in a posteromedial location in the distal thigh. When the vessels are deep because of the patient's body habitus or because of extensive soft tissue swelling, use of a lower-frequency curved array or sector transducer (such as are typically used for abdominal examinations) may improve visualization of the femoropopliteal veins.

Doppler waveform analysis can provide secondary information about a deep venous thrombosis. Asymmetry in respiratory-induced venous flow phasicity can indicate the presence of a proximal obstruction, even when the proximal veins are difficult to visualize (Fig. 21-32). In addition, compression of the distal extremity should produce augmented venous flow in the proximal extremity. Absent flow augmentation indicates the existence of obstruction some place between the site of compression and the site of Doppler sampling. It is generally possible to demonstrate venous flow augmentation in the lower extremity by having the patient plantar flex the foot. This causes the calf muscles to contract and usually eliminates the need for the examiner to squeeze the calf. This self-augmentation maneuver can help eliminate the need for a single examiner to try and compress the calf with one hand while attempting to hold the transducer over the proximal vein with the other hand in order to obtain a venous waveform.

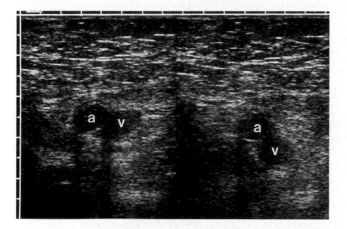

Fig. 21-31 Superficial femoral vein thrombosis. Side-by-side dual images of the superficial femoral artery *(a)* and superficial femoral vein *(v)* obtained with *(left image)* and without *(right image)* compression. The relationship of the two vessels changes with compression, but the venous lumen does not collapse because of the intraluminal thrombus. Note that the echogenicities of the artery and vein are almost identical despite thrombus in the vein.

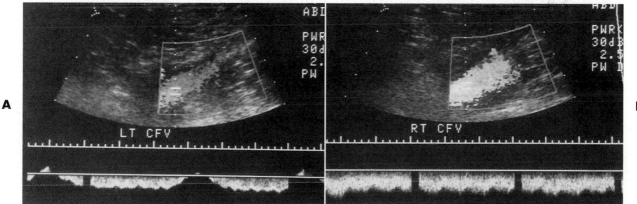

Fig. 21-32 Loss of respiratory phasicity. **A,** Pulsed-Doppler waveform from the left common femoral vein demonstrates respiratory phasicity with decreased flow seen intermittently during the respiratory cycle. **B,** Pulsed-Doppler waveform from the right common femoral vein demonstrates the absence of respiratory phasicity. In this patient a lymphocele was subsequently shown to be compressing the right iliac veins and causing the altered venous signal in the right common femoral vein.

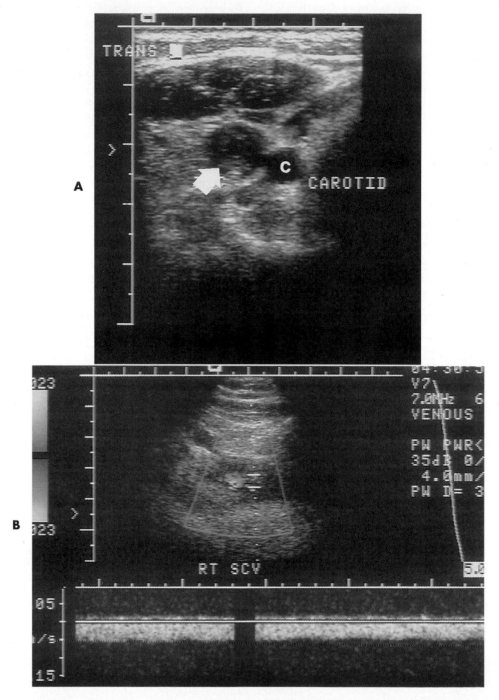

Fig. 21-33   Subclavian vein thrombosis. **A,** Transverse gray-scale view of the right neck shows echogenic material filling the lumen of the internal jugular vein *(arrow).* The normal common carotid *(c)* is also seen. The jugular vein was completely noncompressible, a finding consistent with the appearance of thrombosis. **B,** Pulsed-Doppler waveform from the distal right subclavian vein shows a dampened venous waveform with no pulsatility. Proximal subclavian thrombosis is highly likely in such a case, even if the actual thrombus is not visualized.

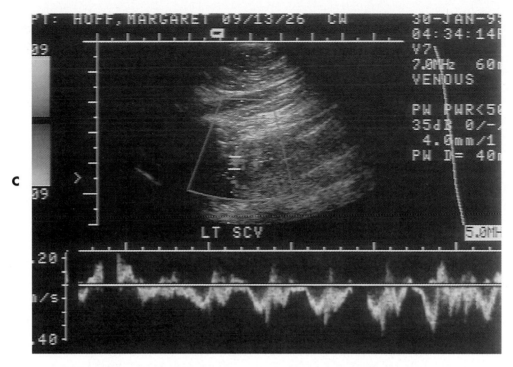

Fig. 21-33, cont'd.   C, Pulsed-Doppler waveform from the normal left subclavian vein shows normal venous pulsatility.

Similar techniques are used to evaluate the upper extremity veins. However, the overlying clavicle makes it impossible to apply compression to the subclavian vein. Therefore detection of subclavian venous thrombosis depends on the gray-scale or color-Doppler detection of filling defects within the venous lumen. Pulsed-Doppler analysis of the venous waveform is also useful. In general the subclavian venous waveform should demonstrate pulsations related to the cardiac cycle. When these are unilaterally dampened, a proximal obstruction of some type should be suspected (Fig. 21-33). Internal jugular vein thrombosis frequently coexists with subclavian vein thrombosis, so evaluation of the jugular vein should be a routine part of an upper extremity venous Doppler examination.

Key Features

Arteries supplying parenchymal organs have a low resistance–type waveform.

Extremity arteries have a high-resistance, triphasic waveform.

Velocity measurements should be obtained at Doppler angles of 60 degrees or less.

Velocity measurements and velocity ratios of the carotid artery are reliable in detecting and quantitating stenoses that narrow the diameter by more than 50%.

Gray-scale and color-Doppler sonography are reliable in detecting stenoses that narrow the diameter by less than 50%.

Pseudoaneurysms are characterized by a swirling internal flow and a to-and-fro waveform at the neck.

Arteriovenous fistulas produce localized hemodynamic changes in the artery and vein but no abnormalities are detected by gray-scale imaging.

It should be possible to completely compress normal extremity veins. Incomplete compressibility indicates the presence of venous thrombosis.

SUGGESTED READINGS

Altin RS, Flicker S, Naidech HJ: Pseudoaneurysm and arteriovenous fistula after femoral artery catheterization: association with low femoral punctures, *AJR* 152:629, 1989.

Bluth EI et al: Sonographic characterization of carotid plaque: detection of hemorrhage, *AJR* 146:1061, 1986.

Bluth EI et al: Carotid duplex sonography: a multicenter recommendation for standardized imaging and Doppler criteria, *Radiographics* 8:487, 1988.

Cardoso TJ, Middleton WD: Duplex and color Doppler ultrasound of the carotid arteries, *Semin Intervent Radiol* 7:1-8, 1990.

Carroll BA: Carotid sonography, *Radiology* 178:303, 1991.

Cronan JJ: Venous thromboembolic disease: the role of US, *Radiology* 186:619, 1993.

Cronan JJ, Dorfman GS, Grusmark J: Lower-extremity deep venous thrombosis: further experience with and refinements of US assessment, *Radiology* 168:101, 1988.

Dorfman GS, Cronan JJ: Postcatheterization femoral artery injuries: is there a role for nonsurgical treatment, *Radiology* 178:629, 1991.

Erickson SJ et al: Color Doppler evaluation of arterial stenoses and occlusions involving the neck and thoracic inlet, *Radiographics* 9:389, 1989.

Fellmeth BD et al: Postangiographic femoral artery injuries: nonsurgical repair with US-guided compression, *Radiology* 178:671, 1991.

Gillum RF: Pulmonary embolism and thrombophlebitis in the United States, 1970-1985, *Am Heart J* 114:1262, 1987.

Helvie MA, Rubin J: Evaluation of traumatic groin arteriovenous fistulas with duplex Doppler sonography, *J Ultrasound Med* 8:21, 1989.

Helvie MA et al: The distinction between femoral artery pseudoaneurysms and other causes of groin masses: value of duplex Doppler sonography, *AJR* 150:1177, 1988.

Hunink MG et al: Detection and quantification of carotid artery stenosis: efficacy of various Doppler velocity parameters, *AJR* 160:619, 1993.

Igidbashian VN et al: Iatrogenic femoral arteriovenous fistula: diagnosis with color Doppler imaging, *Radiology* 170:749, 1989.

Knighton RA et al: Techniques for color flow sonography of the lower extremity, *Radiographics* 10:775, 1990.

Kotval PS et al: Doppler sonographic demonstration of the progressive spontaneous thrombosis of pseudoaneurysms, *J Ultrasound Med* 9:185, 1990.

Merritt CR, Bluth EI: The future of carotid sonography, *AJR* 158:37, 1992.

Middleton WD: Duplex and color Doppler sonography of postcatheterization arteriovenous fistulas, *Semin Intervent Radiol* 7:192, 1990.

Murphy TP, Cronan JJ: Evolution of deep venous thrombosis: a prospective evaluation with US, *Radiology* 177:543, 1990.

North American Symptomatic Carotid Endarterectomy Trial Collaborators: Beneficial effect of carotid endarterectomy in symptomatic patients with high-grade carotid stenosis, *N Engl J Med* 325:445, 1991.

O'Leary DH, Polak JF: High-resolution carotid sonography: past, present, and future, *AJR* 153:699, 1989.

Rapoport S et al: Pseudoaneurysm: a complication of faulty technique in femoral arterial puncture, *Radiology* 154:529, 1985.

Ross RS: Arterial complications, *Circulation* 37(suppl):39, 1968.

Sheikh KH et al: Utility of Doppler color flow imaging for identification of femoral arterial complications of cardiac catheterization, *Am Heart J* 117:623, 1989.

Skillman JJ, Kim D, Baim DS: Vascular complications of percutaneous femoral cardiac interventions. Incidence and operative repair, *Arch Surg* 123:1207, 1988.

Vogel P et al: Deep venous thrombosis of the lower extremity: US evaluation, *Radiology* 163:747, 1987.

Zwiebel WJ: Duplex sonography of the cerebral arteries: efficacy, limitations, and indications, *AJR* 158:29, 1992.

INDEX

Page numbers in italics indicate illustrations; *t* indicates tables.